D1562331

IMAGE-GUIDED RADIATION THERAPY OF PROSTATE CANCER

IMAGE-GUIDED RADIATION THERAPY OF PROSTATE CANCER

Edited by

Richard K. Valicenti
Thomas Jefferson University Hospital
Philadelphia, Pennsylvania, USA

Adam P. Dicker
Thomas Jefferson University Hospital
Philadelphia, Pennsylvania, USA

David A. Jaffray
Princess Margaret Hospital
Toronto, Ontario, Canada

informa
healthcare

New York   London

Informa Healthcare USA, Inc.
52 Vanderbilt Avenue
New York, NY 10017

© 2008 by Informa Healthcare USA, Inc.
Informa Healthcare is an Informa business

No claim to original U.S. Government works
Printed in the United States of America on acid-free paper
10 9 8 7 6 5 4 3 2 1

International Standard Book Number-1-4200-6078-3 (hb : alk. paper)
International Standard Book Number-13: 978-1-4200-6078-2 (hb : alk. paper)

Library of Congress Cataloging-in-Publication Data

Image-Guided Radiation Therapy of Prostate Cancer / edited by Richard K.
Valicenti, Adam P. Dicker, David A. Jaffray.
    p. ; cm.
   Includes bibliographical references and index.
   ISBN-13: 978-1-4200-6078-2 (hb : alk. paper)
   ISBN-10: 1-4200-6078-3 (hb : alk. paper)
   1. Prostate—Cancer—Radiotherapy. 2. Image-guided radiation therapy.
I. Valicenti, Richard K. II. Dicker, Adam P. III. Jaffray, David A.
   [DNLM: 1. Prostatic Neoplasms—radiotherapy. 2. Prostatic
Neoplasms—diagnosis. 3. Radiotherapy, Computer-Assisted—methods. WJ
762 P9662 2008]
   RC280.P7P75927 2008
   616.99′4630642—dc22
                                         2008007287

**For Corporate Sales and Reprint Permissions call 212-520-2700 or write to: Sales Department,
52 Vanderbilt Avenue, 16th floor, New York, NY 10017.**

**Visit the Informa Web site at
www.informa.com**

**and the Informa Healthcare Web site at
www.informahealthcare.com**

Preface

Safe and effective radiation dose escalation to the whole or partial prostate target volume is now possible. Because of compelling clinical evidence from large multi-institutional databases as well as multiple clinical trials, this therapeutic approach with a variety of radiation therapy (RT) delivery systems is now part of routine practice for the treatment of localized prostate cancer.

To assure accurate radiation dose delivery with the greatest prospect of maximizing tumor control and minimizing toxicity, image-guided radiation therapy (IGRT) has been developed in both external beam RT and prostate brachytherapy (PBT). Successful execution of prostate IGRT depends on a thorough understanding of a multiplicity of imaging modalities, the criteria for target and normal tissue volume definition, methods of real-time monitoring of prostate gland motion, and the potential of on-line radiation dose verification. There is an increasing demand from the radiation oncology community to have a compilation of this information in the form of a single textbook to assist in the practical issues of implementing IGRT into clinical practice.

This book meets this demand by focusing primarily on new techniques of IGRT and provides detailed treatment guidelines for prostate cancer. It is also intended as an overview and offers a guide for radiation oncologists and other professionals in the field to implement new techniques of IGRT. At the same time, it may serve to highlight areas that need advancement and define a roadmap for future research and development. Many of the contributing authors constantly receive requests from their radiation oncology colleagues all over the world to provide treatment guidelines for IGRT for prostate cancer.

Image-guided radiation therapy opens a new era of RT delivery systems for prostate cancer. Focused, hypofractionated, high biologically equivalent dose of RT with IMRT, PBT, or proton beam are promising developments in the field and offers new treatment options for men with prostate cancer. These novel approaches have a unique reliance on IGRT technology, are quickly advancing through clinical evaluation at academic centers, and will soon move out into community practice.

In this book, the reader will find disease stage–specific IGRT guidelines and step-by-step description of current techniques. There is an emphasis on novel approaches using IGRT, particularly megavoltage imaging, cone-beam CT, hypofractionated radiation therapy, IMRT, and proton beam RT. We outline recommended RT doses, fractionation schedules, target volume delineation (including recommended margins in the postoperative setting based on our new cone-beam CT study), and IGRT procedures and policies. We think this is an exciting time to be involved in IGRT and hope this book is of use to the multidisciplinary management of prostate cancer.

Richard K. Valicenti
Adam P. Dicker
David A. Jaffray

Acknowledgements

To Robin, Nicolette, and Tyler. —**Richard K. Valicenti**

To Carolyn, Michal, Shimshon, and Yehuda. —**Adam P. Dicker**

To Stasia, Alexander, Anastasia, and Rosalia. —**David A. Jaffray**

Contents

Contributors

Mitchell S. Anscher Department of Radiation Oncology, Virginia Commonwealth University School of Medicine, Richmond, Virginia, U.S.A.

Gloria P. Beyer Sicel Technologies, Morrisville, North Carolina, U.S.A.

Charles Catton Princess Margaret Hospital, The University of Toronto, Toronto, Ontario, Canada

Fergus V. Coakley Department of Radiology, Helen Diller Family Comprehensive Cancer Center, University of California, San Francisco, California, U.S.A.

Tim Craig Princess Margaret Hospital, The University of Toronto, Toronto, Ontario, Canada

Juanita Crook Department of Radiation Oncology, Princess Margaret Hospital, University Health Network, University of Toronto, Toronto, Ontario, Canada

Joanna E. Cygler Department of Medical Physics, Ottawa Hospital Regional Cancer Centre, Ottawa, Ontario, Canada

Brian J. Davis Department of Radiation Oncology, Mayo Clinic, Rochester, Minnesota, U.S.A.

David P. Dearnaley Academic Department of Radiotherapy, Institute of Cancer Research and Royal Marsden NHS Foundation Trust, Sutton, Surrey, U.K.

Adam P. Dicker Department of Radiation Oncology, Kimmel Cancer Center, Thomas Jefferson University, Philadelphia, Pennsylvania, U.S.A.

Toufik Djemil Cleveland Clinic Foundation, Cleveland, Ohio, U.S.A.

Claudio Fiorino Department of Medical Physics, Istituto Scientifico San Raffaele, Milan, Italy

Michel Ghilezan Department of Radiation Oncology, William Beaumont Hospital Cancer Center, Royal Oak, Michigan, U.S.A.

Leonard G. Gomella Department of Urology, Kimmel Cancer Center, Thomas Jefferson University, Philadelphia, Pennsylvania, U.S.A.

Christopher C. Goulet   Department of Radiation Oncology, Mayo Clinic, Rochester, Minnesota, U.S.A.

Michael G. Herman   Department of Radiation Oncology, Mayo Clinic, Rochester, Minnesota, U.S.A.

Timothy Holmes   St. Agnes Hospital Cancer Center, Baltimore, Maryland, U.S.A.

Eric M. Horwitz   Department of Radiation Oncology, Fox Chase Cancer Center, Philadelphia, Pennsylvania, U.S.A.

Richard Hudes   St. Agnes Hospital Cancer Center, Baltimore, Maryland, U.S.A.

Daniel Indelicato   Department of Radiation Oncology, University of Florida, Proton Therapy Institute, Jacksonville, Florida, U.S.A.

David A. Jaffray   Radiation Medicine Program, Princess Margaret Hospital/ University Health Network, Departments of Radiation Oncology and Medical Biophysics, University of Toronto, Toronto, Ontario, Canada

James Johannes   Department of Urology, Kimmel Cancer Center, Thomas Jefferson University, Philadelphia, Pennsylvania, U.S.A.

Vincent S. Khoo   Urology Oncology Unit, Royal Marsden NHS Foundation Trust and Institute of Cancer Research, Chelsea, London, U.K.

Jon Kruse   Department of Radiation Oncology, Mayo Clinic, Rochester, Minnesota, U.S.A.

Zuofeng Li   Department of Radiation Oncology, University of Florida, Proton Therapy Institute, Jacksonville, Florida, U.S.A.

Alexander Lin   Department of Radiation Oncology, Kimmel Cancer Center, Thomas Jefferson University, Philadelphia, Pennsylvania, U.S.A.

Himu Lukka   Department of Oncology, McMaster University, Hamilton, Ontario, Canada

Cynthia Ménard   Department of Radiation Oncology, Princess Margaret Hospital, University Health Network, University of Toronto, Toronto, Ontario, Canada

Arul Mahadevan   Cleveland Clinic Foundation, Cleveland, Ohio, U.S.A.

Alvaro Martinez   Department of Radiation Oncology, William Beaumont Hospital Cancer Center, Royal Oak, Michigan, U.S.A.

Patrick McLaughlin   Department of Radiation Oncology, University of Michigan, Ann Arbor, Michigan, U.S.A.

Jeff Michalski   Department of Radiation Oncology, Washington University School of Medicine, St. Louis, Missouri, U.S.A.

Martin Murphy   Department of Radiation Oncology, Virginia Commonwealth University School of Medicine, Richmond, Virginia, U.S.A.

Jatinder R. Palta   Department of Radiation Oncology, University of Florida, Proton Therapy Institute, Jacksonville, Florida, U.S.A.

Parag J. Parikh   Department of Radiation Oncology, Washington University School of Medicine, St. Louis, Missouri, U.S.A.

Tarun Podder   Department of Radiation Oncology, Kimmel Cancer Center, Thomas Jefferson University, Philadelphia, Pennsylvania, U.S.A.

Jean Pouliot Department of Radiation Oncology, University of California, San Francisco, NCI-Designated Comprehensive Cancer Center, San Francisco, California, U.S.A.

Tiziana Rancati Prostate Programme, Fondazione IRCCS Istituto Nazionale dei Tumori, Milan, Italy

Mack Roach Department of Radiation Oncology, University of California, San Francisco, NCI-Designated Comprehensive Cancer Center, San Francisco, California, U.S.A.

Habeeb Saleh Department of Radiation Oncology, Virginia Commonwealth University School of Medicine, Richmond, Virginia, U.S.A.

Charles W. Scarantino Sicel Technologies, Morrisville, North Carolina, U.S.A.

Timothy N. Showalter Department of Radiation Oncology, Kimmel Cancer Center, Thomas Jefferson University, Philadelphia, Pennsylvania, U.S.A.

Joshua S. Silverman Department of Radiation Oncology, Fox Chase Cancer Center, Philadelphia, Pennsylvania, U.S.A.

Aaron Spalding Department of Radiation Oncology, University of Michigan, Ann Arbor, Michigan, U.S.A.

Joycelyn L. Speight Department of Radiation Oncology, Helen Diller Family Comprehensive Cancer Center, University of California, San Francisco, California, U.S.A.

Kevin Stephans Cleveland Clinic Foundation, Cleveland, Ohio, U.S.A.

Edouard J. Trabulsi Department of Urology, Kimmel Cancer Center, Thomas Jefferson University, Philadelphia, Pennsylvania, U.S.A.

Riccardo Valdagni Prostate Programme, Fondazione IRCCS Istituto Nazionale dei Tumori, Milan, Italy

Richard K. Valicenti Department of Radiation Oncology, Kimmel Cancer Center, Thomas Jefferson University, Philadelphia, Pennsylvania, U.S.A.

Carlos E. Vargas Department of Radiation Oncology, University of Florida, Proton Therapy Institute, Jacksonville, Florida, U.S.A.

Antonio C. Westphalen Department of Radiology, Helen Diller Family Comprehensive Cancer Center, University of California, San Francisco, California, U.S.A.

Mark Wiesmeyer Department of Radiation Oncology, Virginia Commonwealth University School of Medicine, Richmond, Virginia, U.S.A.

Ping Xia Department of Radiation Oncology, University of California, San Francisco, NCI-Designated Comprehensive Cancer Center, San Francisco, California, U.S.A.

Ying Xiao Department of Radiation Oncology, Kimmel Cancer Center, Thomas Jefferson University, Philadelphia, Pennsylvania, U.S.A.

Di Yan Department of Radiation Oncology, William Beaumont Hospital Cancer Center, Royal Oak, Michigan, U.S.A.

Yan Yu Department of Radiation Oncology, Kimmel Cancer Center, Thomas Jefferson University, Philadelphia, Pennsylvania, U.S.A.

1

Prostate Cancer: Overview and Treatment Guidelines for Image-Guided Radiation Therapy

RICHARD K. VALICENTI AND ALEXANDER LIN

Department of Radiation Oncology, Kimmel Cancer Center, Thomas Jefferson University, Philadelphia, Pennsylvania, U.S.A.

INTRODUCTION

Prostate cancer is one of the leading cause of cancer death among men in the United States (1). With the widespread use of prostate-specific antigen (PSA) screening, most patients present with clinically localized disease, with the majority receiving radiation therapy (RT) as primary treatment. In addition, patients with high-risk features after prostate surgery may also be treated with postoperative RT. According to the National Comprehensive Cancer Network (NCCN)® treatment guidelines, patients in any risk group may be treated with RT as a component of therapy or as the primary form of therapeutic management. The NCCN risk groups are given in Table 1.

In the past two decades several technological innovations have advanced the planning and delivery of RT, thereby allowing for dose escalation to a prostate target resulting in reduced toxicity and better disease-free survival. These benefits have now been demonstrated in several prospective randomized trials, and have resulted from a wide range of RT delivery systems including proton beam therapy (Table 2) (2–6). The current "standard" dose of primary RT for prostate cancer is now between 75 and 80 Gy, which is 10% to 20% higher than what can be safely delivered with conventional RT

techniques. At the same time, there are increasing efforts to precisely locate intraprostatic targets and further escalate radiation dose. There is now evidence that such targeting is achievable with the use of magnetic resonance imaging (MRI) with intensity-modulated radiation therapy (IMRT) so that the RT dose to the treatment target and adjacent critical structures are not compromised (7).

To translate novel therapeutic approaches into safe routine clinical practice, direct imaging of the prostate target and verification of its position is now available during RT, with the ultimate goal of unifying the steps of treatment planning, radiation delivery, and real-time dosimetric verification. To accomplish this goal, image-guided radiation therapy (IGRT) has been developed, to be used in conjunction with external beam RT and prostate brachytherapy (PBT). Successful execution of IGRT depends on a detailed understanding of a multiplicity of imaging modalities, the guidelines for target and organs at risk definition, and the methods of real-time monitoring of prostate target motion. As we will learn in chapter 3, the contribution of accurate target volume delineation and target positioning is postulated to improve tumor control probability by as much as 10% to 20%.

The development of IGRT creates a new era of prostate cancer RT. Electronic portal imaging with intraprostatic

Table 1 NCCN Risk Groupings

- Low risk
    T1-T2a, Gleason $\leq$ 6 and PSA < 10 ng/mL
- Intermediate
    T2b-T2c, Gleason = 7 or PSA 10–20 ng/mL
- High
    T3-T4, Gleason = 8–10 or PSA > 20

National Comprehensive Cancer Network (NCCN) Clinical Practice Guidelines in Oncology v. 1. 2005.

fiducial markers and implanted Beacon® electromagnetic transponder system (Calypso System, Calypso Medical, Seattle, Washington, U.S.A.) may improve targeting accuracy by as much as 25% to 50% (8). In addition, various ultrasound based systems are used to tract prostate movement by the acquisition of transverse and sagittal suprapubic ultrasound images. A new generation of target volume localization and verification methods is based on megavoltage CT and cone-beam CT.

The implementation of IGRT allows the safe testing of focused, hypofractionated, high biological equivalent dose of RT with IMRT or high-dose rate PBT.

Proton beam RT may provide additional therapeutic benefit for localized prostate cancer due to its physical characteristics, which lead to high and conformal dose distribution in the tumor while reducing entrance and exit dose. Similarly, this novel approach also relies heavily on IGRT technology. Since the target dose distribution depends on the proton beam path length, localization and verification methods will need to be specifically developed for this form of RT.

Clearly, there is an increasing need from the radiation oncology community to have a dedicated textbook to address the practical issues of implementing IGRT into routine clinical practice. Thus, our goal in this text was

to meet this need and to develop practical guidelines directed to radiation oncologists, radiologists, urologists, medical physicists, and trainees in these respective disciplines. This work is intended to be a step-by-step approach to apply new techniques of IGRT into clinical practice. At the same time, it may serve as road map for future research and development.

SUMMARY OF DOSE-ESCALATION STUDIES

As noted above, there are historical and prospective data supporting the benefits of radiation dose escalation in localized prostate cancer. Clinical evidence justifies a therapeutic philosophy, in which there is a need to deliver a high radiation dose accurately and precisely to a prostatic clinical target. Technological advances such as IGRT have been made, in part, to assure that the potential benefits of dose escalation are achieved. In addition to reviewing the design and outcome of the published phase III dose-escalation trials, specific treatment and verification techniques used in these trials will be summarized (Table 3).

The first randomized trial to study the effects of radiation dose escalation on prostate cancer was the study by Shipley et al. (2). The investigators set out to determine the effects of high radiation doses (>68 Gy) in patients with clinically localized prostate cancer. In this trial, 202 patients with stage T3-T4 disease were randomized to one of the two treatment arms: a high dose of 75.6 CGE (cobalt Gray equivalent) or the conventional dose of 67.2 Gy. In arm 1, prostate cancer patients received a boost above the 50.4 Gy, via perineal 160-MeV proton boost of 25.2 CGE. The boost was started 7 to 14 days after completion of the 50.4 Gy treatment with conventional RT. This was necessary to allow for sufficient healing since the insertion of a Lucite rectal probe was required to assure

Table 2 Benefits Identified on Radiation Dose–Escalation Trials for Clinically Localized Prostate Cancer

Institution (reference)	Dose levels (n)	Outcome (p value)	Cohort with benefit
Massachusetts General Hospital (2)	75.6 CGE vs. 67.2 Gy (202)	8-yr LC, 84% vs. 19% (p = 0.0014)	Stage T3/T4 with Gleason 4 or 5 of 5
MDACC 93-002 (3)	78 Gy vs. 70 Gy (305)	6-yr FFF, 62% vs. 43% (p = 0.01)	PSA >10 ng/mL
Proton Radiation Oncology Group 95-09 (4)	79.2 GyE vs. 70 GyE (393)	5-yr bNED, 80% vs. 61% (p < 0.001)	Low- and intermediate-risk groups
Netherlands Cancer Institute CKTO 9610 (5)	78 Gy vs. 68 Gy (669)	5-yr FFF, 64% vs. 54% (p = 0.01)	Intermediate- and high-risk groups
Medical Research Council RT 01 (6)	NHT + 74 Gy vs. NHT + 64 Gy (843)	5-yr bPFS, 71% vs. 60% (p = 0.0007)	All risk groups

Abbreviations: n, patient number; CGE, cobalt Gray equivalent; LC, local control (rectal examination and re-biopsy negative; PSA, prostatic-specific antigen; FFF, freedom from failure, which includes clinical and/or biochemical failure defined as three rises in PSA level (9); bNED includes only biochemical failure; NHT, three to six months of neoadjuvant hormonal therapy; bPFS, freedom from biochemical failure defined as an increase in PSA value greater than the nadir by at least 50% and greater than 2 ng/mL (10).

Table 3 Radiation Techniques Used in Radiation Dose–Escalation Trials for Clinically Localized Prostate Cancer

Institution (reference)	Target definition guidelines	CTV to PTV margin	RT planning technique	Immobilization
Massachusetts General Hospital (2)	CTV for conventional RT: GTV + pelvic LNs below iliac bifurcation CTV for proton boost: clinician-defined	Photon boost PTV = CTV + 0.5 cm Proton boost PTV = CTV + 0.5 cm	Conventional (50.4 Gy), boost with lateral photon fields vs. perineal proton field	Endorectal probe for proton therapy; prostate apex fiducial with port films (for protons)
MDACC 93-002 (3)	CTV = prostate + SV	Block edge margin = CTV + 1.25–1.5 cm (anterior and inferior) and 0.75–1.0 cm (posterior and superior)	Conventional ± 3D conformal boost	Verification CT
Proton Radiation Oncology Group 95-09 (4)	Phase 1 photons: CTV = prostate Phase 1 protons: CTV = prostate + 0.5 cm Phase 2 photons: CTV = prostate + SV + 1.0 cm	PTV = CTV + 0.7–1.0 cm	3D Conformal (50.4 Gy) + Proton boost	Body cast; Endorectal balloon with fiducial markers; daily EPID (phase 1) Weekly port films (phase 2)
Netherlands Cancer Institute CKVO 9610 (5)	Group 1: CTV = prostate Group 2: CTV = prostate + SV (SV excluded after 50 Gy) Group 3: CTV = prostate + SV (SV excluded after 68 Gy) Group 4: prostate + SV	PTV_1 = CTV + 1.0 cm for 68 Gy PTV_2 = CTV + 0.5 cm (0.0 cm at rectum) for 10 Gy boost	3D-conformal	Not stated
Medical Research Council RT 01 (6)	GTV = prostate + SV base (low risk) or SV (medium to high risk) CTV = GTV + 0.5 cm	PTV = CTV + 0.5–1.0 cm	Conformal RT	Not stated

Abbreviations: CTV, clinical tumor volume; PTV, planning target volume; RT, radiation therapy.

correct positioning of the prostate target volume. Field alignment was facilitated with fiducials placed in the prostatic apex and the rectal probe. Only in patients with poorly differentiated tumors (Gleason grade 4 or 5 of 5) was there a significant difference in local control rates at five and eight years posttreatment (94% and 84% vs. 64% and 19%; $p = 0.0014$) in arm 1 versus arm 2, respectively. It was also noted that patients randomized to the high-dose arm experienced significantly higher grade 1 and grade 2 rectal bleeding (32% vs. 12%; $p = 0.002$).

Another phase III trial in support of dose escalation for prostate cancer was the study by Pollack et al. in 2002 (3). In this study, 301 patients were randomized to receive either 70 Gy or 78 Gy. All dose prescriptions were specified to the isocenter. For the patients receiving 78 Gy,

three-dimensional conformal RT treatment planning was used and based on a clinical target volume with 0.75 to 1.5 cm margin to the block edge. However, the patients in the 70 Gy arm were treated with a conventional four-field box to 46 Gy, followed by a reduced field boost. To confirm that the prostate and seminal vesicles were in the field pelvic, CT scans were used in the first week of treatment. The primary endpoint was freedom from failure (FFF), i.e., biochemical failure, which was defined as three consecutive increases in PSA according to The American Society for Therapeutic Radiology and Oncology (ASTRO) criteria (9). This study found that prostate cancer patients in the higher dose group achieved significantly better FFF rates at six years, compared to the lower dose arm (70% vs. 64%; $p = 0.03$). However, an analysis based on pretreatment PSA level, concluded that benefit of dose-escalation was restricted to the patients with intermediate- to high-risk prostate cancer as defined by a pretreatment PSA > 10 ng/mL. These patients achieved FFF rates of 62%, compared to only 43% at the lower dose. In fact, patients defined as low-risk (PSA ≤ 10 ng/mL) derived no benefit. Of the 11 patients found to have grade 3 rectal toxicity, all but one was subject to the high-dose arm. Neither the MD Anderson or MGH studies showed a benefit from dose-escalation (>70 Gy) for low-risk prostate cancer patients.

In 2005, Zietman et al. reported on another phase III dose-escalation trial for prostate cancer patients (4). This trial is important because it showed, for the first time, that men with low- to intermediate-risk prostate cancer did benefit from dose-escalated RT. In their study, 393 men were randomized to receive either 70.2 Gray equivalents (GyE) or a higher dose of 79.2 GyE. Patient and prostate immobilization procedures were used throughout treatment and portal images were taken daily during the boost portion of therapy to minimize setup error. Patients were eligible if they had stage T1b-T2b tumors and PSA levels below 15 ng/mL. In contrast to the preceding trials, men had low- to intermediate-risk disease as opposed to more advanced disease. This study found higher rates of FFF at five years in patients receiving 79.2 GyE compared to those in the lower-dose treatment arm (80.4% vs. 61.4%; $p < 0.001$, respectively). The benefit also applied to patients with low-risk disease, defined by stage T1a-T2a tumors, PSA levels below 10 ng/mL, and Gleason scores equal to or below 6. In this cohort, patients receiving 79.2 GyE had a FFF benefit compared to men receiving 70.2 GyE (80.5% vs. 60.1%; $p < 0.001$, respectively). Using the RTOG toxicity scale, only 1% of patients receiving conventional dose (70.2 Gy) and 2% of men treated with high-dose radiotherapy experienced grade 3 or higher toxicity. There were no significant differences in grade 2 acute (42% vs. 49%) or late (18% vs. 20%) genitourinary (GU) toxicity, regardless of dose level. At the higher dose level, there were significant increases in grade 2 acute (41% vs. 57%; $p = 0.004$) and late (8% vs. 17%; $p = 0.005$) gastrointestinal (GI) morbidity.

In 2006, Peeters et al. reported on a Dutch phase III multicenter dose-escalation trial. (5). In this study, 669 patients were randomized to receive either 68 Gy or 78 Gy of dose. Patients were eligible if they had T1b-T4 tumors and PSA less than 60 ng/mL. All patients were treated with 3D-CRT in 2Gy daily fractions. Dose was prescribed to the isocenter. The use of androgen ablation was allowed but not recommended, and left to the discretion of the treating physician. The primary endpoint was FFF, defined as biochemical or clinical failure, whichever occurring first. Biochemical failure was defined according to the ASTRO criteria (9). Freedom from failure was significantly higher at five years in the high-dose arm (64% vs. 54%; $p = 0.01$), largely due to differences in rates of biochemical failure. On subgroup analyses, a significant lower failure rate was seen only for intermediate-risk patients, defined as T1-T2 tumors, with PSA 10–20, or Gleason score 7. No significant differences were seen between the high and low-dose arms for acute GU toxicity ≥ grade 3 (13% vs. 12%) or for late GU toxicity ≥ grade 2 (39% vs. 41%). The high-dose arm had a slightly higher, but nonsignificant, rate of late GI toxicity ≥ grade 2 (32% vs. 27%), but no difference in late GI toxicity ≥ grade 3 (5% vs. 4%).

The most recent dose-escalation study was reported by Dearnaley et al. in 2007 (6). In this study, 843 men with localized prostate cancer were randomized to receive either 64 Gy or 74 Gy external beam radiotherapy. Eligible patients had clinical T1b-T3a disease with PSA under 50 ng/mL. All patients received neoadjuvant androgen ablation for three to six months before the start of radiotherapy. Conformal radiotherapy was used for all patients, with 2 Gy daily fractions prescribed to the intersection point. This trial had five primary endpoints: biochemical progression–free survival (bPFS), freedom from local progression, metastasis-free survival, overall survival, and late toxicity. PSA failure was defined as increase by at least 50% and greater than 2 ng/mL over the nadir, six months or more after start of radiotherapy, which is similar to the current consensus definition, as determined by the RTOG-ASTRO Phoenix Consensus Conference (10). At five years, the high-dose arm had a significantly higher bPFS rate (71% vs. 60%; $p = 0.0007$). The high-dose RT arm had a significantly higher risk of ≥ grade 2 late GI toxicity (33% vs. 24%) reported within five years of treatment. There were no significant differences between the two arms with respect to late GU toxicity.

To date, none of the published studies have been specifically powered to find differences in overall survival. Although the prospective randomized trials have consistently demonstrated improvement in PSA-defined endpoints, this does not necessarily imply a reduction in cancer-specific mortality. However, one secondary analysis of prospectively treated patients did suggest a survival advantage when the outcome was stratified according to radiation dose. Valicenti et al. analyzed 1465 men with clinically localized prostate cancer from four RTOG phase III randomized trials (11). The authors were able to demonstrate that Gleason score was an independent predictor of both disease-specific survival and overall survival. Furthermore, when outcome was broken down by Gleason score and radiation dose, patients receiving doses greater than 66 Gy had an improved cancer-specific and overall survival, though the benefit was restricted to men with Gleason score 8 or higher tumors.

Prospective randomized studies are needed to determine whether dose-escalation above 70 Gy leads to improved survival in any risk group. The Radiation Therapy Oncology Group Trial 0126 was designed to test this hypothesis of dose escalation for men with intermediate-risk prostate cancer (T1b-T2b with Gleason 2–6, but PSA > 10 ng/mL and < 20 ng/mL; T1b-T2b, Gleason of 7 and PSA < 15 ng/mL). This study was sufficiently powered to detect a significant difference in overall survival.

TECHNICAL CONSIDERATIONS IN THE DOSE-ESCALATION TRIALS

A careful examination of the techniques of radiation planning and daily immobilization in the five randomized trials of dose escalation illustrates the evolving nature of prostate RT. Conventional radiation fields are now rarely used, yielding to ever-increasing conformal techniques (3D CRT, IMRT, proton beam therapy). The earliest dose-escalation studies, from Shipley et al. (2) and Pollack et al. (3), used conventional four-field box for the initial portion of therapy. The Massachusetts General Hospital (MGH) Study used opposed photon beams for boost in the low-dose arm, and a perineal proton boost in the high-dose RT arm. The MD Anderson Study used conformal methods for boost only in the high-dose arm. The remaining dose-escalation studies (4–6) all required 3D CRT to be used from the onset of treatment, and PROG 95-09 (6) used conformal proton beams for the boost portion of therapy. The advancement of radiation techniques to highly conformal methods, as witnessed in the dose-escalation randomized trials, has been mirrored in standard clinical practice. Techniques such as IMRT are now commonly used for prostate radiotherapy in most academic and community centers.

The implementation of conformal radiation requires effective patient immobilization. Again, examination of the dose-escalation trials reveals a variety of methods. For patients receiving proton boost in the MGH study, positioning was verified via the use of an endorectal probe, a prostate apex fiducial, and daily port films (2). Patients in the MD Anderson study had a verification pelvic CT scan during the first week of treatment, which was used to make any necessary adjustments (3). PROG 95-09 used a body cast for patient immobilization. An endorectal balloon was utilized for prostate immobilization. Setup error was minimized via the use of daily EPID during the proton boost, and weekly portal images during delivery of photons (4). The emergence of IGRT has helped to create new techniques for treatment verification and to improve the quality of prostate IMRT.

In an era where technological advances have allowed for highly conformal therapy, with immobilization and

verification techniques permitting the reduction of the planning target volume (PTV) margin, it is vital that these advances are applied in a judicious manner. Specifically, the issue of accurate target volume definition becomes of paramount importance in radiation treatment planning.

THE DEFINITION OF TARGET VOLUMES

The goal of IGRT is to direct the radiation treatments (beams) according to specific positional data of the planned and actual treatment targets for an individual patient in such a manner that there is acceptable reproducibility (<5–10 mm) of the treatment plan with that of each individually delivered treatment. To accomplish this task, it is imperative that there is a minimum standard for definitions of target and organ at risk (OAR) structures as it applies to the steps linking the radiation treatment planning, verification, and radiation dose delivery. The nomenclature as published by the International Commission on Radiation Units and Measurements (ICRU) (12) and the supplement ICRU 62 serve as essential guides to define target volumes and OAR (13).

Normal tissues identified on CT or MRI imaging dataset constitute OAR, and may include the walls of the rectum and bladder, the femoral heads, penile bulb, and the outer skin surface. Portions of the small bowel or sigmoid colon within 1 cm of the PTV are also taken into consideration, if necessary, during planning. In addition, the central diameter portion of the prostate encompassing the prostatic urethra may be defined for dosimetric consideration.

Overview of Clinical Tumor Volume Definition in Prostate IGRT

In men undergoing IGRT for prostate cancer, the clinical tumor volume (CTV) ultimately depends on the intrinsic biological aggressiveness of the tumor and its likelihood to spread locally and regionally. Several risk classification schemes exist and are commonly used to assist in prostate CTV definition. The Partin nomograms predict pathologic stage [organ confinement, extracapsular extension (ECE), seminal vesicle invasion (SVI)], involvement of pelvic lymph nodes based on clinical T stage, Gleason score, and pretreatment PSA (14,15). Patients are commonly classified by "risk" category, based on the work by D'Amico et al. (16). Guidelines useful for CTV determination in IGRT treatment planning by the NCCN risk groups are summarized in Table 4.

For low-risk patients, in the absence of secondary risk factors [i.e., percent core positive biopsies and perineural invasion (PNI)], the risk of ECE or SVI is sufficiently low

Table 4 Prostate Target Guidelines by Risk Group for Definitive RT

Risk group	CTV	PTV	Additional concerns
Low	Prostate only	1.0 cm	May add SV for PNI
Low-intermediate	Prostate + 0.5 cm	<1.0 cm with image guidance	Pelvic LN optional. Consider short-term androgen suppression
High-intermediate	Prostate + 0.5 cm + 1.0 cm of SV	<1.0 cm with image guidance	Pelvic LN optional. Consider short-term androgen suppression
High	Prostate + 0.5 cm + 2 cm of SV + pelvic LN	1.0 cm	Consider long-term androgen suppression

Abbreviations: RT, radiation therapy; CTV, clinical tumor volume; PTV, planning target volume; SV, seminal vesicle; PNI, perineural invasion; LN, lymph node.

to reliably exclude these structures from the CTV (17,18). Therefore, the definition of the prostate alone for the CTV is reasonable. However, the presence of one or more of the secondary risk factors may warrant modification of the treatment target. A higher percent positive biopsy has been found to correlate with higher prostate cancer-specific mortality (19), time to PSA failure (20), and increased risk of SVI and ECE (21). The presence of PNI should also be taken into account in CTV definition, as it has been associated with ECE and biochemical failure (22), and consideration of adding the seminal vesicles in the CTV may be justified in low-risk patients with PNI.

The presence of ECE is another important factor in CTV definition for prostate RT. Pathological evaluation of patient undergoing prostatectomy has demonstrated a significant relationship between ECE and rising clinical tumor stage, Gleason score, and pretreatment PSA (23–25). The addition of a 0.5 cm margin for periprostatic extension is recommended for intermediate- and high-risk patients.

Invasion of the seminal vesicles also affects target delineation. Kestin et al. found that the risk of SVI was 1% in low-risk patients, but increased to 15%, 38%, and 58% for low-intermediate, high-intermediate, and high-risk patients (26). The absolute length of SVI was also evaluated, with only 1% of all patients having a risk of SVI beyond 2 cm. For high- to intermediate-risk patients, we therefore recommend incorporating the proximal 1 cm of seminal vesicles in the CTV, while in high-risk patients, the proximal 2 cm should be incorporated.

Incorporation of pelvic lymph nodes in the CTV is controversial but should be considered for high-risk patients, and this is addressed in detail in chapter 16. Inclusion of pelvic nodes is supported by data that demonstrates improved progression-free survival with pelvic RT and neoadjuvant hormonal therapy (27,28). What is not known is whether the same is true when long-term androgen ablation is used. The decision of whether to include pelvic lymph nodes in a separate CTV should ultimately be determined by the estimated risk of lymph node involvement, balanced by the potential toxicity of including the whole pelvis in the radiation field.

Overview of PTV Definition in Prostate IGRT

The planning target volume (PTV) is defined as the CTV with a margin to account for physical uncertainties including setup reproducibility, inter- and intra-fractional organ motion. At Thomas Jefferson University, a 0.7 mm margin is added to the CTV to form the PTV in all directions. This planning margin may be modified depending on the patient's relational pelvic anatomy. For example, at the interface with the rectum, the margin may be reduced to 0.5 mm if the prostate is in close proximity to both the anterior and posterior rectal walls.

Traditionally, PTV margins were based on serial CT scan studies evaluating organ motion during a course of RT (29). Typically, in such population-based approaches, additional margins to account for daily setup error and internal organ motion of the CTV are derived from studies in groups of patients. A disadvantage of this statistical approach is that, by definition, the positional variation of the CTV of an individual patient is unknown, and that a generalized PTV must be created to achieve adequate dose coverage in the majority of patients.

In order to customize radiation treatments to individual patients, IGRT approaches have been created and depend on the individual localization of the CTV by using online imaging data to determine and correct the CTV position for an individual patient (30–35). For prostate cancer patients, established systems to accomplish this goal have consisted of regional irradiation of implanted radio-paque fiducial markers and real-time ultrasonographic monitoring of pelvic anatomy. Recently, cone-beam (CB) imaging technology with kilovoltage (kV) or mega-voltage (MV) X rays has also been developed. Limitations to these IGRT methods are the potential for excessive radiation exposure and the inability to continuously image during actual treatment delivery. The specifics of the various localization methods will be discussed throughout this textbook.

SUMMARY OF PERTINENT CONCLUSIONS

- Prostate cancer radiotherapy is a constantly evolving field. Recent advances such as dose-escalated RT and IMRT have allowed the treatment of clinical targets with increased conformality and efficacy, with low risks of morbidity.
- IGRT, with daily imaging and repositioning, can only increase the efficacy and safety of therapy, by maximizing the accuracy and precision of our therapy, and minimizing the risk of treatment-related toxicity.
- These advances require judicious application of clinical acumen with respect to delineation of clinical target volumes and organs at risk.
- Emerging treatment modalities, such as proton beam therapy, hold great promise in improving therapy. At the same time, such advances will bring up additional challenging issues in the era of IGRT.
- The principles and practices of IGRT, as well as the promise and challenges of emerging modalities, are the subjects of the remainder of this textbook.

REFERENCES

1. Jemal A, Siegel R, Ward E, et al. Cancer statistics 2006. J Clin 2006; 56(2):106–130.
2. Shipley WU, Verhey U, Munzenrider JE, et al. Advanced prostate cancer: the results of a randomized comparative trial of high-dose irradiation boosting with conformal protons compared with conventional dose irradiation using photons alone. Int J Radiat Oncol Biol Phys 1995; 32:3–12.
3. Pollack A, Zagars GK, Smith LG, et al. Preliminary results of a randomized radiotherapy dose-escalation study comparing 70 Gy with 78 Gy for prostate cancer. J Clin Oncol 2000; 18:3904–3911.
4. Zietman AL, DeSilvio ML, Slater JD, et al. Comparison of conventional-dose vs. high-dose conformal radiation therapy in clinically localized adenocarcinoma of the prostate. JAMA 2005; 294:1233–1239.
5. Peeters STH, Heemsbergen WD, Koper PCM, et al. Dose-response in radiotherapy for localized prostate cancer: results of the Dutch Multicenter Randomized Phase III Trial comparing 68 Gy of radiotherapy with 78 Gy. J Clin Oncol 2006; 24:1990–1996.
6. Dearnaley DP, Sydes MR, Graham JD, et al. Escalated-dose versus standard-dose conformal radiotherapy in pros-
tate cancer: first results from the MRC RT01 randomised controlled trial. Lancet Oncol 2007; 8:475–487.
7. De Meerleer G, Villeirs G, Bral S, et al. The magnetic resonance detected intraprostatic lesion in prostate cancer: planning and delivery of intensity-modulated radiotherapy. Radiother Oncol 2005; 75:325–333.
8. Willoughby TR, Kupelian PA, Pouliot J, et al. Target localization and real-time tracking using the calypso 4D localization system in patients with localized prostate cancer. Int J Radiat Oncol Biol Phys 2006; 65:528–534.
9. American Society for Therapeutic Radiology and Oncology. American Society for Therapeutic Radiology and Oncology consensus panel consensus statement: guidelines for PSA following radiation therapy. Int J Radiat Oncol Biol Phys 1997; 37:1035–1041.
10. Roach M III, Hanks G, Thames H Jr., et al. Defining biochemical failure following radiotherapy with or without hormonal therapy in men with clinically localized prostate cancer: recommendations of the RTOG-ASTRO Phoenix Consensus Conference. Int J Radiat Oncol Biol Phys 2006; 65:965–974.
11. Valicenti R, Lu J, Pilepich M, et al. Survival advantage from higher-dose radiation therapy for clinically localized prostate cancer treated on the Radiation Therapy Oncology Group trials. J Clin Oncol 2000; 18(14):2740–2746.
12. International Commission on Radiation Units and Measurement. ICRU 50 Report 50. Prescribing, recording, and reporting photon beam therapy. Bethesda, MD: ICRU, 1993.
13. International Commission on Radiation Units and Measurements. ICRU Report 62. Prescribing, recording, and reporting photon beam therapy. Bethesda, MD: ICRU, 1999.
14. Khan MA, Partin AW. Partin tables: past and present. Br J Urol Int 2003; 92:7–11.
15. Partin AW, Mangold LA, Lamm DM, et al. Contemporary update of prostate cancer staging nomograms (Partin Tables) for the new millennium. Urology 2001; 58:843–848.
16. D'Amico AV, Desjardin A, Chung A, et al. Assessment of outcome prediction models for patients with localized prostate carcinoma managed with radical prostatectomy or external beam radiation therapy. Cancer 1998; 82:1887–1896.
17. D'Amico AV, Whittington R, Kaplan I, et al. Equivalent 5-year bNED in select prostate cancer patients managed with surgery or radiation therapy despite exclusion of the seminal vesicles from the CTV. Int J Radiat Oncol Biol Phys 1997; 39:335–340.
18. Lieberfarb ME, Schultz D, Whittington R, et al. Using PSA, biopsy Gleason score, clinical stage, and the percentage of positive biopsies to identify optimal candidates for prostate-only radiation therapy. Int J Radiat Oncol Biol Phys 2002; 53:898–903.
19. D'Amico AV, Renshaw AA, Cote K, et al. Impact of the percentage of positive prostate cores on prostate cancer-specific mortality for patients with low or favorable intermediate-risk disease. J Clin Oncol 2004; 22:3726–3732.
20. D'Amico AV, Whittington R, Malkowicz SB, et al. Utilizing predictions of early prostate-specific antigen failure to optimize patient selection for adjuvant systemic therapy trials. J Clin Oncol 2000; 18:3240–3246.

21. Lieberfarb ME, Schultz D, Whittington R, et al. Using PSA, biopsy Gleason score, clinical stage, and the percentage of positive biopsies to identify optimal candidates for prostate-only radiation therapy. Int J Radiat Oncol Biol Phys 2002; 53:898–903.

22. Beard CJ, Chen MH, Cote K, et al. Perineural invasion is associated with increased relapse after external beam radiotherapy for men with low-risk prostate cancer and may be a marker for occult, high-grade cancer. Int J Radiat Oncol Biol Phys 2004; 73:61–64.

23. Teh BS, Bastasch MD, Mai WY, et al. Predictors of extracapsular extension and its radial distance in prostate cancer: implications for prostate IMRT, brachytherapy, and surgery. Cancer J 2003; 9:454–460.

24. Teh BS, Bastasch MD, Wheeeler TM, et al. IMRT for prostate cancer: defining target volume based on correlated pathologic volume of disease. Int J Radiat Oncol Biol Phys 2003; 56:184–191.

25. Wheeler TM, Dillioglugil O, Kattan MW, et al. Clinical and pathological significance of the level and extent of capsular invasion in clinical stage T1-2 prostate cancer. Hum Pathol 1998; 29:856–862.

26. Kestin L, Goldstein N, Vicini F, et al. Treatment of prostate cancer with radiotherapy: should the entire seminal vesicles be included in the clinical target volume? Int J Radiat Oncol Biol Phys 2002; 54:686–697.

27. Roach M III. Hormonal therapy and radiotherapy for localized prostate cancer: who, where and how long? J Urol 2003; 170:S35–S40.

28. Roach M III, DeSilvio M, Lawton C, et al. Phase III trial comparing whole-pelvic versus prostate-only radiotherapy and neoadjuvant versus adjuvant combined androgen-suppression: Radiation Therapy Oncology Group 9413. J Clin Oncol 2003; 21:1904–1911.

29. Zelefsky MJ, Crean D, Mageras GS, et al. Quantification and predictors of prostate position variability in 50 patients evaluated with multiple CT scans during conformal radiotherapy. Radiother Oncol 1999; 50:225–234.

30. Bel A, van Herk M, Bartelink H, et al. A verification procedure to improve patient set-up accuracy using portal images. Radiother Oncol 1993; 29:253–260.

31. Langen KM, Jones DT. Organ motion and its management. Int J Radiat Oncol Biol Phys 2005; 50:265–278.

32. Litzenberg DW, Balter JM, Lam KL, et al. Retrospective analysis of prostate cancer patients with implanted gold markers using off-line and adaptive therapy protocols. Int J Radiat Oncol Biol Phys 2005; 63:123–133.

33. Lattanzi J, McNeeley S, Hanlon A, et al. Ultrasound-based stereotactic guidance of precision conformal external beam radiation therapy in clinically localized prostate cancer. Urology 2000; 55:73–78.

34. Balter JM, Wright JN, Newell LJ, et al. Accuracy of a wireless localization system for radiotherapy. Int J Radiat Oncol Biol Phys 2005; 61:933–937.

35. Yan D, Lockman D, Brabbins D, et al. An off-line strategy for constructing a patient-specific planning target volume in adaptive treatment process for prostate cancer. Int J Radiat Oncol Biol Phys 2000; 48:289–302.

2

The Use of Imaging Modalities in the Evaluation and Treatment of Prostate Cancer

JOYCELYN L. SPEIGHT

Department of Radiation Oncology, Helen Diller Family Comprehensive Cancer Center, University of California, San Francisco, California, U.S.A.

ANTONIO C. WESTPHALEN AND FERGUS V. COAKLEY

Department of Radiology, Helen Diller Family Comprehensive Cancer Center, University of California, San Francisco, California, U.S.A.

INTRODUCTION

Conformal radiotherapy treatment approaches like intensity modulated radiation therapy (IMRT) continue to gain in popularity and their use is becoming more widespread. These new technologies have resulted in more targeted, conformal treatment plans that deliver higher doses to the target, while sparing neighboring normal tissues. Accordingly, a premium has been placed on accurate definition of all relevant volumes [i.e., gross tumor volume (GTV), clinical treatment volume (CTV), planning treatment volume (PTV), organ at risk (OAR)]. As more sophisticated treatment planning systems were developed, imaging played a progressively larger role in prostate cancer management, from diagnosis to treatment and follow-up.

The general acceptance of prostate-specific antigen (PSA) screening has led to a well-documented downward stage migration of prostate cancer (1). Accompanying the lower stages seen at diagnosis is a decline in the incidence of high-risk disease and an increase in the rate of diagnosis of clinically undetectable low-risk and intermediate-risk disease. Conventional anatomic imaging modalities have become somewhat limited in their prognostic and diagnostic utility as earlier, often clinically unapparent disease

stages have become more common. Functional imaging techniques that take advantage of cellular biology and metabolism to detect tumor presence, assess tumor extent, and characterize tumor location are finding an expanding role in treatment planning. An additional potential role for functional imaging techniques is the assessment of treatment response. To date, no consensus exists regarding what are the best imaging approaches for the detection, pretreatment and posttreatment evaluation of prostate cancer. This chapter reviews several imaging techniques relevant to the detection and diagnosis of prostate cancer and their role in prostate cancer evaluation and management.

RISK STRATIFICATION MODELS FOR PROSTATE CANCER

The American Joint Cancer Center (AJCC) TNM staging system (Table 1A) has limited utility in predicting outcome and directing therapy, particularly in men with intermediate risk disease (2). Clinical staging is insufficiently accurate to rely on as the sole determinant of treatment approach; clinical understaging is reported in up to 60% of cases. Several independent prognostic factors other than AJCC stage including patient age, Gleason score, PSA at diagnosis, PSA velocity during two years before diagnosis, the number of positive biopsy cores, and the percentage of tumor within the positive biopsy cores have been demonstrated to influence outcome. The Gleason score appears to correlate with disease extent and prognosis and is the single best predictor of biologic activity and tumor stage (3). Higher Gleason scores are associated with increased probability of disease extension to the prostate capsule, seminal vesicles, lymph nodes, and distant sites. Partin and others developed series of nomograms, mostly using Gleason score, PSA level, and T stage to predict the probability of extracapsular extension (ECE), seminal vesicle invasion (SVI), and lymph node involvement (LN+) as well as to predict treatment outcomes, including PSA failure and survival. Several risk classification schemes have been proposed based on grouping of patients with different prognostic features and similar clinical outcomes (4–10). Many physicians have adopted these simplified approaches to make treatment recommendations.

Perhaps the most widely used risk classification scheme is the one proposed by D'Amico et al. (9), which stratifies patients with clinically localized prostate cancer into three groups. Low risk is defined as T1c to T2a, PSA ≤10 ng/mL, and Gleason score ≤6. Intermediate-risk prostate cancer is defined as T2b, PSA >10 ng/mL but ≤20 ng/mL, or Gleason score 7. High-risk prostate cancer has any one of the following features: ≥T2c, PSA ≥20 ng/mL, or Gleason score 8 to 10. Ten-year PSA failure–free survival rates for low-, intermediate-, and high-risk prostate cancer are approximately 80%, 50%, and 33%, respectively. This risk stratification scheme has been validated and found to predict for prostate cancer–specific mortality following radiotherapy treatment (11).

IMAGING FOR THE DETECTION AND STAGING OF PROSTATE CANCER

The accurate assessment of disease stage at the time of initial diagnosis or extent of disease at the time of recurrence is critical for the selection of the most appropriate treatment and for the management of all stages of prostate cancer. The mainstay anatomic imaging techniques are somewhat limited in their ability to accurately describe the volume and location of tumor within the prostate at the time of diagnosis. Yet, tumor localization has become more important as focal therapies are more widely used. Anatomic imaging also has limited utility in follow-up evaluation and the early detection of posttreatment recurrences.

Prostate adenocarcinoma is often multifocal, most frequently originating within the peripheral zone of the prostate gland, though lesions within the central zone do infrequently occur (12). A detailed discussion of prostate anatomy is covered in chapter 4 "Advances in Imaging and Anatomical Considerations for Prostate Cancer Treatment Planning." Historically, anatomic imaging modalities, including transrectal ultrasound (TRUS), computed tomography (CT) imaging, magnetic resonance (MR) imaging, and radionuclide bone scintigraphy have been the primary diagnostic imaging approaches used to stage prostate cancer. The AJCC however incorporates only TRUS and bone scintigraphy in the determination of clinical stage. The current TNM staging system and stage grouping for prostate cancer are shown in Tables 1A and B.

Table 1A AJCC Tumor-Node and Metastasis (TMN) Staging System (6th Edition)

TX		Primary tumor cannot be assessed
T0		No evidence of primary
T1		Clinically inapparent tumor neither palpable nor visible by imaging
	T1a	Tumor incidental histologic finding in 5% or less tissue resected
	T1b	Tumor incidental histologic finding in more than 5% of tissue resected
	T1c	Tumor identified by needle biopsy
T2		Tumor confined within the prostate
	T2a	Tumor involves one-half of one lobe or less
	T2b	Tumor involves more than one-half of one lobe but not both lobes
	T2c	Tumor involves both lobes
T3		Tumor extends through the prostate capsule
	T3a	Extracapsular extension (unilateral or bilateral)
	T3b	Tumor invades seminal vesicle(s)
T4		Tumor is fixed or invades adjacent structures other than seminal vesicles: bladder neck, external sphincter, rectum, levator muscles and/or pelvic wall
NX		Regional lymph nodes were not assessed
N0		No regional lymph node metastasis
N1		Metastasis in regional lymph nodes
MX		Distant metastases cannot be assessed
M0		No distant metastasis
M1		Distant metastasis

Table 1B AJCC Stage Grouping

Stage I	T1a N0 M0 grade 1
Stage II	T1a N0 M0 grade 1
	T1b, T1c N0 M0 any grade
	T2 N0 M0 any grade
Stage III	T3 N0 M0 any grade
Stage IV	T4 N0 M0 any grade
	Any T, N1, M0 any grade
	Any T, any N, M1 any grade

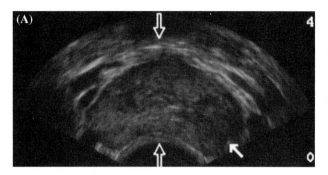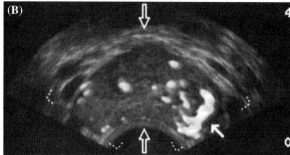

Figure 1 (**A**) Gray scale TRUS image of the prostate at the level of the mid gland. A hypoechoic area may be seen (*solid arrow*), suggesting the presence of prostate cancer at that location. (**B**) Power color Doppler demonstrating hypervascularity in the same hypoechoic region identified in **A**. *Abbreviation*: TRUS, transrectal ultrasound.

Transrectal Ultrasound

Ultrasound relies on reflected sound waves to generate an image. The image identifies the boundaries between structures that have different acoustic properties. TRUS is the most commonly used detection and staging imaging technique for prostate cancer, with a primary role in tumor assessment and biopsy guidance. However, TRUS has proven unsatisfactory for local staging of prostate cancer. A significant limitation is the effect of operator dependence and imaging technique on image quality and reproducibility. In addition, limitations exist in the ability of TRUS imaging to accurately and quantitatively identify prostate cancer location and volume within the prostate gland. The sonographic characteristics of prostate cancer within the prostate gland are nonspecific, and can appear as hypoechoic, isoechoic, and in some instances, hyperechoic areas (Fig. 1A) (13). Furthermore, the limited resolution of standard gray scale TRUS reliably detects cancers only within the peripheral zone; detection of anterior and transitional zone cancers is poor (14). Concern also exists regarding the inability of TRUS to detect capsular invasion and ECE (15–18). TRUS has marginally higher sensitivity and specificity for the detection of seminal vesicle invasion. Overall, the low positive predictive value (PPV) of standard gray scale TRUS makes it inappropriate for prostate cancer screening (15,19).

Color and power Doppler ultrasonography have increased ability to detect lesions and appear to increase the detection rate for targeted biopsy cores (20), however, this has not translated into increased staging accuracy (21,22). Figure 1B shows the corresponding image to Figure 1A with color Doppler demonstrating hypervascularity in the same hypoechoic region identified in Figure 1A. Color Doppler TRUS does appear superior in two situations (*i*) the detection of higher Gleason score tumors, which are significantly more hypervascular than low-grade tumors and (*ii*) the detection of tumors less than 3 mm in size.

Contrast enhanced ultrasonography (CEU), which uses intravenous microbubble agents in conjunction with color and power Doppler, has also been shown to improve the detection rates of prostate cancer. One study suggests that it may be useful for the identification of local recurrences in cases of postprostatectomy PSA failure (23). Yi et al. showed that CEU enhanced sensitivity of directed biopsies in men with indeterminate PSA levels and negative findings on digital rectal examination when compared with gray scale or color Doppler ultrasound (24). Three-dimensional ultrasound techniques are also available. European investigators have reported 91% staging accuracy when staging three-dimensional TRUS images were correlated with postprostatectomy histopathologic staging (25,26). Sensitivity and specificity were 84% and 96%, respectively. Positive and negative predictive values were 93% and 91%, respectively.

Computed Tomography

CT scanning had been considered a mainstay for the identification of nodal and distant metastases as part of the evaluation of diseases extent. Low sensitivity for the detection of ECE (27) limits its utility for staging. Because of insufficient soft tissue resolution to identify intraprostatic cancer, CT offers no advantage over TRUS for biopsy guidance. The primary use for CT in prostate cancer evaluation has become the detection of gross tumor extension into the periprostatic fat or adjacent organs, seminal vesicle invasion, and lymph node involvement. However, CT, which relies predominantly on size criteria for diagnosis of metastatic nodal involvement, is suboptimal for the detection of nodal metastasis (28,29). Lymph nodes greater than or equal to 1-cm diameter in short axis

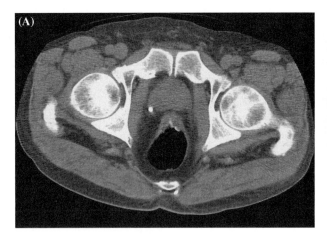
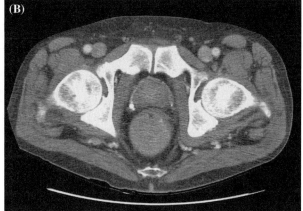

Figure 2 Axial noncontrast and contrast CT scan images of the pelvis and prostate gland. The homogeneous attenuation of all regions of the prostate gland on the noncontrast image (**A**) prevents distinction between the prostate gland itself and periprostatic vessels and muscle. These features are better seen on the contrast image (**B**).

are considered suspicious for metastatic involvement. False-negative results can occur when metastases are present in normal size nodes. False-positive results can occur with inflammation or benign nodal hyperplasia. The sensitivity and specificity of detecting nodal metastases are approximately 30% to 70% and 77% to 97%, respectively (30–32).

Due to its three-dimensional spatial capabilities, CT has been the most commonly used anatomic imaging modality in radiotherapy treatment planning for prostate cancer. Nonetheless, significant limitations include the homogeneous attenuation of all regions of the prostate gland and difficulty in distinguishing between normal prostate tissue, cancerous regions of the gland, and surrounding normal musculature. The location of urethra within the prostate gland is also difficult to identify. Axial noncontrast and contrast images of the prostate gland are shown in Figure 2A, B. The unusual finding of a visible prostate cancer on a contrast-enhanced CT scan can be seen in Figure 3.

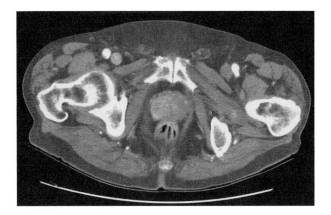

Figure 3 Axial cut from a contrast-enhanced CT scan showing a large tumor within the prostate gland.

Magnetic Resonance Imaging

MR imaging relies on the resonance properties of atomic nuclei with unmatched neutrons or protons for image generation. Resonance characteristics are influenced by the intracellular environment such as water content or fat content. Nuclear magnetic resonance (NMR or MR) signals are generated by nuclear protons when a strong magnetic field that induces coherent spinning of hydrogen protons is applied followed by the application of radiofrequency (RF) pulses. When the field is removed and the protons "spin down" returning to their base state or equilibrium, radio waves are emitted and detected as the MR signal. Spatial mapping of multiple MR signals of varying intensity yields the MR image. The time between the application of successive RF pulses (TR time) and the time to echo (TE) can be varied; images generated with short TR and TE times are designated as T1-weighted images. The time delay between the application of the RF magnetic field and the detection of the MR signal is called TE time. Images generated with a long TR and TE times are called T2-weighted images. Examples of T1- and T2-weighted images of the prostate gland are shown in Figure 4.

Image resolution is optimized with the use of an endorectal coil in association with a pelvic phase–arrayed coil (erMRI) on 1.5 tesla (T) or greater magnet. With the use of an endorectal coil, the signal-to-noise ratio is increased, allowing a smaller field of view and increased spatial resolution. Endorectal magnetic resonance imaging (erMRI) appears to be the best imaging modality for identifying the zonal anatomy of the prostate (33,34). Compared with CT, erMRI also permits localization of the neurovascular bundles, delineation of the prostatic apex from surrounding muscle of the pelvic floor, and

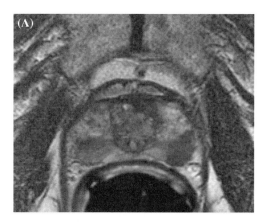 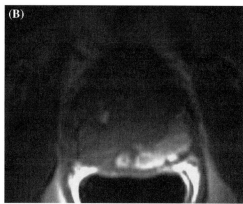

Figure 4 (**A**) An axial T2-weighted erMRI of the prostate at mid gland level. Zonal anatomy is well differentiated with the peripheral zone appearing as an area on increased signal intensity. BPH nodules are seen within the central gland. An area of low signal intensity in the left peripheral zone is suspicious for the presence of PCa. (**B**) An axial T1-weighted image. Note the area of high signal intensity within the peripheral zone, suggesting the presence postbiopsy hemorrhage. *Abbreviations*: erMRI, endorectal magnetic resonance image; BPH, benign prostatic hyperplasia; PCa, prostate cancer.

identification of ECE. Seminal vesicle invasion can also be detected with erMRI (35,36).

The zonal anatomy of the prostate gland is better seen on T2-weighted images. The transition zone, prostate capsule, and neurovascular bundles can be clearly identified. The peripheral zone has higher signal intensity than the transition and central zones, which are indistinguishable from each other. The prostate capsule appears as a peripheral area of low signal intensity. The proximal prostatic urethra is poorly visualized with erMRI, however the distal urethra appears as a ring of low T2 signal near the apex of the prostate gland. The veramontanum is a centrally located high T2-signal intensity structure at the level of the mid gland.

Prostate cancer is best seen on T2-weighted images. It appears as an area of decreased signal intensity relative to the high signal intensity of normal peripheral zone tissue (34,37). The finding of low signal regions is sensitive but not specific. Androgen deprivation, prostatitis, and prior radiotherapy treatment can also cause low signal areas on T2 images. Blood from post-biopsy hemorrhage also appears as an area of low T2-signal intensity. Blood can be differentiated from tumor by evaluating the corresponding T1-weighted image; blood will appear as an area of high-signal intensity on T1-weighted MRI. Figure 4A shows an axial T2-weighted MRI, with an area of low signal intensity in the left peripheral zone. Also apparent are benign prostatic hyperplasia (BPH) nodules within the central gland. Figure 4B shows an axial T1-weighted image. The high-intensity areas are because of blood. It is recommended that at least four weeks be allowed between biopsy and imaging (33,38–43). It must be kept in mind,

however, that the absence of an abnormal appearing peripheral zone does not exclude the presence of prostate cancer. Specific radiographic criteria exist for the diagnosis of early ECE and seminal vesicle invasion (44).

Low sensitivity and PPV for prostate cancer detection and cost make erMRI inappropriate for cancer screening (33,39). However, it has found some use for cancer detection in cases where a high index of suspicion exists for the presence of cancer despite negative TRUS imaging and biopsy results (45–47). Reports of accuracy range from approximately 50% to 90% (15,36,40,48). However, its use in PCa staging is gaining in acceptance (44,49). MRI is more accurate than digital rectal exam (DRE), and when interpreted in conjunction with TRUS, there is a trend toward increased staging accuracy. MRI seems to be most beneficial for the evaluation of intermediate- and high-risk patients with clinically localized prostate cancer (37,44,48,50,51).

The detection of lymph node metastases is not significantly better with unenhanced MR imaging than with CT scans (34). However, the addition of ultra small iron oxide particle contrast is reported to significantly enhance the sensitivity and specificity for detection of nodal involvement (52). Functional MRI imaging techniques will be discussed later in this chapter.

Because of superior image quality, erMRI is being investigated as an alternative to CT imaging for treatment planning (53–56). MRI alone may not be sufficient, as it does not provide anatomic information in a format suitable for dose calculation. However, the coregistration and fusion of MRI with CT images greatly enhances treatment planning.

ANATOMIC IMAGING AND RADIOTHERAPY TREATMENT PLANNING

Contemporary radiotherapy planning, verification, and delivery are based on a variety of imaging techniques. The integration of CT imaging into radiotherapy treatment planning introduced three-dimensional conformal radiotherapy (3DCRT). Accompanying advances in imaging combined with sophisticated dose calculation algorithms led to greatly improved tumor localization and the generation of highly conformal treatment plans. Target volumes and organs at risk could be defined with accuracy. Dose calculations performed at multiple points within the defined treatment volumes, use of beam's eye view to shape the radiation beams, and design treatment portals improved target coverage and minimized the radiation exposure to the rectum and surrounding normal tissues (57). Higher radiation doses could be delivered to the prostate with acceptable rectal and normal tissue toxicity (58–61). The demonstration that radiation dose is an independent determinant of biochemical control highlights the significance of dose escalation (62–66). Using 3DCRT, doses up to 78 Gy can be safely delivered to the prostate (66–68).

IMRT is a technically more sophisticated form of 3DCRT. Inverse treatment planning algorithms and iterative computer optimizations produce treatment volumes throughout which radiation intensity can be varied. The result is the ability to create highly conformal dose distributions, with steep dose gradients at the interface with normal structures. Though no studies yet confirm an overall survival benefit for doses greater than 78 to 79 Gy in the treatment of prostate cancer, radiation doses greater than or equal to 81 Gy can be safely delivered with IMRT, which significantly improves disease-free survival (60,69). In addition, the ability to deliver non-uniform radiotherapy doses within a treatment volume can be used to selectively escalate the dose to a portion of the target volume, such as a dominant intraprostatic lesion (70,71).

A necessary adjunct to the delivery of higher radiation doses to complicated contours is the need for precise target localization. The challenge of achieving geographic accuracy is well recognized (72,73), as is the need for recognition and correction of geometric uncertainties inherent to treatment delivery (i.e., setup error or interfraction variation and/or prostate motion during treatment: intrafraction variation). The clinical consequences of positional uncertainties have been reported (74–76). Several advanced image-based approaches to address these uncertainties, both before and during treatment, have been developed and are currently in use. The integration of these techniques with sophisticated radiotherapy treatment systems characterizes image guided radiation therapy (IGRT). Chapter 5 specifically considers target and organ motion, chapters 8 through 10 and 12 look at specific techniques for prostate IGRT.

FUNCTIONAL IMAGING

The incorporation of functional imaging into conformal radiotherapy treatment planning is an important step along the path to true image-guided, adaptive radiation therapy. The ability to modify treatment plans based not only on alterations in target size or location but also considering treatment response or the likelihood of response holds tremendous promise. The clinical concept of the International Commission on Radiation Units and Measurement (ICRU) reports 50 and 62 (77–80) entail the inclusion of all microscopic disease extent. Functional imaging aids in the detection and definition of these volumes. The integration of functional images and fused or hybrid anatomic-functional images into treatment planning may facilitate the definition of a more clinically significant target, the so-called "biologic target volume" (BTV) (81–83). The ability to identify a BTV may facilitate the identification of more biologically aggressive, and therefore, perhaps more clinically significant prostate cancers, from those likely to be more indolent.

The following section will review the role of several functional imaging modalities including endorectal magnetic resonance spectroscopy (MRS), positron emission tomography (PET), single-photon emission tomography (SPECT), and bone scintigraphy in the evaluation and treatment of prostate cancer.

Endorectal Magnetic Resonance Spectroscopic Imaging

Three-dimensional endorectal magnetic resonance spectroscopic imaging (MRSI) provides metabolic information about the prostate gland. It is an added sequence to an MRI scan, which when performed as part of the same exam allows direct correlation of the metabolic data with the anatomic data. The addition of MRS to MRI increases the specificity in the detection and localization of prostate cancer and improves staging accuracy (84–86). MRS takes advantage of the different resonance characteristics. During standard MRI, the signals from all hydrogen protons are combined, although the signals from the hydrogen protons in different molecules have distinct frequencies, a property known as chemical shift. MRS utilizes this property to produce a map of signal intensity versus frequency that reflects the relative concentration of different metabolites in different regions of the prostate gland.

In prostate cancer, the relevant metabolic information is the intracellular levels of creatine, choline, and citrate.

Choline is a constituent of normal cell membranes that is elevated in many tumors, and citrate is a constituent of normal prostate tissue. Spectroscopic evaluation of the levels of the three cellular metabolites is used to distinguish between normal prostate tissue, which has elevated citrate levels and areas of prostate cancer, which has elevated choline levels and reduced citrate levels. These variations are thought to represent differences in cell membrane turnover associated with normal cell functioning and the increased rates of cell proliferation and growth seen with tumor cells (87,88). A ratio of choline-creatine to citrate greater than 3 standard deviations compared with normal peripheral zone tissue is suggestive of the presence of prostate cancer (33,39–43). Figure 5A shows an axial T2-weighted MR image of the prostate gland from a patient with prostate cancer. The regions of cancer appear as hypointense areas in the left peripheral zone. Figure 5B shows the MRS study performed at the same level.

The combination of erMRI and MRS spatially identifies the abnormalities in cellular biochemistry that occur with the change to the malignant phenotype and differentiates normal and altered tissue metabolism. The biochemical changes associated with prostate cancer are detectable, even in the absence of anatomic or adiographic abnormalities. This makes erMRI/MRS a powerful tool in situations where a high index of suspicion exists, but multiple biopsies have been non-diagnostic. Studies suggest that concordant findings of the presence of prostate cancer on both scans significantly improve the specificity of cancer detection and localization (84,85,89). A combined positive result has a PPV of 88% to 92%. Similarly, a negative result on both scans has a high negative predictive value (NPV) (80%). The combination of erMRI and MRS also significantly enhances the detection of ECE (44,48) and can provide information relative to Gleason grade. Investigators have shown that changes in the choline to citrate ratios appear to be relative to Gleason score (87). A study comparing MRI and MRS results with the pathologic evaluation of step-sectioned prostate tissue obtained at radical prostatectomy indicated that MRS imaging was dependent on Gleason grade. Tumor

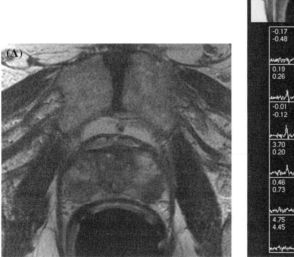
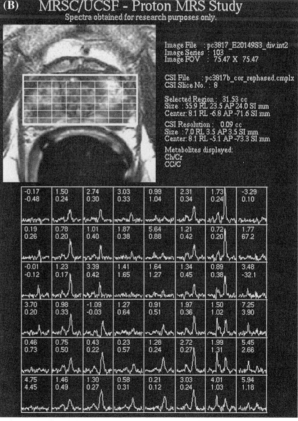

Figure 5 (**A**) Axial endorectal MRSI. Combined erMRI and three-dimensional proton MRS study in a patient with prostate cancer. (**B**) The overlaying 8 × 6 spectroscopy grid with the obtained spectra. The spectra show areas of increased choline and decreased citrate in the left peripheral zone, which is concordant with T2 hypointense regions at the left peripheral zone. *Abbreviations*: erMRSI, endorectal magnetic resonance spectroscopic imaging; MRSC, magnetic resonance science center; UCSF, University of California, San Francisco; MRS, magnetic resonance spectroscopy.

identification increased from approximately 45% to 90% with progression from Gleason grade 6 to 8 and 9 (90).

The suggestion that MRS provides information about tumor aggressiveness fostered several evaluations of the potential predictive capability of erMRI-MRS. D'Amico et al. evaluated the role of MR imaging for predicting the time to postprostatectomy PSA failure. For the majority of patients evaluated, MR imaging did not add clinically meaningful information. However, for intermediate-risk patients, erMRI-MRS appears to provide a clinically and statistically relevant stratification of PSA outcome at five years, based on the presence or absence of ECE (35).

Less is known about the preradiotherapy predictive value of erMRI-MRS. McKenna et al. have presented results suggesting that pretreatment erMRI-MRS findings are predictive of outcome (85). Their data suggest that the presence and extent of ECE is a strong predictor for the development of metastases. An earlier study by Nguyen et al. suggested that the identification of SVI in patients with clinically localized prostate cancer was associated with an increased risk of biochemical failure. In these patients, the risk of PSA failure was commensurate with that of patients with locally advanced disease (91). erMRI-MRS may also be useful to evaluate clinically low-risk cancers in an effort to discern which are likely to remain clinically indolent and therefore suitable for active surveillance protocols (92). In one retrospective study, the addition of erMRI-MRS data to a nomogram model for clinically insignificant prostate cancer significantly improved the accuracy of the model compared to earlier models that only incorporated clinical information (92).

erMRI-MRS may also have an expanding role in radiotherapy treatment planning. For example, the addition of MRS to erMRI improves the sensitivity and specificity for identifying sites of dominant intraprostatic lesions (DIL) (93). In theory, by using this information radiotherapy treatment planning can be modified to insure that the areas with the highest concentration of tumor receive the highest dose.

A significant area of strength for erMRI-MRS appears to be posttreatment follow-up and the detection of recurrence (89,94,95). Alone, MRI has limited value for tumor detection in the prostate gland after radiotherapy treatment, due to the development of diffuse low T2-signal intensity and inability to distinguish normal zonal anatomy (96–98). The addition of MRS, which detects abnormal metabolism rather than abnormal anatomy, diminishes the effect of these limitations. A small study by Coakley et al. examined patients with biochemical failure after external beam radiotherapy. erMRI-MRS had an area under the receiver operating curve (AUROC) of 81%, which was significantly better than for erMRI alone (94). A prospective study by Pucar et al. correlated MRI-MRS findings with pathologic findings after external beam radiotherapy treatment. MRSI had an AUROC of 88% for discriminating between benign and malignant tissue (99). Menard et al. showed that the sensitivity and specificity of erMRI-MRS for detecting posttreatment recurrence were 89% and 92%, respectively, with accuracy of 91% (100). Pickett et al. have shown that the determination of time to metabolic atrophy as assessed by erMRI-MRS may provide a tool for early evaluation of treatment response for patients treated with external beam radiotherapy and brachytherapy (101–103). Posttreatment erMRI-MRS increased the level of confidence of local control assessment, helping to differentiate benign posttreatment PSA spikes from PSA increases due to local failure. In response to treatment with androgen deprivation therapy, chemotherapy can also be assessed with erMRI-MRS.

Positron Emission Tomography

PET has become an important diagnostic tool in cancer diagnosis, staging, restaging, and management of many cancers. The overall utility of its role in the evaluation of new and recurrent prostate cancer is under evaluation (104–107). Cancers exhibit increased metabolism via the glycolytic pathway leading to increased uptake of the injected radiolabeled glucose analogues. PET images detect the distribution of two 511-keV gamma rays that are emitted after an annihilation reaction between injected positron emitting radiopharmaceuticals and intracellular electrons. PET is quantified by estimating a parameter called the specific uptake value (SUV). The SUV is an estimate of relative concentrations of radiotracer uptake in the area of interest compared with the average uptake throughout the remainder of the body. Comparisons of relative SUV values may be helpful to assess disease response to treatment as well as residual or recurrent disease. The most commonly used PET radiopharmaceutical is fluorine-18-deoxyglucose. Combining the anatomic imaging capabilities of CT with the metabolic assessment of PET can provide the data needed to more accurately determine disease extent as well as assess treatment efficacy.

In contrast to other sites, prostate uptake of the most commonly used tracer, ^{18}F-2-fluoro-D-deoxy-glucose (^{18}FDG), is highly variable, likely due to low glucose uptake by the prostate. There is little difference in tracer uptake between benign hyperplasia and prostate carcinoma (108–110) making the use of PET for screening purposes inappropriate. The use of ^{18}FDG PET in the management of prostate cancer has been largely limited to patients with hormone refractory prostate cancer (111,112). There maybe a use for the detection of local recurrence or distant metastases in the setting of biochemical failure (107).

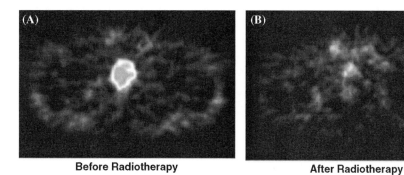

Before Radiotherapy   **After Radiotherapy**

Figure 6 [^{11}C]choline PET images of the prostate gland.

Other radiotracers including ^{18}F-fluoride, ^{11}C- and ^{18}F-labeled choline, and ^{11}C-acetate derivatives appear to be more useful than ^{18}FDG (113–119). Table 2 summarizes the results of several recent studies that have evaluated the role of PET in prostate cancer imaging. The better specificity of these newer agents in part, may be explained by their pattern of excretion. In contrast to ^{18}FDG, ^{11}C-acetate is not excreted in the urine and appears to have lower physiologic uptake in pelvic organs, removing the problem of obstructed visualization caused by ^{18}F-FDG accumulation in the bladder. Consequently, ^{11}C-acetate appears to be better suited for assessing pelvic recurrences after radical prostatectomy (RP) (113,114). In addition, the metabolic characteristics of prostate cancer cells, specifically the transformation to citrate-oxidizing cells, may account for greater tracer uptake and higher sensitivity. ^{11}C-choline and ^{18}F-fluorocholine have also been shown to be useful for localizing disease within the prostate gland (116,117). Figure 6 shows a [^{11}C]choline PET image of the prostate gland before and after radiotherapy treatment.

Table 2 Selected Studies Addressing the Role of PET for Men with Prostate Cancer

First author, year (reference)	Imaging agent (country)	Conclusions of selected studies
Sandblom, 2006 (115)	^{11}C-acetate (Sweden)	Post-RP with rising PSA median 2 ng/mL and PSADT 12 mo. PET scanning with ^{11}C-acetate is promising for detection of recurrences but high false positive rate is limiting.
Wachter, 2006 (114)	^{11}C-acetate (Austria)	CT and MRI image fusion with ^{11}C-AC PET for recurrences post-RP or -RT. Image fusion (CT-PET, MRI-PET) defined abnormal uptake in 37 (73%) of 51 sites. ^{11}CAC PET and CT/MRI fusion may be useful in pts with ^{11}C-AC uptake in the prostate bed & in pelvic nodes.
Langsteger, 2006 (118)	^{18}FDG, ^{18}FCH (Austria)	Sensitivity of ^{18}FDG for bone mets no better than bone scans. ^{18}FCH may to be useful in the staging of prostate cancer.
Reske, 2006 (116)	^{11}C-choline (Germany)	^{11}C-choline PET and CT prior to RP, and correlated with histopathology. SUV of ^{11}C-choline in PCa tissue 3.5 times higher than benign tissue ($p < 0.001$).
Martorana, 2006 (117)	^{11}C-choline (Italy)	^{11}C-choline PET/CT prior to biopsy sensitivity/specificity of PET/CT and MRI compared for prediction of ECE. PET/CT showed 83% sensitivity for localizing nodules >5 mm. PET/CT has comparable sensitivity to TRUS/Bx but was less specific (84% vs. 97%, $p = 0.008$). PET/CT lower sensitivity than MRI (22% vs. 63%, $p < 0.001$).
Hacker, 2006 (119)	^{18}F-fluorocholine (Germany)	Preoperative ^{18}F-fluorocholine PET/CT and intraoperative lap radioisotope guided sentinel PLND in men with a PSA >10 and/or a Gleason score >7. Sentinel PLND preceded extended PLND. In 50% points node mets detected. Mets would have been missed with standard PLND. Extended PLND reveals more mets. ^{18}F-fluorocholine and PET/CT are not useful for occult nodal mets.

Abbreviations: PSA, prostate-specific antigen; PSADT, prostate-specific antigen doubling time; PET, positron emission tomography; RP, radical prostatectomy; RT, radiation therapy; FDG, fluorodeoxyglucose; AC, Acetate; FCH, ^{18}F-choline ^{18}F-fluoride; SUV, specific uptake value; TRUS, transrectal ultrasound; CT, computed tomography; MRI, magnetic resonance imaging; PLND, pelvic lymph node dissection; mets, metastases.

18-Fluorodihydrotestosterone (^{18}F-FDHT) has been studied as a possible means to quantify androgen deprivation receptors in patients with metastatic prostate cancer. ^{18}F-FDHT PET imaging was positive in 63% of advanced prostate cancer patients (120).

SPECT and Radioimmunoscintigraphy

SPECT imaging is based on the same biologic principle as PET imaging. The distinguishing feature relative to PET is the utilization of radioisotopes that emit a single photon rather than positron.

The most commonly used SPECT agent for prostate cancer is Capromab pendetide, an Indium-111 (^{111}In) radiolabeled monoclonal antibody against an intracellular domain of the prostate-specific membrane antigen (PSMA). Studies have shown some efficacy for this approach in detecting lymph node metastases (121–123). There may also be a use for the detection of metastases in patients with posttreatment PSA failure (124). A major limitation of this type of scan is the somewhat low and highly variable rates of sensitivity and specificity. This may be due to the intracellular binding site for the antibody and the expression of PSMA by nonprostate tissues (125). A more limited experience has been reported for using SPECT for treatment planning (126). Ellis and coworkers have been most active in this area (127). They described a technique that involves fusing a radioactive SPECT imaging agent with pelvic CT images for the purpose of designing brachytherapy that targets areas at high risk for treatment failure. They correlated areas of increased intensity seen on SPECT-CT fusion images with biopsy results and reported an overall accuracy of 80%. More studies are needed to confirm these findings. Newer antibody-based imaging methods that target the extracellular domains of the PSMA are being evaluated (128).

Radionuclide Bone Scintigraphy

Nuclear bone scans are a standard component of the staging evaluation for prostate cancer. They have greater sensitivity than plain radiographs or CT scans for the detection of osteoblastic bone metastases. Bone scans are less sensitive than MRI for metastases; however, they have the advantage of evaluating the entire skeleton. Bone scans are also less sensitive than CT scans for osteolytic and mixed osteolytic-osteoblastic bone metastases. Bone scintigraphy does suffer from low specificity; infection, old and new healing fractures, benign bone islands, and degenerative changes can all lead to increased radiotracer uptake.

The sensitivity of bone scans varies with PSA and Gleason score. Studies have suggested that asymptomatic patients with low PSA levels ($\leq$10 ng/mL) are highly unlikely to have a positive bone scan. Patients with PSA $\leq$20 ng/mL and Gleason score $<$8 have a 1% to 13% rate of positive bone scans (129,130). The positive bone scan rate increases to about 50% with a PSA level $\geq$50 ng/mL (131). The American College of Radiology (ACR) appropriateness criteria recommend radionuclide bone scintigraphy for patients with PSA $\geq$20 ng/mL, T3-T4 disease, Gleason score $\geq$8, and symptomatic patients.

Imaging and Pelvic Nodal Disease

The poor prognostic significance of pelvic nodal disease in prostate cancer is well documented. Studies have suggested that the incidence of pelvic lymph node involvement in men with clinically localized prostate cancer is much higher than previously recognized, because most estimates of nodal positivity are based on patients who underwent standard lymph node dissection. Up to 40% of histopathologically positive nodes would be missed if a standard lymph node sampling were performed. In addition, lymph nodes that were removed and considered negative by routine histopathologic evaluation may harbor occult disease (132–134). The significance of occult lymph node involvement is tied to recent studies indicating that patients with a risk of lymph involvement of 15% or higher benefit from prophylactic irradiation of pelvic lymph nodes (135). Targeting, treatment indications, and techniques of pelvic lymph nodes are discussed in detail in chapter 16 by Roach, Xia, and Pouliot. The group at University of California, San Francisco (UCSF) previously published on the benefit of IMRT for pelvic lymph node coverage (136); however, the problem of accurate identification of involved nodes remains a formidable one. Two novel approaches for the detection of lymph node metastases are described below.

Nanoparticle-Enhanced MRI for Pelvic Nodal Disease

A number of studies have suggested that PET/CT with ^{18}F-fluorocholine may not be as sensitive as an extended pelvic lymph node dissection or laproscopic, radioisotope guided, sentinel lymph node dissection for identifying metastases to pelvic lymph nodes (Table 2). As previously discussed, reliance on size criteria is suboptimal for the detection of nodal metastasis (28,29). Sentinel lymph node studies using radiolabeled colloids injected transrectally, preoperatively into the prostate gland have demonstrated 96% sensitivity for detecting nodal micrometastatses

(137–141). While these agents appear to function well, some investigators suggest that some of the features of the radio-colloids may pose technical problems for their use.

Other studies have shown that using a contrast agent containing lymphotropic superparamagnetic nanoparticles consisting of densely packed dextran-coated iron oxide cores with MRI may dramatically improve the sensitivity and specificity of MRI (52,142). Iron oxide nanoparticles are phagocytosed by macrophages, via which they are deposited in normal lymph nodes. Malignant nodes are unable to take up the particles, providing a means of distinguishing involved from uninvolved lymph nodes. This technique is particularly useful in identifying involved nodes that on other forms of imaging would not meet size criteria. Sensitivity and specificity for the detection of nodal metastases were significantly higher for MRI with lymphotrophic superparamagnetic nanoparticles compared with standard MRI, 90.5% and 97.8% and 35.4% and 90.4% respectively. This technology is likely to prove useful for designing radiation fields to insure that lymph node areas at risk are adequately covered (143). Unfortunately, this compound is not currently commercially available in the United States.

A preclinical study of an alternative sentinel lymph node mapping agent [^{99M}TC]Diethylenetetramine Penta-acetic Acid-Manosyl-Dextran (Lymphoseek™) has been reported by investigators at the University of California, San Diego. The particular characteristics of this agent make intraoperative injection feasible (as opposed to pre-operative injection) and prolonged time of accumulation in the sentinel lymph node with less diffusion out of the node to other sites. Clinical phase I studies are underway (144).

SPECT Imaging for Lymph Node Disease

There is an extensive but controversial body of literature evaluating the role of [^{111}]In-capromab Pendetide Scan (ProstaScint® Scan, Cyt-356) in the determination of lymph node status of patients being considered for definitive therapy. Several recent reviews suggest that this imaging modality may be of value in identifying pelvic lymph nodes and treatment planning for radiotherapy (125,145). However, other studies question its use. It is now clear that CT or MRI imaging should be combined with SPECT scanning to optimize accuracy. More work is needed to define the role of this modality in the management of patients with clinically localized prostate cancer.

IMAGE REGISTRATION AND FUSION

The optimum utilization of functional images in radiotherapy treatment planning requires them to be combined with anatomical images, usually from CT and/or MRI scans. The goal of incorporating information from multiple image studies is to have access to the most comprehensive anatomic and functional data about a treatment area. Ultimately, the objective is to facilitate radiotherapy treatment planning. Fusion of serial imaging studies can also be useful for assessment of tumor response to treatment, detection of residual disease post-therapy, evaluation of organ motion, and uncertainties in patient setup. More recently, Italian researchers have reported that image fusion between color Doppler TRUS and erMRI improves the accuracy of pathologic staging (accuracy 92%, sensitivity 71%, specificity 100%, PPV 100%, NPV 90%) (146).

The process of combining and transferring data from different imaging modalities is called image fusion. Image registration is the process of defining a coordinate system for matching or mapping like areas between different images that will allow accurate translation of information between multiple images. Different methods for image registration exist depending on the nature of the coordinate transformation. Rigid body transformations are the simplest and combine images of structures that move as a rigid uniform structure (i.e., the spinal cord). More complex warping approaches are required to register images in which the shape of anatomic tissues varies between scans, either because of body position or changes in organ size, contour, or location. Differences in image volumetric and pixel intensity can also be used for matching and image registration. Most commonly, patient anatomy is used as the basis for registration (intrinsic registration) via matching homologous anatomical areas on the different images. Discrete points such as bony landmarks can be used for matching images as can contiguous curved structures such as the anterior rectal wall. Extrinsic coordinate systems, such as stereotactic frames, can also be used. Several excellent references are available for a detailed discussion of image registration and fusion (147).

Sophisticated image registration and fusion software permits single modality (i.e., CT to CT) and multimodality (i.e., PET to CT or PET to TRUS) image fusion. Since image guided radiotherapy depends on accurate target delineation, high fidelity of image registration and fusion is critical. For this reason, the development of hybrid scanners that permit concurrent acquisition of scans is believed by many clinicians to be more advantageous than separately acquired scans.

IMAGING IN POSTTREATMENT FOLLOW-UP

The role of imaging following radiotherapy for prostate cancer is largely determined by the results of serial PSA testing. Exceptions to this are the use of CT scan for postimplant dosimetry or symptom development, such as bone pain in a patient with locally advanced or high-risk prostate cancer. Postimplant CT scans are typically performed three to four weeks postimplantation and are used to evaluate implant quality. Evaluation of new onset bone pain typically consists of plain radiographs of the involved area or bone scan. If suspicious, a CT scan or MRI scan are often requested for further evaluation. No indication exists for routine imaging evaluation in the absence of a rising PSA or clinical signs or symptoms.

In the setting of biochemical failure, the primary impetus is to differentiate between local and metastatic relapse. Clinical stage at diagnosis, Gleason score, timing of posttreatment relapse, and PSA doubling time provide prognostic information regarding the probable location of recurrence, and have been relied on more than imaging. When imaging is performed, TRUS is the most frequently used imaging modality. It is more sensitive, but less specific than DRE, and appears to be more sensitive than CT in detecting postprostatectomy tumor recurrence (148,149). One might anticipate that functional imaging studies would hold more promise for the evaluation and localization of recurrences, particularly if similar pretreatment scans are available for comparison. Standard MRI has excellent sensitivity and specificity for the detection of postprostatectomy recurrence (150,151). erMRI-MRS appears helpful for the evaluation of recurrence following external beam radiotherapy and brachytherapy seed implantation (101–103). Once radiotracer selection for prostate cancer is optimized, PET/CT may have a larger role in posttreatment imaging.

SUMMARY OF PERTINENT CONCLUSIONS

- Multiple imaging modalities are used to characterize prostate cancer throughout diagnosis, evaluation, and treatment.
- Radiotherapy treatment of prostate cancer is an imaging intensive process across all disease stages.
- Stage-specific appropriateness criteria by the ACR address the appropriate use of the variety of imaging modalities in prostate cancer management (152) (available at www.acr.org).
- The most recent guidelines were updated in 2007. These criteria are an excellent guideline for decision making regarding the use of radiologic imaging for prostate cancer.
- In low-risk disease TRUS is used for diagnosis and biopsy guidance.
- Imaging has a larger role in patients with intermediate-risk prostate cancer for staging and directing therapy. It has been suggested that imaging may

find its greatest use in intermediate-risk prostate cancer.
- A need for posttreatment follow-up imaging studies can be anticipated in patients with high-risk prostate cancer.
- The development of a standard protocol (Digital Imaging and Communications in Medicine, DICOM-RT) to communicate imaging information between imaging devices and treatment planning computers was a critical achievement that has allowed progressively greater integration of imaging into radiotherapy treatment.
- Further integration and refinement in imaging and radiotherapy techniques, continued development of novel imaging approaches and the discovery of new radiotracers and molecular markers can be expected.

REFERENCES

1. Cooperberg MR, Grossfeld GD, Lubeck DP, et al. National practice patterns and time trends in androgen ablation for localized prostate cancer. J Natl Cancer Inst 2003; 95:981–989.
2. Roach MR, Weinberg V, Sandler H, et al. Staging for prostate cancer: time to incorporate pretreatment prostate-specific antigen and Gleason score? Cancer 2007; 109(2): 213–220.
3. Gleason DF, Mellinger GT. Prediction of prognosis for prostatic adenocarcinoma by combined histological grading and clinical staging. J Urol 1974; 111:58–64.
4. D'Amico AV, Cote K, Loffredo M, et al. Determinants of prostate cancer-specific survival after radiation therapy for patients with clinically localized prostate cancer. J Clin Oncol 2002; 20:4567–4573.
5. Kattan MW, Zelefsky MJ, Kupelian PA, et al. Pretreatment nomogram for predicting the outcome of three-dimensional conformal radiotherapy in prostate cancer. J Clin Oncol 2000; 18:3352–3359.
6. Roach M, Weinberg V, McLaughlin P, et al. Serum prostate specific antigen (PSA) and survival following external beam radiotherapy for carcinoma of the prostate. Urology, 2003; 61(4):730–735.
7. Partin AW, Mangold LA, Lamm DM, et al. Contemporary update of prostate cancer staging nomograms (Partin Tables) for the new millennium. Urology 2001; 58:843–848.
8. Kattan MW, Zelefsky MJ, Kupelian PA, et al. Pretreatment nomogram that predicts 5-year probability of metastasis following three-dimensional conformal radiation therapy for localized prostate cancer. J Clin Oncol 2003; 21:4568–4571.
9. D'Amico AV, Whittington R, Malkowicz SB, et al. Biochemical outcome after radical prostatectomy, external beam radiation therapy, or interstitial radiation therapy for clinically localized prostate cancer. JAMA 1998; 280: 969–974.

10. Zelefsky MJ, Leibel SA, Gaudin PB, et al. Dose escalation with three-dimensional conformal radiation therapy affects the outcome in prostate cancer. Int J Radiat Oncol Biol Phys 1998; 41:491–500.

11. D'Amico AV, Moul J, Carroll PR, et al. Cancer-specific mortality after surgery or radiation for patients with clinically localized prostate cancer managed during the prostate-specific antigen era. J Clin Oncol 2003; 21:2163–2172.

12. McNeal JE. Normal histology of the prostate. Am J Surg Pathol 1988; 12:619–633.

13. Dahnert WF, Hamper UM, Eggleston JC, et al. Prostatic evaluation by transrectal sonography with histopathologic correlation: the echopenic appearance of early carcinoma. Radiology 1986; 158:97–102.

14. Oesterling JE, Suman VJ, Zincke H, et al. PSA-detected (clinical stage T1c or B0) prostate cancer. Pathologically significant tumors. Urol Clin North Am 1993; 20:687–693.

15. Rifkin MD, Zerhouni EA, Gatsonis CA, et al. Comparison of magnetic resonance imaging and ultrasonography in staging early prostate cancer. Results of a multi-institutional cooperative trial. N Engl J Med 1990; 323:621–626.

16. Lorentzen T, Nerstrom H, Iversen P, et al. Local staging of prostate cancer with transrectal ultrasound: a literature review. Prostate Suppl 1992; 4:11–16.

17. Smith JA Jr., Scardino PT, Resnick MI, et al. Transrectal ultrasound versus digital rectal examination for the staging of carcinoma of the prostate: results of a prospective, multi-institutional trial. J Urol 1997; 157:902–906.

18. Yoon F, Rodrigues G, D'Souza D, et al. Assessing the prognostic significance of transrectal ultrasound extracapsular extension in prostate cancer. Clin Oncol (R Coll Radiol) 2006; 18:117–124.

19. Rifkin M. Comparison of magnetic resonance imaging and ultrasonography in staging early prostate cancer. Results of a multi-institutional cooperative trial. Invest Radiol 1991; 26:1024–1025.

20. Pelzer A, Bektic J, Berger AP, et al. Prostate cancer detection in men with prostate specific antigen 4 to 10 ng/ml using a combined approach of contrast enhanced color Doppler targeted and systematic biopsy. J Urol 2005; 173:1926–1929.

21. Cornud F, Hamida K, Flam T, et al. Endorectal color doppler sonography and endorectal MR imaging features of nonpalpable prostate cancer: correlation with radical prostatectomy findings. AJR Am J Roentgenol 2000; 175:1161–1168.

22. Sauvain JL, Palascak P, Bourscheid D, et al. Value of power doppler and 3D vascular sonography as a method for diagnosis and staging of prostate cancer. Eur Urol 2003; 44:21–30; discussion 30–31.

23. Drudi FM, Giovagnorio F, Carbone A, et al. Transrectal colour Doppler contrast sonography in the diagnosis of local recurrence after radical prostatectomy–comparison with MRI. Ultraschall Med 2006; 27:146–151.

24. Yi A, Kim JK, Park SH, et al. Contrast-enhanced sonography for prostate cancer detection in patients with indeterminate clinical findings. AJR Am J Roentgenol 2006; 186:1431–1435.

25. Mitterberger M, Horninger W, Pelzer A, et al. A prospective randomized trial comparing contrast-enhanced targeted versus systematic ultrasound guided biopsies: impact on prostate cancer detection. Prostate 2007; 67:1537–1542.

26. Mitterberger M, Pelzer A, Colleselli D, et al. Contrast-enhanced ultrasound for diagnosis of prostate cancer and kidney lesions. Eur J Radiol 2007; 64:231–238.

27. Engeler CE, Wasserman NF, Zhang G. Preoperative assessment of prostatic carcinoma by computerized tomography. Weaknesses and new perspectives. Urology 1992; 40:346–350.

28. Wolf JS Jr., Cher M, Dall'era M, et al. The use and accuracy of cross-sectional imaging and fine needle aspiration cytology for detection of pelvic lymph node metastases before radical prostatectomy. J Urol 1995; 153:993–999.

29. Tiguert R, Gheiler EL, Tefilli MV, et al. Lymph node size does not correlate with the presence of prostate cancer metastasis. Urology 1999; 53:367–371.

30. Oyen RH, Van Poppel HP, Ameye FE, et al. Lymph node staging of localized prostatic carcinoma with CT and CT-guided fine-needle aspiration biopsy: prospective study of 285 patients. Radiology 1994; 190:315–322.

31. Weinerman PM, Arger PH, Coleman BG, et al. Pelvic adenopathy from bladder and prostate carcinoma: detection by rapid-sequence computed tomography. AJR Am J Roentgenol 1983; 140:95–99.

32. Golimbu M, Morales P, Al-Askari S, et al. CAT scanning in staging of prostatic cancer. Urology 1981; 18:305–308.

33. Hricak H, Dooms GC, McNeal JE, et al. MR imaging of the prostate gland: normal anatomy. AJR Am J Roentgenol 1987; 148:51–58.

34. Hricak H, Dooms GC, Jeffrey RB, et al. Prostatic carcinoma: staging by clinical assessment, CT, and MR imaging. Radiology 1987; 162:331–336.

35. Wang L, Mullerad M, Chen HN, et al. Prostate cancer: incremental value of endorectal MR imaging findings for prediction of extracapsular extension. Radiology 2004; 232:133–139.

36. Cornud F, Flam T, Chauveinc L, et al. Extraprostatic spread of clinically localized prostate cancer: factors predictive of pT3 tumor and of positive endorectal MR imaging examination results. Radiology 2002; 224:203–210.

37. Vapnek JM, Hricak H, Shinohara K, et al. Staging accuracy of magnetic resonance imaging versus transrectal ultrasound in stages A and B prostatic cancer. Urol Int 1994; 53:191–195.

38. Ikonen S, Kivisaari L, Vehmas T, et al. Optimal timing of post-biopsy MR imaging of the prostate. Acta Radiol 2001; 42:70–73.

39. Hricak H, White S, Vigneron D, et al. Carcinoma of the prostate gland: MR imaging with pelvic phased-array coils versus integrated endorectal—pelvic phased-array coils. Radiology 1994; 193:703–709.

40. Schnall MD, Bezzi M, Pollack HM, et al. Magnetic resonance imaging of the prostate. Magn Reson Q 1990; 6:1–16.

41. Rifkin MD, Dahnert W, Kurtz AB. State of the art: endorectal sonography of the prostate gland. AJR Am J Roentgenol 1990; 154:691–700.

42. Ellis WJ, Brawer MK. The significance of isoechoic prostatic carcinoma. J Urol 1994; 152:2304–2307.

43. Shinohara K, Wheeler TM, Scardino PT. The appearance of prostate cancer on transrectal ultrasonography: correlation of imaging and pathological examinations. J Urol 1989; 142:76–82.

44. Yu KK, Hricak H, Alagappan R, et al. Detection of extracapsular extension of prostate carcinoma with endorectal and phased-array coil MR imaging: multivariate feature analysis. Radiology 1997; 2023:697–702.

45. Beyersdorff D, Taupitz M, Winkelmann B, et al. Patients with a history of elevated prostate-specific antigen levels and negative transrectal US-guided quadrant or sextant biopsy results: value of MR imaging. Radiology 2002; 224: 701–706.

46. Perrotti M, Han KR, Epstein RE, et al. Prospective evaluation of endorectal magnetic resonance imaging to detect tumor foci in men with prior negative prostastic biopsy: a pilot study. J Urol 1999; 162:1314–1317.

47. Costouros NG, Coakley FV, Westphalen AC, et al. Diagnosis of prostate cancer in patients with an elevated prostate-specific antigen level: role of endorectal MRI and MR spectroscopic imaging. AJR Am J Roentgenol 2007; 188: 812–816.

48. Outwater EK, Petersen RO, Siegelman ES, et al. Prostate carcinoma: assessment of diagnostic criteria for capsular penetration on endorectal coil MR images. Radiology 1994; 193(2):333–339.

49. Sala E, Akin O, Moskowitz CS, et al. Endorectal MR imaging in the evaluation of seminal vesicle invasion: diagnostic accuracy and multivariate feature analysis. Radiology 2006; 238:929–937.

50. Tempany CM, Zhou X, Zerhouni EA, et al. Staging of prostate cancer: results of Radiology Diagnostic Oncology Group project comparison of three MR imaging techniques. Radiology 1994; 192:47–54.

51. Huch Boni RA, Boner JA, Debatin JF, et al. Optimization of prostate carcinoma staging: comparison of imaging and clinical methods. Clin Radiol 1995; 50:593–600.

52. Harisinghani MG, Barentsz J, Hahn PF, et al. Noninvasive detection of clinically occult lymph-node metastases in prostate cancer. N Engl J Med 2003; 348:2491–2499.

53. Payne GS, Leach MO. Applications of magnetic resonance spectroscopy in radiotherapy treatment planning. Br J Radiol 2006; 79 Spec No 1:S16–S26.

54. McLaughlin PW, Narayana V, Meriowitz A, et al. Vessel-sparing prostate radiotherapy: dose limitation to critical erectile vascular structures (internal pudendal artery and corpus cavernosum) defined by MRI. Int J Radiat Oncol Biol Phys 2005; 61:20–31.

55. Buyyounouski MK, Horwitz EM, Uzzo RG, et al. The radiation doses to erectile tissues defined with magnetic resonance imaging after intensity-modulated radiation therapy or iodine-125 brachytherapy. Int J Radiat Oncol Biol Phys 2004; 59:1383–1391.

56. Buyyounouski MK, Horwitz EM, Price RA, et al. Intensity-modulated radiotherapy with MRI simulation to reduce doses received by erectile tissue during prostate cancer treatment. Int J Radiat Oncol Biol Phys 2004; 58: 743–749.

57. McShan DL, Fraass BA, Lichter AS. Full integration of the beam's eye view concept into computerized treatment planning. Int J Radiat Oncol Biol Phys 1990; 18:1485–1494.

58. Dearnaley DP, Khoo VS, Norman AR, et al. Comparison of radiation side-effects of conformal and conventional radiotherapy in prostate cancer: a randomised trial. Lancet 1999; 353:267–272.

59. Hanks GE, Schultheiss TE, Hunt MA, et al. Factors influencing incidence of acute grade 2 morbidity in conformal and standard radiation treatment of prostate cancer. Int J Radiat Oncol Biol Phys 1995; 31:25–29.

60. Zelefsky MJ, Fuks Z, Hunt M, et al. High-dose intensity modulated radiation therapy for prostate cancer: early toxicity and biochemical outcome in 772 patients. Int J Radiat Oncol Biol Phys 2002; 53:1111–1116.

61. Nutting CM, Convery DJ, Cosgrove VP, et al. Reduction of small and large bowel irradiation using an optimized intensity-modulated pelvic radiotherapy technique in patients with prostate cancer. Int J Radiat Oncol Biol Phys 2000; 48:649–656.

62. Pollack A, Zagars GK, Smith LG, et al. Preliminary results of a randomized radiotherapy dose-escalation study comparing 70 Gy with 78 Gy for prostate cancer. J Clin Oncol 2000; 18:3904–3911.

63. Pollack A, Zagars GK, Starkschall G, et al. Prostate cancer radiation dose response: results of the M. D. Anderson phase III randomized trial. Int J Radiat Oncol Biol Phys 2002; 53:1097–1105.

64. Hanks GE, Lee WR, Hanlon AL, et al. Conformal technique dose escalation for prostate cancer: biochemical evidence of improved cancer control with higher doses in patients with pretreatment prostate-specific antigen > or = 10 NG/ML. Int J Radiat Oncol Biol Phys 1996; 35: 861–868.

65. Roach M, Meehan S, Kroll S, et al. Radiotherapy for high-grade clinically localized adenocarcinoma of the prostate. J Urol 1996; 156:1719–1723.

66. Peeters ST, Heemsbergen WD, van Putten WL, et al. Acute and late complications after radiotherapy for prostate cancer: results of a multicenter randomized trial comparing 68 Gy to 78 Gy. Int J Radiat Oncol Biol Phys 2005; 61:1019–1034.

67. Michalski JM, Winter K, Purdy JA, et al. Toxicity after three-dimensional radiotherapy for prostate cancer with RTOG 9406 dose level IV. Int J Radiat Oncol Biol Phys 2004; 58:735–742.

68. Michalski JM, Winter K, Purdy JA, et al. Toxicity after three-dimensional radiotherapy for prostate cancer on RTOG 9406 dose Level V. Int J Radiat Oncol Biol Phys 2005; 62:706–713.

69. Shu HK, Lee TT, Vigneualt E, et al. Toxicity following high-dose three-dimensional conformal and intensity modulated radiation therapy for clinically localized prostate cancer. Urology 2001; 57:102–107.

70. Xia P, Pickett B, Vigneault E, et al. Comparison of intensity modulated treatment plans for multiple dominant tntra-prostatic lesions of prostate cancer. In: Cox J ed. Proceedings of the American Society for Therapeutic Radiology and Oncology, 40th Annual Meeting. Phoenix, AZ: Elsevier, 1998:208.

71. Xia P, Pickett B, Vigneault E, et al. Forward or inversely planned segmental multileaf collimator IMRT and sequential tomotherapy to treat multiple dominant intraprostatic lesions of prostate cancer to 90 Gy. Int J Radiat Oncol Biol Phys 2001; 51:244–254.

72. Huang E, Dong L, Chandra A, et al. Intrafraction prostate motion during IMRT for prostate cancer. Int J Radiat Oncol Biol Phys 2002; 53:261–268.

73. Ten Haken RK, Forman JD, Heimburger DK, et al. Treatment planning issues related to prostate movement in response to differential filling of the rectum and bladder. Int J Radiat Oncol Biol Phys 1991; 20:1317–1324.

74. Trichter F, Ennis RD. Prostate localization using trans-abdominal ultrasound imaging. Int J Radiat Oncol Biol Phys 2003; 56:1225–1233.

75. Millender LE, Aubin M, Pouliot J, et al. Daily electronic portal imaging for morbidly obese men undergoing radiotherapy for localized prostate cancer. Int J Radiat Oncol Biol Phys 2004; 59:6–10.

76. de Crevoisier R, Tucker SL, Dong L, et al. Increased risk of biochemical and local failure in patients with distended rectum on the planning CT for prostate cancer radiotherapy. Int J Radiat Oncol Biol Phys 2005; 62:965–973.

77. Stroom JC, Korevaar GA, Koper PC, et al. Multiple two-dimensional versus three-dimensional PTV definition in treatment planning for conformal radiotherapy. Radiother Oncol 1998; 47:297–302.

78. Bourland JD. ICRU 50 revisited. Health Phys 1995; 69:580–581.

79. Purdy JA. Current ICRU definitions of volumes: limitations and future directions. Semin Radiat Oncol 2004; 14:27–40.

80. Muren LP, Karlsdottir A, Kvinnsland Y, et al. Testing the new ICRU 62 'Planning Organ at Risk Volume' concept for the rectum. Radiother Oncol 2005; 75:293–302.

81. Ling CC, Humm J, Larson S, et al. Towards multidimensional radiotherapy (MD-CRT): biological imaging and biological conformality. Int J Radiat Oncol Biol Phys 2000; 47:551–560.

82. Levin-Plotnik D, Hamilton RJ. Optimization of tumour control probability for heterogeneous tumours in fractionated radiotherapy treatment protocols. Phys Med Biol 2004; 49:407–424.

83. Tepper J. Form and function: the integration of physics and biology. Int J Radiat Oncol Biol Phys 2000; 47: 547–548.

84. Zelefsky MJ, Fuks Z, Hunt M, et al. High-dose intensity modulated radiation therapy for prostate cancer: early toxicity and biochemical outcome in 772 patients. Int J Radiat Oncol Biol Phys 2002; 535:1111–1116.

85. McKenna DA, Coakley FV, Westphalen AC, et al. Prostate Cancer; Role of pre-treatment MR in predicting outcome after External Beam Radiation Therapy—Initial Experience. Radiology 2008 (Epub ahead of print).

86. Rasch C, Barillot I, Remeijer P, et al. Definition of the prostate in CT and MRI: a multi-observer study. Int J Radiat Oncol Biol Phys 1999; 43(1):57–66.

87. Kurhanewicz J, Vigneron D, Hricak H, et al. Three-dimensional H-1 MR spectroscopic imaging of the in situ human prostate with high (0.24-0.7-cm3) spatial resolution. Radiology 1983; 795–805.

88. Jung JA, Coakley FV, Vigneron DB, et al. Prostate depiction at endorectal MR spectroscopic imaging: investigation of a standardized evaluation system. Radiology 2004; 233(3):701–708.

89. Scheidler J, Hricak H, Vigneron DB, et al. Prostate cancer: localization with three-dimensional proton MR spectroscopic imaging—clinicopathologic study. Radiliogy 1999; 213(2):473–480.

90. Zakian KL, Sircar K, Hricak H, et al. Correlation of proton MR spectroscopic imaging with gleason score based on step-section pathologic analysis after radical prostatectomy. Radiology 2005; 234:804–814.

91. Nguyen P, Whittington R, Koo S, et al. Quantifying the impact of seminal vesicle invasion identified using endorectal magnetic resonance imaging on PSA outcome after radiation therapy for patients with clinically localized prostate cancer. Int J Radiat Oncol Biol Phys 2004; 59 (2):400–405.

92. Shukla-Dave A, Hricak H, Kattan MW, et al. The utility of magnetic resonance imaging and spectroscopy for predicting insignificant prostate cancer: an initial analysis. BJU Int 2007; 99:786–793.

93. Pickett B, Vigneault E, Kurhanewicz J, et al. Static field intensity modulation to treat a dominant intra-prostatic lesion to 90 Gy compared to seven field 3-dimensional radiotherapy. Int J Radiat Oncol Biol Phys 1999; 44:921–929.

94. Coakley FV, Kurhanewicz J, Lu Y, et al. Prostate cancer tumor volume: measurement with endorectal MR and MR spectroscopic imaging. Radiology 2002; 2231:91–97.

95. Coakley FV, Teh HS, Qayyum A, et al. Endorectal MR imaging and MR spectroscopic imaging for locally recurrent prostate cancer after external beam radiation therapy: preliminary experience. Radiology 2004; 233:441–448.

96. Susii R, Camphausen K, Choyke P, et al. System for prostate brachytherapy and biopsy in a standard 1.5 T MRI scanner. Magn Reson Med 2004; 474:1085.

97. Zaider M, Zelefsky M, Lee E, et al. Treatment planning for prostate implants using magnetic-resonance spectroscopy imaging. Int J Radiat Oncol Biol Phys 2000; 47(4): 1085–1096.

98. Chan T, Kressel H. Prostate and seminal vesicles after irradiation: MR appearance. J Magn Reson Imaging 1991; 15:503.

99. Pucar D, Shukla-Dave A, Hricak H, et al. Prostate cancer: correlation of MR imaging and MR spectroscopy with pathologic findings after radiation therapy-initial experience. Radiology 2005; 236(2):545–553.

100. Menard C, Smith IC, Somorjai RL, et al. Magnetic resonance spectroscopy of the malignant prostate gland after

radiotherapy: a histopathologic study of diagnostic validity. Int J Radiat Oncol Biol Phys 2001; 50:317–323.

101. Pickett B, Kurhanewicz J, Fein B, et al. Use of magnetic resonance imaging and spectroscopy in the evaluation of external beam radiation therapy for prostate cancer. Int J Radiat Oncol Biol Phys 2003; 57:S163–S164.

102. Pickett B, Ten Haken RK, Kurhanewicz J, et al. Time course to metabolic atrophy following permanent prostate seed implantation based on magnetic resonance spectroscopic imaging. In: Cox JD, ed. Proceeding of the 44th Annual ASTRO Meeting. New Orleans, LA: Elsevier, 2003:31–32.

103. Pickett B, Kurhanewicz J, Coakley F, et al. Use of MRI and spectroscopy in evaluation of external beam radiotherapy for prostate cancer. Int J Radiat Oncol Biol Phys 2004; 60:1047–1055.

104. Kumar R, Zhuang H, Alavi A. PET in the management of urologic malignancies. Radiol Clin North Am 2004; 42:1141–1153, ix.

105. Peterson JJ, Kransdorf MJ, O'Connor MI. Diagnosis of occult bone metastases: positron emission tomography. Clin Orthop Relat Res 2003; S120–S128.

106. Sanz G, Rioja J, Zudaire JJ, et al. PET and prostate cancer. World J Urol 2004; 22:351–352.

107. Schoder H, Larson SM. Positron emission tomography for prostate, bladder, and renal cancer. Semin Nucl Med 2004; 34:274–292.

108. Effert PJ, Bares R, Handt S, et al. Metabolic imaging of untreated prostate cancer by positron emission tomography with 18fluorine-labeled deoxyglucose. J Urol 1996; 155:994–998.

109. Hofer C, Laubenbacher C, Block T, et al. Fluorine-18-fluorodeoxyglucose positron emission tomography is useless for the detection of local recurrence after radical prostatectomy. Eur Urol 1999; 36:31–35.

110. Liu IJ, Zafar MB, Lai YH, et al. Fluorodeoxyglucose positron emission tomography studies in diagnosis and staging of clinically organ-confined prostate cancer. Urology 2001; 57:108–111.

111. Morris MJ, Akhurst T, Osman I, et al. Fluorinated deoxyglucose positron emission tomography imaging in progressive metastatic prostate cancer. Urology 2002; 59:913–918.

112. Morris MJ, Akhurst T, Larson SM, et al. Fluorodeoxyglucose positron emission tomography as an outcome measure for castrate metastatic prostate cancer treated with antimicrotubule chemotherapy. Clin Cancer Res 2005; 11:3210–3216.

113. Morris MJ, Scher HI. (11)C-acetate PET imaging in prostate cancer. Eur J Nucl Med Mol Imaging 2007; 34:181–184.

114. Wachter S, Tomek S, Kurtaran A, et al. 11C-acetate positron emission tomography imaging and image fusion with computed tomography and magnetic resonance imaging in patients with recurrent prostate cancer. J Clin Oncol 2006; 24:2513–2519.

115. Sandblom G, Sorensen J, Lundin N, et al. Positron emission tomography with C11-acetate for tumor detection and localization in patients with prostate-specific antigen relapse after radical prostatectomy. Urology 2006; 67:996–1000.

116. Reske SN, Blumstein NM, Neumaier B, et al. Imaging prostate cancer with 11C-choline PET/CT. J Nucl Med 2006; 47:1249–1254.

117. Martorana G, Schiavina R, Corti B, et al. 11C-choline positron emission tomography/computerized tomography for tumor localization of primary prostate cancer in comparison with 12-core biopsy. J Urol 2006; 176:954–960; discussion 960.

118. Langsteger W, Heinisch M, Fogelman I. The role of fluorodeoxyglucose, 18F-dihydroxyphenylalanine, 18F-choline, and 18F-fluoride in bone imaging with emphasis on prostate and breast. Semin Nucl Med 2006; 36:73–92.

119. Hacker A, Jeschke S, Leeb K, et al. Detection of pelvic lymph node metastases in patients with clinically localized prostate cancer: comparison of [18F]fluorocholine positron emission tomography-computerized tomography and laparoscopic radioisotope guided sentinel lymph node dissection. J Urol 2006 176:2014–2018; discussion 2018–2019.

120. Dehdashti F, Picus J, Michalski JM, et al. Positron tomographic assessment of androgen receptors in prostatic carcinoma. Eur J Nucl Med Mol Imaging 2005; 32:344–350.

121. Hinkle GH, Burgers JK, Olsen JO, et al. Prostate cancer abdominal metastases detected with indium-111 capromab pendetide. J Nucl Med 1998; 39:650–652.

122. Manyak MJ, Hinkle GH, Olsen JO, et al. Immunoscintigraphy with indium-111-capromab pendetide: evaluation before definitive therapy in patients with prostate cancer. Urology 1999; 54:1058–1063.

123. Ponsky LE, Cherullo EE, Starkey R, et al. Evaluation of preoperative ProstaScint scans in the prediction of nodal disease. Prostate Cancer Prostatic Dis 2002; 5:132–135.

124. D'Amico AV, Whittington R, Malkowicz B, et al. Endorectal magnetic resonance imaging as a predictor of biochemical outcome after radical prostatectomy in men with clinically localized prostate cancer. J Urol 2000; 164(3 pt.1):759–763.

125. O'Keefe DS, Bacich DJ, Heston WD. Comparative analysis of prostate specific membrane antigen (PMSA) versus a prostate specific membrane antigen-like gene. Prostate 2004; 58(2):200–210.

126. Sodee DB, Ellis RJ, Samuels MA, et al. Prostate cancer and prostate bed SPECT imaging with ProstaScint: semiquantitative correlation with prostatic biopsy results. Prostate 1998; 37:140–148.

127. Ellis RJ, Kaminsky DA. Fused radioimmunoscintigraphy for treatment planning. Rev Urol 2006; 8(suppl 1):S11–S19.

128. Yao D, Trabulsi EJ, Kostakoglu L, et al. The utility of monoclonal antibodies in the imaging of prostate cancer. Semin Urol Oncol 2002; 20:211–218.

129. Oesterling JE. Using PSA to eliminate the staging radionuclide bone scan. Significant economic implications. Urol Clin North Am 1993; 20:705–711.

130. Albertsen PC, Hanley JA, Harlan LC, et al. The positive yield of imaging studies in the evaluation of men with newly diagnosed prostate cancer: a population based analysis. J Urol 2000; 163:1138–1143.

131. Lin K, Szabo Z, Chin BB, et al. The value of a baseline bone scan in patients with newly diagnosed prostate cancer. Clin Nucl Med 1999; 24:579–582.

132. Heidenreich A, Varga Z, Von Knobloch R. Extended pelvic lymphadenectomy in patients undergoing radical prostatectomy: high incidence of lymph node metastasis. J Urol 2002; 167:1681–1686.

133. Shariat SF, Kattan MW, Erdamar S, et al. Detection of clinically significant, occult prostate cancer metastases in lymph nodes using a splice variant-specific rt-PCR assay for human glandular kallikrein. J Clin Oncol 2003; 21:1223–1231.

134. Ferrari AC, Stone NN, Eyler JN, et al. Prospective analysis of prostate-specific markers in pelvic lymph nodes of patients with high-risk prostate cancer. J Natl Cancer Inst 1997; 89:1498–1504.

135. Roach M III, DeSilvio M, Lawton C, et al. Phase III trial comparing whole-pelvic versus prostate-only radiotherapy and neoadjuvant versus adjuvant combined androgen suppression: Radiation Therapy Oncology Group 9413. J Clin Oncol 2003; 21:1904–1911.

136. Wang-Cheseboro A, Coleman J, Xia P, et al. IMRT improves plevic lymph node (PLN) coverage and dose to critical structures compared with standard four field (4F) whole pelvis (WP) radiation therapy (RT) in prostate cancer (PC). In: J Cox ed. ASTRO. Denver, CO: Elsevier, 2005.

137. Wawroschek F, Vogt H, Wengenmair H, et al. Prostate lymphoscintigraphy and radio-guided surgery for sentinel lymph node identification in prostate cancer. Technique and results of the first 350 cases. Urol Int 2003; 70:303–310.

138. Wawroschek F, Vogt H, Weckermann D, et al. Radioisotope guided pelvic lymph node dissection for prostate cancer. J Urol 2001; 166:1715–1719.

139. Rudoni M, Sacchetti GM, Leva L, et al. Recent applications of the sentinel lymph node concept: preliminary experience in prostate cancer. Tumori 2002; 88:S16–S17.

140. Weckermann D, Wawroschek F, Harzmann R. Is there a need for pelvic lymph node dissection in low risk prostate cancer patients prior to definitive local therapy? Eur Urol 2005; 47:45–50; discussion 50–51.

141. Weckermann D, Dorn R, Trefz M, et al. Sentinel lymph node dissection for prostate cancer: experience with more than 1,000 patients. J Urol 2007; 177:916–920.

142. Harisinghani MG, Barentsz JO, Hahn PF, et al. MR lymphangiography for detection of minimal nodal disease in patients with prostate cancer. Acad Radiol 2002; 9 (suppl 2):S312–S313.

143. Shih HA, Harisinghani M, Zietman AL, et al. Mapping of nodal disease in locally advanced prostate cancer: rethinking the clinical target volume for pelvic nodal irradiation based on vascular rather than bony anatomy. Int J Radiat Oncol Biol Phys 2005; 63:1262–1269.

144. Salem CE, Hoh CK, Wallace AM, et al. A preclinical study of prostate sentinel lymph node mapping with [99mTC] diethylenetetramine pentaacetic acid-mannosyl-dextran. J Urol 2006; 175:744–748.

145. Schettino CJ, Kramer EL, Noz ME, et al. Impact of fusion of indium-111 capromab pendetide volume data sets with those from MRI or CT in patients with recurrent prostate cancer. AJR Am J Roentgenol 2004; 183:519–524.

146. Selli C, Caramella D, Giusti S, et al. Value of image fusion in the staging of prostatic carcinoma. Radiol Med (Torino) 2007; 112:74–81.

147. Maintz JB, Viergever MA. A survey of medical image registration. Med Image Anal 1998; 2:1–36.

148. Leventis AK, Shariat SF, Slawin KM. Local recurrence after radical prostatectomy: correlation of US features with prostatic fossa biopsy findings. Radiology 2001; 219:432–439.

149. Kramer S, Gorich J, Gottfried HW, et al. Sensitivity of computed tomography in detecting local recurrence of prostatic carcinoma following radical prostatectomy. Br J Radiol 1997; 70:995–999.

150. Silverman JM, Krebs TL. MR imaging evaluation with a transrectal surface coil of local recurrence of prostatic cancer in men who have undergone radical prostatectomy. AJR Am J Roentgenol 1997; 168:379–385.

151. Sella T, Schwartz LH, Swindle PW, et al. Suspected local recurrence after radical prostatectomy: endorectal coil MR imaging. Radiology 2004; 231:379–385.

152. Israel G, Francis IR, al. RMe: ACR Appropriateness Criteria, 2007.

3

Modeling Outcome After Prostate IGRT

CLAUDIO FIORINO

Department of Medical Physics, Istituto Scientifico San Raffaele, Milan, Italy

TIZIANA RANCATI AND RICCARDO VALDAGNI

Prostate Programme, Fondazione IRCCS Istituto Nazionale dei Tumori, Milan, Italy

INTRODUCTION

This chapter begins with a brief review of tumor control probability (TCP) and normal tissue complication probability (NTCP) models as it applies to the treatment of prostate cancer. It is important to note that biological models aim to represent an extremely complex reality using simplistic equations and a few parameters. The use of such models for clinical decision making should, therefore, be approached with caution.

Modeling of NTCP and TCP requires reliable recording of precise and accurate dosimetric and clinical outcome information, and for this purpose appropriately designed studies should be performed. Furthermore, radiobiological modeling is a complicated process when it is based on accurate clinical/dosimetric data. As a matter of fact, the information usually covers only a limited region of the dose-response curve since the clinical data are derived from radiation treatments, which aim to achieve tumor control with minimum normal tissue complication. This means that the part of the dose-response relation outside the therapeutical range is based on the shape

(i.e., the mathematical equation) of the model's curve and cannot be experimentally verified by clinical observations in that particular region. Consideration of this limitation is critical when the models are applied to a dose range outside the original clinical data.

For these reasons, the main goal of TCP/NTCP models is not to predict an absolute individual response of human tissue to radiation but to give a quantitative measure of the relative impact of different dose distributions and, maybe, for selection, improvement, or optimization of treatment plans. Controversies and pitfalls of such models have been widely discussed by Schultheiss (1).

In the second part of this chapter, the potential benefit from image-guided radiation therapy (IGRT) on TCP and NTCP is examined.

This will be discussed in four main topics: (*i*) safe delivery of three-dimensional conformal radiotherapy/intensity-modulated radiation therapy (3DCRT/IMRT) at conventional doses, (*ii*) dose escalation, (*iii*) hypofractionation, and (*iv*) intraprostatic subvolume boosting. On each topic, we will briefly review the literature addressing important issues and how they are affected by IGRT.

TCP MODELS

General Considerations

TCP models are mathematical/biophysical methods describing the probability of killing all tumor clonogenic cells in the defined tumor volume after irradiating the target to a selected dose.

From a theoretical point of view, since one single surviving clonogenic cell is able to repopulate the tumor, TCP models postulate that all clonogenic cells need to be eradicated to achieve tumor control (2).

Animal experiments and clinical studies show that the tumor dose-response curve has a sigmoidal shape. One important difference between clinical and animal data is that the dose-response curve is very steep for clinical experiments and shallower for clinical data. Literature data strongly suggest that the shallow clinical slope is due to a considerable interpatient heterogeneity in the radio-sensitivity of human tumor cells (3).

Two main TCP models have been developed in the last decades, the Niemierko and Goitein model (4) and the Webb-Nahum-Tait model (3,5). These two tools are very similar: they both assume that the dose response for tumor has a sigmoidal shape and take into account interpatient heterogeneity in cell sensitivity. Furthermore, both models assume that the number of surviving clonogens follows Poisson statistics coupled with the linear quadratic (LQ) model (6) of cell killing. We will discuss the Webb-Nahum-Tait model in detail in the next section.

Webb-Nahum-Tait TCP Model (3,5)

Let us suppose to start with a target tumor volume composed of N_0 clonogenic cells and to treat it with n radiation therapy (RT) fractions of single dose d and total dose $D = nd$. Applying the LQ model (6) of cell killing, at the end of RT, the number of surviving cells (N_S) will be

$$N_S = N_0 \cdot e^{-\alpha D \left(1 + \frac{\beta}{\alpha} d\right)} \qquad (1)$$

The probability that no single clonogenic cell survives is obtained by inserting equation (1) into the expression of Poisson statistics. Thus, the expression of TCP becomes

$$\text{TCP} = e^{-N_S} \qquad (2)$$

The interpatient variation of tumor sensitivity is incorporated into the model by assuming that α is normally distributed with a mean value α_{mean} and a standard deviation σ_α. The final TCP is calculated as the average of the TCPs of patients with different tumor radiosensitivity:

$$\text{TCP} = \text{TCP}_{\text{mean}} = \sum_i g_i \cdot \text{TCP}_i(\alpha_i, \beta, D, N_0) \qquad (3)$$

where g_i is the normal distribution of the parameter α, $g_i = e^{-(\alpha - \alpha_{\text{mean}})^2 / 2\sigma_\alpha^2}$ and TCP_i is calculated using equations (1) and (2), and explicitly depends on α_i (which is extracted from the g_i distribution), β, D, and N_0. The model assumes that the parameter β is constant.

The above written equations are derived under the hypotheses of homogeneous irradiation of the whole tumor target. If inhomogeneous irradiation is considered, a straightforward generalization of equations (1)–(3) is necessary: $N_{0,j}$ cells receive a fractional dose d_j, total dose D_j. Through equations (1) and (2) $\text{TCP}_{j,i}$ can be calculated, and the total TCP is given by the product of the $\text{TCP}_{j,i}$:

$$\text{TCP}_{\text{total}} = \prod_j \sum_i g_i \cdot \text{TCP}_{j,i}(\alpha_i, \beta, D_j, N_{0,j}) \qquad (4)$$

TCP formula depends on several parameters (α_{mean}, σ_α, α/β, $N_{0,j}$) that have to be estimated for each human tumor through the fit of clinical data. The estimation of $N_{0,j}$ is usually replaced by the estimation of clonogenic cell density ρ and $N_{0,j} = \rho V_i$, where V_i is the tumor volume irradiated at dose D_i.

It is worth to remember that TCP models are derived in the framework of the LQ model, and they are valid if they are not used with extremely low or extremely high doses per fraction, where different mechanisms of tissue injury may appear.

TCP Parameters for Prostate Carcinoma

Data on TCP parameters for prostate carcinoma are scarce. The main difficulty in collecting tumor control data and relating them to dose, volume, and clonogenic cell density is that they are only available when (*i*) the dose distribution in the whole target is calculated and recorded, (*ii*) the volume of the target is measured, and (*iii*) the patient population has an adequate follow-up. If clinical control is considered, the follow-up period should be long (7–10 yr) in prostate cancer. A way to shorten the follow-up period is to consider biochemical control as a surrogate for clinical control; however, note that the definition of biochemical failure cannot separate between distant metastases and local failure, thus introducing a confounding factor in TCP parameter estimation (7,8). Other potential biases relate to androgen deprivation (9) and T staging (8) since tumor burden is strongly related to the chance of controlling the disease. For this reason, data derived from different populations and TCP parameters for these different groups are strongly required. Tumor stage may also influence the density of clonogenic cells or their sensitivity, or more realistically both parameters.

The first estimate of prostate TCP parameters was carried out by Webb (10): $\alpha_{mean} = 0.305$ Gy^{-1}, $\sigma_\alpha = 0.08$ Gy^{-1}, and $\rho = 10^7$ cm^{-3}.

Sanchez-Nieto and Nahum (11) also estimated the cell sensitivity for prostate carcinoma: $\alpha_{mean} = 0.29$ Gy^{-1}, $\sigma_\alpha = 0.07$ Gy^{-1}, and $\rho = 10^7$ cm^{-3}. TCP calculations using these parameters reproduce reasonably well the clinical data (freedom from recurrence at 7 yr) published by Hanks et al. (12) for the subset of stage B and C prostate cancer patients.

Levergrün et al. (13) fit TCP models to biopsy outcome. The study involved 103 patients with stage T1c to T3 clinically localized adenocarcinoma of the prostate treated with 3DCRT (doses from 64.8 to 81 Gy) at the Memorial Sloan-Kettering Cancer Center. Posttreatment biopsies were performed at least 2.5 years after the end of RT (range 2.5–6.3 yr). No androgen deprivation was prescribed. The estimate of TCP parameters was performed by splitting the population in different groups: low-risk patients (T stage < T2c and Gleason score ≤ 6), intermediate-risk patients (either T stage ≥ T2c and low Gleason score or Gleason score > 6 and low T stage), and high-risk group (patients with T stage ≥ T2c and Gleason score > 6). For all patients the dose distribution information was derived from the dose-volume histogram (DVH) of the planning target volume (PTV). Best fitted parameters for the Webb-Nahum-Tait TCP model were (i) $\alpha_{mean} = 0.105$ Gy^{-1}, $\sigma_\alpha = 0.0053$ Gy^{-1}, and $\rho = 10.55$ cm^{-3} for the low-risk group; (ii) $\alpha_{mean} = 0.120$ Gy^{-1}, $\sigma_\alpha = 0.000054$ Gy^{-1}, and $\rho = 53.53$ cm^{-3} for the intermediate-risk group, and (iii) $\alpha_{mean} = 0.107$ Gy^{-1}, $\sigma_\alpha = 0.000006$ Gy^{-1}, and $\rho = 54.51$ cm^{-3} for the high-risk group. Levergrün et al. point out that TCP calculations based on such estimated parameters underestimate the real tumor control rate, and this is probably due to the use of DVH of the PTV, which includes cold spots. These cold spots are mainly located in the periphery of the PTV, and probably even after accounting for organ motion and setup uncertainties, most of the time the low-dose region does not coincide with gross tumor location. This study deserves attention for the selection of the outcome, which is clinically relevant, and for the choice of stratifying the patient population through clinical prognostic factors. Another crucial point is the emphasis to the dose distribution that has to be related to TCP: DVH of the clinical target volume (CTV) are surely more representative than DVH of the PTV.

A further estimate of α_{mean} and σ_α can be derived from studies involving irradiation of human prostate cancer cell lines. A review of the available studies is given in Nahum et al. (14) and from these results $\alpha_{mean} = 0.26$ Gy and $\sigma_\alpha = 0.06$ Gy are obtained.

An essential parameter to be considered is α/β, which determines how sensible the tissue is to fractionation

effects. Tumors are acute responding tissues, and their α/β value is generally assumed to be 10 Gy (6). This was also the case of prostate tumor (15), until a study by Brenner and Hall (16) reported α/β values substantially lower than the traditionally accepted value of 10 Gy.

Work by Brenner and Hall (16) triggered a series of studies aiming at the definition of α/β value (17–22); published estimates give values ranging from 1 to 5 Gy with an average value of 1.5 Gy. However, the main limit of all these values for the fractionation sensitivity of prostate cancer is that they consider together outcomes derived from brachytherapy and external beam RT (23).

Furthermore, α/β estimates higher than 4 Gy are reported in the literature. Valdagni and coworkers (24) compared standard fractionation and hyperfractionation (two daily fractions of 1.2 Gy) results (330 patients, median dose 74 and 79.2 Gy in the standard and hyperfractionation group, respectively) and obtained a point estimate of $\alpha/\beta = 8.3$ Gy. In a recent published work (25), Williams et al. analyzed a total of 3756 patients treated with radiation monotherapy in three institutions, including 185 high-dose-rate brachytherapy (HDRB). HDBR data were corrected using a homogeneity correction factor considering the fact that the effective tumor dose for the HDR fraction was higher than the dose specified at the periphery of the gland. For the intermediate-risk group, α/β ratio estimates of 6.5 and 8.7 Gy for early prostate-specific antigen (PSA) control and substantial PSA control were reported.

Another important topic to be discussed is the effect of the presence of hypoxic regions in the tumor. Severe hypoxia in prostate regions of a significant number of patients has been shown (26–31), and this variable might limit overall cure rates by conventional radiotherapy (32,33). Nahum et al. (14) demonstrated that neither α/β nor the density of clonogenic cells need to be extremely low to explain prostate cancer response to brachytherapy and external beam RT. They incorporated new hypoxia measurements from prostate cancer into the TCP model and produced a good fit for brachytherapy and external beam RT outcomes using $\alpha/\beta = 8.4$ Gy for normal cells and $\alpha/\beta = 15.5$ Gy for the hypoxic fraction. α/β for the hypoxic cells is calculated starting from α/β for oxygenated cells and correcting it through a factor taking the oxygenating effect into account, namely oxygen enhancement ratio (OER$_\alpha$) = 1.75 and OER$_\beta$ = 3.25.

This chapter is entirely dedicated to the hypofractionation issue. In this section, we want to remark that more research is needed to reach a good understanding of fractionation sensitivity of prostate cancer cells, and that it is important to consider all important radiobiological and tumor physiology parameters to accurately predict TCP in a self-consistent way.

NTCP MODELS

General Considerations

NTCP models are mathematical/biophysical methods describing the probability that a certain percentage of the patient population will exhibit unfavorable reactions in healthy tissues surrounding the target. NTCP is calculated from nonuniform dose distribution throughout the organ of interest using its related DVH. A number of models have been proposed to predict the NTCP of critical organs, and an extensive review on this issue is given by Yorke (34).

All models predict an increase in NTCP when increasing the dose and the irradiated volume, and they describe the dose-NTCP relationship through a sigmoid shaped curve. The dose-volume relationship differs for each organ considered. It is generally a mixture of two extreme situations of cell organization patterns (35): (*i*) *serial organs,* where reaching a well-determined dose level severely conditions the organ functionality, meaning that a poor volume effect is present and (*ii*) *parallel organs,* whose functionality is highly impaired causing complication when irradiating a significant percentage of their total volume.

All NTCP model parameters are generally derived for standard 2 Gy/day fractionation. For inhomogeneous irradiation of normal tissues, the dose per fraction is consequently inhomogeneous and for this reason, physical doses should be converted into equivalent doses at 2 Gy/fr (LQD2) using the LQ model formalism (6):

$$\text{LQD2} = D \cdot \frac{1 + d/(\alpha/\beta)}{1 + 2/(\alpha/\beta)} \qquad (5)$$

where D is the total dose, d is dose per fraction, and α and β are the LQ parameters for the organ under consideration. If different treatment phases are present, different doses per fraction and consequently different LQD2 are to be considered.

Some details on most popular NTCP models are given in the section here below.

Models

The Lyman-EUD model (36–39)

The Lyman-EUD (LEUD) model is a strictly phenomenological model which uses the probit formula to describe the dose-response relationship for normal tissues. The standard format uses two parameters as descriptors: $D_{50}(\nu)$, i.e., the dose that causes 50% probability of injury when a fraction ν of the organ volume is uniformly irradiated, and the slope of the response curve at D_{50}, the steepest part of the curve, which is named m.

NTCP for uniform irradiation of a fraction ν of the organ at dose D can be calculated by

$$\text{NTCP} = \frac{1}{\sqrt{2\pi}} \int_{-\infty}^{t} e^{-\frac{x^2}{2}} dx \qquad (6)$$

where $t = \frac{D - D_{50}(\nu)}{m \cdot D_{50}(\nu)}$, $D_{50}(\nu) = D_{50} \cdot \nu^{-n}$, and n is a parameter describing the importance of the volume effect (higher values correspond to more resistant organ or parallel architecture).

When considering nonuniform dose distributions (characterized by their DVH), the DVH has to be converted or reduced to an equivalent uniform dose distribution. Here the DVH is reduced to an equivalent uniform dose (EUD) to total volume [DVH $\rightarrow$ (D = EUD, $\nu = 1$)]. The EUD algorithm uses the power-law relationship:

$$\text{EUD} = \left(\sum_i \nu_i \cdot D_i^{\frac{1}{n}} \right)^n \qquad (7)$$

where D_i and ν_i correspond to a point of the differential DVH (the sum is performed through the entire DVH) and n is a parameter that, for every organ, describes the volumetric dependence of the dose-response relationship. For small n ($n \rightarrow 0$), the EUD tends to the maximum dose, while for $n = 1$ the EUD is the average dose.

This definition of EUD can also be derived from the Kutcher-Burnam (KB) DVH reduction scheme (40): the KB reduction algorithm reduces the DVH to a partial organ irradiation of an effective volume which receives the maximum dose of the original DVH [DVH $\rightarrow$ ($D = D_{\max}$, $\nu = \nu_{\text{EFF}}$)]. This is accomplished through the following calculation:

$$\nu_{\text{EFF}} = \sum_i \nu_i \left(\frac{D_i}{D_{\max}} \right)^{\frac{1}{n}} \qquad (8)$$

where D_i, ν_i, and n have the same meaning as in equation (7). From equations (7) and (8) the relation between EUD and ν_{EFF} is

$$\text{EUD} = \nu_{\text{EFF}}{}^{n} \cdot D_{\max} \qquad (9)$$

For this reason, LEUD model is equivalent to the classical Lyman-Kutcher-Burnam model.

The logit-EUD model (36,39,41)

This is also a phenomenological model that uses the logit formula coupled with the generalized EUD reduction algorithm (Eq. 7). The logit formula describes the dose-response relationship for normal tissues through D_{50} and k (the slope of the response curve at D_{50}):

$$\text{NTCP}(D) = \frac{1}{1 + \left(\frac{D_{50}}{D} \right)^{k}} \qquad (10)$$

k is related to the parameter m of the probit formula (Eq. 6) through the relation $k = \frac{1.6}{m}$ (42).

This model is very attractive because of its simplicity in calculations.

The relative seriality model (43)

Relative seriality (RS) is a more radiobiologically based model. It describes cell inactivation through Poisson statistics, and it accounts for the architecture of the organ through the parameter of relative seriality, s. The relative seriality is derived from the ratio of serial subunits to all subunits in the organ: $s = 1$ for a serial organs and $s = 0$ for parallel organs.

For a heterogeneous dose distribution, the complication probability is given by

$$NTCP = \left\{ 1 - \prod_{i=1}^{M} [1 - P(D_i)^s]^{\Delta \nu_i} \right\}^{\frac{1}{s}} \quad (11)$$

where M is the number of calculation subvolumes in the dose calculation volume, D_i is the dose in the subvolume considered, and $\Delta \nu_i = v_i/V$, where v_i is the volume of each subvolume in the DVH and V is the total volume of the organ. $P(D)$ is the Poisson dose-response relationship:

$$P(D) = 2^{-\exp\left(e\gamma\left(1 - \frac{D}{D_{50}}\right)\right)} \quad (12)$$

where D_{50} is the uniform dose that causes 50% probability of injury and γ is the slope of the response curve at D_{50} γ is related to the parameter m of the probit formula (Eq. 6) through the relation $\gamma = \frac{0.4}{m}$ (42).

Determination of Model Parameters

Model parameters must be derived either from fitting clinical/dosimetric individual data or considering literature-based complication rates. In the past, all models were challenged by the lack of availability of accurate clinical/dosimetric data usable for the calculation of these parameters.

The widespread use of CT-based three-dimensional planning and treatment, as well as the effort of establishing precise procedures for clinical endpoint determination and recording, greatly improved the parameterization of such NTCP models in recent years.

The next section reports on the recent evidence pertaining to NTCP model parameters of critical organs involved in prostate cancer irradiation.

Late Rectal Syndrome

The first parameters describing rectal complications (44) (rectal necrosis, $D_{50} = 80$ Gy, $n = 0.12$, $m = 0.15$, Lyman model) suggested that the rectum is a highly serial organ.

It is worth to remember that this parameterization was derived from few clinical data referring to the whole organ irradiation. NTCP predictions on the basis of this estimate constituted a good tool for plan comparison for more than a decade; however, today parameterizations on the basis of different endpoints have been published (45–47).

In all recent studies, the determination of the best estimate of the model parameters was performed fitting radiobiological models to individual clinical and dosimetric data and, to this purpose, the Maximum Likelihood method is generally used.

Rancati et al. (45) reviewed the rectal DVHs and clinical records of 547 prostate cancer patients from five institutions (retrospective study, doses between 64 and 79.2 Gy). The investigated endpoint was G2–G3 late rectal bleeding [defined through a slightly modified Radiation Therapy Oncology Group/European Organization for Research and Treatment of Cancer (RTOG/EORTC) scoring system]. DVHs were calculated for the rectum including filling, and rectum contouring was started just above the anal verge and continued till the point at which it turns into the sigmoid colon. For the LEUD model they found $D_{50} = 81.9$ Gy, $n = 0.23$, $m = 0.19$, and $D_{50} = 82.2$ Gy, $n = 0.24$, $k = 7.85$ for the LOGEUD model. When only G3 late bleeding was considered, the best-fitted parameterization was $D_{50} = 78.6$ Gy, $n = 0.06$, $m = 0.06$ for the LEUD model and $D_{50} = 76.8$ Gy, $n = 0.06$, $k = 33.6$ for the LOGEUD model. These n values suggest that the rectum is less serial than previously reported for G2 bleeding, but more serial when G3 events are considered.

Peeters et al. (46) analyzed prospective data from 468 patients in four institutions participating in a randomized trial comparing 68 with 78 Gy. They considered the LEUD model and three severe complications: (i) late rectal bleeding requiring laser treatment or blood transfusion, (ii) fecal incontinence requiring use of pads more than twice a week, and (iii) high stool frequency (more than 6 times per day). In this study, DVHs were calculated for the anorectal wall (for bleeding and stool frequency) and for the anal canal wall (for incontinence). The anorectum was defined from the anal verge until the lower gastrointestinal tract was no longer adjacent to the sacrum, while the anal canal was defined as the caudal 3 cm of the anorectum, measured in the craniocaudal direction. The fitted parameters were $D_{50} = 81$ Gy, $n = 0.13$, $m = 0.14$ for severe bleeding; $D_{50} = 105$ Gy, $n = 7.48$, $m = 0.46$ for severe fecal incontinence; and $D_{50} = 84$ Gy, $n = 0.39$, $m = 0.24$ for high stool frequency. This study strengthens the finding that rectum acts as a fairly serial organ for severe bleeding and gives a first quantification of the rectal volume effect for high stool frequency and incontinence.

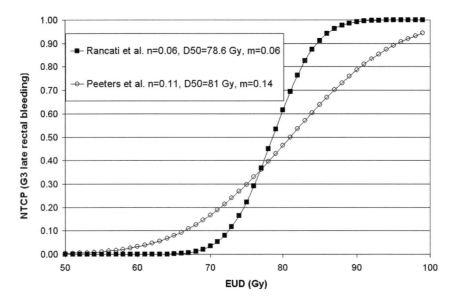

Figure 1 NTCP curves derived from best-fitted parameters of Rancati et al. and Peteers et al. for severe late rectal bleeding (LEUD model).

Figure 1 presents the NTCP curves derived from best-fitted parameters of Rancati et al. and Peeters et al. for severe late rectal bleeding (LEUD model).

Söhn et al. (47) analyzed data of 319 patients participating at a dose escalation study from 70.2 to 79.2 Gy. The clinical endpoint was G2-G3-G4 late rectal bleeding, with complication graded through the Common Terminology Criteria for Adverse Events (CTCAE) scale. DVHs were calculated for the rectal wall, with rectum contoured from the anal verge or ischial tuberosities (whichever was anatomically more cranial) to the sacroiliac joints or rectosigmoid junction (whichever was anatomically more caudal). For the LEUD model they found $D_{50} =$ 78.4 Gy, $n = 0.08$, $m = 0.11$ and $D_{50} = 78.1$ Gy, $n = 0.08$, $k = 15.4$ for the LOGEUD model.

Figure 2 presents the NTCP curves derived from best-fitted parameters of Rancati et al. and Söhn et al. for moderate/severe late rectal bleeding (LOGEUD model).

Very recently, Tucker et al. (48) analyzed data of 1023 patients enrolled on protocol RTOG 94-06. The parameter estimates obtained from fitting the generalized Lyman model to the rectal toxicity data were: $D_{50} = 78$ Gy, $m = 0.14$, and $n = 0.08$. Their clinical endpoint was G2-G3 rectal toxicity.

Peeters et al. (49,50) and Fiorino et al. (51) showed that some previously ignored variables (e.g., history of

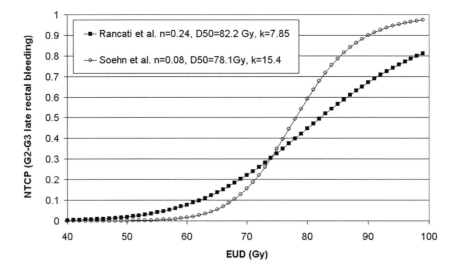

Figure 2 NTCP curves derived from best-fitted parameters of Rancati et al. and Söhn et al. for moderate/severe late rectal bleeding (LOGEUD model).

abdominal surgery) are predisposing for the development of late rectal complications. To further analyze this effect, Peeters et al. (46) tested a modified NTCP model where predisposing clinical features can be taken into account. They fitted the LEUD model with four parameters: n, m, D_{50} for patients without clinical risk factor (D_{50N}) and D_{50} for patients with clinical risk factors (D_{50Y}). For rectal bleeding and fecal incontinence they considered patient's history of abdominal surgery as a risk factor, and for high stool frequency, acute G2–G3 GI toxicity was considered as a predisposing variable. The fitting procedure leads to the following parameters: $D_{50N} = 85$ Gy, $D_{50Y} = 78$ Gy, $n = 0.11$, $m = 0.14$ for bleeding; $D_{50N} = 172$ Gy, $D_{50Y} = 60$ Gy, $n = 10.0$, $m = 0.47$ for incontinence; and $D_{50N} = 106$ Gy, $D_{50Y} = 80$ Gy, $n = 0.44$, $m = 0.26$ for high stool frequency.

It is important to underline that different DVHs were used in the above-mentioned studies. Generally speaking, the question of whether the DVHs of the rectum including filling are sufficiently reliable compared to dose-wall histograms (DWHs) or normalized dose-surface/volume histograms (NDSHs, NDVHs) is still unanswered (52–56). In principle, the rectum wall should be considered as the "true" organ; however, due to the difficulty in contouring the rectal wall, most institutions either prefer or are required to draw the rectum including filling and use the related DVH as a "surrogate" of the DWH. Nonetheless, the common practice of emptying the rectum before simulation and therapy is helpful in keeping the deviation between DVHs and DWHs within an acceptable level for most patients (52). Recent studies also demonstrated that the empty rectum minimizes the movements of internal organs and reduces the risk of geographic miss of the target (57,58).

Bladder and Genitourinary Injury

Due to different reasons, data on DVH constraints and consequently on NTCP modeling for genitourinary (GU) toxicities are scarce and poorly understood.

The first limit is represented by bladder dose-volume information, which is significantly unreliable. DVHs and DWHs are usually obtained from planning CT, while daily filling of the bladder may clearly not be uniform. Obviously, this may generate discrepancy between CT calculated and real bladder volume, consequently impacting the actual dose distribution. The time required to the onset of GU toxicity represents another important limiting factor: late urinary toxicity increases continuously with time and can become a significant morbidity in longer-term study (59–61). For this reason reliable clinical data require a long follow-up.

Last urethral dose suggested to be important specifically in brachytherapy studies (62,63), has not been considered in 3DCRT/IMRT planning; this is due to problems in contouring and to the inability to "dig" the dose distributions around the urethra, which locates in the RT target.

At this time more research is still needed, and hopefully IGRT techniques will be able to enlighten this issue.

The first report dealing with the parameterization of bladder complications was published in 1991 (44), $D_{50} = 80$ Gy, $n = 0.5$, $m = 0.11$ (Lyman model). This set of parameters has been used for a long time for the comparison and the optimization of treatment planning.

In contrast to the fist historical findings, a very recent study (64) suggests that maximal doses and hotspots in bladder wall are significantly related to bladder toxicity. Cheung and coworkers analyzed DVHs and clinical data of 128 patients conformally treated at a total dose of 78 Gy. The endpoint for NTCP analysis was grade ≥ 1 GU toxicity (RTOG/EORTC, 19/128 events) within two years after the end of RT. LEUD best fit parameter estimates were as follows: $D_{50} = 77.6$ Gy, $n = 0.01$, and $m = 0.022$. Being the parameter n very close to zero, it is clear that the maximum dose to the bladder is a strong determinant for GU toxicity. The main limitation of this study is represented by the choice of grouping together mild, moderate, and severe events, while from a clinical point of view only grade ≥ 2 side effects are of major concern for RT optimization.

POTENTIAL BENEFITS FROM IGRT ON TCP AND NTCP

General Considerations

Although the use of IGRT is expected to significantly contribute to improved outcome with respect to reduced toxicities and increased local control rates, very few studies deal with the estimate of the amount of such potential gain. The lack of investigations on this issue is quite surprising; on the other hand, the large uncertainties associated with a number of parameters describing the biology of prostate tumors and of the surrounding organs at risk, as discussed in the previous sections, may in part justify the present poor interest in this topic. The impact of geometrical uncertainties and the way IGRT could take them into account might also dramatically affect the results of studies assessing TCP and NTCP quantitative estimates. The question *if we really need such estimates of geometrical uncertainties* is still open and deserves some discussion.

The availability of tools like TCP and NTCP or other surrogates of the expected radiation effect, like EUD, might address in a more appropriate way the resources in implementing IGRT in clinical trials.

In this section, several examples concerning estimates of the expected clinical gains in using IGRT with different approaches will be discussed and a brief review of the literature on this topic will be presented. The potential approach of IGRT for treating prostate cancer has been split in four different categories, each of them presenting peculiar problems with different potential impacts on IGRT clinical practice.

IGRT for a Safe Delivery of 3DCRT/IMRT at Conventional Doses

The need for IGRT in treating prostate cancer patients originates from anatomical reasons: the proximity of the prostate to organs at risk, primarily the rectum, in a "moving" organ scenario. It is well recognized that the prostate moves, and this is due to the variable rectal and bladder filling. Consequently, the most obvious application of IGRT is to guarantee that we are not missing the prostate target.

Many authors theoretically analyzed the potential impact of prostate motion on TCP reduction (65,66). In particular, a possible systematic difference between the average position of the prostate during treatment and at the planning CT scan has been suggested as a significant event potentially conditioning local control rates. This difference can be maximized when a planning CT scan with a "full" rectum is followed by several treatment fractions with an empty rectum.

The reduced local control probability has been clinically detected on a cohort of 128 patients treated at the M.D. Anderson Cancer Center (MDACC) at 78 Gy (58), where the rectal distension at the planning scan was found to be the most predictive parameter for local relapse. On the whole population, the local control rate was reduced by about 25% in patients with distended rectum compared to patients with empty rectum at the planning CT scan. Rectal distension was also found to be the most predictive parameter for local control, being superior to the risk class stratification variable. These results have been recently confirmed in two independent series of patients: (i) De Crevoisier found a significant impact on biochemical control in a group of approximately 200 patients treated at the IGR in Paris at 70 Gy (67), with a detrimental effect on control in the distended rectum group similar to that found in the MDACC group; (ii) in a randomized trial conducted at Nederland Kanker Instituut (NKI) (559 patients treated at 68 or 78 Gy), a 15% reduction in local control was reported in the group of patients with distended rectum (volume > 90 cc) compared to patients without rectal distension (57). The reported clinical evidence of a significant impact on local control due to systematic difference of prostate position at the planning scan and during treatment strongly confirms the importance of IGRT in limiting the risk of geographically missing the prostate target. It is also important to under-

line that a careful rectal emptying procedure should have the potential to significantly improve treatment accuracy. Nonetheless, the application of anisotropic margins is useful and should be considered: choosing a larger anterior margin, which takes into account the possible shift of the prostate, is reasonable when coupled to the prescription of carefully emptying the rectum before the planning scan.

Other evidences of the reduced prostate motion with rectal emptying derive from recently published experiences (68,69).

In agreement with these findings, the analysis of daily megavoltage CT (MVCT) data of IGRT of prostate cancer, using tomotherapy at San Raffaele Hospital, clearly shows a reduced motion of the prostate due to the careful emptying of the rectum (i.e., with rectal enema before simulation and treatment) (70), being the standard deviation of organ motion relative to bony structures within 1 mm.

Estimates of the gain due to daily correction of prostate position by IGRT show up to 10% TCP decrement if IGRT is not applied when a 5 mm posterior margin is added to CTV (71), in agreement with the clinical data previously discussed. Song et al. (72) reported similar findings with an increment of up to 15% in TCP due to IGRT.

Another potential approach not exploiting IGRT for dose escalation purposes is the possibility to safely reduce PTV margins and in particular the posterior one, with a consequent decrease of NTCP without any detrimental effect on TCP. A number of critical issues should be addressed in this context. First, when considering severe toxicity, rectum behaves as a serial-like organ with minimum volume effect (45–47). This means that, when compared with conventional non-IGRT radiotherapy, it could be hard to detect a significant reduction of severe toxicity through the application of IGRT with reduced margin, if the overlap between the rectum and the PTV is "handled" in the same way in the two treatment modalities, i.e., without establishing a maximum "safe" dose to the overlap area.

Furthermore, another important point concerns the impact of intrafraction motion, so that in the case of an important reduction of margins (for instance from 10 mm without IGRT to 3 mm with IGRT), there might be a significant and negative impact on TCP due to prostate intrafraction motion. Intrafraction motion can be as large as 4 to 5 mm in many patients, as recently underlined by Litzenberg et al. (73) using the Calipso system; similar or slightly lower impact has been reported by several investigations using fiducial markers (74–76). In conclusion, it is necessary to be very careful in reducing the margin below 5 to 6 mm even when IGRT techniques are utilized; however, both intrafraction motion and the intrinsic uncertainty of the available IGRT systems should always be carefully assessed.

IGRT for Dose Escalation

Reducing the margin as a consequence of the application of IGRT techniques may potentially allow to safely escalate the dose to the prostate. However, when the overlap between the PTV and the rectum receives the same dose, this approach implies intrinsic limitations because of the evidence that the rectum behaves as an almost serial-like organ when severe bleeding is considered as the endpoint. Reasonably, a reduction from 8–10 mm to 5–6 mm due to IGRT seems to be a safe limit because of the intrinsic uncertainties of the IGRT systems and of intrafraction motion.

The unavoidable irradiation of small but clinically not insignificant portions of the rectal wall at the prescribed dose limits the possibility to escalate the dose to the very high doses probably needed in high-risk patients. Recently, Song et al. (77) estimated an expected average increase of about 4% in TCP for a patient population when using a 5 mm margin due to the application of IGRT (compared to conventional patient setup) for a conventional dose of 70 Gy. In this case the NTCP values calculated with LKB model and Emami parameters were around 2% with or without IGRT. For higher doses (say more than 80 Gy), a lower gain in TCP may be expected because of the less steep shape of the TCP curve at high doses with no difference in NTCP of the rectum between IGRT and non-IGRT techniques (72). Note, however, that this limited improvement in TCP is due to the combination of a significant gain (>10%) for a small fraction of patients and no gain for most patients.

Because of these intrinsic limitations, a generally accepted strategy for dose escalation is to limit the dose in the overlap PTV-rectal wall region. On the other hand, the choice of reducing the dose to the overlap area is more sensitive to organ motion and setup errors, thus potentially reducing TCP in a significant number of patients, once geometrical uncertainties are taken into account in the planning (65, 66). IGRT should therefore be a valid tool to reduce the risk of underdosing parts of the CTV because of the rapid dose gradient existing in the overlap region in the proximity of the rectal wall. However, no definitive estimates of the expected gains in terms of TCP/NTCP in using IGRT (i.e., a reduced impact of interfraction geometrical uncertainties) have been reported for this specific situation. In the contest of limiting the dose in the overlap between rectum and PTV, an interesting result was reported by Ghilezan et al. (78), using EUD-based optimization. They showed an average increase in the deliverable dose of 13% when applying online IGRT compared to conventional treatment, while keeping the EUD of the rectal wall at the same "safe" level; nonetheless, for about one-third of patients, the gain was small (<5%) while for one-third it was greater than 15% with a maximum increase of 41% of dose increment.

Because of the shape of the dose-volume curve, a 15% to 20% increase of the dose in the range of 70 Gy should correspond to an increase in TCP as high as 20%. This interesting "biological-based" investigation suggests both a high potential of online IGRT in the case of inversely optimized IMRT, and the need to carefully select patients who might really benefit from IGRT in terms of dose escalation.

IGRT for Hypofractionation

The debate around the value of α/β for prostate cancer is still open; however, on the basis of the suggestion that this value might be low (<2 Gy), several trials have been activated to explore hypofractionated regimens. Different approaches are under clinical testing using from slight hypofractionated schemes (2.3–2.6 Gy/fr in 25–28 fractions) (79, 80), to moderate regimens (3–3.3 Gy/fr in 16–20 fractions) (81), to extreme hypofractionation in the case of low-risk patients (6–8 Gy/fr in 5–7 fractions) (82, 83). Beside the intrinsic risk related to the uncertainties in calculating biological equivalent doses with the LQ model with the assumption of a low α/β value for prostate cancer clonogens, it is quite intuitive that the lower the number of fractions, the higher the impact of geometrical uncertainties on the delivered dose (77, 84, 85). For this reason IGRT should be considered as mandatory when exploring hypofractionated regimens.

Few investigators tried to estimate the impact of geometrical uncertainties in hypofractionated treatments. Song et al. (77) showed a larger impact of geometrical uncertainties on TCP (when keeping the same biological equivalent dose and assuming $\alpha/\beta = 3$ Gy) in hypofractionation compared to conventional fractionation, if IGRT is not utilized. They also suggest that, in the case the α/β value of prostate clonogens is low (<2 Gy), the loss of TCP due to geometrical uncertainties is more than compensated by the increase of biological dose, when keeping rectal toxicity at the same level of a conventionally fractionated treatment. Similar findings were also reported by Craig et al. (84).

It is important to underline how this positive potential of hypofractionation is strongly depending on the assumption of an α/β value below 2 Gy. The above-cited paper by Craig et al. shows that a 4.4 Gy $\times$ 10 schedule, which is equivalent to 2 Gy $\times$ 37 when $\alpha/\beta = 1.5$ Gy, would result in a detrimental effect in TCP of about 30% when the α/β value is equal to 3 Gy.

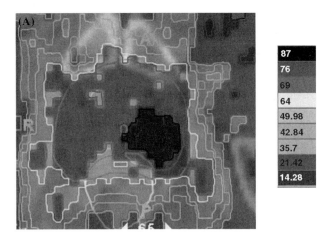

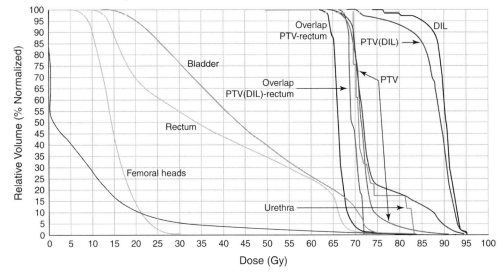

(B) **Dose Volume Histogram—Cumulative Mode Relative**

Figure 3 IGRT for boosting DIL using helical tomotherapy: (**A**) color-wash map and (**B**) dose-volume histograms: large fractions of DIL and of PTV(DIL), obtained with a 5-mm expansion, may receive doses as high as 90 Gy while the remaining portion of the prostate receives 71.4 Gy, and the rectum is well protected through hard constraints in the overlap between PTV and rectum and between PTV (DIL) and rectum. Also the portion of urethra receiving more than 75 Gy could be drastically limited. These simulations were performed at San Raffaele Hospital considering a 28 fractions regimen. The 2-Gy equivalent dose received by DIL is equal to 96 to 99 Gy for an α/β value ranging between 10 and 15, in the hypothesis of hypoxic radioresistant cells. *Abbreviation*: DIL, dominant intraprostatic lesion.

IGRT for Intraprostatic Subvolume Boosting

Although prostate cancer is a multifocal disease (86), there is a growing consensus on the fact that local failure is depending on the radioresistance of one or more local intraprostatic foci (87) named dominant intraprostatic lesion (DIL). Several investigations highlighted the evidence of radioresistant hypoxic regions within the DIL using a number of methods like electrode measurements (26, 27, 30), pimonidazole (28), and fluoromisonidazole using PET (31). Preliminary data also showed a correla-

tion between pre-RT tumor hypoxia and local failure (32, 33). Transrectal ultrasonography (TRUS), MRI spectroscopy (88, 89), and T2-weighted MRI (90, 91) have been investigated as appropriate imaging modalities to visualize DILs for most patients.

On the basis of a quite large experience using T2-weighted MRI to detect DILs in the peripheral zone of the prostate (corresponding to about three-fourth of the cases) (92), a mean 10 cc DIL volume (15 patients, range 1–95 cc) was reported by De Meerleer and coworkers (91). The mean distance of the DIL to the anterior rectal wall was 3 mm (range 0–12 mm), for 13/15 patients, the distance was lower than 5 mm.

IGRT may offer the possibility of selectively escalating the dose to the DIL to very high levels while delivering differential doses to the rest of the PTV. Xia et al. (93) showed the feasibility to concomitantly deliver 90 Gy while keeping the dose to the rectal wall to a safe level (less than 20% of the rectal wall receiving 70 Gy or higher dose).

More recently, van Lin et al. (89) confirmed these preliminary findings. An important limit of this approach is the lack of knowledge about rectal side effects [and of other organs at risk (OARs) like urethra and bladder] to very high doses (>85–90 Gy). As reported by De Meerleer et al. (91) in their clinical experience on 15 patients using T2-weighted MRI, the dose escalation to the DIL was limited by the hard constraints for the rectal dose.

On the other hand and based on the assumption that the DIL is characterized by the presence of hypoxic cells, TCP models including hypoxia (14, 94) suggest that dose values as high as 100 to 120 Gy might be necessary to sterilize cancer cells in a large hypoxic region. However, Popple et al. indicate that boosting just a portion of DIL might be sufficient to significantly increase the TCP (94). Further investigations are necessary to better assess potentials and limits of using IGRT to boost the DIL.

An example of this approach is reported in Figure 3. A dose escalation up to 90 Gy to a single DIL in a 28-fraction regimen (3.21 Gy/fr) could be obtained by using helical tomotherapy while delivering 71.4 Gy (2.55 Gy/fr) to the remaining portion of the prostate, if "safe" constraints are applied to the overlap between the PTV(DIL) and the rectum ($D_{max} < 76$ Gy; V70 < 1%); the prescribed dose to the overlap between PTV (excluding DIL) and rectum was kept equal to 65.5 Gy (2.34 Gy/fr, equivalent to 70 Gy, 2 Gy/fr for $\alpha/\beta = 3$ Gy). In this case, the DIL was drawn just for this exercise, in agreement with the findings of De Meerleer et al. (91), concerning volume and distance from the rectal wall.

SUMMARY OF PERTINENT CONCLUSIONS

- The reported clinical evidence of a significant impact on local control because of systematic difference of prostate position at the planning scan and during treatment strongly confirms the importance of IGRT in limiting the risk of geographically missing the prostate target.
- Increases in TCP up to 10% to 15% might be expected when using IGRT at conventional treatment doses with respect to standard techniques.
- IGRT may allow a safe reduction of PTV margins and in particular the posterior one, with a consequent decrease of NTCP for moderate toxicity without any detrimental effect on TCP.
- Because of the serial-like behavior of the rectum with respect to G3 injury, it could be hard to detect a significant reduction of severe toxicity through the application of IGRT with reduced margin without establishing a maximum "safe" dose to the overlap area.
- Due to the impact of intrafraction motion and the intrinsic uncertainty of the available IGRT systems a margin reduction below 5 to 6 mm seems to be unlikely.
- IGRT potentially allows a safe escalation of the dose to the prostate. To reduce rectal NTCP for severe toxicity, a possible strategy could be to limit the dose in the PTV-rectal wall overlap region. On the other hand, the choice of reducing the dose to the overlap area is more sensitive to organ motion and setup errors, thus potentially reducing TCP in a significant number of patients.
- Due to a reduction in the number of fractions, hypofractionation increases the impact of geometrical uncertainties on the delivered dose. For this reason, IGRT should be considered as mandatory when exploring hypofractionated regimens.
- The positive potential of hypofractionation strongly depends on the assumption that the α/β value for prostate cancer is below 2 Gy. If the α/β ratio is higher, significant detrimental effects in TCP could be expected for many fractionation schemes under investigation in a number of clinical trials.
- In the hypothesis that the local control is critically depending on the presence of hypoxic subvolumes (DIL), IGRT may offer the possibility of selectively escalate the dose to the DIL to very high doses while delivering differential doses to the rest of the PTV. Even boosting just a portion of the DIL might be sufficient to significantly increase the TCP.

REFERENCES

1. Schultheiss TE. The controversies and pitfall in modeling normal tissue radiation injury/damage. Semin Radiat Oncol 2001; 11(3):210–214.
2. Steel GG. Cell survival as a determinant of tumor response. In: Steel GG, ed. Basic Clinical Radiobiology. 3rd ed. London: Arnold, 2002:52–63.
3. Webb S, Nahum AE. A model for calculating tumour control probability in radiotherapy including the effects of inhomogeneous distributions of dose and clonogenic cell density. Phys Med Biol 1993; 38(6):653–666.
4. Niemierko A, Goitein M. Implementation of a model for estimating tumor control probability for an inhomogeneously irradiated tumor. Radiother Oncol 1993; 29(2):140–147.

5. Nahum AE, Sanchez-Nieto B. Tumor control probability modeling: basic principles and applications in term of planning. Phys Med 2001; 17(suppl 2):13 23.

6. Joiner MC, Bentzen SM. Time-dose relationships: the linear-quadratic approach. In: Steel GG, ed. Basic Clinical Radiobiology. 3rd ed. London: Arnold, 2002:120–133.

7. Morgan PB, Hanlon AL, Horwitz EM, et al. Radiation dose and late failures in prostate cancer. Int J Radiat Oncol Biol Phys 2007; 67(4):1074–1081.

8. Morgan PB, Hanlon AL, Horwitz EM, et al. Timing of biochemical failure and distant metastatic disease for low-, intermediate-, and high-risk prostate cancer after radiotherapy. Cancer 2007; 110(1):68–80.

9. Milosevic M, Chung P, Parker C, et al. Androgen withdrawal in patients reduces prostate cancer hypoxia: implications for disease progression and radiation response. Cancer Res 2007; 67(13):6022–6025.

10. Webb S. Optimum parameters in a model for tumour control probability including interpatient heterogeneity. Phys Med Biol 1994; 39(11):1895–1914.

11. Sanchez-Nieto B, Nahum AE. The delta-TCP concept: a clinically useful measure of tumor control probability. Int J Radiat Oncol Biol Phys 1999; 44(2):369–380.

12. Hanks GE, Martz KL, Diamond JJ. The effect of dose on local control of prostate cancer. Int J Radiat Oncol Biol Phys 1988; 15(6):1299–1305.

13. Levergrün S, Jackson A, Zelefsky MJ, et al. Fitting tumor control probability models to biopsy outcome after three-dimensional conformal radiation therapy of prostate cancer: pitfalls in deducing radiobiologic parameters for tumors from clinical data. Int J Radiat Oncol Biol Phys 2001; 51(4):1064–1080.

14. Nahum AE, Movsas B, Horwitz EM, et al. Incorporating clinical measurements of hypoxia into tumor local control modeling of prostate cancer: implications for the alpha/beta ratio. Int J Radiat Oncol Biol Phys 2003, 57(2):391–401.

15. Fowler J. Radiobiological principles guiding the management of prostate cancer. In: Greco C, Zelefsky J, eds. Radiotherapy of Prostate Cancer. Amsterdam: Harwood Academic Publisher, 2000:131–141.

16. Brenner DJ, Hall EJ. Fractionation and protraction for radiotherapy of prostate carcinoma. Int J Radiat Oncol Biol Phys 1999; 43(5):1095–1101.

17. Fowler J, Chappell R, Ritter M. Is alpha/beta for prostate tumors really low? Int J Radiat Oncol Biol Phys 2001; 50(4):1021–1031.

18. Wang JZ, Guerrero M, Li XA. How low is the alpha/beta ratio for prostate cancer? Int J Radiat Oncol Biol Phys 2003; 55(1):194–203.

19. King CR, Mayo CS. Is the prostrate alpha/beta ratio of 1.5 from Brenner & Hall a modeling artefact? Int J Radiat Oncol Biol Phys 2000; 47(2):536–538.

20. Brenner DJ, Hall EJ. In response to Drs. King and Mayo: low alpha/beta values for prostate appear to be independent of modeling details. Int J Radiat Oncol Biol Phys 2000; 47(2):538–539.

21. Kal HB, Van Gellekom MP. How low is the alpha/beta ratio for prostate cancer? Int J Radiat Oncol Biol Phys 2003; 57(4):1116–1121.

22. King CR, Fowler JF. A simple analytic derivation suggests that prostate cancer alpha/beta ratio is low. Int J Radiat Oncol Biol Phys 2001; 51(1):213–214.

23. Lindsay PE, Moiseenko VV, Van Dyk J, et al. The influence of brachytherapy dose heterogeneity on estimates of alpha/beta for prostate cancer. Phys Med Biol 2003; 48(4):507–522.

24. Valdagni R, Italia C, Montanaro P, et al. Is the alpha-beta ratio of prostate cancer really low? A prospective, non-randomized trial comparing standard and hyperfractionated conformal radiation therapy. Radiother Oncol 2005; 75(1):74–82.

25. Williams SG, Taylor JM, Liu N, et al. Use of individual fraction size data from 3756 patients to directly determine the alpha/beta ratio of prostate cancer. Int J Radiat Oncol Biol Phys 2007; 68(1):24–33.

26. Movsas B, Chapman JD, Horwitz EM, et al. Hypoxic regions exist in human prostate carcinoma. Urology 1999; 53(1):11–18.

27. Movsas B, Chapman JD, Hanlon AL, et al. Hypoxia in human prostate carcinoma: an Eppendorf PO2 study. Am J Clin Oncol 2001; 24(5):458–561.

28. Carnell DM, Smith RE, Daley FM, et al. An immunohistochemical assessment of hypoxia in prostate carcinoma using pimonidazole: implications for radioresistance. Int J Radiat Oncol Biol Phys 2006; 65(1):91–99.

29. Hoskin PJ, Carnell DM, Taylor NJ, et al. Hypoxia in prostate cancer: correlation of BOLD-MRI with pimonidazole immunohistochemistry-initial observations. Int J Radiat Oncol Biol Phys 2007; 68(4):1065–1071.

30. Parker C, Milosevic M, Toi A, et al. Polarographic electrode study of tumor oxygenation in clinically localized prostate cancer. Int J Radiat Oncol Biol Phys 2004; 58(3):750–757.

31. Rasey JS, Koh WJ, Evans ML, et al. Quantifying regional hypoxia in human tumors with positron emission tomography of [18F]fluoromisonidazole: a pretherapy study of 37 patients. Int J Radiat Oncol Biol Phys 1996; 36(2):417–428.

32. Movsas B, Chapman JD, Greenberg RE, et al. Increasing levels of hypoxia in prostate carcinoma correlate significantly with increasing clinical stage and patient age: an Eppendorf pO(2) study. Cancer 2000; 89(9):2018–2024.

33. Movsas B, Chapman JD, Hanlon AL, et al. Hypoxic prostate/muscle pO2 ratio predicts for biochemical failure in patients with prostate cancer: preliminary findings. Urology 2002; 60(4):634–639.

34. Yorke ED. Modelling the effects of inhomogeneous dose distributions in normal tissues. Semin Radiat Oncol 2001; 11(3):197–209.

35. Travis EL. Organizational response of normal tissues to irradiation. Semin Radiat Oncol 2001; 11(3):184–196.

36. Deasy J, Niemierko A, Herbert D, et al. Methodological issues in radiation dose-volume outcome analyses: summary of a joint AAPM/NIH workshop. Med Phys 2002; 29(9):2109–2127.

37. Fowler JF. Brief summary of radiobiological principles in fractionated radiotherapy. Semin in Radiat Oncol 1992; 2(1):16–21.

38. Lyman JT. Complication probability as assessed from dose-volume histograms. Radiat Res Suppl 1985; 104 (suppl 8):S13–S19.

39. Niemierko A. A generalized concept of equivalent uniform dose (EUD). Med Phys 1999; 26(6):1100.

40. Kutcher GJ, Burman C, Brewster L, et al. Histogram reduction method for calculating complication probabilities for three-dimensional treatment planning evaluations. Int J Radiat Oncol Biol Phys 1991; 21(1):137–146.

41. Mohan R, Mageras GS, Baldwin B, et al. Clinically relevant optimization of 3-D conformal treatments. Med Phys 1992; 19(4):933–944.

42. Kallman P, Agren A, Brahme A. Tumor and normal tissue responses to fractionated non-uniform dose delivery. Int J Radiat Biol 1992; 62(2):249–262.

43. Fowler J. Normal tissue complication probabilities: how well do the models work? Phys Med 2001; 17(suppl 2): 24–34.

44. Burman C, Kutcher GJ, Emami B, et al. Fitting of normal tissue tolerance data to an analytic function. Int J Radiat Oncol Biol Phys 1991; 21(1):123–135.

45. Rancati T, Fiorino C, Gagliardi G, et al. Fitting late rectal bleeding data using different NTCP models: results from an Italian multi-centric study (AIROPROS0101). Radiother Oncol 2004; 73(1):21–32.

46. Peeters ST, Hoogeman MS, Heemsbergen WD, et al. Rectal bleeding, fecal incontinence, and high stool frequency after conformal radiotherapy for prostate cancer: normal tissue complication probability modeling. Int J Radiat Oncol Biol Phys 2006; 66(1):11–19.

47. Söhn M, Yan D, Liang J, et al. Incidence of late rectal bleeding in high-dose conformal radiotherapy of prostate cancer using equivalent uniform dose-based and dose-volume–based normal tissue complication probability models. Int J Radiat Oncol Biol Phys 2007; 67(4): 1066–1073.

48. Tucker SL, Dong L, Bosch WR, et al. Fit of a generalized Lyman normal-tissue complication probability (NTCP) model to grade ≥2 late rectal toxicity data from patients treated on protocol RTOG 94-06. Int J Radiat Oncol Biol Phys 2007; 69(suppl 3):S8–S9.

49. Peeters ST, Lebesque JV, Heemsbergen WD, et al. Localized volume effects for late rectal and anal toxicity after radiotherapy for prostate cancer. Int J Radiat Oncol Biol Phys 2006; 64(4):1151–1561.

50. Peeters ST, Heemsbergen WD, Koper PC, et al. Dose-response in radiotherapy for localized prostate cancer: results of the Dutch multicenter randomized phase III trial comparing 68 Gy of radiotherapy with 78 Gy. J Clin Oncol 2006; 24(13):1990–1996.

51. Fiorino C, Fellin G, Rancati T, et al. Clinical and dosimetric predictors of late rectal syndrome after 3DCRT for localized prostate cancer: preliminary results of a multicenter prospective study. Int J Radiat Oncol Biol Phys 2008; 70:1130–1137.

52. Fiorino C, Gianolini S, Nahum AE. A cylindrical model of the rectum: comparing dose-volume, dose-surface and dose-wall histograms in the radiotherapy of prostate cancer. Phys Med Biol 2003; 48(16):2603–2616.

53. Lebesque JV, Bruce AM, Kroes AP, et al. Variation in volumes, dose-volume histograms and estimated normal tissue complication probabilities of rectum and bladder during conformal radiotherapy of T3 prostate cancer. Int J Radiat Oncol Biol Phys 1995; 33(5):1109–1119.

54. Lu Y, Song PY, Li SD, et al. A method of analyzing rectal surface area irradiated and rectal complications in prostate conformal radiotherapy. Int J Radiat Oncol Biol Phys 1995; 33(5):1121–1125.

55. MacKay RI, Hendry JH, Moore CJ, et al. Predicting late rectal complications following prostate conformal radiotherapy using biologically effective doses and normalized dose-surface histograms. Brit J Radiol 1997; 70(833):517–526.

56. Meijer GJ, van den Brink M, Hoogeman MS, et al. Dose-wall histograms and normalized dose-surface histograms for the rectum: a new method to analyse the dose distribution over the rectum in conformal radiotherapy. Int J Radiat Oncol Biol Phys 1999; 45(4):1073–1080.

57. Heemsbergen WD, Hoogeman MS, Witte MG, et al. Increased risk of biochemical and clinical failure for prostate patients with a large rectum at radiotherapy planning: results from the Dutch trial of 68 GY versus 78 Gy. Int J Radiat Oncol Biol Phys 2007; 67(5):1418–1424.

58. de Crevoisier R, Tucker SL, Dong L, et al. Increased risk of biochemical and local failure in patients with distended rectum on the planning CT for prostate cancer radiotherapy. Int J Radiat Oncol Biol Phys 2005; 62(4):965–973.

59. Marks LB, Carroll PR, Dugan TC, et al. The response of the urinary bladder, urethra, and ureter to radiation and chemotherapy. Int J Radiat Oncol Biol Phys 1995; 31(5): 1257–1280.

60. Gardner BG, Zietman AL, Shipley WU, et al. Late normal tissue sequelae in the second decade after high dose radiation therapy with combined photons and conformal protons for locally advanced prostate cancer. J Urol 2002; 167(1): 123–126.

61. Zelefsky MJ, Cowen D, Fuks Z, et al. Long term tolerance of high dose three-dimensional conformal radiotherapy in patients with localized prostate carcinoma. Cancer 1999; 85(11):2460–2468.

62. Allen ZA, Merrick GS, Butler WM, et al. Detailed urethral dosimetry in the evaluation of prostate brachytherapy-related urinary morbidity. Int J Radiat Oncol Biol Phys 2005; 62(4):981–987.

63. Albert M, Tempany CM, Schultz D, et al. Late genitourinary and gastrointestinal toxicity after magnetic resonance image-guided prostate brachytherapy with or without neoadjuvant external beam radiation therapy. Cancer 2003; 98(5):949–954.

64. Cheung MR, Tucker SL, Dong L, et al. Investigation of bladder dose and volume factors influencing late urinary toxicity after external beam radiotherapy for prostate cancer. Int J Radiat Oncol Biol Phys 2007; 67(4):1059–1965.

65. Happerset L, Mageras GS, Zelefsky MJ, et al. A study of the effects of internal organ motion on dose escalation in conformal prostate treatment. Radiother Oncol 2003; 66: 263–270.

66. Bos LJ, van der Geer J, van Herk M, et al. The sensitivity of dose distributions for organ motion and set-up uncertainties in prostate IMRT. Radiother Oncol 2005; 76:18–26.

67. De Crevoisier R. Variations anatomique en cours d'irradiation conformationnelle puor cancer de la prostate: quantification, impact dosimetrique et clinicque, rationnel pour une radiotherapie guideè par l'image. PhD thesis. Universite Paris XI, Paris, 2007.

68. Stasi M, Munoz F, Fiorino C, et al. Emptying the rectum before treatment delivery limits the variations of rectal dose-volume parameters during 3DCRT of prostate cancer. Radiother Oncol 2006; 80(3):363–370.

69. Nijkamp J, Pos FJ, Nuver TT, et al. Adaptive radiotherapy for prostate cancer using kilovoltage cone-beam computed tomography: first clinical results. Int J Radiat Oncol Biol Phys 2008; 70(1):75–82.

70. Fiorino C, Di Muzio N, Broggi S, et al. Evidence of limited motion of the prostate by careful emptying of the rectum as assessed by daily MVCT image-guidance with Helical Tomotherapy. Int J Radiat Oncol Biol Phys 2008 (in press).

71. Orton NP, Tomè WA. The impact of daily shifts on prostate IMRT dose distributions. Med Phys 2004; 31(10): 2845–2848.

72. Song W, Schaly B, Bauman G, et al. Image-guided adaptive radiation therapy (IGART): Radiobiological and dose escalation considerations for localized carcinoma of the prostate. Med Phys 2005; 32(7):2193–2203.

73. Litzenberg DW, Balter JM, Hadley SW, et al. The influence of intra-fraction motion on margins for prostate radiotherapy. Int J Radiat Oncol Biol Phys 2006; 65:548–553.

74. Nederveen A, Lagendijk J, Hofman P. Detection of fiducial gold markers for automatic on-line megavoltage position verification using a marker extraction kernel (MEK). Int J Radiat Oncol Biol Phys 2000; 47:1435–1442.

75. Nederveen AJ, van der Heide UA, Dehnad H, et al. Measurements and clinical consequences of prostate motion during a radiotherapy fraction. Int J Radiat Oncol Biol Phys 2002; 5:206–214.

76. Kitamura K, Shirato H, Seppenwoolde Y, et al. Three-dimensional intrafractional movement of prostate measured during real-time tumor-tracking radiotherapy in supine and prone treatment positions. Int J Radiat Oncol Biol Phys 2002; 53:1117–1123.

77. Song WY, Schaly B, Bauman G, et al. Evaluation of image-guided radiation therapy (IGRT) technologies and their impact on the outcomes of hypofractionated prostate cancer treatments: a radiobiologic analysis. Int J Radiat Oncol Biol Phys 2006; 64(1):289–300.

78. Ghilezan M, Yan D, Liang J, et al. Online image-guided intensity-modulated radiotherapy of prostate cancer: how much improvement can we expect? A theoretical assessment of clinical benefits and potential dose escalation by improving precision and accuracy of radiation delivery. Int J Radiat Oncol Biol Phys 2004; 60(5):1602–1610.

79. Kupelian PA, Reddy CA, Carlson TP, et al. Preliminary observations on biochemical relapse-free survival rates after short-course intensity-modulated radiotherapy (70 Gy at 2.5 Gy/fraction) for localized prostate cancer. Int J Radiat Oncol Biol Phys 2002; 53:904–912.

80. Pollack A, Hanlon AL, Horwitz EM, et al. Dosimetry and preliminary acute toxicity in the first 100 men treated for prostate cancer on a randomized hypofractionation dose escalation trial. Int J Radiat Oncol Biol Phys 2006; 64(2): 518–526.

81. Soete G, Arcangeli S, De Meerleer G, et al. Phase II study of a four-week hypofractionated external beam radiotherapy regimen for prostate cancer: report on acute toxicity. Radiother Oncol 2006; 80(1):78–81.

82. Madsen BL, Hsi RA, Pham HT, et al. Stereotactic hypofractionated accurate radiotherapy of the prostate (SHARP), 33.5 Gy in five fractions for localized disease: first clinical trial results. Int J Radiat Oncol Biol Phys 2007; 67(4):1099–1105.

83. Hara W, Patel D, Pawlicki T, et al. Hypofractionated stereotactic radiotherapy for prostate cancer: early results. Int J Radiat Oncol Biol Phys 2006; 66(3):S324–S325.

84. Craig T, Moiseenko V, Battista J, et al. The impact o geometric uncertainty on hypofractionated external beam radiation therapy of prostate cancer. Int J Radiat Oncol Biol Phys 2003; 57(3):833–842.

85. Van Herk M, Witte M, van der Geer J, et al. Biological and physical fractionation effects of random geometric errors. Int J Radiat Oncol Biol Phys 2003; 57(5):1460–1471.

86. Djavan B, Milani S, Remzi M. Prostate biopsy: who, how and when. An update. Can J Urol 2005; 12(suppl 1):44–48.

87. Cellini N, Morganti AG, Mattiucci GC, et al. Analysis of intraprostatic failures in patients treated with hormonal therapy and radiotherapy: implications for conformal therapy planning. Int J Radiat Oncol Biol Phys 2002; 53: 595–599.

88. Schiebler ML, Schnall MD, Pollack HM, et al. Current role of MR Imaging in the staging of adenocarcinoma of the prostate. Radiology 1993; 189:339–352.

89. van Lin EN, Futterer JJ, Heijmink SW, et al. IMRT boost dose planning on dominant intraprostatic lesions: gold marker-based three-dimensional fusion of CT with dynamic contrast-enhanced and ^{1}H-spectroscopic MRI. Int J Radiat Oncol Biol Phys 2006; 65(1):291–303.

90. Cruz M, Tsuda K, Narumi Y, et al. Characterization of lowsignal-intensity lesions in the peripheral zone of prostate on pre-biopsy endorectal coil imaging. Eur Radiol 2002; 12: 357–365.

91. De Meerleer G, Villeirs G, Bral S, et al. The magnetic resonance detected intraprostatic lesion in prostate cancer: planning and delivery of intensity-modulated radiotherapy. Radiother Oncol 2005; 75(3):325–333.

92. McNeal JE, Redwine EA, Freiha FS, et al. Zonal distribution of prostatic adenocarcinoma: correlation with histopathologic pattern and direction of spread. Am J Surg Pathol 1988; 12:897–906.

93. Xia P, Pickett B, Vigneault E, et al. Forward or inversely planned segmental multileaf collimator IMRT and sequential tomotherapy to treat multiple dominant intraprostatic lesions of prostate cancer to 90 Gy. Int J Radiat Oncol Biol Phys 2001; 51(1):244–254.

94. Popple RA, Ove R, Shen S. Tumor control probability for selective boosting of hypoxic subvolumes, including the effect of reoxygenation. Int J Radiat Oncol Biol Phys 2002; 54(3):921–927.

4

Advances in Imaging and Anatomical Considerations for Prostate Cancer Treatment Planning

AARON SPALDING AND PATRICK McLAUGHLIN

Department of Radiation Oncology, University of Michigan, Ann Arbor, Michigan, U.S.A.

INTRODUCTION

The modern standard of successful prostate cancer treatment includes both cancer control and quality of life preservation. Realizing the full potential of advanced treatment planning such as intensity-modulated radiation therapy (IMRT) and image-guided delivery depend on improved imaging and target definition. T2 MRI imaging and time-of-light MRI angiography allow improved definition of the prostate and multiple critical structures, not visualized on CT. Integration of MRI requires physician training in pelvic functional anatomy to take full advantage of the improved imaging. Correlation of dose and toxicity of critical adjacent structures made possible by MRI-based planning will ultimately complement the correlation of prostate dose and biochemical control to improve the therapeutic ratio and fulfill the modern standard of successful prostate cancer radiotherapy.

Recent advances in prostate cancer therapy from IMRT to image-guided radiation therapy (IGRT) have improved the capacity to deliver high dose conformal treatments with a previously impossible precision. Taking full advantage of this technology requires accurate definition of target and critical adjacent structures. All studies to date suggest that variance in prostate contouring remains extreme, especially when CT imaging is

employed (1,2). CT planning for prostate cancer results in interobserver and intraobserver variation in target definition, and limited definition of critical adjacent structures impacting quality of life. Currently there are no objective guidelines to assure accurate target definition or consensus. This leaves open the possibility of high cost, highly conformal dose delivery to a grossly overestimated or underestimated target, effectively negating the potential gain of IMRT and IGRT.

Improved target definition and contouring consensus is possible with MRI imaging (3), but multiple structures not visible on CT create confusion and necessitate training in pelvic MRI and functional anatomy to take advantage of this potential (4). Full integration of MRI imaging requires registration, a potential source of error that can diminish the advantage of MRI imaging (5,6). Multiple complementary methods of registration are available, and no single method is without potential error. In spite of caution about registration error, the clarity of MRI imaging is compelling, and there is little doubt that integration of a variety of functional scans will be routine in the future.

For the immediate future, there is a vital need to define competence in MRI contouring and registration, create education modules to teach the necessary skills, and to establish testing methods to validate competence. This chapter will focus on the current state-of-the-art in MRI

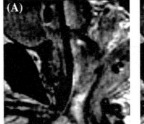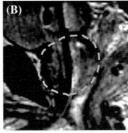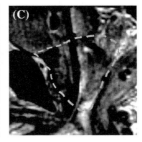

Figure 1 Sagittal MRI demonstrating (**A**) circular or globular shape of prostate, (**B**) contour of prostate on MRI, (**C**) CT contours cut onto MRI demonstrating projection from the globular form due to influence of unclear boundaries with adjacent structures. Also note the length of rectum (rectal volume) in the high dose region is doubled by overestimation of prostate on CT.

imaging and registration for prostate cancer treatment planning. In particular, it will be discussed in the context of the identification of specific prostatic and other pelvic anatomical structures.

LIMITATION OF CT-BASED PROSTATE TREATMENT PLANNING

The vast majority of prostate cancer radiation treatment planning in the modern era is CT based. Limitations of CT scans in prostate definition have been well documented, and are due to merging of the prostate with adjacent tissues. The normal globular prostate, as defined by MRI (Fig. 1A, B) or ultrasound, may acquire a host of projections (Fig. 1C) due to contouring of adjacent tissues as prostate. Such projections are recognizable on lateral beam's eye view of the prostate contours. In addition, underestimation is possible on CT due to poor visualization of intralumen extension and merging of the prostate apex with the genitourinary diaphragm (GUD).

Common projections from the globular prostate are presented in Figure 2, as they would appear from a lateral beam's eye view projection. At the base of the prostate, the anterior fibromuscular stroma (AFS) is contiguous with the bladder muscle and no clear demarcation is possible. Inclusion of this extension of the bladder from the AFS results in a sharp anterior protrusion (Fig. 2B). The prostate seminal vesicle interface is also difficult to define on CT and inclusion of seminal vesicle is relatively common, resulting in a posterior superior projection (Fig. 2C). The posterior surface of the prostate is convex on MRI, but because of poor definition at the apex, contouring may continue anterior to the rectum resulting in a concave posterior surface (Fig. 2D), especially when combined with seminal vesicle inclusion as prostate. Other patterns at the apex include the "pedestal" wherein the lack of clarity is compensated by repeat of a same small area contour in an effort to avoid underestimating the prostate (Fig. 2E),

as well as including GUD elements as prostate resulting in an inferior anterior projection (Fig. 2F).

Underestimation of the prostate extent is possible and may be recognized on beam's eye view as excessively flat superior or inferior prostate contour on lateral beam's eye view resulting from failure to contour the full extent of the prostate. A median lobe is a unique form of hypertrophy which projects into the bladder lumen, and is the one normal projection from the globular prostate form. Depending on patient size and technique, this may be clearly visible on CT or barely visible (Fig. 3A). Conversely, in patients with small prostates and an intact bladder neck, the bladder neck may appear as a solid intralumen structure contiguous with the prostate and result in overestimation of the prostate extent (Fig. 3B).

In the past, adjacent structures clearly defined on CT have been used to define the prostate. The penile bulb was used as a reference in defining the apex position. It was

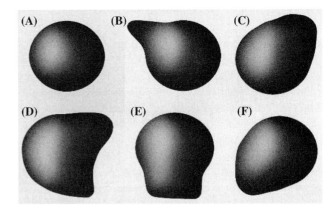

Figure 2 Lateral beam's eye view of prostate contour: (**A**) globular prostate, (**B**) anterior superior projection secondary to including bladder as prostate, (**C**) posterior superior projection due to including seminal vesicle as prostate, (**D**) inferior posterior projection from use of rectum as reference, (**E**) pedestal projection due to repeat of lowest contour, (**F**) inferior anterior projection due to including GUD as prostate. *Abbreviation*: GUD, genitourinary diaphragm.

Intra-lumen Extension

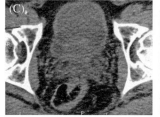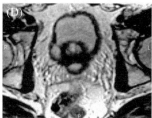

Figure 3 Intraluminal prostate: (**A**) CT with unclear boundaries of extension from prostate, (**B**) MRI with clear definition, (**C**) CT with bladder neck appearing as intralumen projection, (**D**) MRI demonstrating hollow bladder neck.

thought that the distance from the penile bulb to the prostate apex was fixed at 1.5 cm. Later studies disclosed that this distance varies from 0.6 to 2.3 cm, and use of the 1.5-cm rule may result in overestimation or underestimation of the prostate apex position (7). Because of such variation, contouring rules based on distance from a defined structure should be abandoned. What has proven useful in defining the prostate extent is the recognition of critical adjacent structures on CT after viewing such structures clearly on MRI. For example, the GUD layers from the penile bulb through the triangular and circular shaped levels may be visible on CT (Fig. 4) after MRI training (Fig. 5). Recognition of GUD elements on CT can dramatically improve apex level definition to within 0.5 cm of the MRI-defined prostate (8), with no risk of underestimation when properly applied.

MRI IN PROSTATE TREATMENT PLANNING

MRI imaging has been employed to improve prostate definition. T2 imaging results in clear demarcation of the prostate relative to adjacent structures. Especially clear is the distinction of prostate and muscle, whether bladder muscle above or levator ani and external sphincter below. Structures not ordinarily visualized as distinct entities on CT are clearly seen on MRI, which can be incorporated into IGRT planning and assigned a cost function. Variation in prostate size and shape due to variable hypertrophy, variation in GUD thickness and elements, and variation in prostate to bladder connection may result in confusion to the uninitiated, but ultimately

GUD Recognition on CT

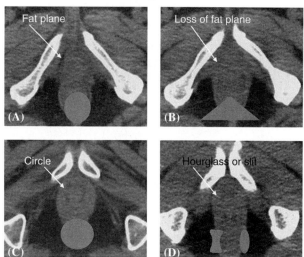

Figure 4 GUD recognition on CT: (**A**) penile bulb layer visible by fat plane separation of medial and lateral structures, (**B**) triangle layer with connection of central and lateral structures, (**C**) circular mid-GUD, (**D**) slit or hourglass shape just below prostate apex. *Abbreviation*: GUD, genitourinary diaphragm.

MRI-based planning may improve the therapeutic ratio relative to CT-based planning by improved definition of both prostate and normal tissues.

Zonal Anatomy and Interface with Bladder and External Sphincter

The prostate increases in size over a man's lifetime, but not all tissue within the prostate increases proportionally. The principal area of hypertrophy is the transition zone (TZ), which is visualized on MRI as a dark central area (Fig. 6) relative to the lighter peripheral zone (PZ). The PZ is the origin of the majority of prostate cancers, which may appear dark within the PZ, and may visibly disrupt the prostate capsule when advanced. The AFS is also highly variable and distinct on MRI as darker than the TZ. The AFS is contiguous with the bladder above and the external sphincter below, a contiguity that may be responsible for coordinating the internal sphincter at the bladder neck and the external sphincter. Although the prostate may be visualized in a chain from bladder to prostate to external sphincter and GUD, both bladder and external sphincter elements extend into the prostate (Fig. 7). The bladder mucosa extends to the veromontanum, which is in the lower half of the prostate in older men. The veromontanum is an expansion of the urethra within the prostate and is the point where prostate and seminal vesicle secretions enter the urethra. To treat the entire bladder mucosa, one must treat almost the entire prostate.

GUD Levels on MRI

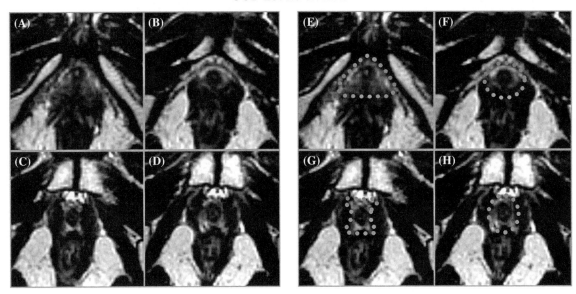

Figure 5 GUD levels on MRI: (**A**) triangle, (**B**) circle, (**C**) hourglass (convex levator ani), (**D**) apex (concave levator ani), (**E–H**) contours of recognizable levels. *Abbreviation*: GUD, genitourinary diaphragm.

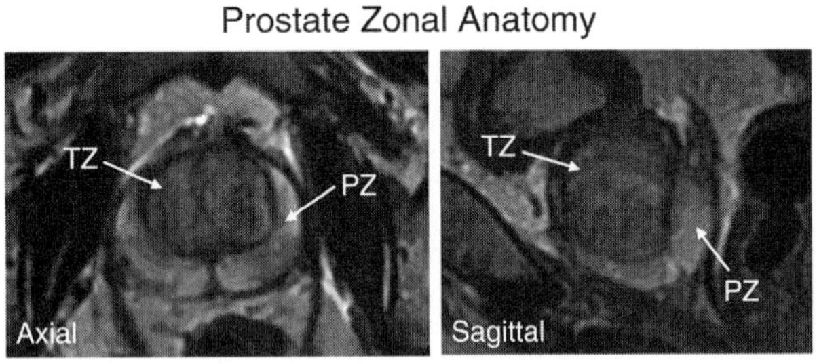

Prostate Zonal Anatomy

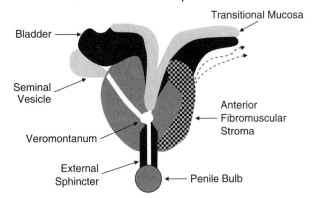

Figure 6 Zonal anatomy: (**A**) axial view with TZ and PZ, (**B**) sagittal view of TX and PZ. *Abbreviations*: PZ, peripheral zone; TZ, transition zone.

Bladder and External Sphincter Interface

Figure 7 (*See color insert.*) Prostate interface with bladder and external sphincter. Note the bladder mucosa extends to the veromontanum and the external sphincter extends to just below the veromontanum.

Inferiorly the external sphincter extends into the prostate to the veromontanum. In younger men with minimal TZ hypertrophy, the internal sphincter is nearly adjacent to the external sphincter (above and below the veromontanum). With age, there is an increasing separation of the internal and external sphincter as well as obstruction and distortion of the internal sphincter by hypertrophy, with a host of consequences. It is not possible to predict that consequence from the anatomy; men may have marked enlargement of the prostate with minimal impact on urinary function, or may have minimal change and lack of coordination of the internal and external sphincters resulting in a range of obstructive and irritative symptoms.

The Prostatic Apex

The apex is clearly visualized on T2 MRI by the change in the shape of the levator ani from a concave shape cupping the prostate to a convex shape below the prostate (Fig. 5). This pelvic muscle is clearly distinguished from the prostate and cradles the prostate. Below the apex, the muscle itself bows in creating a part of the GUD through which the urethra passes below the prostate. In addition to the levator, the external sphincter is visible within the GUD as a dark central circular structure. However, it must be noted that the external sphincter passes into the body of the prostate, and therefore the appearance of the external sphincter on axial MRI is not a sign of the prostate apex. The clearest definition of the prostate apex/GUD interface

Apex/GUD Interface

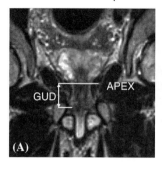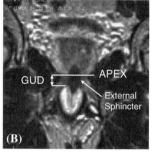

Figure 8 Wide variation in GUD thickness: (**A**) coronal MRI of patient with thin GUD, (**B**) patient with a wide GUD. Note the extension of the external sphincter into the prostate and penile bulb, especially clear in (**B**). *Abbreviation*: GUD, genitourinary diaphragm.

is on coronal MRI. The clarity of the apex and GUD interface on coronal MRI as well as the variation in GUD thickness is apparent in Figure 8.

The Base of the Prostate

At the base, the variations in prostate anatomy have been documented. In young men before prostate TZ enlargement, there is a distinct bladder neck or funnel formed as the bladder empties into the prostate (Fig. 9A). With enlargement of the transition zone, there is expansion of the bladder neck and ultimately obliteration of the bladder neck (Fig. 9B). Intralumen extension of the prostate can occur, especially dramatic with median lobe formation (Fig. 9C). The full appreciation of the bladder neck encroachment by prostate is visualized on sagittal MRI, but again, once initiated, the T2 axial MRI is sufficient to allow definition of the prostate.

It has been argued that proper definition of the prostate is sufficient in accomplishing most of the normal tissue sparing possible with prostate cancer treatment. By conforming to a well-defined prostate volume, there is a de facto sparing of critical adjacent structures related to

sexual, genitourinary, and rectal function. On the other hand, an advantage of MRI planning is definition of such critical adjacent structures that can be included in treatment planning. Because of the wide variation in the relationship of these structures to the prostate and the capacity of IMRT-based planning to apply cost function and selectively limit dose to such structures, inclusion of critical adjacent structures in treatment planning is now possible.

CRITICAL ADJACENT STRUCTURES VISIBLE ON MRI

GUD and Corporal Bodies

The MRI provides full detail of the GUD structure. The external sphincter is a distinct muscle that passes through the GUD. It originates at the veromontanum, approximately in the lower one-third of the prostate and extends into the penile bulb. In addition, the levator ani anatomy is clearly depicted. Finally, the penile bulb and corpus cavernosum are much more clearly defined on the MRI than CT. The cavernosal nerves, which are the terminal branches of the neurovascular bundle, are not visible on MRI, but can be defined by their relationship to the external sphincter. They proceed from a 5- and 7-o'clock position at the prostate apex to an 11- and 1-o'clock position above the penile bulb. The cavernosal nerves represent the termination of the neurovascular bundle.

Neurovascular Bundle and Plexus

The neurovascular bundle has been defined on MRI as well as CT on the basis of its posterior-lateral position. In fact, recent pathology studies call into question the nature of the neurovascular bundle (9). In 50% of patients, the nerves pass along the entire lateral surface rather than in a distinct bundle (Fig. 10). Thus, correlation of dose to the neurovascular bundle as previously defined may be inaccurate, and sexual function studies must be updated to include dose to the common neurovascular plexus configurations.

Prostate/Bladder Neck Variation

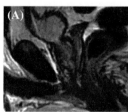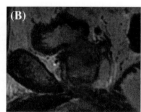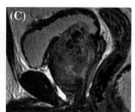

Figure 9 Progressive bladder neck expansion by prostate: (**A**) intact bladder neck, (**B**) expanded bladder neck, (**C**) bladder neck expansion with extensive intralumen component (median lobe).

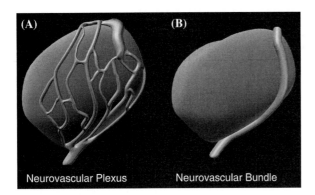

Figure 10 Variation in neurovascular anatomy: (**A**) lateral prostate plexus, (**B**) posterior-lateral bundle (classic configuration).

Current surgical literature suggests that marked improvement in postsurgical sexual function is possible by sparing
the entire plexus, employing the "veil of Aphrodite"
technique (10).

Bladder and Rectum

The anatomy of the base and seminal vesicle prostate
junction is well defined on T2 MRI. This is especially
helpful in intraluminal disease that is not always visible on
CT. The outer rectal wall is clearly delineated on CT and
distinct layers of the rectal wall, including muscle and
mucosa, are visible on T2 MRI. The rectal wall is, on
average, 0.5 cm in thickness, regardless of the diameter of
the rectum and the immediate area adjacent to the prostate
(11). Although with extreme expansion there is thinning of
the rectal wall for the region adjacent to the prostate,
variation in rectal wall thickness is minimal. Therefore,
deexpansion of a CT rectum to 0.5 cm is a very reliable
means to simulate the actual rectal wall. The definition of
rectal muscle versus rectal mucosa does open the path for
potential mucosal sparing therapy, but given the minimal
thickness of the rectal muscle wall (2–3 mm), improved
prostate immobilization and improved IMRT delivery
would be necessary to accomplish mucosal sparing. In
most patients, the rectal mucosa is included in a 3- to
5-mm posterior expansion of the prostate.

Internal Pudendal Artery

Novel targets such as the internal pudendal artery are
visible on MR studies by a time-of-flight sequence. This
can be accomplished in less than 10 minutes and does not
require contrast. Both patency of the internal pudendal
artery as well as definition of its termination in the corpus
cavernosum is possible (Fig. 11). The most terminal
branches may not be depicted on the angiogram and
may require use of coronal imaging for optimal definition.
At present, this is a research question, but with the ever-
increasing technical improvements in MR sequencing, it is
quite likely that a number of studies will be performed by
MRI, including both functional studies as well as imaging
studies, and these will likely be incorporated in the future.

   In this chapter, we have not discussed intraprostatic
definition and functional imaging to delineate the prostate
cancer relative to normal tissues. This is best accomplished at present with a rectal probe that distorts
the prostate and makes registration with a standard anatomic position difficult. With 3-T and higher MR scans,
the possibility of MR spectroscopy of the prostate using
a pelvic coil has been entertained and pursued, and in
all likelihood such imaging will be possible within the
next few years (12). Figure 12 is a summary of structures
definable on MRI.

INTEGRATION AND REGISTRATION

Three levels of integration of MRI and CT are possible.
Improved CT contouring is possible after training in MRI
anatomy, specifically by improved recognition of critical
adjacent structures recognizable on CT after training in
MRI. The next level is parallel MRI and CT scans. Side by
side analysis with correlation by a radiation oncologist can
improve the interpretation of CT at the base and apex.
Finally, registration of MRI and CT represents full integration, but requires a significant commitment to registration, given the moment-to-moment variation in prostate
position relative to bony anatomy. Three methods for
registration are available; mutual information, seed to
seed, and contour to contour. Competence in all methods

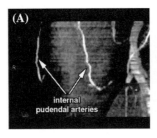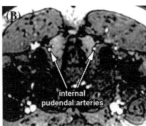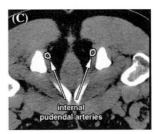

Figure 11 Internal pudendal artery: (**A**) posterior-lateral view of a time-of-flight angiogram of the IPA, (**B**) axial MRI view of IPA,
(**C**) CT scan with IPA contour from MRI angio registered. *Abbreviation*: IPA, interal pudendal arteries.

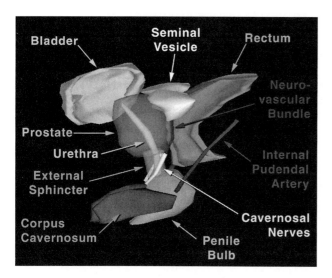

Figure 12 Prostate and critical adjacent structures definable on MRI.

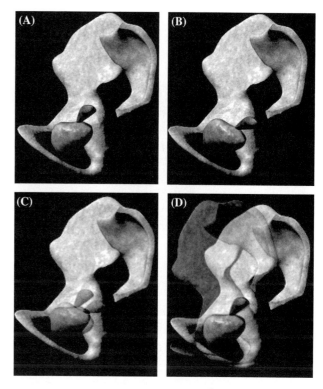

Figure 13 Registration by mutual information. (**A,B**) The same patient with differing prostate positions. (**C**) Full pelvis registration by mutual information. Bones dominate the match at the expense of accurate prostate registration. (**D**) With cropping of the registration to the prostate it is possible to accurately register prostate to prostate, with resultant bone mismatch.

is necessary due to the failure of any single method to work reliably in all patients.

Mutual information provides the most rapid registration of data sets. Commonly, the pelvic bones dominate the match and are extremely well matched by mutual information of full pelvic CT to full pelvic MRI. The prostate is a relatively small volume organ within the pelvis and its position may change and not influence the mutual information match. It is necessary to crop the data set to the area of interest, specifically the prostate and immediate adjacent areas, to improve the match of the prostate to the CT prostate. With cropping, it is possible to accurately register a majority of patients. The effect of cropping on the prostate versus pelvis registration is demonstrated in Figure 13. However, this is operator dependent and experience dependent. Error in the z-axis remains possible because the prostate diameter is constant throughout its mid levels, and error in the z-axis may not be detectable by visual inspection in spite of review of registered images.

A second option for registration is seed to seed match. With the common use of fiducial markers and the use of sequences highlighting such markers on MRI, it is possible to match seed to seed. It should be noted, however, that seed to seed registration has approximately the same potential for error in the z-axis as mutual information. This is due to the uncertainty of seed position due to slice thickness artifact introduced by CT and MRI. This is demonstrated in Figure 14A. In addition, seed position on MRI is more difficult to define due to a tailing effect, wherein a seed may appear on several slices that in total are a greater length than the actual seed. Paradoxically, the thinner the MR slice, the greater confusion about seed position is created. With thicker slices, the seed position is less ambiguous, but obviously less

well defined relative to actual position in space. With any seed to seed imaging by sliced-base imaging (CT/MRI), as opposed to orthogonal X-ray images, there is some displacement by the slice scanning which in turn prevents a perfect match of seeds, unless the slices began in identical location within the patient (Fig. 14B–D).

Registration of contours is a third option. This, of course, depends on accurate contouring and as contouring on CT varies so dramatically, this may be the least desirable approach. However, it is very clear that some patients matched by mutual information or seed to seed have differences in prostate position, obvious by difference in position of the prostate/rectum interface. In such patients, registration of contours or the rectum interface is a useful strategy to refine the registration. Caution must be applied in this approach because of the complex nature of prostate movement. With filling of the rectum, the prostate moves superior and anterior. There may be greater movement at the base than at the apex, as the apex serves as a point of rotation in some patients. Contouring studies suggest that MRI and CT contours vary least at mid-prostate, and verifying match at this level is often useful when mutual information or seed to seed matching does

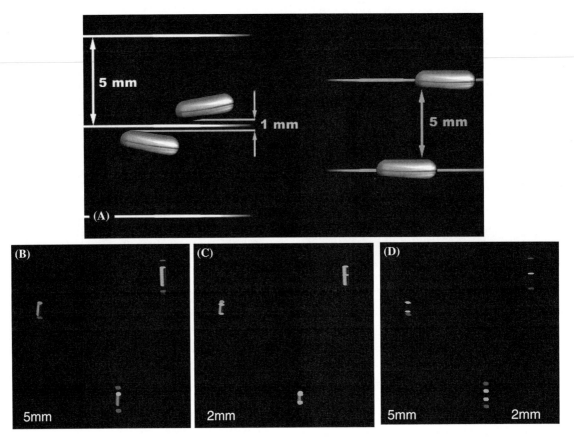

Figure 14 Effect of slice thickness on seed position. (**A**) Seeds 1 mm apart will appear 5 mm apart when scanned with 5-mm slice thickness. (**B,C**) Identical three-dimensional seed phantom scanned at 2- and 5-mm slice thickness. (**D**) Seed match of 2 and 5 mm demonstrates impossibility of actual seed to seed match.

not accomplish an acceptable registration. Because the fascia surrounding the prostate is often included as prostate on CT contouring, it is useful to define the "fascial prostate" as a structure on MRI and this may improve the contour to contour checking of registration (Fig. 15). Otherwise, predictably, the MR prostate is smaller than the CT prostate and will only match in its posterior surface at the rectum/bladder interface.

The discussion of registration also applies to daily imaging. Cone beam CT matching of the prostate has the same limitations of registration of CT and MR. Z-axis error is possible. Even matching CT data sets to CT data sets offers the possibility of error. Fiducial markers with orthogonal X-ray images provide the most accurate means for daily alignment, but for actual alignment, full range of motion adjustment is necessary, including x-, y-, and z-axes. Such refinement is increasingly available in the modern era.

SUMMARY OF PERTINENT CONCLUSIONS

- Taking full advantage of advances in high-dose conformal radiation therapy including IMRT and IGRT

depend on accurate definition of both prostate and critical adjacent structures affecting genitourinary, rectal, and sexual function.
- The current limiting factor for improvement of prostate cancer radiation therapy is imaging and consensus on contouring, especially when CT-based imaging is employed.
- T2 MRI sequences employing a pelvic coil and noncontrast time-of-flight sequence angiography allow definition of prostate and critical adjacent structures and inclusion of such structures in IMRT treatment planning.
- Correlation of toxicity to dose to critical adjacent structures will ultimately allow refinement of cost functions for IMRT treatment planning and improved quality of life outcomes.
- Physician training in regional pelvic anatomy and contouring must continue to keep pace with the improved imaging.
- Educational modules and competency testing will be necessary to limit the wide variability in contouring and improve multi-institutional studies.

Contour Match at Mid Prostate

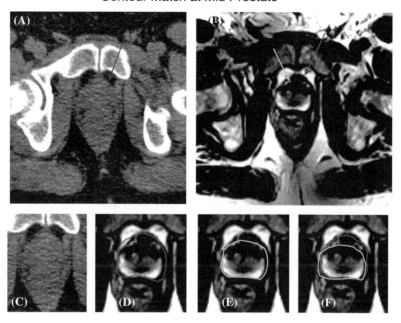

Figure 15 Contour match at mid prostate. Although contours at mid-prostate match more reliably than base and apex contours (uncertain on CT), the fascia around the prostate merge with prostate on CT (**A**) but are distinct from the prostate on MRI (**B**). To match contours, it is useful to contour the "prostate with fascia on MRI" to allow match at posterior and anterior prostate surface rather than matching at the posterior surface alone. (**C**) Prostate contour on CT (includes fascia). (**D**) MRI with prostate plus fascia contour. (**E**) MRI with prostate contour alone. (**F**) MRI with both prostate contour and prostate plus fascia contour.

REFERENCES

1. Roach M III, Faillace-Akazawa P, Malfatti C, et al. Prostate volumes defined by magnetic resonance imaging and computerized tomographic scans for three-dimensional conformal radiotherapy. Int J Radiat Oncol Biol Phys 1996; 35(5):1011–1018.
2. Rasch C, Barillot I, Remeijer P, et al. Definition of the prostate in CT and MRI: a multi-observer study. Int J Radiat Oncol Biol Phys 1999; 43(1):57–66.
3. Debois M, Oyen R, Maes F, et al. The contribution of magnetic resonance imaging to the three-dimensional treatment planning of localized prostate cancer. Int J Radiat Oncol Biol Phys 1999; 45(4):857–865.
4. McLaughlin PW, Troyer S, Narayana V, et al. Functional anatomy of the prostate: implications for treatment planning. Int J Rad Oncol Biol Phys 2005; 63(2):479–491.
5. Roberson PL, McLaughlin PW, Narayana V, et al. Use and uncertainties of mutual information for CT/MR registration post permanent implant of the prostate. Med Phys 2005; 32:473–482.
6. McLaughlin PW, Narayana V, Kessler M, et al. The use of mutual information in registration of CT and MRI datasets post permanent implant. Brachytherapy 2004; 3(2):61–70.
7. McLaughlin PW, Narayana V, Meriowitz A, et al. Vessel sparing prostate radiotherapy: dose limitation to critical erectile vascular structures (internal pudendal artery and corpus cavernosum) defined by MRI. Int J Rad Oncol Biol Phys 2005; 61(1):20–31.
8. McLaughlin P, Feng M, Berri S, et al. Improved CT prostate apex definition by genitourinary diaphragm recognition. Int J Rad Oncol Biol Phys 2006; 66(3):S336.
9. Kiyoshima K, Yokomizo A, Yoshida T, et al. Anatomic features of periprostatic tissue and its surroundings: a histological analysis of 79 radical retropubic prostatectomy specimens. Jpn J Clin Oncol 2004; 34:463–468.
10. Kaul S, Savera A, Badani K, et al. Functional outcomes and oncological efficacy of Vattikuti Institute prostatectomy with Veil of Aphrodite nerve-sparing: an analysis of 154 consecutive patients. BJU Int 2006; 97:467–472.
11. McLaughlin P, Berri S, Narayana V. Determination of rectal muscle, rectal mucosa, and rectal wall dimension: dosimetric implications in prostate brachytherapy. Brachytherapy 2007; 6(2):105.
12. Manenti G, Squillaci E, Carlani M, et al. Magnetic resonance imaging of the prostate with spectroscopic imaging using a surface coil. Initial clinical experience. Radiol Med (Torino) 2006; 111(1):22–32.

5

Target and Organ Motion Considerations

CHARLES CATTON AND TIM CRAIG

Princess Margaret Hospital, The University of Toronto, Toronto, Ontario, Canada

INTRODUCTION

Five randomized trials have shown improved biochemical relapse free rates (bRFR) with radiation dose escalation for localized prostate cancer (1–5). These randomized trials and other nonrandomized prospective trials of dose escalation were designed and implemented relatively early in the development of conformal and intensity-modulated radiotherapy (IMRT) techniques, and the planning target volume (PTV) margins employed were not optimized by current standards. The reported rates of grade 2 or greater rectal toxicity in these trials are between 17% and 33% (1–6). In comparison, more recent toxicity data using either highly conformal IMRT techniques or a more optimized PTV with image-guided radiotherapy (IGRT) shows improved grade 2 or greater rectal toxicity rates of 2% to 3% (7–9).

More importantly, indirect evidence from two sources suggests that employing an unoptimized PTV for prostate cancer treatment may result in inferior disease control. de Crevoisier et al. (10) reported the MD Anderson Hospital experience showing that patients planned with a distended rectum had 62% five-year bRFR compared with 94% for patients planned with an empty rectum. The implication is that over the course of treatment, rectal decompression caused the prostate to move outside the planned treatment volume, resulting in target underdosing. A similar finding was made in patients treated in the Dutch randomized trial

of dose escalation (11). Patients with a greater than 25% risk of seminal vesicle involvement had a 15% lower biochemical control rate at five years if they were planned with a distended rectum compared with those planned with an empty rectum.

Clinical evidence supports the view that optimizing the PTV for residual uncertainty while minimizing geometric uncertainties in treatment delivery for prostate cancer can maximize tumor control and minimize treatment related toxicity.

Various strategies may be employed to minimize the uncertainties of radiation planning and delivery. Alternate imaging techniques may be brought into the planning process to assist target delineation. Bowel and bladder protocols may be employed to reduce inter- and intrafraction motion and deformation, and pelvic immobilization may be used to reduce patient intrafraction motion, as may prostate immobilization using an intrarectal balloon.

Image guidance (IG) is an important component of any strategy designed to optimize treatment accuracy and minimize treatment related uncertainties. This may be as basic as a day-1 port film of bony anatomy to identify and correct systematic setup errors, or as complex as online daily soft-tissue imaging and correction that can identify and potentially correct random and systematic setup errors, and errors arising from target and normal tissue deformation. Imaging implanted prostate fiducial markers is an intermediate IG strategy that can identify random and systematic setup errors, but cannot identify target and normal tissue deformation, or seminal vesicle motion.

A very interesting and novel IG technique for prostate cancer involves implanting passive microtransponders into the prostate gland (12). These markers allow real-time tracking of the target organ during treatment, and could permit correction of intrafractional positional uncertainty and perhaps allow for a small optimized PTV if coupled with appropriate treatment delivery gating technology.

PTV optimization requires an understanding of the major sources of error in treatment planning and delivery. Identification of correctable errors and uncertainties with appropriate modification and adjustment of radiation planning techniques and treatment delivery will keep the PTV as small as possible, and minimize treatment related toxicity. Accounting for the residual uncertainty with an adequate PTV will keep the risk of target underdosing to a minimum.

The main sources of geometric uncertainty in prostate cancer planning and delivery are in the interobserver target delineation error, interfraction prostate motion and deformation, and intrafraction prostate motion and deformation. The causes and magnitude (where known) of these sources of uncertainty will be discussed in detail in this chapter. We will propose two means of accounting for uncertainty in an adequate PTV by using population-based margins, or using an adaptive strategy to better tailor the PTV to the individual patient.

TARGETING ERROR IN PROSTATE RADIOTHERAPY

Delineation Errors

Delineation uncertainty refers to the disagreement between observers (or with a single observer on sequential trials) on the location of the interface between the target and adjacent soft tissues. Like all sources of error, it has both a random and systematic component, although delineation is generally considered to act as a systematic uncertainty, since it "burns in" a target position that may not represent the true target. The magnitude of this uncertainty relates to the experience of the delineator and to the level of contrast between the target and surrounding tissues on the images provided. This in turn relates to both the imaging modality employed and the quality of the images generated.

The magnitude of systematic delineation uncertainty for prostate between expert observers measured on computed tomography (CT) images has been shown to be in the order of 3.0 to 3.6 mm at the apex (13,14) and 3.5 mm

at the seminal vesicles (14). Alternate imaging modalities, such as magnetic resonance imaging (MRI), can provide higher contrast between the prostate and adjacent tissues than does CT, and it has been proposed that using these images to delineate the prostate may reduce interobserver delineation error (15–18).

Studies that have compared CT with MRI for target delineation have shown reduced interobserver variability with MRI in terms of identifying the position of the prostatic apex (18) and in identifying the prostate rectal interface (13). The tendency is to contour a larger prostate on CT images than on MRI. Rasch et al. (14) demonstrated that the CT-derived prostate was 8 mm larger at the base on CT compared with MRI and 6 mm larger at the apex. Kagawa et al. (19) reported the average CT-derived prostate volume to be 63.0 mL compared with the MRI derived average volume of 50.9 mL. The discrepancies were usually at the prostate base and apex.

A similar effect is seen by observers attempting to match soft-tissue images of the prostate to a reference image during IG. One recent study (20) showed that the group systematic error between five therapist observers for matching cone-beam CT images to a reference CT image was 2.21 mm in the superior-inferior (SI) plane, 1.61 mm in the anterior-posterior (AP) plane, and 0.61 mm in the left-right plane. The systematic matching error was no more than 0.36 mm in any plane when the same observers were asked to match an unambiguous high-contrast image of a fiducial marker with a reference image.

Setup Error and Patient Immobilization

Rigid immobilization has a well-established history in radiotherapy and is intended to improve the day-to-day reproducibility of treatment setup. The patient repositioning rate was reduced from 23.1% to 17.4% with the use of rigid hemibody immobilization in one study of prostate irradiation (21), and another nonrandomized study of prostate irradiation demonstrated that the simulator to treatment variability rate of 5 mm or greater was significantly reduced from 66% to 43% (22). This study also showed that the mean simulation to treatment variability was 4 mm with immobilization and 6 mm without immobilization. Soffen et al. (23), in one of the first reports of the effect of immobilization for prostate radiotherapy reported that a rigid alpha cradle reduced the total median daily setup error for all fields from 3 mm to 1 mm without immobilization. Similarly, Catton et al. (24) reported that leg immobilization compared with free setup reduced the overall positioning error (random plus systematic) on lateral fields from 3.9 to 2.6 mm.

Several randomized trials have compared the effects of immobilization with no immobilization for radiotherapy of prostate cancer. Kneebone et al. (25) reported on patients treated for bladder and prostate cancer in the prone position with or without rigid immobilization and showed that the average simulator to treatment deviation was significantly reduced from 8.5 mm without immobilization to 6.2 mm with immobilization. Major setup deviations of 10 mm or more were reduced from 30.9% to 10.6% with immobilization, and the greatest benefit of immobilization was in reducing variability the AP and SI directions.

Rattray et al. (26) showed that a pelvic cradle reduced the mean lateral deviation and mean craniocaudal deviation to 2 and 2.5 mm, respectively compared with 3.8 and 3.9 mm without immobilization.

Fiorino et al. (27) compared pelvic immobilization to pelvic and leg immobilization and found that leg immobilization significantly improved the overall simulator to treatment variability in all three planes. The difference for pelvic and leg immobilization in the left-right plane was 2.4 mm versus 3.6 mm, in the posteroanterior plane 2.6 mm versus 4.4 mm, and in the craniocaudal plane 2.7 mm versus 3.3 mm. Interestingly, although leg immobilization offered an improvement in this study, pelvic immobilization actually increased the positioning uncertainty when compared with no immobilization at all.

The largest randomized trial was reported by Nutting et al. (28). They evaluated over 1600 portal images and failed to show any significant improvement in simulation to treatment variability for patients irradiated for prostate cancer, whether they were treated supine with soft leg support only, or supine in an evacuated cushion immobilization device. In each instance, the simulator to treatment variability was less than or equal to 2 mm in all planes. The very small setup error demonstrated for all the patients investigated in this study with or without immobilization compared with other reports suggests that other center-specific factors may affect simulator to treatment variability as much or more than the use of pelvic immobilization. These factors could include treatment setup policies, time spent on individual setups, and the experience of the treating staff. It also implies that the overall benefit a policy of immobilization may vary from institution to institution, and that acquiring some knowledge of the magnitude and sources of simulator to treatment variability within individual centers would be an asset when establishing radiation treatment setup and immobilization policies for prostate cancer.

Pelvic immobilization is widely employed for prostate radiotherapy, but it is limited by the fact that the target organ moves independently of the pelvic bony structures. Certain types of rigid immobilization have actually been shown to increase prostate motion (29), presumably by exaggerating the respiratory motion caused by increasing intra-abdominal pressure in the prone position (30,31). While accurate targeting of the prostate is best achieved by direct or indirect visualization of the organ, intrafractional motion error and rotational setup error cannot be easily corrected with current image-guided techniques. Rigid immobilization has been shown to reduce intrafractional translational error in one study (32). Rotational errors were reported in one of the aforementioned randomized trials (28). This trial reported that serious rotational errors were uncommon for all patients, and that rotational error in the anterior and lateral planes was 2° or less for 90% of cases. The use of immobilization statistically significantly reduced the mean systematic rotational error only in the anterior plane, where the difference was between 0.0° and –0.2°.

Three studies of interfractional prostate motion (33–35) reported large rotational errors in the right-left (RL) axis with standard deviations (SDs) ranging from 4.0° to 6.8°. Rotational errors in the other planes were smaller, with a range of 1.3° to 4.8°. None of these measurements were taken with the subjects immobilized, and this may account for the large rotational errors seen in the RL axis.

Intrarectal balloons have been employed in an attempt to immobilize the prostate directly. Gerstner et al. (36) reported that a 40-mL air-filled rectal balloon reduced prostate motion of 4 mm or more in the AP plane from 6 of 10 patients without the balloon to 1 of 10 patients with the balloon, measured on serial CT scans. No difference was seen in the other planes. Ciernik et al. (37) reported on nine patients treated for prostate cancer with a 40-mL air-filled rectal balloon in place. Sequential CT scans over the course of treatment demonstrated a range of prostate motion of 1.8 to 7.6 mm in the lateral direction, 2.2 to 16.8 mm in the anteroposterior direction, and 5.8 to 29.9 mm in the craniocaudal direction. In contrast, Teh et al. (38) reported on 10 patients who underwent twice weekly CT scanning over a five-week course of prostate radiotherapy using a 100-mL air-filled rectal balloon in place. AP prostate motion was no more than 1 mm. The SD of SI prostate movement was 1.78 mm.

The same group (39) has reported that the 100-mL balloon was tolerated by 393 of 396 (99.2%) treated patients, and that 17 of 396 (4.3%) required topical lidocaine anesthesia for insertion. Ronson et al. (40) reported that only 2.4% of 3561 patients who underwent proton irradiation for prostate cancer declined the rectal balloon for one or more treatment fractions.

Sanghani et al. (41) reported that a comparison of conformal treatment plans to 75.6 Gy for patients planned with and without a rectal balloon in place demonstrated that the use of a rectal balloon for some or all of the treatment course significantly reduced the volume of rectal wall exposed to more than 70 Gy. A similar finding was reported by Teh et al. (42) who found that none of their patients received more than 70 Gy to more than 25% of the rectal wall, when treated to 76-Gy IMRT using rectal balloon immobilization. D'Amico et al. (43) reported clinical outcome for a cohort of 57 patients treated to 75.6 Gy using conformal techniques and balloon prostate immobilization for the initial 15 fractions. They identified 10% grade 3 rectal bleeding at a median follow-up of 1.8 years, although all grade 3 bleeding was also associated with the use of anticoagulants. van Lin et al. (44) reported that a cohort of 24 patients treated with rectal balloon and three-dimensional conformal radiotherapy showed significantly less high-grade rectal mucosal telangiectasia at two-years post treatment than a cohort of 27 patients similarly treated but without a rectal balloon.

The limited literature on rectal balloon immobilization for prostate cancer indicates that most patients tolerate a rectal balloon, and that a 100-mL balloon is more effective for immobilization than a 40-mL balloon.

There is some evidence that prostate immobilization with a rectal balloon improves dose sparing of the anterior rectal wall, although significant rates of grade 3 rectal bleeding were seen in one study.

INTER- AND INTRAFRACTIONAL MOTION

The prostate gland has long been recognized as a mobile organ (45) whose positional variability within the bony pelvis must be taken into account to accurately target the gland during radiation treatment (46). Initial studies have shown that prostate positional variability is largely influenced by changes in bladder and rectal filling (45,47), there is greater potential for movement at the base of the gland because of tethering at the apex, and movement in the lateral plane is limited by the pelvic sidewall (48). Furthermore, the seminal vesicles may move independently of the prostate. More detailed studies have subsequently shown that rectal volume changes have a greater impact on prostate motion than do bladder volume changes (33,49,50) (Fig. 1), and that respiratory artifact can be observed (29,31). Cine-MRI studies have also demonstrated that the prostate gland has the capacity to deform significantly (50–52). All of these changes in prostate contour and position may take place over a course of treatment or during any given treatment fraction and must be adequately accounted for in the PTV to minimize the risk of underdosing the target. The safe treatment volume required is much larger than the CTV, and there is value in adopting measures designed to minimize the impact of inter- and intrafractional motion, where possible, to allow for a smaller PTV and improved normal tissue protection.

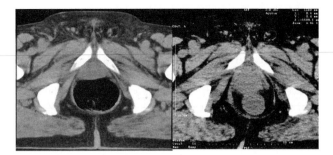

Figure 1 An extreme example of prostate translation and deformation due to rectal distension from transiting bowel gas. The pelvic CT scans were taken two days apart.

Interfractional variation in prostate position has been studied using implanted fiducial markers and sequential CT scans. Prostate motion over the time course of a single fraction (intrafractional motion) has been studied with cine-MRI, portal image cine-loops of implanted fiducials, transabdominal ultrasound, and implanted passive transponders.

Interfractional Prostate Motion

Studies of interfractional prostate motion are summarized in Table 1. These studies demonstrate that prostate motion occurs in all three planes but tends to be greatest in the AP and SI axes, and least in the RL axis, where movement is confined by the pelvic sidewalls. The potential for movement in the AP and SI axes is large, with ranges for all studies being between -17.9 and $+16.3$ mm for AP and -16.3 and $+10.8$ mm for SI, respectively. The systematic error has the largest effect on the appropriate margin requirements and is not generally reported. Two recent studies (34,35) have reported this component of error separately, and report a systematic SD of 3.5 to 4.8 mm for AP, 2.3 to 3.5 mm for SI axis, and 2.0 to 3.3 mm for the RL axis. These two studies did not use routine pelvic immobilization and included standard setup error in the measurements, which may account for the unusually large RL movement identified. Studies that report only the overall SD of overall prostate motion show SD that range in the AP axis from 2.1 to 6.4 mm, in the SI axis from 2.1 to 5.9 mm, and in the RL axis from 0.9 to 3.6 mm.

Rotational errors have been reported in only three studies of interfractional prostate movement (33–35). These tend to show that rotational errors are greatest in the RL axis: SD 4.0°, SD 4.7° (systematic), and SD 6.8° (systematic). Rotational errors in the AP and SI axes were less. For the AP plane they were SD 1.3°, SD 2.0° (systematic), and SD 2.8° (systematic), respectively. For the SI axis they were SD 1.7°, SD 3.5° (systematic), and SD° 2.8 (systematic), respectively. Again, the greater magnitude of rotational errors seen in the RL axis may reflect the absence of immobilization during the measurements.

Table 1 Studies Reporting Interfractional Prostate Motion

Author Technique	Point of measurement	Anterior-posterior (mm)	Superior-inferior (mm)	Right-left (mm)
Crook et al., 1995 (53) Markers	Base	SD 5.3 range (−17.9 to 3.6)	SD 5.4 range (−16.3 to 6.9)	SD 18 range (−3.6 to 3.7)
	Apex	SD 4.4 (−16.7 to 1.9)	SD 5.9 (−13.7 to 6.6)	SD 1.5 (−2.2 to 4.8)
Van Herk et al., 1995 (33) CT	Center of mass	SD 2.7 Rotation SD 1.3	SD 1.7 Rotation SD 2.1	SD 0.9 Rotation SD 4.0
Roeske et al., 1995 (47) CT	Center of mass prostate	Range (−5.3 to 5.0)	Range (−4.2 to 6.3)	Range (−1.2 to 0.2)
	Center of mass Seminal vesicles	Range (−9.3 to 7.6)	Range (−11.7 to 9.0)	Range (−4.3 to 5.5)
Rudat et al., 1996 (54) CT	Center of mass (combined positioning and target motion)	SD 6.1	Not stated	SD 3.6
Melian et al., 1997 (55) **CT**		SD 4.0	SD 3.1	SD 1.2
Dawson et al., 1998 (49) CT	Prostate	SD 6.3 95% CI (12.4 to 12.2)	SD 4.0 95% CI (5.4 to 10.3)	SD 2.1 95% CI (5.6 to 2.4)
	Seminal vesicles	SD 6.4 95% CI (11.3 to 13.8)	SD 3.1 95% CI (5.2 to 8.6)	SD 1.9 95% CI (3.9 to 3.9)
Wu et al., 2001 (48) Markers	Base	SD 2.9 range (−11.8 to 16.4)	SD 2.1 range (−6.8 to 10.8)	
	Apex	SD 2.1 range (−7.9 to 9.4)	2.1 range (−6.7 to 7.2)	
Chung et al., 2004 (56) Markers	Base	SD 4.8 range (−12.2 to 14.1)	SD 3.2 range (−8.5 to 7.9)	
	Apex	SD 3.5 range (−10.4 to 10.3)	SD 2.7 range (−7.5 to 8.6)	
Schallenkamp et al., 2005 (57) Markers	Center of mass	Median 3.7 range (0 to 16.3)	Median 2.5 range (0 to 9.1)	Median 1.9 range (0 to 15.2)
Dehnad et al., 2005 (34) Markers	Center of mass	Random SD 3.2 Rotational SD 1.7 Systematic SD 4.8 Rotational SD 2.0	Random SD 2.2 Rotational SD 1.9 Systematic SD 3.5 Rotational SD 2.7	Random SD 2.1 Rotational SD 3.6 Systematic SD 3.3 Rotational SD 4.7
van der Heide et al., 2007 (35) Markers	Center of mass	Random SD 4.8 Rotational SD 1.7 Systematic SD 3.5 Rotational SD 2.8	Random SD 2.9 Rotational SD 2.0 Systematic SD 2.3 Rotational SD 2.8	Random SD 2.2 Rotational SD 3.1 Systematic SD 2.0 Rotational SD 6.8

All linear measurement are in millimeter (mm) and all rotational measurements are in degrees (°).

Intrafractional Prostate Motion

Intrafractional motion occurs between the completion of setup procedures and completion of delivery of the intended radiation fraction. This interval is typically 5 to 15 minutes for standard prostate radiotherapy but may be longer with very complex treatment protocols (20). Clearly, the longer the patient is kept on the treatment couch, the greater the probability that some deviation will occur during any given fraction.

Intrafractional pelvic motion is usually addressed by immobilization of the bony pelvis (32). Apart from this, independent intrafractional prostate motion has been observed with cine-MRI (50,51,58), cine-fluoroscopy of implanted fiducial markers (56, 59–61), transabdominal ultrasound (62), or by tracking implanted transponders (12). These prostate movements may include rhythmic translations related to respiratory excursions, a gradual translation related to bladder filling, and an abrupt translation and deformation of the gland due to the rapid transit of large gas bubbles through the lower rectum.

As described earlier the magnitude of respiratory excursion transferred to the prostate is small, and is related to the type of immobilization and positioning of the patient. Rigid immobilization in the prone position, for example, appears to produce more respiratory-induced motion (29,31). The importance of changes in bladder volume as a significant contributor to intra- and interfractional prostate motion has been variably described, but may not be as significant as initially believed (45,47,49,50).

The intrafractional uncertainty caused by abrupt passage of gas through the lower rectum is most significant, since it is the most unpredictable and has the greatest potential for large magnitude deviations (50,51). As discussed above, intrarectal balloons are an invasive but effective method for limiting this type of intrafractional motion, provided a 100 mL balloon is used and is properly positioned.

Imaging patients with an empty rectum (50) or with the use of a peristalsis inhibitor (58) has been shown to reduce intrafractional prostate motion. Instructing patients on a daily bowel preparation protocol to ensure that they present daily for treatment with an empty rectum may limit intrafractional prostate motion. A randomized trial of such a bowel regimen (63) showed that patients experienced fewer prostate displacements of greater than 3 mm (10.1% of patients vs. 5.4%) while on the protocol than off the protocol during nine minutes of cine-MRI scanning. However, the trial was not sufficiently powered to show a statistically significant advantage to the regimen.

The recent introduction of implantable passive transponders (64) provides an opportunity to accurately measure intrafractional motion throughout a course of treatment. Techniques to use this information to reduce the PTV remain to be developed, but could include gating strategies for radiation delivery, or the use of adaptive radiotherapy.

Studies investigating intrafractional prostate motion are summarized in Table 2.

The number of reports investigating intrafractional motion is less than for interfractional motion, however the trends observed are unsurprisingly similar. These reports show that the probability of identifying significant prostate deviation is related to the length of time that the patient is imaged, and that large deviations of up to

Table 2 Studies Reporting Intrafractional Prostate Motion

Author/technique	Point of measurement	Anteroposterior (mm)	Superoinferior (mm)	Right-left (mm)
Padhani et al., 1999 (58) cine-MRI 7 min	Center of mass	Median 4.2 (−5 to 14)	Not reported	Not reported
Huang et al., 2002 (62) Ultrasound	Prostate borders	SD 1.3 (−4.6 to 6.8)	SD 1.0 (−6.8 to 3.5)	SD 0.4 (−2.4 to 2.5)
Mah et al., 2002 (51) cine-MRI 9 min	Center of mass	SD 1.19 (−4.0 to 3.6)	SD 0.73 (−1.3 to 1.9)	SD 0.65 (−4 to 3.6)
Nederveen et al., 2002 (60) Fluroscopy fiducials 2–3 min	Center of mass	Median 1.0 Maximum 7.0 8% > 3	Median 2.0 Maximum 9.5 21% > 3	Median 0.5 Maximum 1.5
Britton et al., 2005 (59) Image fiducials at start and finish of fraction	Center of mass	Median 0.2 (−1.7 to 2.0)	Median 0.2 (−2.1 to 1.1)	Median 0.1 (−1.2 to 0.7)
Ghilezan et al., 2005 (50) cine-MRI	11 points of interest Full rectum	Apex SD 1.26 Mid-posterior SD 1.72 Posterior base SD 1.44 Seminal vesicles SD 1.56	Not reported	Not reported
	Empty rectum	Apex SD 1.04 Mid-posterior SD 0.79 Posterior base SD 0.85 Seminal vesicles SD 0.68	Not reported	Not reported
Nichol et al., 2004 (63) cine-MRI 9 min	Posterior mid-prostate	10% probability of >3 displacement Maximum 10.7	Not reported	Not reported
Willoughby et al., 2006 (64) Implanted transponders 8 min	Center of mass	Maximum 13.9	Maximum 9.9	Maximum 1.4
Kupelian et al., 2007 (12) Implanted transponders 8 min	Center of mass	All axes combined 41% probability of excursion >3 15% probability of excursion > 5 (for >30 sec)	Not reported	Not reported

13.9 mm have been recorded (64). The direction of large movements is similar to what has been observed in the interfractional situation, and is predominantly in the AP and SI axes. Reports indicate that the probability of prostate movement greater than 3 mm during a fraction is between 8% and 41% (12,60,63), and two reports indicate that deviations are either more frequently observed (63) or of a significantly greater magnitude (50) in patients imaged with a full rectum compared with an empty rectum.

ICRU TARGET VOLUME DEFINITIONS

The International Commission on Radiological Units and Measurements (ICRU) Reports 50 (65) and 62 (66) are the basis for target volume definition in modern radiation therapy. Report 50 defines the most common volumes: the gross tumor volume (GTV), clinical target volume (CTV), and planning target volume (PTV). The GTV is the demonstrable extent of disease, and in modern practice, is represented by evident gross tumor on medical images. Because of the difficulty in imaging gross prostate tumor, the GTV is rarely defined for prostate cancer. The CTV is defined as a volume that includes gross tumor plus microscopic disease to be treated to the prescription dose. The prostate cancer CTV is almost always defined as the prostate gland.

The PTV is defined by adding a margin to the CTV. This margin accounts for the impact of geometric uncertainties and ensures the intended dose is actually delivered to the CTV. The uncertainties in target delineation, patient positioning, and internal organ motion described above must be considered when defining the PTV.

ICRU Report 62 proposes a separation of the PTV margin into an internal margin that accounts for physiologic uncertainties (e.g., rectum and bladder filling) and a setup margin that accounts for patient positioning uncertainty. The addition of the internal margin to the CTV defines a volume named the internal target volume (ITV). While the use of an ITV, in conjunction with 4DCT, has proven popular for the management of respiratory motion in lung cancer, reports of its application to prostate cancer are rare. For the remainder of this discussion, it is assumed that the PTV is generated by adding a margin to the CTV, without the definition of an ITV.

CONSIDERATIONS FOR AN OPTIMAL PLANNING VOLUME

The PTV margin in prostate cancer should ensure that the planned dose to the PTV represents the delivered dose to the CTV in the presence of treatment-related uncertainties. However, unnecessarily large PTV margins will require the irradiation of large volumes of rectum and bladder. Therefore, an optimal PTV margin is the smallest margin that maintains an acceptable CTV dose. Almost all PTV margins in clinical use are based on the uncertainty for a population of patients. A topic of considerable research and some novel clinical application is the extension to adaptive radiation therapy approaches where individualized PTV margins are produced.

Population-Based Delivery

Population-based PTV margins are the standard for nearly all patients and all sites in radiation therapy. When patient-specific data does not exist for positioning uncertainty, intrafractional motion, and other uncertainties, the best estimate will come from the data describing similar previously treated patients.

Calculation of the appropriate population-based margin requires data for each uncertainty to be considered and a model to determine the appropriate margin. Multiple models have been proposed. The simplest "data-based" model is to assume a Gaussian distribution of uncertainties and to multiply the SD by 2 for a geometric coverage of 95% (67). More involved modeling has been used to calculate different multipliers (68). The simplicity of this approach is appealing; however, this simplicity comes at the cost of some assumptions. Most importantly, this simple calculation does not separate uncertainties into random and systematic components.

The class of PTV "margin recipes" (69–71) is generally considered to represent the best compromise between complexity and a robust and accurate margin calculation. These margin recipes require the uncertainties to be quantified as SDs of random (σ) and systematic (Σ) uncertainty. SDs from different sources are generally assumed to be independent and added in quadrature. The most popular formalism determines the margin by a weighted sum of the total random and systematic uncertainty using $2.5\Sigma + 0.7\sigma$. These recipes have the advantage of separating random and systematic components and adding an element of a clinical intent in the margin derivation (e.g., 90% of patients to receive a CTV minimum dose of 95%).

An example is presented using published uncertainty data (14,20,50,72) and the popular margin recipes to demonstrate the role of image-guided processes in target position and PTV margin reduction (Fig. 2).

First, a scenario is considered with conventional patient positioning and no IG. In this case, systematic positioning uncertainty is the largest uncertainty. It dominates the margin calculation and requires PTV margins of 7 to 13 mm (AP largest). The introduction of IG with a simple off-line correction strategy is able to reduce systematic positioning uncertainty enough that CTV delineation

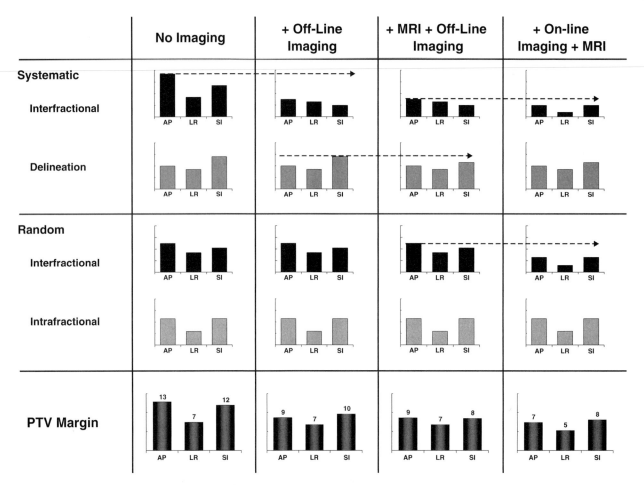

Figure 2 The effect on PTV margins of interventions intended to minimize uncertainty for prostate radiotherapy. The measurements for these calculations are taken from the literature and are described in the accompanying text. *Abbreviation*: PTV, planning target volume.

uncertainty is now the dominant uncertainty, and 7- to 10-mm margins (SI largest) are appropriate. IG at the treatment unit is not able to reduce this delineation uncertainty. However, it may be reduced through improved imaging, such as MRI, at the time of planning. Addition of MRI reduces the SI delineation uncertainty, and 7- to 9-mm margins (AP largest) are achieved. Finally, introduction of an online IG correction protocol further reduces the systematic positioning uncertainty and also reduces random positioning uncertainty. The margin can now be reduced to 5 to 8 mm (SI largest), representing a substantial improvement achieved through improvements in imaging at the time of planning and treatment.

Adaptive Therapy

The term "adaptive" is currently applied to a range of activities in radiation therapy. For this discussion, adaptive radiation therapy will refer to description of Yan et al. (73) as "a closed-loop radiation treatment process where

the treatment plan can be modified using a systematic feedback of measurements." This treatment modification allows an evolution from population-based to patient-specific models through highly coordinated processes that acquire patient-specific imaging information, apply an algorithm to determine an appropriate treatment intervention, and apply that intervention. There are only a few reports of clinical implementations for prostate cancer; however, these results demonstrate promising uncertainty reduction and clinical outcomes.

The most mature and widely reported adaptive prostate program is from William Beaumont Hospital. In the initial clinical implementation, patients were imaged using portal imaging for the first four to nine treatment fractions (74). A sophisticated algorithm estimated random and systematic positioning uncertainty. Treatment plan adaptation was performed by modification of multileaf collimator (MLC) leaf positions to account for these estimated uncertainties. This procedure reduced the mean systematic displacement from 4 to 0.5 mm. The initial work was followed by the description (75) and initial clinical implementation (76) of a process to modify the PTV and replan treatments with patient-specific dose escalation. This very advanced system uses measurements from portal imaging and CT scans acquired during the first four fractions.

An algorithm estimates the uncertainty and determines a PTV. The mean PTV volume reduction was 24%, and dose escalation of 5% and 7.5% of the prescription dose was achievable in patients treated with three-dimensional conformal radiotherapy (3DCRT) and IMRT, respectively. Ten percent of the patients had increased PTV volumes, underscoring the point that adaptive procedures aim to design appropriate margins, not just smaller margins. Two further reports have shown that chronic toxicity is not significantly different between patients treated to different dose levels, implying that this adaptive approach appropriately selects patients for dose escalation (77,78).

Toronto-Sunnybrook Regional Cancer Center has reported a different adaptive approach (79). The first treatment phase uses a 3DCRT technique and a 10-mm margin. During this phase, fluoroscopy and pre- and posttreatment portal imaging of implanted fiducial markers were acquired to quantify intrafractional motion. In contrast to the complexity of the previous method, a simple equation uses intrafractional motion and residual patient positioning uncertainty to calculate a patient-specific PTV using geometric coverage concepts. Phase 2 uses an online correction protocol and IMRT technique with the patient-specific PTV margin. The margin decreases were dramatic, with an average margin of 4 mm AP, and 3 mm LR and SI. The simplicity of this approach greatly facilitates clinical implementation, although it omits the separation of random and systematic uncertainty components that are valuable in margin calculation.

The Netherlands Cancer Institute has reported the clinical implementation of their adaptive method (80). It builds upon off-line IG correction protocols, using kilovoltage (kV) cone-beam computed tomography (CBCT) for soft-tissue guidance. The patient is imaged for the first four fractions and treated with a 10-mm margin. Translations and rotations are used to determine an average prostate and rectum. PTV margins for all patients are reduced from a 10-mm expansion of the planning CT CTV to a 7-mm expansion of the average CTV.

These implementations vary in the uncertainties that they consider. Intrafractional motion is not explicitly considered by some methods. None of the studies consider delineation uncertainty, which would dramatically increase the adapted margin size. Some of these authors cite pathological and imaging evidence that the prostate CTV is overestimated from CT imaging. This argument

may require further substantiation as modern MRI and other imaging improvements are added to pretreatment imaging.

ISSUES OF REAL-TIME IMAGING, EVALUATION, AND LOCALIZATION

Image-guided radiotherapy (IGRT) is defined as frequent imaging during a course of treatment as used to direct radiation therapy. Optimally, IGRT will improve both the accuracy and precision of radiation delivery by reducing the uncertainty related to systematic and random setup errors and interfraction organ motion. Through continuous monitoring, IGRT will facilitate interventions, such as gating or adaptive therapy, designed to mitigate the effects of intrafraction organ motion and organ deformation.

Increased precision in therapy offers the potential for better treatment outcomes through reduced severity, risk of complications, and improved tumor control and provides opportunities for exploiting alternate radiation strategies such as hypofractionation for prostate cancer (81,82).

The ideal IGRT system does not yet exist, although its properties have been described by Mageras (83). It will be both accurate and precise, and allow for explicit interpretation, and be both operator friendly and operator independent. It will be well integrated with the treatment unit for rapid image acquisition, interpretation, and intervention and will have a low impact on resources. It should have a small cost in extra radiation dose delivered, provide images that are useful for both planning and evaluation, and permit real-time continuous monitoring. It should have enough flexibility to be useful for a variety of clinical sites, which usually means providing a large field of view.

Systems currently available for IGRT of prostate cancer include kV radiography or fluoroscopy on implanted fiducial markers, kV or megavoltage (MV) tomography, CBCT or X-ray volume imaging, transabdominal ultrasound, implantable sensors, and optical imaging.

Each of these systems can potentially provide information about target motion in three planes, but tracking fiducial markers or implanted sensors is a surrogate for prostate position that provides no information about target organ deformation, seminal vesicle motion, or critical normal tissue motion and deformation. Furthermore, marker implantation is an invasive procedure with potential for bleeding and infection and inducing prostate edema.

It is possible to continuously monitor intrafractional movement with fluoroscopy of implanted markers, but the cost in additional dose is substantial. Implanted sensors permit continuous monitoring of prostate motion at no cost in extra radiation dose and may lead to gating strategies to mitigate the effect of intrafractional prostate motion. Optical sensors allow for continuous monitoring of surface movement, but provide a remote surrogate for prostate motion. Optical sensing is most useful for gating respiratory movements when used in conjunction with a more direct system of prostate imaging.

Transabdominal ultrasound, tomography, and CBCT image pelvic anatomy and provide the most direct evaluation of prostate and seminal vesicle motion, and target and normal tissue deformation. These systems do not provide for continuous monitoring, and provide anatomic information at only one point in time, usually just before the delivery of a treatment fraction. The cost in extra dose for these X-ray systems can be from 0 to 9 cGy/fraction depending on the system and technique employed and the level of resolution required. Transabdominal ultrasound has a clear advantage in this regard, but the effectiveness ultrasound guidance has been shown to have significant operator dependence (84) and can be affected by patient body habitus (85), and excessive probe pressure on the abdomen has been shown to displace the prostate up to 10 mm (86). Systematic differences in prostate position have been observed in comparison of transabdominal ultrasound with imaged fiducial markers (84,87), and a larger PTV is required with ultrasound IG (88).

The quality of tomographic and CBCT images are influenced by the photon energy, acquisition speed and resolution of the detector system, dose delivered, and field of view employed. Even under optimal conditions, these images will not be of diagnostic quality. The advantage gained in visualizing anatomy is counterbalanced by less precision in matching soft tissues to reference images. Moseley et al. (20) demonstrated that therapists could match CBCT images of an unambiguous object (an implanted fiducial) to a reference image with an accuracy of 0.12 mm; however, the same therapists demonstrated an accuracy of 2.2 mm when matching CBCT images of soft tissues to a reference CT image. This study also compared orthogonal MV imaging of fiducial markers with soft-tissue CBCT matching and demonstrated that the cost in dose was 8 cGy/fraction for MV imaging versus 2.1 to 3.3 cGy/fraction for CBCT. Image acquisition time was 20 seconds for MV imaging versus 132 seconds for CBCT, and accuracy was 0.36 mm for MV imaging versus 2.2 mm for CBCT.

In situations where both very high precision and full anatomic information is desirable, consideration may be given to using a cross-sectional X-ray imaging technique with implanted markers.

The Princess Margaret Hospital implemented, in 1997, an IG radiation technique for low- and intermediate-risk prostate cancer utilizing implanted fiducial markers.

Patients are immobilized supine in an evacuated polystyrene ball-filled bag and are planned and treated with rectum empty and bladder comfortably full to limit intrafractional pelvic and prostate movement. Orthogonal MV images are taken daily and the fiducials are matched to a reference image and a translation correction in three planes is calculated. Rotational corrections are not performed, and when a rotational error is identified, therapists use a visual "best-fit" match marker manually. A 3-mm action level (along any cardinal axis) is in place, which limits the need for correction to less than 28% of setups (56). The 8 cGy/fraction imaging dose is included in the total dosage calculation.

Published evaluations of this technique (20,48,56) have shown that therapists can match MV images of fiducials to a reference image with a residual error of 0.36 mm. Allowing for a 3-mm action level, the employed margins of 7 mm posteriorly and 10 mm in other planes are more than adequate to account for residual setup error, but are retained to account for other sources of error, such as intrafractional motion and delineation uncertainty.

The use of CBCT to localize fiducial markers is now used on those treatment machines where it is available. Since the CBCT image is used to localize high-contrast markers, not soft tissue, it has been possible to use a fast, low-dose (0.5 cGy/fraction) image acquisition for this purpose. This approach has the advantages of lower dose, simplified matching of fiducial markers, and the production of a volumetric patient image, although the dose from a kV scan, while lower, cannot be included in the treatment plan and is spread over a larger volume of the normal tissue.

The reported physician and patient assessed late rectal toxicity has been very modest for patients treated with this IGRT technique and 3DCRT or IMRT to 75.6 Gy or 79.8 Gy to prostate alone (7,9). The rates of grade 2 and 3 toxicity are 2.5% and 0.7%, respectively.

The introduction of a remotely adjustable treatment couch will improve the precision of this technique by allowing the implementation of a 0-mm action level without imposing a significant time penalty.

Our comparison of CBCT soft-tissue matching to MV fiducial matching has been described above. The advantages of soft-tissue visualization with CBCT are offset by a small loss of precision compared with MV fiducials. This can be overcome by using CBCT images of fiducials to perform an initial match and then make additional corrections using the information provided in the soft-tissue images. This is currently under investigation at our center and suggests that future guidance strategies may require utilization of more than one technique to take full advantage of the precision that may be achieved with IGRT.

SUMMARY OF PERTINENT CONCLUSIONS

- Systematic positioning errors are the main source of inaccuracy in radiation treatment planning and delivery and may be accounted for with off-line or online imaging strategies.
- The three main sources of imprecision in radiation planning and delivery for prostate cancer are target delineation uncertainty, intrafractional prostate motion, and interfractional prostate motion.
- Improved accuracy leads to improved tumor control.
- Improved precision leads to smaller PTV margins and an improved toxicity profile.
- Smaller margins permit investigation and implementation of alternate treatment strategies, such as hypofractionation.
- Including alternate imaging modalities in the treatment planning process, such as MRI, can mitigate delineation uncertainty.
- Intrafractional motion can be mitigated by
  a. using bowel and bladder filling protocols to limit variability in bladder and rectal distension,
  b. immobilizing the pelvis in a rigid immobilization device,
  c. immobilizing the prostate with an intrarectal balloon, and
  d. future strategies to track intrafractional prostate motion in real time coupled with gating techniques to deliver treatment.
- Interfractional motion can be mitigated by
  a. using bowel and bladder filling protocols to limit variability in bladder and rectal distension and
  b. daily online IG techniques to identify and correct for interfractional movement of the prostate.
- PTV optimization can be achieved by
  a. limiting the sources of uncertainty as much as possible, and incorporating the residual uncertainty into a population-based PTV. This will be adequate for most patients, but will be larger or smaller than required for some patients and
  b. using adaptive treatment planning techniques to custom-tailor the PTV to the individual patient.

REFERENCES

1. Zietman AL, DeSilvio ML, Slater JD, et al. Comparison of conventional-dose vs. high-dose conformal radiation therapy in clinically localized adenocarcinoma of the prostate: a randomized controlled trial. JAMA 2005; 294:1233–1239.
2. Peeters ST, Heemsbergen WD, Koper PC, et al. Dose-response in radiotherapy for localized prostate cancer: results of the Dutch multicenter randomized phase III trial comparing 68 Gy of radiotherapy with 78 Gy. J Clin Oncol 2006; 24:1990–1996.
3. Pollack A, Zagars GK, Starkschall G, et al. Prostate cancer radiation dose response: results of the M. D. Anderson phase III randomized trial. Int J Radiat Oncol Biol Phys 2002; 53:1097–1105.
4. Sathya JR, Davis IR, Julian JA, et al. Randomized trial comparing iridium implant plus external-beam radiation therapy with external-beam radiation therapy alone in node-negative locally advanced cancer of the prostate. J Clin Oncol 2005; 23:1192–1199.
5. Dearnaley DP, Sydes MR, Graham JD, et al. Escalated-dose versus standard-dose conformal radiotherapy in prostate cancer: first results from the MRC RT01 randomised controlled trial. Lancet Oncol 2007; 8(6):475–487.
6. Zelefsky MJ, Cowen D, Fuks Z, et al. Long term tolerance of high dose three-dimensional conformal radiotherapy in patients with localized prostate carcinoma. Cancer 1999; 85:2460–2468.
7. Nichol A, Chung P, Lockwood G, et al. A phase II study of localized prostate cancer treated to 75.6 Gy with 3D conformal radiotherapy. Radiother Oncol 2005; 76:11–17.
8. Zelefsky MJ, Fuks Z, Hunt M, et al. High-dose intensity modulated radiation therapy for prostate cancer: early toxicity and biochemical outcome in 772 patients. Int J Radiat Oncol Biol Phys 2002; 53:1111–1116.
9. Skala M, Rosewall T, Dawson L, et al. Patient-assessed late toxicity rates and principal component analysis following image guided radiation therapy for prostate cancer. Int J Radiat Oncol Biol Phys 2007; 68:690–698.
10. de Crevoisier R, Tucker SL, Dong L, et al. Increased risk of biochemical and local failure in patients with distended rectum on the planning CT for prostate cancer radiotherapy. Int J Radiat Oncol Biol Phys 2005; 62:965–973.
11. Heemsbergen WD, Hoogeman MS, Witte MG, et al. Increased risk of biochemical and clinical failure for prostate patients with a large rectum at radiotherapy planning: results from the Dutch trial of 68 GY versus 78 Gy. Int J Radiat Oncol Biol Phys 2007; 67:1418–1424.
12. Kupelian P, Willoughby T, Mahadevan A, et al. Multi-institutional clinical experience with the Calypso System in localization and continuous, real-time monitoring of the prostate gland during external radiotherapy. Int J Radiat Oncol Biol Phys 2007; 67:1088–1098.
13. Parker CC, Damyanovich A, Haycocks T, et al. Magnetic resonance imaging in the radiation treatment planning of localized prostate cancer using intra-prostatic fiducial markers for computed tomography co-registration. Radiother Oncol 2003; 66:217–224.
14. Rasch C, Barillot I, Remeijer P, et al. Definition of the prostate in CT and MRI: a multi-observer study. Int J Radiat Oncol Biol Phys 1999; 43:57–66.
15. Khoo VS, Padhani AR, Tanner SF, et al. Comparison of MRI with CT for the radiotherapy planning of prostate cancer: a feasibility study. Br J Radiol 1999; 72:590–597.
16. Khoo VS, Dearnaley DP, Finnigan DJ, et al. Magnetic resonance imaging (MRI): considerations and applications in radiotherapy treatment planning. Radiother Oncol 1997; 42(1):1–15 (review).

17. Kagawa K, Lee WR, Schultheiss TE, et al. Initial clinical assessment of CT-MRI image fusion software in localization of the prostate for 3D conformal radiation therapy. In J Radiat Oncol Biol Phys 1997; 38:319–325.

18. Milosevic M, Voruganti S, Blend R, et al. Magnetic resonance imaging (MRI) for localization of the prostatic apex: comparison to computed tomography (CT) and urethrography. Radiother Oncol 1998; 47:277–284.

19. Kagawa K, Lee WR, Schultheiss TE, et al. Initial clinical assessment of CT-MRI image fusion software in localization of the prostate for 3d conformal radiation therapy. Int J Radiat Oncol Biol Phys 1997; 38(2):319–325.

20. Moseley DJ, White EA, Wiltshire KL, et al. Comparison of localization performance with implanted fiducial markers and cone-beam computed tomography for on-line image-guided radiotherapy of the prostate. Int J Radiat Oncol Biol Phys 2007; 67:942–953.

21. Bentel GC, Marks LB, Sherouse GW, et al. The effectiveness of immobilization during prostate irradiation. Int J Radiat Oncol Biol Phys 1995; 31:143–148.

22. Rosenthal SA, Roach M III, Goldsmith BJ, et al. Immobilization improves the reproducibility of patient positioning during six-field conformal radiation therapy for prostate carcinoma. Int J Radiat Oncol Biol Phys 1993; 27:921–926.

23. Soffen EM, Hanks GE, Hwang CC, et al. Conformal static field therapy for low volume low grade prostate cancer with rigid immobilization. Int J Radiat Oncol Biol Phys 1991; 20:141–146.

24. Catton C, Lebar L, Warde P, et al. Improvement in total positioning error for lateral prostatic fields using a soft immobilization device. Radiother Oncol 1997; 44:265–270.

25. Kneebone A, Gebski V, Hogendoorn N, et al. A randomized trial evaluating rigid immobilization for pelvic irradiation. Int J Radiat Oncol Biol Phys 2003; 56:1105–1111.

26. Rattray G, Hopley S, Mason N, et al. Assessment of pelvic stabilization devices for improved field reproducibility. Australas Radiol 1998; 42:118–125.

27. Fiorino C, Reni M, Bolognesi A, et al. Set-up error in supine-positioned patients immobilized with two different modalities during conformal radiotherapy of prostate cancer. Radiother Oncol 1998; 49:133–141.

28. Nutting CM, Khoo VS, Walker V, et al. A randomized study of the use of a customized immobilization system in the treatment of prostate cancer with conformal radiotherapy. Radiother Oncol 2000; 54:1–9.

29. Bayley A, Haycocks T, Alasti H, et al. A randomised trial of supine vs. prone positioning for patients undergoing escalated dose conformal radiotherapy for prostate cancer. Radiother Oncol 2004; 70:37–44.

30. Bentel GC, Munley MT, Marks LB, et al. The effect of pressure from the table-top and patient position on pelvic organ location in patients with prostate cancer. Int J Radiat Oncol Biol Phys 2000; 47:247–253.

31. Dawson LA, Litzenberg DW, Brock KK, et al. A comparison of ventilatory prostate movement in four treatment positions. Int J Radiat Oncol Biol Phys 2000; 48:319–323.

32. Serago CF, Buskirk SJ, Igel TC, et al. Comparison of daily megavoltage electronic portal imaging or kilovoltage imaging with marker seeds to ultrasound imaging or skin marks for prostate localization and treatment positioning in patients with prostate cancer. Int J Radiat Oncol Biol Phys 2006; 65:1585–1592.

33. van Herk M, Bruce A, Guus Kroes AP, et al. Quantification of organ motion during conformal radiotherapy of the prostate by three dimensional image registration. Int J Radiat Oncol Biol Phys 1995; 33:1311–1320.

34. Dehnad H, Nederveen AJ, van der Heide UA, et al. Clinical feasibility study for the use of implanted gold seeds in the prostate as reliable positioning markers during megavoltage irradiation. Radiother Oncol 2003; 67:295–302.

35. van der Heide U, Kotte A, Dehnad H, et al. Analysis of fiducial marker-based position verification in the external beam radiotherapy of patients with prostate cancer. Radiother Oncol 2007; 82:38–45.

36. Gerstner N, Wachter S, Dorner D, et al. Significance of a rectal balloon as internal immobilization device in conformal radiotherapy of prostatic carcinoma. Stralenther Onkol 1999; 175:232–238.

37. Ciernik IF, Baumert BG, Egli P, et al. On-line correction of beam portals in the treatment of prostate cancer using an endorectal balloon device. Radiother Oncol 2002; 65:39–45.

38. Teh BS, McGary JE, Dong L, et al. The use of rectal balloon during the delivery of intensity modulated radiotherapy (IMRT) for prostate cancer: more than just a prostate gland immobilization device? Cancer J 2002; 8:476–483.

39. Bastasch MD, Teh BS, Mai WY, et al. Tolerance of endorectal balloon in 396 patients treated with intensity-modulated radiation therapy (IMRT) for prostate cancer. Am J Clin Oncol 2006; 29:8–11.

40. Ronson BB, Yonemoto LT, Rossi CJ, et al. Patient tolerance of rectal balloons in conformal radiation treatment of prostate cancer. Int J Radiat Oncol Biol Phys 2006; 64:1367–1370.

41. Sanghani MV, Ching J, Schultz D, et al. Impact on rectal dose from the use of a prostate immobilization and rectal localization device for patients receiving dose escalated 3D conformal radiation therapy. Urol Oncol 2004; 22:165–168.

42. Teh BS, Dong L, McGary JE, et al. Rectal wall sparing by dosimetric effect of rectal balloon used during intensity-modulated radiation therapy (IMRT) for prostate cancer. Med Dosim 2005; 30:25–30.

43. D'Amico AV, Manola J, McMahon E, et al. A prospective evaluation of rectal bleeding after dose-escalated three-dimensional conformal radiation therapy using an intrarectal balloon for prostate gland localization and immobilization. Urology 2006; 67(4):780–784.

44. van Lin EN, Kristinsson J, Philippens ME, et al. Reduced late rectal mucosal changes after prostate three-dimensional conformal radiotherapy with endorectal balloon as observed in repeated endoscopy. Int J Radiat Oncol Biol Phys 2007; 67:799–811.

45. Ten Haken RK, Foreman JD, Heimburger DK, et al. Treatment planning issues related to prostate movement in response to differential filling of the rectum and bladder. Int J Radiat Oncol Biol Phys 1991; 20:1317–1324.

46. Pickett B, Roach M III, Verhey L, et al. The value of nonuniform margins for six-field conformal irradiation of

localized prostate cancer. Int J Radiat Oncol Biol Phys 1995; 32:211–218.

47. Roeske JC, Forman JD, Mesina CF, et al. Evaluation of changes in the size and location of the prostate, seminal vesicles, bladder, and rectum during a course of external beam radiation therapy. Int J Radiat Oncol Biol Phys 1995; 33(5):1321–1329.

48. Wu J, Haycocks T, Alasti H, et al. Portal film analysis of an escalated dose conformal prostatic irradiation protocol using fiducial markers and portal images to confirm target organ and isocentre position. Radiother Oncol 2001; 61(2): 127–135.

49. Dawson LA, Mah K, Franssen E, et al. Target position variability throughout prostate radiotherapy. Int J Radiat Oncol Biol Phys 1998; 42:1155–1161.

50. Ghilezan MJ, Jaffray DA, Siewerdsen JH, et al. Prostate gland motion assessed with cine-magnetic resonance imaging (cine-MRI). Int J Radiat Oncol Biol Phys 2005; 62:406–417.

51. Mah D, Freedman G, Milestone B, et al. Measurement of intrafractional prostate motion using magnetic resonance imaging. Int J Radiat Oncol Biol Phys 2002; 54:568–575.

52. Nichol AM, Brock KK, Lockwood GA, et al. A magnetic resonance imaging study of prostate deformation relative to implanted gold fiducial markers. Int J Radiat Oncol Biol Phys 2007; 67:48–56.

53. Crook JM, Raymond Y, Yang H, et al. Prostate motion during radiotherapy as assessed by fiducial markers. Radiother Oncol 1995; 37:35–42.

54. Rudat V, Schraube P, Oetzel D, et al. Combined error of patient positioning variability and prostate motion uncertainty in 3D conformal radiotherapy of localized prostate cancer. Int J Radiat Oncol Biol Phys 1996; 35:1027–1034.

55. Melian E, Mageras GS, Fuks Z, et al. Variation in prostate position quantitation and implications for three-dimensional conformal treatment planning. Int J Radiat Oncol Biol Phys 1997; 38:73–81.

56. Chung PW, Haycocks T, Brown T, et al. On-line aSI portal imaging of implanted fiducial markers for the reduction of interfraction error during conformal radiotherapy of prostate carcinoma. Int J Radiat Oncol Biol Phys 2004; 60: 329–334.

57. Schallenkamp JM, Herman MG, Kruse JJ, et al. Prostate position relative to pelvic bony anatomy based on intra-prostatic gold markers and electronic portal imaging. Int J Radiat Oncol Biol Phys 2005; 63:800–811.

58. Padhani AR, Khoo VS, Suckling J, et al. Evaluating the effect of rectal distension and rectal movement on prostate gland position using cine MRI. Int J Radiat Oncol Biol Phys 1999; 44(3):525–533.

59. Britton K, Takai Y, Mitsuya M, et al. Evaluation of inter- and intrafraction organ motion during intensity modulated radiation therapy (IMRT) for localized prostate cancer measured by a newly developed on-board image-guided system. Radiat Med 2005; 23:14–24.

60. Nederveen AJ, van der Heide UA, Dehnad H, et al. Measurements and clinical consequences of prostate motion during a radiotherapy fraction. Int J Radiat Oncol Biol Phys 2002; 53:206–214.

61. Vigneault E, Pouliot J, Laverdière J, et al. Electronic portal imaging device detection of radioopaque markers for the evaluation of prostate position during megavoltage irradiation: a clinical study. Int J Radiat Oncol Biol Phys 1997; 37:205–212.

62. Huang E, Dong L, Chandra A, et al. Intrafraction prostate motion during IMRT for prostate cancer. Int J Radiat Oncol Biol Phys 2002; 53:261–268.

63. Nichol AM, Jaffray D, Catton C, et al. A cohort study using milk of magnesia for the reduction of intra-fraction prostate motion (abstract). Radiother Oncol 2004; 72(suppl 1):S53.

64. Willoughby TR, Kupelian PA, Pouliot J, et al. Target localization and real-time tracking using the Calypso 4D localization system in patients with localized prostate cancer. Int J Radiat Oncol Biol Phys 2006; 65:528–534.

65. International Commission on Radiation Units and Measurements. ICRU Report 50: Prescribing, Recording, and Reporting Photon Beam Therapy. Bethesda, MD: International Commission on Radiation Units and Measurements, 1993.

66. International Commission on Radiation Units and Measurements. ICRU Report 62: Prescribing, Recording and Reporting Photon Beam Therapy (Supplement to ICRU Report 50). Bethesda, MD: International Commission on Radiation Units and Measurements, 1999.

67. Tinger A, Michalski JM, Cheng A, et al. A critical evaluation of the planning target volume for 3-D conformal radiotherapy of prostate cancer. Int J Radiat Oncol Biol Phys 1998; 42:213–221.

68. Antolak JA, Rosen II, Childress CH, et al. Prostate target volume variations during a course of radiotherapy. Int J Radiat Oncol Biol Phys 1998; 42:661–672.

69. Stroom JC, de Boer HC, Huizenga H, et al. Inclusion of geometrical uncertainties in radiotherapy treatment planning by means of coverage probability. Int J Radiat Oncol Biol Phys 1999; 43:905–919.

70. van Herk M, Remeijer P, Rasch C, et al. The probability of correct target dosage: dose population histograms for deriving treatment margins in radiotherapy. Int J Radiat Oncol Biol Phys 2000; 47:1121–1135.

71. van Herk M, Remeijer P, Lebesque J. Inclusion of geometric uncertainties in treatment plan evaluation. Int J Radiat Oncol Biol Phys 2002; 52:1407–1422.

72. de Boer H, van Os MJ, Jansen PP, et al. Application of the no action level (NAL) protocol to correct for prostate motion based on electronic portal imaging of implanted markers. In J Radiat Oncol Biol Phys 2005; 61:969–983.

73. Yan D, Vicini F, Wong J, et al. Adaptive radiation therapy. Phys Med Biol 1997; 42:123–132.

74. Yan D, Ziaja E, Jaffray D, et al. The use of adaptive radiation therapy to reduce setup error: a prospective clinical study. In J Radiat Oncol Biol Phys 1998; 41:715–720.

75. Yan D, Lockman D, Brabbins D, et al. An off-line strategy for constructing a patient-specific planning target volume in adaptive treatment process for prostate cancer. In J Radiat Oncol Biol Phys 2000; 48:289–302.

76. Martinez AA, Yan D, Lockman D, et al. Improvement in dose escalation using the process of adaptive radiotherapy combined with three-dimensional conformal or intensity-modulated

beams for prostate cancer. In J Radiat Oncol Biol Phys 2001; 50:1226–1234.

77. Brabbins D, Martinez A, Yan D, et al. A dose-escalation trial with the adaptive radiotherapy process as a delivery system in localized prostate cancer: analysis of chronic toxicity. Int J Radiat Oncol Biol Phys 2005; 61:400–408.

78. Vargas C, Yan D, Kestin LL, et al. Phase II dose escalation study of image-guided adaptive radiotherapy for prostate cancer: use of dose-volume constraints to achieve rectal isotoxicity. Int J Radiat Oncol Biol Phys 2005; 63:141–149.

79. Cheung P, Sixel K, Morton G, et al. Individualized planning target volumes for intrafractional motion during hypofractionated intensity-modulated radiotherapy boost for prostate cancer. Int J Radiat Oncol Biol Phys 2005; 62:418–442.

80. Nuver T, Hoogeman M, Remeijer P, et al. An adaptive off-line procedure for radiotherapy of prostate cancer. Int J Radiat Oncol Biol Phys 2007; 67:1559–1567.

81. Martin JM, Rosewall T, Baylcy A, ct al. Phase II Trial of Hypofractionated Image-guided Intensity-modulated Radiotherapy for Localized Prostate Adenocarcinoma. Int J Radiat Oncol Biol Phys 2007; 69(4):1084–1089.

82. Kupelian P, Thakkar V, Khuntia D, et al. Hypofractionated intensity-modulated radiotherapy (70 gy at 2.5 Gy per fraction) for localized prostate cancer: long-term outcomes. Int J Radiat Oncol Biol Phys 2005; 63:1463–1468.

83. Mageras GS. Introduction management of target localization uncertainties in external-beam therapy. Semin Radiat Oncol 2005; 15(3):133–135.

84. Langen KM, Pouliot J, Anezinos C, et al. Evaluation of ultrasound-based prostate localization for image-guided radiotherapy. Int J Radiat Oncol Biol Phys 2003; 57: 635–644.

85. Morr J, DiPetrillo T, Tsai JS, et al. Implementation and utility of a daily ultrasound-based localization system with intensity-modulated radiotherapy for prostate cancer. Int J Radiat Oncol Biol Phys 2002; 53:1124–1129.

86. Dobler B, Mai S, Ross C, et al. Evaluation of possible prostate displacement induced by pressure applied during transabdominal ultrasound image acquisition. Strahlenther Onkol 2006; 182:240–246.

87. McNair HA, Mangar SA, Coffey J, et al. A comparison of CT- and ultrasound-based imaging to localize the prostate for external beam radiotherapy. Int J Radiat Oncol Biol Phys 2006; 65:678–687.

88. Scarbrough TJ, Golden NM, Ting JY, et al. Comparison of ultrasound and implanted seed marker prostate localization methods: implications for image-guided radiotherapy. Int J Radiat Oncol Biol Phys 2006; 65:378–387.

6

Overview of Image-Guided Localization Modalities

PARAG J. PARIKH AND JEFF MICHALSKI

Department of Radiation Oncology, Washington University School of Medicine, St. Louis, Missouri, U.S.A.

INTRODUCTION

Various strategies may be employed to minimize the uncertainties of radiation planning and delivery. Alternate imaging techniques may be brought into the planning process to assist target delineation. Bowel and bladder protocols may be employed to reduce inter- and intrafraction motion and deformation, and pelvic immobilization may be used to reduce patient intrafraction motion, as may prostate immobilization using an intrarectal balloon.

Image guidance (IG) is an important component of any strategy designed to optimize treatment accuracy and minimize treatment related uncertainties. This may be as basic as a day-1 port film of bony anatomy to identify and correct systematic setup errors, or as complex as online daily soft-tissue imaging and correction that can identify and potentially correct random and systematic setup errors, and errors arising from target and normal tissue deformation. Imaging implanted prostate fiducial markers is an intermediate IG strategy that can identify random and systematic setup errors, but cannot identify target and normal tissue deformation, or seminal vesicle motion. In this Chapter, we will give an overview of several widely used IG modalities for targeted prostate cancer radiation therapy.

SURROGATES OF PROSTATE MOTION

The current tradeoffs between modalities available today are between spatial resolution and temporal resolution.

Spatial resolution is best on an MRI, followed by fan-beam (simulation) CT, onboard imaging [kilovoltage (kV) cone-beam computed tomography (CBCT), megavoltage (MV) CBCT, and MV helical CT], and ultrasound. Fiducials give the least spatial resolution. On the other hand, temporal resolution is best with the Calypso® 4D Localization System, followed by the Accuray CyberKnife® and then other radiographic fiducial measurement systems. Volumetric imaging cannot be logistically performed more than once during a radiation therapy fraction.

The effect of the temporal resolution on measuring intrafraction fiducial motion was recently investigated by Noel et al. (1). In this study, the continuous electromagnetic tracking by the Calypso 4D Localization System was used to track the prostate isocenter (at a rate of 10 Hz) of 35 patients over 1157 total fractions, representing 195 hours of tracking information. Intermittent imaging was simulated by sampling each tracking session at predetermined intervals, from every 15 seconds to every 5 minutes. The sensitivity of the intermittent imaging in predicting prostate motion events greater than 3 mm that lasted for at least 30 seconds was evaluated. Results showed that imaging every 5 minutes only detected 57% of the intrafraction motion events, and one had to image every 30 seconds to achieve a sensitivity greater than 92% (Fig. 1). Moreover, the sensitivity varied per patient, and even imaging every 15 seconds did not achieve a sensitivity of 95% in 95% of the patients in the study. This

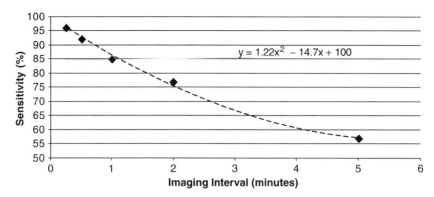

Figure 1 Relationship between imaging frequency and detection of intrafraction prostate motion. Each diamond represents the sensitivity of intermittent imaging in the detection of intrafraction prostate motion events of 3 mm for 30 seconds or more.

shows that high temporal fidelity is essential in accurately measuring intrafraction prostate motion.

INTRODUCTION OF AVAILABLE DEVICES

The ideal prostate localization device would (*i*) cost very little, (*ii*) visualize both the prostate and critical normal structures, (*iii*) perform both before (interfraction) and during (intrafraction) therapy, and (*iv*) be compatible with a standard linear accelerator configuration. Thus far, there is no device that satisfies all of these considerations. We will introduce the localization technologies that are currently available and discuss the details of each later in this volume.

Rectal Balloons

Rectal balloons are small balloons filled with water or air and are placed in the rectum and inflated to push the prostate against the pubic symphysis. In theory, this should reduce the anteroposterior movement of the prostate and reduce the amount of the posterior rectal wall in the irradiated field. Rectal balloons are inexpensive and are compatible with use in a standard linear accelerator configuration. They can be used to decrease both inter- and intrafraction prostate motion. Many studies have been used to show that the balloon is effective in reducing the amount of anteroposterior movement of the prostate, radiation to the prostate wall, and variability of the rectal volume (2–7). Its use has been commonly integrated in proton radiation therapy, but it is not clear that this practice results in significant reduction of dose to critical structures (8). Though many radiation oncologists doubt that daily rectal balloons can be tolerated by prostate cancer patients, the data suggests otherwise. A review of 3561 patients by the physicians at Loma Linda showed that over 97% of patients were able to complete radiation therapy with daily rectal balloons (9). A similar study

looking at 396 patients from Baylor had similar results (10). The dose reduction to the rectal wall that a rectal balloon causes seems more important in three-dimensional conformal radiation therapy (3DCRT) than intensity-modulated radiotherapy (IMRT), since IMRT allows dose to "bend" over the rectum whereas 3DCRT normally uses some opposed lateral fields. In addition, the rectal balloon is most effective when the prostate alone is the radiation target; inclusion of the seminal vesicles results in much higher radiation doses to the rectum as it is pushed anteriorly between these structures (7). Also, quality assurance of the rectal balloon placement is mandatory (6). Though no clinical study has assessed the effectiveness of a rectal balloon in a randomized fashion, many have indicated a possibility of a reduction of rectal toxicity (5,11,12). Rectal balloons represent a low cost method of reducing prostate motion with the cost of patient and staff tolerance, and the questionable dosimetric benefit in the era of IMRT.

Radiographic Fiducials

Portal imagers show good bony pelvic anatomy but do not show the prostate. Implantation of radiopaque markers into the prostate, such as gold seeds or coils, allows visualization of these makers on standard portal imagines, and thus indirectly the prostate target. The position of the markers on near-orthogonal portal images are compared with the positions obtained at planning, and a shift is applied based on the results of manual comparison or stereoscopic projection. The technique is inexpensive and compatible with a standard linear accelerator configuration. This technique has also been described for custom floor mounted kV imaging systems, such as the Novalis system (BrainLAB AG, Germany). The technique is normally used just before each radiation therapy fraction, though it is theoretically possible to image before each beam. The disadvantage is that the technique is invasive (and exposes the patients to the same risks as prostate biopsy) and only tracks the prostate and not the critical normal structures. The prostatic fiducials are well visualized on portal imaging, though oblique angles are sometimes used to avoid imaging the fiducials through the femurs (13,14). The fiducials have not been shown to migrate, and interfiducial measurements have shown stability with standard deviations of 0.67 to 1.68 mm (13–17). Though much research has been conducted on automated image analysis for prostate fiducial localization (18), the majority of the clinical systems rely on the therapist to identify the fiducials on each image. The interobserver variability seems low, with one study measuring a mean $\pm$ standard deviation error of 0.9 ± 0.7 mm (19). Studies on prostate motion using fiducials have led to guidelines on suggested margins (14,20–22) when there is no fiducial localization, but the adequacy of these margins over intrafraction prostate motion is still being investigated (23). Prostate fiducials may also facilitate "biological" targeting by acting as points to fuse pretherapy MRI spectroscopic imaging or other MRI sequences to facilitate focal areas of the prostate to boost (24).

In summary, prostate fiducial placement is an inexpensive method of prostate localization that is compatible with a standard linear accelerator installation and is most commonly used for pretherapy setup.

Radiographic Fiducials—the CyberKnife System

The CyberKnife[TM] System (Accuray Inc., Sunnyvale, California, U.S.) was developed initially for intracranial stereotactic radiosurgery. It uses a miniature linear accelerator mounted on a robotic arm with six degrees of freedom, which allows for a large amount of noncoplanar beams to be delivered with excellent spatial precision. Orthogonal kV sources and imagers are positioned to allow continuous monitoring of implanted radiographic fiducials with images taken every 90 to 120 seconds. Unlike all other implementations of radiographic fiducials, the CyberKnife System integrates intrafraction imaging with correction of the beam via linear accelerator retargeting and couch movements, if necessary. A recently developed clinical trial is being undertaken at Stanford University to treat prostate cancer patients in an extremely hypofractionated regimen using the intermittent kV imaging to localize the prostate (25). Each fraction takes about 40 minutes or longer, causing some investigators to look into how this could be implemented on the linear accelerator (26). The CyberKnife is expensive, requires a special vault design and custom installation, and does not visualize adjacent normal structures. It does perform both inter- and intrafraction monitoring of the prostate position with automatic correction of therapy.

Ultrasound Localization

Ultrasound localization technologies for prostate cancer radiation uses the "brightness mode" acquisition to visualize changes in acoustic impedance found in tissue planes. In the product from NOMOS Corporation (BAT), the prostate is localized via two orthogonal images (saggital and transverse plane). The planning contours from the CT simulation are overlaid on the ultrasound images and can be moved manually such that they create a best match. The BAT Software calculates a shift that can be then applied to the table. The process takes three to seven minutes. Newer ultrasound products, such as the SonArray by Varian Medical Systems and the I-Beam by CMS give 3D ultrasound images, which may allow better visualization than 2D approaches. Also, a new product from Resonant Medical allows baseline localization to be done at the time of CT simulation, so that subsequent daily localization can be compared with ultrasound images at the time of simulation. At least one study shows that "intramodality verification" may be superior to "cross-modality verification" when comparing Resonant to another ultrasound system (27). Ultrasound is inexpensive and can be used for interfraction localization. It does not require an invasive procedure to implant fiducials and does not deliver ionizing radiation like that needed to localize radiographic fiducials. However, comparisons between ultrasound and CT or ultrasound and fiducials have shown systematic differences (28,29). These differences range from 3 to 6 mm and probably represent some inherent inaccuracies with ultrasound localization. There are inter- and intraobserver variations, as well as technical problems with obese patients, bladder filling, and shadowing of the prostate by the pubic symphysis. Ultrasound localization is inexpensive and efficient but has residual inaccuracies that need to be accounted for in planning target volume margins.

CT on Rails

CT on rails represents a custom linear accelerator setup where the treatment table can be moved directly into a CT scanner. This allows the patient to have regular high quality imaging that could also be used for daily replanning. Studies using this modality have supported the use of a 5-mm margin to encompass inter- and intrafraction prostate motion (30). The high cost and large vault requirements, as well as the lack of standardized software have made the number of these installations very small. Moreover, the advent of onboard volumetric imaging has made these systems obsolete. Studies using CT-on-rails have shown that daily replanning is possible but takes over an hour per day (31).

Onboard Volumetric Imaging

Onboard volumetric imaging is quickly becoming a standard installation piece on new linear accelerators. Elekta and Varian have pursued CBCT with an orthogonally mounted kV energy source with an opposed flat panel imager, while Siemens has developed a CBCT system with the MV delivery beam. Tomotherapy uses a helical MV scan technique that also produces daily images for both alignment and adaptive treatment planning. All these images allow visualization of both the soft-tissue and bony anatomy, albeit at a lower quality than kV multi-detector fan-beam CT. Each imaging technique delivers a significant amount of radiation (1.5–8 cGy) and takes anywhere from one to five minutes to acquire. The advantages of onboard volumetric imaging over fiducial localization are the ability to detect prostate deformation, allow real-time replanning, and visualize normal adjacent critical structures. Disadvantages include the inter/intra-observer segmentation error and the increased time to process and store these large datasets. Though work is being performed to improve autosegmentation on these images (32), these are not yet universally available. Initial comparisons between onboard volumetric imaging for soft-tissue localization show that there is increased uncertainty in determining the required shifts when relying on observers' segmentation of the images compared with observers' using the images of implanted fiducials. This has been shown for both kV CBCT (33) and helical MV imaging (34). The use of the daily imaging of the critical structures in adaptive planning is actively being investigated. Onboard volumetric imaging will have increased availability over the next several years as both large and small centers replace older linear accelerators. The cost will be incorporated into new linear accelerator purchases. Work is ongoing to determine if onboard volumetric imaging can be used during treatment delivery (26).

Electromagnetic Tracking Systems

The Calypso 4D Localization System is a Food and Drug Administration (FDA)-approved continuous tracking system for prostate cancer. It represents a high precision, objective, real-time inter- and intrafraction monitoring system. It consists of implantable passive transponders whose positions are continuously measured at 10 Hz during radiation by an electromagnetic array placed over the patient (35). The transponders are implanted with the same technique as other prostate fiducials. The implanted transponders have very little prostate migration, similar to radiographic fiducials (36). The continuous measurements are obtainable in all but obese men, equaling 35 of 41 men in a multiinstitutional trial (37). Isocenter

displacements greater than 3 mm and greater than 5 mm for cumulative durations of at least 30 seconds were observed during 41% and 15%, respectively, of the continuously tracked radiation therapy fractions. In individual patients, the number of fractions with displacements greater than 3 mm ranged from 3% to 87% whereas the number of fractions with displacements greater than 5 mm ranged from 0% to 56%. Efforts to measure the dosimetric impact of this motion are still ongoing. The Calypso System is unique in its ability to continuously track the prostate both before and during radiation therapy without the use of ionizing radiation and is compatible with standard linear accelerators. It is moderately expensive and, like other fiducial-based systems, only tracks the prostate and not adjoining critical structures.

SUMMARY OF PERTINENT CONCLUSIONS

- The ideal prostate localization device does not yet exist
- Each localization modality has a balance between spatial and temporal resolution
- Spatial resolution: MRI > CT > onboard volumetric imaging > ultrasound >> fiducials
- Temporal resolution: Calypso 4D Localization System > Accuray CyberKnife > fiducials >> volumetric imaging
- High temporal resolution is necessary to appropriately measure intrafraction prostate motion
- Each available modality has pros and cons, which are summarized in Table 1

Table 1 Summary of Characteristics of the Various Image-Guided Localization Modalities

Device	Expense	Interfraction or intrafraction use	Standard linear accelerator compatible	Visualizes critical structures
Rectal balloon	$	Inter/intra	Yes	No
Radiographic fiducials	$	Inter	Yes	No
Accuray CyberKnife	$$$$$	Inter/intra	No	No
Ultrasound	$$	Inter	Yes	Yes
CT on rails	$$$$$	Inter	No	Yes
Onboard volumetric imaging	$$$$	Inter	Varies	Yes
Calypso 4D Localization System	$$$	Inter/intra	Yes	No

REFERENCES

1. Noel C, Parikh PJ, Roy M, et al. Are pre and post imaging sufficient to assess intrafraction prostate motion? Int J Radiat Oncol Biol Phys 2007; 69(3):S22–S23 (abstr).

2. Ciernik IF, Baumert BG, Egli P, et al. On-line correction of beam portals in the treatment of prostate cancer using an endorectal balloon device. Radiother Oncol 2002; 65:39–45.

3. D'Amico AV, Manola J, Loffredo M, et al. A practical method to achieve prostate gland immobilization and target verification for daily treatment. Int J Radiat Oncol Biol Phys 2001; 51:1431–1436.

4. Hille A, Schmidberger H, Tows N., et al. The impact of varying volumes in rectal balloons on rectal dose sparing in conformal radiation therapy of prostate cancer a prospective three-dimensional analysis. Strahlenther Onkol 2005; 181:709–716.

5. Sanghani MV, Ching J, Schultz D, et al. Impact on rectal dose from the use of a prostate immobilization and rectal localization device for patients receiving dose escalated 3D conformal radiation therapy. Urol Oncol 2004; 22:165–168.

6. van Lin EN, Hoffmann AL, van Kollenburg P, et al. Rectal wall sparing effect of three different endorectal balloons in 3D conformal and IMRT prostate radiotherapy. Int J Radiat Oncol Biol Phys 2005; 63:565–576.

7. Wachter S, Gerstner N, Dorner D, et al. The influence of a rectal balloon tube as internal immobilization device on variations of volumes and dose-volume histograms during treatment course of conformal radiotherapy for prostate cancer. Int J Radiat Oncol Biol Phys 2002; 52:91–100.

8. Kagawa K, Murakami M, Hishikawa Y, et al. Immobilization and dose-sparing effects of a rectal balloon in conformal proton radiotherapy of the prostate. Int J Radiat Oncol Biol Phys 2002; 54:184.

9. Ronson BB, Yonemoto LT, Rossi CJ, et al. Patient tolerance of rectal balloons in conformal radiation treatment of prostate cancer. Int J Radiat Oncol Biol Phys 2006; 64:1367–1370.

10. Bastasch MD, Teh BS, Mai WY, et al. Tolerance of endorectal balloon in 396 patients treated with intensity-modulated radiation therapy (IMRT) for prostate cancer. Am J Clin Oncol 2006; 29:8–11.

11. D'Amico AV, Manola J, McMahon E, et al. A prospective evaluation of rectal bleeding after dose-escalated three-dimensional conformal radiation therapy using an intrarectal balloon for prostate gland localization and immobilization. Urology 2006; 67:780–784.

12. Teh BS, Dong L, McGary JE, et al. Rectal wall sparing by dosimetric effect of rectal balloon used during intensity-modulated radiation therapy (IMRT) for prostate cancer. Med Dosim 2005; 30:25–30.

13. Kupelian PA, Willoughby TR, Meeks SL, et al. Intra-prostatic fiducials for localization of the prostate gland: monitoring intermarker distances during radiation therapy to test for marker stability. Int J Radiat Oncol Biol Phys 2005; 62:1291–1296.

14. Schallenkamp JM, Herman MG, Kruse JJ, et al. Prostate position relative to pelvic bony anatomy based on intra-prostatic gold markers and electronic portal imaging. Int J Radiat Oncol Biol Phys 2005; 63:800–811.

15. Poggi MM, Gant DA, Sewchand W, et al. Marker seed migration in prostate localization. Int J Radiat Oncol Biol Phys 2003; 56:1248–1251.

16. Pouliot J, Aubin M, Langen KM, et al. (Non)-migration of radiopaque markers used for on-line localization of the prostate with an electronic portal imaging device. Int J Radiat Oncol Biol Phys 2003; 56:862–866.

17. Litzenberg D, Dawson LA, Sandler H, et al. Daily prostate targeting using implanted radiopaque markers. Int J Radiat Oncol Biol Phys 2002; 52:699–703.

18. Harris EJ, McNair HA, Evans PM. Feasibility of fully automated detection of fiducial markers implanted into the prostate using electronic portal imaging: a comparison of methods. Int J Radiat Oncol Biol Phys 2006; 66:1263–1270.

19. Ullman KL, Ning H, Susil RC, et al. Intra- and inter-radiation therapist reproducibility of daily isocenter verification using prostatic fiducial markers. Radiat Oncol 2006; 1:2.

20. Alasti H, Petric MP, Catton CN, et al. Portal imaging for evaluation of daily on-line setup errors and off-line organ motion during conformal irradiation of carcinoma of the prostate. Int J Radiat Oncol Biol Phys 2001; 49:869–884.

21. Wu J, Haycocks T, Alasti H, et al. Positioning errors and prostate motion during conformal prostate radiotherapy using on-line isocentre set-up verification and implanted prostate markers. Radiother Oncol 2001; 61:127–133.

22. Soete G, De Cock M, Verellen D, et al. X-ray-assisted positioning of patients treated by conformal arc radiotherapy for prostate cancer: comparison of setup accuracy using implanted markers versus bony structures. Int J Radiat Oncol Biol Phys 2007; 67:823–827.

23. Kupelian P, Willoughby T, Mahadevan A, et al. Multi-institutional clinical experience with the Calypso System in localization and continuous, real-time monitoring of the prostate gland during external radiotherapy. Int J Radiat Oncol Biol Phys 2007; 67:1088–1098.

24. van Lin EN, Futterer JJ, Heijmink SW, et al. IMRT boost dose planning on dominant intraprostatic lesions: gold marker-based three-dimensional fusion of CT with dynamic contrast-enhanced and 1H-spectroscopic MRI. Int J Radiat Oncol Biol Phys 2006; 65:291–303.

25. King CR, Presti J, Harcharan G, et al. Hypofractionated Radiotherapy for Localized Prostate Cancer. Vol. Protocol ID 79432, Stanford University IRB Panel, 2004.

26. Pawlicki T, Kim GY, Hsu A, et al. Investigation of linac-based image-guided hypofractionated prostate radiotherapy. Med Dosim 2007; 32:71–79.

27. Cury FL, Shenouda G, Souhami L, et al. Ultrasound-based image guided radiotherapy for prostate cancer: comparison of cross-modality and intramodality methods for daily localization during external beam radiotherapy. Int J Radiat Oncol Biol Phys 2006; 66:1562–1567.

28. Langen KM, Pouliot J, Anezinos C, et al. Evaluation of ultrasound-based prostate localization for image-guided radiotherapy. Int J Radiat Oncol Biol Phys 2003; 57:635–644.

29. Lattanzi J, McNeeley S, Pinover W, et al. A comparison of daily CT localization to a daily ultrasound-based system in prostate cancer. Int J Radiat Oncol Biol Phys 1999; 43: 719–725.

30. de Crevoisier R, Dong L, Bonnen MO, et al. Quantification and volumetric change and internal organ motion during radiotherapy for prostate carcinoma using an integrated CT/linear accelerator system. Int J Radiat Oncol Biol Phys 2004; 60:227–228.

31. Geinitz H, Zimmermann FB, Kuzmany A, et al. Daily CT planning during boost irradiation of prostate cancer. Feasibility and time requirements. Strahlenther Onkol 2000; 176:429–432.

32. Smitsmans MH, de Bois J, Sonke JJ, et al. Automatic prostate localization on cone-beam CT scans for high precision image-guided radiotherapy. Int J Radiat Oncol Biol Phys 2005; 63:975–984.

33. Moseley DJ, White EA, Wiltshire KL, et al. Comparison of localization performance with implanted fiducial markers and cone-beam computed tomography for on-line image-guided radiotherapy of the prostate. Int J Radiat Oncol Biol Phys 2007; 67:942–953.

34. Langen KM, Zhang Y, Andrews RD, et al. Initial experience with megavoltage (MV) CT guidance for daily prostate alignments. Int J Radiat Oncol Biol Phys 2005; 62: 1517–1524.

35. Balter JM, Wright JN, Newell LJ, et al. Accuracy of a wireless localization system for radiotherapy. Int J Radiat Oncol Biol Phys 2005; 61:933–937.

36. Litzenberg DW, Willoughby TR, Balter JM, et al. Positional stability of electromagnetic transponders used for prostate localization and continuous, real-time tracking. Int J Radiat Oncol Biol Phys 2007; 68:199–206.

37. Kupelian P, Willoughby T, Mahadevan A, et al. Multi-institutional clinical experience with the Calypso System in localization and continuous, real-time monitoring of the prostate gland during external radiotherapy. Int J Radiat Oncol Biol Phys 2007; 67:1088–1098.

7

Targeted Therapies for Localized Prostate Cancer: The Urologist's Perspective

JAMES JOHANNES, LEONARD G. GOMELLA, AND EDOUARD J. TRABULSI
Department of Urology, Kimmel Cancer Center, Thomas Jefferson University, Philadelphia, Pennsylvania, U.S.A.

INTRODUCTION

There have been great advances in both detection and treatment of prostate cancer over the past 20 years. Largely, because of the application of routine prostate-specific antigen (PSA) screening, cancer-specific mortality from prostate cancer has decreased over this time period (1). With early detection and modern treatment modalities, prostate cancer five-year survival in the United Stated is now greater than 99% for all patients (2). In addition to these improvements, routine PSA screening has led to a marked stage migration with the majority of newly diagnosed patients presenting with localized disease. These epidemiological changes are prompting a reexamination of prostate cancer risk stratification and treatment algorithms. Patients with low-risk localized disease are eager to pursue minimally invasive, targeted therapies to avoid radical surgery or radiation therapy, because of the side effects and complications commonly seen with traditional treatment options.

Treatment options for localized prostate cancer are expanding. Historically, patients decided among radical surgery, radiotherapy, or active surveillance (watchful waiting) (3). Treatment direction should be made after a personalized discussion, ideally, in a multidisciplinary fashion (4). With the advent of laparoscopic and robotic radical prostatectomy, much of the perioperative morbidity of the procedure is minimized while offering the benefits of a curative procedure with improved convalescence and cosmesis. Despite the technical advantages of laparoscopy, patients still face similar postoperative functional and quality of life side effects as with standard open radical prostatectomy. In a recent review of robotic-assisted laparoscopic prostatectomy (RALP), between 82% and 96% of patients required 0 to 1 pad daily for incontinence and only between 38% and 66% were able to perform sexual intercourse six months after surgery (5).

Three-dimensional conformal external beam radiotherapy (3DCRT), intensity-modulated radiotherapy (IMRT), and prostate brachytherapy are targeted radiotherapeutic options for the treatment of localized prostate cancer. Technological improvements in modern radiotherapy have improved the accurate targeting of prostate cancer. These advances have decreased the dose administered to the adjacent tissues such as the bladder and rectum, significantly reducing toxicity, while concomitantly allowing a higher and potentially more efficacious dose administered to the target (prostate) tissue (6). However, there exists a significant number of patients who fail to get localized treatment from presumed understaging or radioresistant tumors (7). Finally, active surveillance in the correct patient population avoids the morbidity of treatment and may not affect their prostate cancer–specific mortality (8). However, many of these patients eventually opt for treatment or progress to advanced disease.

Today is an exciting time for prostate cancer specialists, both in the refinement of older technologies and development of new approaches for prostate cancer. Clinicians today have new minimally invasive treatment options including cryotherapy and high-intensity-focused ultrasound (HIFU) ablation. By implanting fiducial markers to improve radiation therapy, multimodality approaches to prostate cancer are expanding into treatment. Although these modalities are not yet widely available, tomorrow's urologist will likely see these technologies become mainstream.

CRYOTHERAPY

History

The first use of freezing for the treatment of cancer in medical literature dates to 1850 (9). The first closed cryosurgical system was reported in 1938 when hollow bore instruments carried an ice mixture to treat metastatic tumors (10). Following the development of liquid nitrogen closed system technology, cryosurgery of the human prostate was described as a treatment for benign prostatic hyperplasia (BPH) and cancer (11,12). Innovations in cryotherapy over the past several decades have marked milestones in the improvement of this treatment modality (Table 1).

First Generation

Early cryosurgery of the prostate was used only on nonsurgical candidates. In the late 1960s and 1970s, a direct transurethral or transperineal approach using liquid nitrogen was used (13,14). In these early techniques, cystoscopic and digital rectal monitoring of the freeze sought to minimize injury or damage to periprostatic tissues. The morbidity from these procedures was extreme by modern standards. Despite the high risks of incontinence, severe urethral sloughing, and stricture, first generation cryosurgery compared favorably to the radiation and radical surgery morbidity of the era (15).

Second Generation

Several technological advancements in the 1980s prompted reinvestigation in prostatic cryosurgery. Transrectal

ultrasound proved to be an improved method of observing the extent of ice ball formation (16). Constant flow urethral warming catheters marked a major breakthrough in limiting cryotherapy morbidity. By keeping the urethral tissue from freezing, the rate of postsurgical urethral sloughing, stricture, and fistula improved greatly (17). The use of multiple cryoprobes improved the uniformity of freeze and improved efficacy by simultaneously freezing the entire gland (18). These technical advances were made in the setting of modern PSA testing. PSA screening identified prostate cancer earlier and provided a valuable method of monitoring treatment response. It proved that cryotherapy was efficacious in properly selected patients with localized cancer (19).

Third Generation

Although cryotherapy is described in three generations, the modifications in technique and equipment were added as they became available, ultimately evolving into what is commonly described as the third generation of cryosurgery. A major limitation of liquid nitrogen is the requirement of relatively large bore needles. Utilizing the Joule-Thompson effect of gas compression, a new cryogen using argon and helium gasses made cryotherapy through small-bore needles possible. These thin needles now allow a direct percutaneous approach and multiple needle placements providing a more exact freeze.

Multiple small cryoprobes are inserted percutaneously in the perineum through holes in a brachytherapy-like template. Several coordinated systems optimize the treatment while seeking to minimize injury to nontarget tissues. The edge of the advancing ice ball is monitored not only by transrectal ultrasound but also by thermocouplers placed at the target margins. Urethral warmers prevent excessive urethral sloughing and its side effects. Finally, optimal treatment plans are calculated using computer modeling. Together with better patient selection, these advances culminating in today's cryosurgical technique have minimized the morbidity and optimized the efficacy of prostate cryosurgery.

Tissue Destruction Physiology

Refinements in cryoablative surgery have improved the ability to efficiently kill cancer cells. Optimizing the

Table 1 Evolution of Cryotherapy

Generation	Cryogen	Probe size	Ultrasound guidance	Urethral warmer	Temperature monitoring
1st (1960s)	Liquid nitrogen	6.3 mm	No	No	Manual
2nd (1990s)	Liquid nitrogen	3.4 mm	Yes	Yes	Manual
3rd (current)	Argon/helium	17 gauge	Yes	Yes	Thermocouplers

freeze temperature, duration of freeze, speed of cooling, and the number of cycles maximizes tumor death. The lethality of extreme cold to prostate tissue is due to both direct cell effects and secondary vascular causes. A rapid and prolonged freeze with a slow thaw maximizes lethality by a combination of intracellular ice crystal formation and disruption of normal osmotic gradients (20). Furthermore, a double freeze-thaw cycle has been shown to have lower posttreatment positive biopsy rates and fewer PSA recurrences (21). In addition to intracellular effects, the freeze-thaw cycle destroys prostatic microvasculature that contributes to a delayed necrosis (22).

Patient Selection

Careful patient selection is crucial for all treatment modalities for prostate cancer and is particularly important for cryotherapy. As the indications for cryotherapy of prostate cancer continue to evolve, its applications are broadening. Most commonly, it is used as a primary treatment in patients who are nonsurgical candidates and are eligible for radiation therapy and decide against active surveillance or watchful waiting. Although use as a salvage therapy is controversial, secondary cryotherapy may have a promising future as a surgical option for local recurrence after initial radiotherapy treatment.

Clinical risk stratification in patients with presumed organ-confined prostate cancer is a primary determinant of treatment options. With routine PSA screening, the majority of patients with localized cancer present with clinical stage T1c disease (23). Risk stratification is estimated by pretreatment PSA, Gleason score on TRUS biopsy, and clinical stage on digital rectal exam. Several nomograms are used routinely by urologists and radiation oncologists to estimate pathological stage and recurrence rates on the basis of these variables (23–30).

Primary cryotherapy for localized prostate cancer is an option, in general, for patients with clinical T1c to T3 disease. However, patients with periurethral disease are poor candidates as urethral warmers prevent an adequate kill temperature from reaching this tissue zone. Furthermore, high impotency rates associated with cryotherapy makes patients interested in preserving potency poor candidates.

Prostate size is an important consideration in offering cryotherapy. Patients with large pretreatment volumes (larger than 50 cm^3) or those with a serum PSA level >10 ng/mL, may benefit from neoadjuvant hormone blockade (21,31). After hormonally induced size reduction, the entirety of the gland is more reliably treated. Additionally, shrinking the prostate can help separate it from the rectum, preventing rectal wall damage (32).

Despite these limitations, cryotherapy offers advantages over primary radiation therapy or surgery. First, it is administered in a single day as compared to the several week course of treatment for radiation therapy. Due to the minimal blood loss, shorter operative time, and quick recovery, patients with a prohibitive operative risk can typically undergo cryotherapy safely, even under spinal anesthesia. In patients with high-risk disease, a pretreatment laparoscopic pelvic lymph node dissection can help determine the status of lymphatic metastasis (33). Patients with evidence of extraprostatic involvement should not be offered cryotherapy, but counseled on other treatment options. Finally, cryotherapy is safe to repeat, improving local control of locally recurrent disease.

Follow-up After Cryotherapy

Patient follow-up after cryotherapy is based on PSA surveillance. Initially, PSA is checked every three months for the first year and every six months thereafter for the first few years. Due to cell necrosis, there is an initial bump in serum PSA that falls over time to a nadir (34). Unlike the postprostatectomy setting, in which the PSA should nadir to undetectable, and similar to radiation therapy, there is no consensus postcryotherapy nadir PSA indicative of biochemical failure. Biochemical failure has been variably defined in a range from 0.3 up to 1.0 ng/mL (35,36). Others advocate the use of the accepted American Society for Therapeutic Radiology and Oncology (ASTRO) criteria of three consecutive PSA rises following nadir (37).

There have been several studies describing five-year follow-up of patients treated with cryotherapy (Table 2). For low-risk patients, the biochemical recurrence–free range from 60% to 80% (36,38,39). The largest single institution experience reported cryotherapy outcomes in 590 consecutive patients with seven-year follow-up (36). Although the first 350 patients were treated with a second generation machine, the results are consistent with other smaller more recent series (Table 2). Overall, 15.9%, 30.3%, and 53.7% were low-, intermediate-, and high-risk patients, respectively. All patients were followed with both PSA measurements and routine biopsies at 6, 12, 24, and 60 months postoperatively. Using the ASTRO criteria, the seven-year actuarial biochemical disease–free survival (DFS) was approximately 90% for all risk groups. Overall, 13% of patients had a positive posttreatment positive biopsy although the authors did not stratify these patients according to preoperative risk. Together, these results suggest there were some recurrences or treatment failures identified by biopsies that were not identified by PSA recurrence. Although definitions of recurrence vary,

Table 2 Outcomes in Modern Prostate Cryotherapy Series

Series	Year	Number of patients	Generation	Length of follow-up	PSA recurrence criteria (ng/mL)	PSA recurrence-free rate % (risk)
Han et al. (45)	2003	122	3rd	12 mo	≥0.4	76 (low)
						73 (all)
Donnelly et al. (39)	2002	76	2nd	5 yr	>1.0	75 (low)
						89 (intermediate)
						76 (high)
					>0.3	60 (low)
						77 (intermediate)
						48 (high)
Ellis (44)	2002	75	3rd	3 mo	>0.4	84
Bahn et al. (36)	2002	590	2nd/3rd	7 yr	ASTRO	92 (low)
						92 (intermediate)
						89 (high)
					>1.0	87 (low)
						79 (intermediate)
						71 (high)
					>0.3	61 (low)
						68 (high)
						61 (high)
Long et al. (38)[a]	2001	975	2nd/3rd	5 yr	>1.0	76 (low)
						71 (intermediate)
						61 (high)
					>0.5	60 (low)
						61 (intermediate)
						36 (high)

[a]Pooled analysis of five series.
Abbreviations: ASTRO, American Society for Therapeutic Radiology and Oncology; PSA, prostate-specific antigen.
Source: From Ref. 81.

patients generally undergo biopsy once recurrence is suspected.

A smaller series reporting results of 65 men with high-risk prostate cancer defined as a preoperative PSA >10 ng/mL or Gleason score ≥8 utilizing the ASTRO criteria for PSA recurrence shows that cryotherapy is a viable primary option for high-risk cancer (40). Eighty three percent of their patients were free of biochemical recurrence at a median of 35-month follow-up. Moreover, only one of the eight patients who underwent biopsy had histological evidence of cancer. This highlights the difficulty in using both the ASTRO criteria to screen for recurrence and reliability of the small sample prostate biopsy to confirm recurrence. Although these numbers are promising, ten-year follow-up data with modern cryotherapy is awaited to determine the long-term recurrence-free rates.

Although cryotherapy is often a secondary option for many patients who cannot be offered radical surgery and choose against radiotherapy, the cryotherapy cancer control rates are comparable to reported rates for radical prostatectomy and radiotherapy. A representative study of 743 patients receiving dose escalation conformational

radiation therapy were followed prospectively for PSA recurrence (41). These patients were stratified into favorable risk (stage T1 or T2, Gleason score 6 or less, PSA 10 or less), intermediate risk [one adverse feature or unfavorable (two adverse features)]. The five-year PSA-free recurrences were 85%, 65%, and 35%, respectively. For patients treated with brachytherapy, similar results are seen. One study of brachytherapy with a long mean follow-up period of 82 months showed PSA-free recurrence rates according to ASTRO criteria in low-, intermediate-, and high-risk patients of 91%, 80%, and 66%, respectively (42). Unfortunately, a randomized trial comparing cryotherapy and radiotherapy options that could compare the oncological efficacy of these modalities has not been performed, and most clinicians shy away from cryotherapy for higher-risk patients.

Cryotherapy as an Option for Recurrent Disease

Cryotherapy has an emerging role as salvage therapy for local recurrence or progression following primary radiotherapy modalities, based on PSA or biopsy data.

Radiation therapy has long been a salvage therapy for patients with biochemical failure and presumed local recurrence after prostatectomy. Similarly, cryotherapy is a potential salvage therapy for local recurrence after radiation failure. Once residual cancer is confirmed by biopsy and evidence of systemic disease is excluded, curative options for these patients are limited. Salvage cryotherapy offers an attractive alternative to salvage prostatectomy, which is technically difficult and carries significant risk and morbidity than primary radical prostatectomy.

Salvage cryotherapy, in properly selected patients, may be an appropriate choice for radiotherapy failures. In the largest cohort of patients failing primary radiotherapy, salvage cryotherapy showed a five-year 79% disease-specific survival (DSS) and 40% DFS rate (43). Examining the relatively modest five-year DFS, it is clear that patient selection is paramount, since the majority of patients will fail despite additional local therapy, indicative of likely micrometastatic disease at the time of salvage treatment. Several factors predictive of a durable response to salvage cryotherapy were identified, including hormone-sensitive prostate cancer, PSA <10 ng/mL, Gleason score 8 or less, and preradiation treatment clinical stage of T1 to T2. However, further studies are needed to compare salvage cryotherapy with other salvage treatment modalities.

Complications of Cryotherapy and Effect on Quality of Life

Potential complications and quality of life side effects weigh heavily in the decision process for treatment of localized prostate cancer. Cryotherapy in the past was limited by its high complication rates. However, current third generation technical improvement has limited much of the morbidity associated with treatment. Complication rates are summarized in Table 3.

Despite the improvements of third generation cryotherapy, erectile dysfunction remains the most common complication of cryotherapy. Several recent series measured the rate of erectile dysfunction to be between 82% and 95% (36,44,45). The high rate of postoperative impotence

is attributed to extension of the ice ball to the neurovascular bundles. Although lower rates of impotence have been reported to be as low as 53% with the help of erectile aids (46), patients wishing to preserve erectile function should consider other therapy.

Urinary side effects are not eliminated by the current third generation machinery. Cryotherapy can lead to stress or urge incontinence by a number of putative mechanisms, including damage to the striated sphincter, urethral sloughing, nerve damage, and subsequent detrusor instability. Variable definitions of incontinence make direct comparisons among published series difficult. Recent series report incontinence rates between 4.3% and 7.5% (36,38). Although these relatively low rates reflect the advantages of third generation cryotherapy, patients requiring a postoperative transurethral resection of the prostate (TURP) appear to have a significantly higher stress incontinence rate of almost 50% compared to 4% of those not requiring TURP (21).

Several complications unique to cryotherapy are also seen less frequently today. Urethral sloughing from damage or urethral mucosa can cause intermittent obstruction, stricture, or calcification necessitating intermittent catheterization, dilation, or transurethral resection. Representative modern series show a low rate of sloughing between 5.8% and 6.7% (44,45). Although these low rates reflect refinement in technique, there should be a low index of suspicion to evaluate patients for these complications both in perioperative and long-term follow-up period.

Complaints of pelvic pain or perineal sensation alterations are common after cryotherapy. In a large multicenter experience, pelvic pain was a relatively infrequent complication occurring in 6% of patients treated with cryotherapy (45). This same study reports penile numbness occurring in 2% of patients. All of these patients experienced resolution of their symptoms with conservative management.

Fistula formation between the rectum and prostate, bladder, or urethra can be a catastrophic complication after cryotherapy. In older generation cryotherapy machines, this dreaded complication was unfortunately much more common. Fortunately, it is a rare complication

Table 3 Complication Rates in Modern Prostate Cryotherapy Series

Series	Year	Number of patients	Erectile dysfunction (%)	Fistula rate	Incontinence (%)	Urethral sloughing and/or TURP (%)
Han et al. (45)	2003	122	87	0	4.30	5.80
Donnelly et al. (39)	2002	76	47	0	1.3	3.9
Ellis (44)	2002	75	82.40	0	5.50	6.70
Long et al. (38)	2001	975	93	0.50%	7.50	13
Bahn et al. (36)	2002	590	94.90	<0.1	4.30	5.50

Abbreviation: TURP, transurethral resection of the prostate.

today. Han et al. (45) reported no rectourethral fistulas in their experience of 106 patients, although a larger experience of 975 patients showed an overall incidence of 0.5% at a five-year follow-up (38). Although conservative treatment with catheter drainage can be successful, often a fecal or urinary diversion is required, with subsequent complex reconstructive procedures. Fistulas can be especially problematic in previously irradiated fields when cryotherapy is used as local salvage therapy.

Using the Functional Assessment of Cancer Treatment-Prostate (FACT-P) and Sexuality Follow-up Questionnaire (SFQ), standardized metrics of patients' quality of life after treatment for prostate cancer have been measured. In a single cohort, cryotherapy patients reported no significant changes in their quality of life between one and three years postoperatively with the exception of sexual function (46,47). Moreover, the FACT-P scores in cryotherapy patients are very similar at one year after treatment to patients undergoing radical prostatectomy, external beam radiation, or brachytherapy (48,49).

HIGH-INTENSITY-FOCUSED ULTRASOUND

History

Together with the newest generation of cryotherapy, HIFU offers another minimally invasive option to prostate cancer patients. It is an older technology that has shown promise in a limited but expanding international experience. The first clinical applications of HIFU date back to the middle of the twentieth century as it was first used to selectively ablate brain lesions (50). Earlier techniques, however, were severely limited as there was no reliable way to image in three dimensions and monitor the ablation. Advances in the past twenty years in computed tomography (CT) and transrectal ultrasound have allowed a minimally invasive application of this technology to ablate prostatic tissue. The eagerness of both patients and practitioners to have minimally invasive nonsurgical treatment of localized prostate cancer is advancing HIFU into the arena of mainstream prostate cancer therapeutics.

The first use of HIFU specifically for prostate cancer was reported in 1995 (51). In this study, 29 patients with cT2 prostate cancer underwent treatment to study the in vivo effect of varying focal length and intensity. All of these patients underwent immediate radical prostatectomy under the same anesthesia. Pathological examination confirmed coagulative necrosis in every specimen, although the extent of tissue ablation was dependent of focal length and higher intensities.

Shortly thereafter, HIFU was investigated in a feasibility study where a small cohort of inoperable patients with localized prostate cancer were treated (52). In this study, 50% of the patients had negative posttreatment biopsies and no major complications were observed. Since then broader trials performed on patients with cT1 to cT2 disease as both primary or salvage therapy have confirmed efficacy and defined the future role of HIFU treatment of prostate cancer.

Principles and Physiology of HIFU

HIFU is in principle similar to diagnostic ultrasound. The relatively low intensity and diffuse propagation of ultrasound waves in diagnostic ultrasound do not cause damage to target tissues. Conversely, HIFU uses a high-intensity ultrasound wave that delivers energy many orders of magnitude higher than diagnostic ultrasound. This energy when focused to a small target area causes necrosis of the target tissue.

In prostatic HIFU, tissue destruction results from two main mechanisms, thermal destruction and cavitation (53). Coagulative necrosis has been observed in target tissues at a temperature of 56°C for one second (54). HIFU heats tissue well above that level. Due to the rapid extreme heating, tissue outside the targeted site is spared destruction and has a normal histological appearance (55). Cavitation occurs because of the creation of microbubbles by ultrasound energy absorbed into subcellular organelles and fluids. These bubbles cause mechanical stress and dispersion of energy in the microenvironment, further contributing to direct thermal destruction of tissue.

There are currently two main devices in use for prostatic HIFU, the Sonablate-500 (56) and Ablatherm (57). Although there are design differences, the principles employed in both machines are the same. A rectal probe inserted into the rectum contains the HIFU transducer, a normal diagnostic ultrasound transducer, and a cooling mechanism to protect the rectal wall. Using a combination of computer modeling and real-time imaging, a series of ablation parameters determine the course of treatment. In general, several overlapping ellipses of HIFU energy sequentially ablate the entire prostate. The procedure is performed under spinal or general anesthesia. Newer protocols include a routine TURP prior to therapy to reduce gland volume and have significantly reduced postoperative urinary retention, which has been a common complication (58).

Patient Selection

In general, HIFU has the same indications and patient eligibility as cryotherapy. The current published trials were performed in patients with cT1 or cT2 Nx-0 M0 disease. It should only be considered a primary option for patients who are not suitable candidates for radical surgery. These patients generally cannot receive or refuse radiotherapy.

There are specific contraindications to HIFU therapy. Prostatic size is a crucial factor to the success of the procedure. In general, gland volume should be less than 40 g. To downsize larger glands, urologists either perform a TURP or shrink the gland with hormone deprivation. Further considerations, such as rectal pathology and pelvic anatomy may be contraindications. Prostatic calcifications, which are commonly seen on diagnostic prostate ultrasound, will cause shadowing and interfere with transmission of HIFU waves, which impairs adequate treatment of prostate tissue downstream of the calcification. Calcifications must be removed by TURP prior to therapy, or the patient must be counseled against HIFU treatment.

HIFU Outcomes

With the first American trials investigating HIFU only beginning in 2006, the European experience comprises the published outcome data for HIFU treatment of prostate cancer. Table 4 shows a summary of selected trials. All trials included patients with cT1 to cT2 disease with no evidence of metastatic disease. As in radiotherapy and cryotherapy, PSA nadir is an important marker of outcome. HIFU theoretically ablates the entire prostate and should leave a low PSA nadir. This is reflected in the mean nadir PSA of less than 0.5 ng/mL in most series (Table 4). Since HIFU is a new technology, long-term follow-up data is not yet available. Acknowledging limitations in extrapolating short-term data, PSA recurrence and biopsy results offer insight into the efficacy of HIFU for prostate cancer treatment.

Although there are no broadly accepted criteria for determining biochemical recurrence after HIFU, most studies use the ASTRO criteria. The study with the longest follow-up to date is of 227 patients treated with HIFU (59). Based on both ASTRO PSA criteria and postoperative biopsy, the authors report a five-year disease-free rate of 66%. This is comparable to the other selected studies (Table 4). Interestingly, clinical stage, Gleason score, or neoadjuvant hormone therapy were not significant predictors of DFS. However, improved DFS was noted for patients with lower pretreatment PSA values, with DFS for preoperative PSA <4.0, 4.1 to 10, and >10 of 90%, 57%, and 61% at five years, respectively (59). The authors postulated that these observations were indicative that HIFU effectively destroyed all treated tissues, with Gleason score or more aggressive tumors being equally susceptible to HIFU treatment. Additionally, the lack of effect of pretreatment with hormonal therapy may be indicative of lack of synergy between hormonal ablation and HIFU, unlike that seen with hormonal therapy and radiotherapy.

In 2003, the results from the European Multicentric Study of HIFU for prostate cancer were reported (60). This multiinstitutional nonrandomized clinical trial is one of the largest HIFU series published. The results reported were preliminary, with a median follow-up of slightly less than one year. Additionally, the treatment protocols were heterogeneous between centers, and retreatments were allowed, with a mean of 1.5 HIFU treatments per patient. This study showed an overall posttreatment negative biopsy rate of 87%. In low-, medium-, and high-risk patients, the negative biopsy rate was 92%, 86%, and 82%, respectively. In patients available for follow-up for a period greater than six months, the mean nadir PSA was 1.8 ng/mL. This relatively high mean is skewed higher due to inclusion of nonresponders. To further emphasize the importance of patient selection, patients with a gland size less than 40 cc had a median nadir PSA of 0.4 (60). Because of the short follow-up and heterogeneous treatment plans used in this study, conclusions about efficacy

Table 4 Outcomes in Current Prostate HIFU Series

Series	Year	Number of patients	Mean or median PSA follow-up (mo)	Median nadir PSA (ng/mL)	PSA recurrence criteria (ng/mL)	Cancer-free survival (%) (risk)
Poissonnier et al. (59)	2007	227	27	0.1	Routine biopsy and ASTRO	66.00
Vallancien et al. (58)	2004	30	20	0.9	Routine biopsy and PSA < 0.9	73.30
Blana et al. (82)	2004	146	22.5	0.07	PSA < 1.0	84.00
Chaussy and Thuroff (62)	2003	271	14.8	0	ASTRO	82.10
Thuroff et al. (60)	2003	402	13.1	0.6	Routine biopsy	92 (low) 86 (medium) 82 (high)
Uchida et al. (83)	2003	63	23	1	ASTRO	75.0

Abbreviations: ASTRO, American Society for Therapeutic Radiology and Oncology; PSA, prostate-specific antigen.

must be confirmed with future prospective studies with longer follow-up.

A recent small retrospective study examined the nadir PSA after HIFU treatment (61). One hundred three patients with a median follow-up of 4.9 years after HIFU treatment were stratified according to the PSA nadir achieved for each patient. Using PSA nadir levels <0.2 ng/mL, 0.2 to 1.0 ng/mL, and >1 ng/mL, the actuarial five-year DFS rates were 95%, 55%, and 0%, respectively. Therefore, in addition to the ASTRO definition, absolute PSA nadir achieved after HIFU may be an accurate assessment of treatment efficacy and allows quicker implementation of salvage therapy or HIFU retreatment to improve long-term oncological outcomes.

It is important to emphasize that very little long-term data is available for evaluating HIFU for prostate cancer. This should be emphasized when counseling patients on treatment options for prostate cancer. Starting in 2006, a multicenter American equivalency trial was initiated to compare the outcomes of HIFU and cryotherapy. Select centers offering either HIFU or cryotherapy will enroll patients with localized disease who are not surgical candidates. This will be a landmark study directly comparing the outcomes between these two modalities and largely determine the future of HIFU beyond an experimental treatment in the United States.

HIFU Complications and Effects on Quality of Life

Complication rates are well documented in all HIFU trials to date. Table 5 summarizes the adverse events seen in several HIFU trials. Urinary retention is a common complication and will be present in almost all patients immediately following treatment. Urinary retention can be caused by a number of treatment-specific mechanisms, including tissue sloughing and prostate edema. All patients require postoperative catheter drainage with a Foley catheter or suprapubic tube. The duration of catheter drainage is not easy to predict, because of the multiple

machine prototypes and treatment plans used in the various published studies. Concomitant TURP with HIFU has made a significant improvement in urinary retention rates. One study comparing two cohorts of HIFU and TURP with HIFU alone shows a marked difference in the duration of urinary catheterization, with a median of 40 and 7 days, respectively (62). Patients receiving a TURP had a lower rate of incontinence, 15.6% versus 6.9%, respectively, and postoperative urinary tract infection, 47.9% and 11.4%, respectively. For these reasons, a TURP is considered the current standard of care in Europe for HIFU unless contraindicated. One concern with the current American trial is that TURP is not allowed in the HIFU cohort, and the duration of urinary catheterization will be closely analyzed.

Incontinence rates in HIFU are low in the later reported series and a result of improved technique. Stress urinary incontinence is observed in 0.6% to 16% of patients (Table 5). Refinements in administration of HIFU, specifically leaving a 6-mm safety margin at the prostate apex, have been credited with significantly reducing stress incontinence (59). However, the long-term effect on oncological outcome from leaving this portion of viable prostatic tissue is worrisome. In the European Multicentric Study, grade I or II incontinence was seen in 10.6% and 2.5%, respectively and only six cases of grade 3 incontinence requiring invasive treatment (60). Impotency rates in HIFU are similar to the high rates observed in other targeted therapies. Different definitions of potency show varying impotency rates in HIFU (Table 5). A nerve-sparing approach has been proposed that limits the lateral extent of the ablation (63). By sparing the contralateral neurovascular bundle in unilateral disease, these authors preserved potency in almost two-thirds of patients but had a 15% higher recurrence rate. Patients should be carefully counseled as the long-term effect on survival of this recurrence risk is unknown.

The risk of bladder outlet obstruction from stricture has greatly improved in the era of TURP and HIFU. Previously, in HIFU alone, stricture rates were as high 22% (64),

Table 5 Complication Rates in Current Prostate HIFU Series

Series	Year	Number of patients	Impotence	Incontinence	Urinary retention	Bladder outlet obstruction	Fistula (%)
Poissonnier et al. (59)	2007	227	39.0%	13.0%	Not reported	12.0%	0.0
Vallancien et al. (58)	2004	30	21.4%	3.0%	6.0%	0.0%	0.0
Blana et al. (82)	2004	146	49.8%	7.6%	Not reported	19.7%	0.5
Chaussy and Thuroff (62)	2003	271	35.9%	15.4/6.9%[a]	Not reported	Not reported	0.0
Thuroff et al. (60)	2003	402	8.7%[b]	14.6%	8.6%	3.6%	1.2
Uchida et al. (83)	2006	63	20.0%	0.6%	0.6%	22.0%	1.0

[a]HIFU alone/HIFU+TURP.
[b]Pretreatment data potency not recorded.
Abbreviations: HIFU, high-intensity-focused ultrasound; TURP, transurethral resection of the prostate.

but the combination of TURP with HIFU has significantly reduced this risk (62).

Finally, the most serious complication of rectourethral fistula is rare. The universal adoption of rectal cooling devices, better patient selection, and improved technique has driven this risk to a minimum (Table 5).

FIDUCIAL MARKERS—THE UROLOGIST'S ROLE IN EXTERNAL BEAM RADIATION THERAPY

External beam radiation has advanced significantly in the past decade. The concept of dose escalation and subsequent application in the form of conformational radiation therapy and IMRT has had profound effects on the treatment of localized prostate cancer. These technologies allow a higher dose of radiation to be focused on a smaller area. Application of this simple concept using modern technology has decreased the incidence of rectal and bladder complication related to radiation toxicity.

External beam radiotherapy, unlike other targeted therapies such as cryotherapy and HIFU, is a repetitive, sequential treatment repeated multiple times over a course of several weeks. The position of the prostate is not predictably consistent over the course of radiation treatment (65). CT and ultrasound have been used prior to every treatment to better localize the prostate (66,67). The importance of prostate position is highlighted by the study by de Crevoisier et al., examining the effect of rectal distention noted on CT during 3DCRT (68). Patients did not have daily imaging or repositioning during treatment, and those with a distended rectum on planning CT had a significantly higher risk of biochemical failure, indicating that rectal distention at the time of simulation altered the position of the prostate, and subsequent treatments without rectal distention potentially "missed" the prostate. The use of a rectal balloon for each treatment to immobilize the prostate and to allow accurate daily targeting has also been investigated to improve the accuracy of IMRT. These manipulations appear to improve both the accuracy of treatment and lowering the dose to the rectum, and thereby lowering rectal toxicity (69).

Within the past decade, attempts to allow easy identification of the prostate on CT and plain film images during 3DCRT and IMRT led to the development of implantable fiducial markers. This procedure can be performed in the outpatient setting under local anesthesia. Fiducial markers are radiopaque gold seeds that are directly implanted into the prostate by a technique similar to a routine transrectal ultrasound guided prostate biopsy. Typically, three markers are used, at the right and left base laterally and the midline at the apex of the prostate. Combining fiducial markers with an automated realignment system has been shown to both be feasible and reduce treatment margins (70).

Concerns that fiducial markers adversely affect the prostate during treatment have been shown to be clinically insignificant. An initial experience with 10 patients showed there was no significant deformation of the gland secondary to implantation of fiducial markers (71). Moreover, the seeds have been observed to remain aligned and have no significant migration during a complete course of IMRT treatment in 56 patients (72).

Overall, fiducial markers are considered safe with no major complications reported. In our institutional experience with outpatient placement of fiducial markers, no patients have experience of urinary retention, gross hematuria, or infection. Major advances in radiation therapy including innovations in modalities are complimented by improving prostatic localization. Implantation of fiducial markers will play an important role in future advancements in radiation therapy for prostate cancer.

TARGETED FOCAL THERAPY FOR LOCALIZED PROSTATE CANCER

Although refinements in targeted therapies for prostate cancer have improved much of the long-term morbidity, side effects especially impotence are still common. Cryotherapy, brachytherapy, and HIFU were first developed to offer minimally invasive alternatives to radiation therapy in patients who could not tolerate surgery. Since the development of nerve-sparing prostatectomy, many patients maintain erectile function after radical surgery. Similarly, advocates of cryotherapy suggest that partial or focal ablation of the prostate sparing one neurovascular bundle may help prevent the almost definite impotence seen in whole prostate cryotherapy. Similar to the progression from radical mastectomy in women with breast cancer to current standards of lumpectomy, patient advocates have called for similar "partial prostate" treatments to alleviate complications and quality of life side effects. Although published series are limited, they have generated an important discussion on the possibility of focal therapy for prostate cancer, the so-called male lumpectomy.

There are some conceptual limitations to focal therapy for prostate cancer. The majority of prostate cancer is multifocal. Prostate biopsy routinely misses areas of cancer, when compared with the surgical pathology available from radical prostatectomy. Therefore, areas that are untreated after focal therapy may contain an undiagnosed prostate cancer. Moreover, it is thought that patients with prostate cancer in one part of the gland are at a higher risk of developing a second lesion in the remaining normal tissue. These "satellite" lesions, however, may be clinically insignificant, and it has been proposed that as much as 80% of men could undergo focal ablation without leaving clinically significant cancer behind (73). However, there is no follow-up data in patients who have undergone focal ablation to support this claim.

The ability to accurately identify patients with true focal disease is limited using today's technology. Routinely, patients undergo a standard 6 or 12 core TRUS biopsy. False negative rates for TRUS biopsy are high but have been improved by an extended core and saturation biopsy techniques (74,75). In one study, Walz and colleagues found that saturation biopsy found cancer in 41% of patients who previously had two negative prostate biopsies (75). New radiological technologies such as endorectal coil MRI (76), dynamic contrast enhanced MRI (77), and MRI spectroscopy (78) show some promise in identifying prostate cancer nodules. However no radiological technique has had acceptable sensitivity in identifying focal cancer especially with nodules smaller than 1.0 cm. Together, these studies only emphasize the low sensitivity of routine prostate biopsy and current radiological techniques in identifying focal prostate cancer.

The data for focal cryotherapy is scant. In one initial study, nine patients with biopsy-proven unilateral disease underwent focal cryotherapy of the prostate, with preservation of the contralateral neurovascular bundle (79). At a mean follow-up of 36 months, every patient had a stable PSA. Importantly, seven of the nine patients were able to have intercourse. This potency rate of 78% appears significantly improved when compared with whole-gland cryotherapy. Overall morbidity of the procedure was limited as no patient experienced incontinence, obstruction, or fistula formation.

The largest published series to date by Bahn et al. followed 31 patients who were treated with focal cryotherapy (80). At a mean follow-up of 70 months, 92.9% of the patients with postoperative PSA data showed no recurrence according to ASTRO criteria, and only one patient (4%) had evidence of cancer on follow-up biopsy. In terms of postprocedure potency, 48.1% and an additional 40.7% of the patients achieved full potency without and with pharmacological assistance, respectively (80). Therefore, potency was preserved in almost 89% of the patients using pharmacological assistance. These results are very promising; however, additional studies are needed to confirm these results.

Focal HIFU has also been explored in small numbers of patients, again with limited published data. Although the impotency rate after whole-gland HIFU does not appear to be high as cryotherapy, it remains a significant side effect. In an early application of HIFU in 1995, a subset of 10 patients with unilateral disease were focally treated with HIFU and subsequent radical prostatectomy (51). However, on pathological examination of the prostatectomy specimen, 70% of these patients had viable tumor remaining.

As HIFU moves beyond experimental status in both Europe and the North America, application of modern HIFU techniques may show improvement on these initial results.

SUMMARY OF PERTINENT CONCLUSIONS

- Image guided and targeted therapies will assume a larger role in the treatment of localized prostate cancer as technology evolves.
- Cryotherapy and HIFU offer curative, minimally invasive treatment options, previously unavailable to patients. With continued refinements in technique and machinery, these modalities appear to offer acceptably low side effects and complications, with adequate cancer control.
- As demand for minimally invasive therapy increases, patients may be willing to potentially sacrifice some of degree of oncological efficacy in pursuing partial prostate treatments (male lumpectomy), analogous to women with breast cancer.
- Caution must be observed, however, that higher grade, potentially lethal prostate cancers are not missed or undertreated.
- Focal therapies allow an adequate window for curative salvage for inadequately treated primary tumors.

REFERENCES

1. Merrill RM, Stephenson RA. Trends in mortality rates in patients with prostate cancer during the era of prostate specific antigen screening. J Urol 2000; 163:503–510.
2. Penson DF, Chan JM. Prostate cancer. J Urol 2007; 177: 2020–2029.
3. Middleton RG. Counseling patients about therapy for localized prostate cancer. Semin Urol Oncol 1995; 13: 187–190 (review).
4. Valicenti RK, Gomella LG, El-Gabry EA, et al. The multidisciplinary clinic approach to prostate cancer counseling and treatment. Semin Urol Oncol 2000; 18:188–191.
5. Ficarra V, Cavalleri S, Novara G, et al. Evidence from robot-assisted laparoscopic radical prostatectomy: a systematic review. Eur Urol 2007; 51:45–55; discussion 56.
6. Zelefsky MJ, Chan H, Hunt M, et al. Long-term outcome of high dose intensity modulated radiation therapy for patients with clinically localized prostate cancer. J Urol 2006; 176:1415–1419.
7. Mangar SA, Huddart RA, Parker CC, et al. Technological advances in radiotherapy for the treatment of localised prostate cancer. Eur J Cancer 2005; 41:908–921 (review).
8. Kenny LM, Ngan S, Waxman J. 'Time, gentlemen, please' for watchful waiting in prostate cancer? BJU Int 2007; 100: 244–246.

9. Arnott J. Practical illustrations of the remedial efficacy of a very low or anaesthetic temperature. I: In cancer. Lancet 1850; 2:257–259.

10. Fay T, Henry GC. Correlation of body segmental temperature and its relation to the location of carcinomatous metastasis: clinical observations and response to methods of refrigeration. Surg Gynecol Obstet 1938; 66:512–514.

11. Gonder MJ, Soanes WA, Shulman S. Cryosurgical treatment of the prostate. Invest Urol 1966; 3:372–378.

12. Soanes WA. Cryosurgery on prostate reported. JAMA 1966; 196(suppl):29.

13. Flocks RH, Nelson CM, Boatman DL: perineal cryosurgery for prostatic carcinoma. J Urol 1972; 108:933–935.

14. Soanes WA, Gonder MJ. Cryosurgery in benign and malignant diseases of the prostate. Int Surg 1969; 51:104–116.

15. Bonney WW, Fallon B, Gerber WL, et al. Cryosurgery in prostatic cancer: survival. Urology 1982; 19:37–42.

16. Onik G, Cobb C, Cohen J, et al. US characteristics of frozen prostate. Radiology 1988; 168:629–631.

17. Wong WS, Chinn DO, Chinn M, et al. Cryosurgery as a treatment for prostate carcinoma: results and complications. Cancer 1997; 79:963–974.

18. Lee F, Bahn DK, Badalament RA, et al. Cryosurgery for prostate cancer: improved glandular ablation by use of 6 to 8 cryoprobes. Urology 1999; 54:135–140.

19. Derakhshani P, Neubauer S, Braun M, et al. Cryoablation of localized prostate cancer. Experience in 48 cases, PSA and biopsy results. Eur Urol 1998; 34:181–187.

20. Mazur P. Freezing of living cells: mechanisms and implications. Am J Physiol 1984; 247:C125–C142.

21. Shinohara K, Connolly JA, Presti JC Jr., et al. Cryosurgical treatment of localized prostate cancer (stages T1 to T4): preliminary results. J Urol 1996; 156:115–120.

22. Hoffmann NE, Bischof JC. The cryobiology of cryosurgical injury. Urology 2002; 60:40–49 (review).

23. Makarov DV, Trock BJ, Humphreys EB, et al. Updated nomogram to predict pathologic stage of prostate cancer given prostate-specific antigen level, clinical stage, and biopsy Gleason score (Partin tables) based on cases from 2000 to 2005. Urology 2007; 69:1095–1101.

24. Partin AW, Yoo J, Carter HB, et al. The use of prostate specific antigen, clinical stage and Gleason score to predict pathological stage in men with localized prostate cancer. J Urol 1993; 150:110–114.

25. Kattan MW, Eastham JA, Stapleton AM., et al. A preoperative nomogram for disease recurrence following radical prostatectomy for prostate cancer. J Natl Cancer Inst 1998; 90:766–771.

26. Kattan MW, Potters L, Blasko JC, et al. Pretreatment nomogram for predicting freedom from recurrence after permanent prostate brachytherapy in prostate cancer. Urology 2001; 58:393–399.

27. Kattan MW, Stapleton AM, Wheeler TM, et al. Evaluation of a nomogram used to predict the pathologic stage of clinically localized prostate carcinoma. Cancer 1997; 79:528–537.

28. Kattan MW, Zelefsky MJ, Kupelian PA, et al. Pretreatment nomogram that predicts 5-year probability of metastasis following three-dimensional conformal radiation therapy for localized prostate cancer. J Clin Oncol 2003; 21:4568–4571.

29. Kattan MW, Zelefsky MJ, Kupelian PA, et al. Pretreatment nomogram for predicting the outcome of three-dimensional conformal radiotherapy in prostate cancer. J Clin Oncol 2000; 18:3352–3359.

30. Chun FK, Karakiewicz PI, Briganti A, et al. Prostate cancer nomograms: an update. Eur Urol 2006; 50:914–926.

31. Derakhshani P, Zumbe J, Neubauer S, et al. Cryoablation of localized prostate cancer: neoadjuvant downsizing of prostate cancer with LH-RH analogue depot before cryosurgery. Urol Int 1998; 60(suppl) 1:2–8.

32. Ghafar MA, Johnson CW, De La Taille A, et al. Salvage cryotherapy using an argon based system for locally recurrent prostate cancer after radiation therapy: the Columbia experience. J Urol 2001; 166:1333–1337.

33. Raboy A, Adler H, Albert P. Extraperitoneal endoscopic pelvic lymph node dissection: a review of 125 patients. J Urol 1997; 158:2202–2204.

34. Leibovici D, Zisman A, Lindner A, et al. PSA elevation during prostate cryosurgery and subsequent decline. Urol Oncol 2005; 23:8–11.

35. Cresswell J, Asterling S, Chaudhary M, et al. Third-generation cryotherapy for prostate cancer in the UK: a prospective study of the early outcomes in primary and recurrent disease. BJU Int 2006; 97:969–974.

36. Bahn DK, Lee F, Badalament R, et al. Targeted cryoablation of the prostate: 7-year outcomes in the primary treatment of prostate cancer. Urology 2002; 60:3–11.

37. Consensus statement: guidelines for PSA following radiation therapy. American Society for Therapeutic Radiology and Oncology Consensus Panel. Int J Radiat Oncol Biol Phys 1997; 37:1035–1041.

38. Long JP, Bahn D, Lee F, et al. Five-year retrospective, multi-institutional pooled analysis of cancer-related outcomes after cryosurgical ablation of the prostate. Urology 2001; 57:518–523.

39. Donnelly BJ, Saliken JC, Ernst DS, et al. Prospective trial of cryosurgical ablation of the prostate: five-year results. Urology 2002; 60:645–649.

40. Prepelica KL, Okeke Z, Murphy A, et al. Cryosurgical ablation of the prostate: high risk patient outcomes. Cancer 2005; 103:1625–1630.

41. Zelefsky MJ, Leibel SA, Gaudin PB, et al. Dose escalation with three-dimensional conformal radiation therapy affects the outcome in prostate cancer. Int J Radiat Oncol Biol Phys 1998; 41:491–500.

42. Potters L, Morgenstern C, Calugaru E, et al. 12-year outcomes following permanent prostate brachytherapy in patients with clinically localized prostate cancer. J Urol 2005; 173:1562–1566.

43. Izawa JI, Madsen LT, Scott SM, et al. Salvage cryotherapy for recurrent prostate cancer after radiotherapy: variables affecting patient outcome. J Clin Oncol 2002; 20:2664–2671.

44. Ellis DS. Cryosurgery as primary treatment for localized prostate cancer: a community hospital experience. Urology 2002; 60:34–39.

45. Han KR, Cohen JK, Miller RJ, et al. Treatment of organ confined prostate cancer with third generation cryosurgery: preliminary multicenter experience. J Urol 2003; 170:1126–1130.

46. Robinson JW, Donnelly BJ, Saliken JC, et al. Quality of life and sexuality of men with prostate cancer 3 years after cryosurgery. Urology 2002; 60:12–18.

47. Robinson JW, Saliken JC, Donnelly BJ, et al. Quality-of-life outcomes for men treated with cryosurgery for localized prostate carcinoma. Cancer 1999; 86:1793–1801.

48. Robinson JW, Donnelly BJ, Coupland K, et al. Quality of life 2 years after salvage cryosurgery for the treatment of local recurrence of prostate cancer after radiotherapy. Urol Oncol 2006; 24:472–486.

49. Lee WR, Hall MC, McQuellon RP, et al. A prospective quality-of-life study in men with clinically localized prostate carcinoma treated with radical prostatectomy, external beam radiotherapy, or interstitial brachytherapy. Int J Radiat Oncol Biol Phys 2001; 51:614–623.

50. Fry WJ, Mosberg WH Jr., Barnard JW, et al. Production of focal destructive lesions in the central nervous system with ultrasound. J Neurosurg 1954; 11:471–478.

51. Madersbacher S, Pedevilla M, Vingers L, et al. Effect of high-intensity focused ultrasound on human prostate cancer in vivo. Cancer Res 1995; 55:3346–3351.

52. Gelet A, Chapelon JY, Bouvier R, et al. Treatment of prostate cancer with transrectal focused ultrasound: early clinical experience. Eur Urol 1996; 29:174–183.

53. Kennedy JE, Ter Haar GR, Cranston D. High intensity focused ultrasound: surgery of the future? Br J Radiol 2003; 76:590–599.

54. Vaughan MG, ter Haar GR, Hill CR, et al. Minimally invasive cancer surgery using focused ultrasound: a pre-clinical, normal tissue study. Br J Radiol 1994; 67:267–274.

55. Chen L, Rivens I, ter Haar G, et al. Histological changes in rat liver tumors treated with high-intensity focused ultrasound. Ultrasound Med Biol 1993; 19:67–74.

56. Illing R, Emberton M. Sonablate-500: transrectal high-intensity focused ultrasound for the treatment of prostate cancer. Expert Rev Med Devices 2006; 3:717–729.

57. Beerlage HP, Thuroff S, Debruyne FM, et al. Transrectal high-intensity focused ultrasound using the Ablatherm device in the treatment of localized prostate carcinoma. Urology 1999; 54:273–277.

58. Vallancien G, Prapotnich D, Cathelineau X, et al. Transrectal focused ultrasound combined with transurethral resection of the prostate for the treatment of localized prostate cancer: feasibility study. J Urol 2004; 171:2265–2267.

59. Poissonnier L, Chapelon JY, Rouviere O, et al. Control of prostate cancer by transrectal HIFU in 227 patients. Eur Urol 2007; 51:381–387.

60. Thuroff S, Chaussy C, Vallancien G, et al. High-intensity focused ultrasound and localized prostate cancer: efficacy results from the European multicentric study. J Endourol 2003; 17:673–677.

61. Ganzer R, Rogenhofer S, Walter B, et al. PSA Nadir is a significant predictor of treatment failure after high-intensity focussed ultrasound (HIFU) treatment of localised prostate cancer. Eur Urol 2007; 53:547–553.

62. Chaussy C, Thuroff S. The status of high-intensity focused ultrasound in the treatment of localized prostate cancer and the impact of a combined resection. Curr Urol Rep 2003; 4: 248–252.

63. Chaussy C, Thuroff S. Results and side effects of high-intensity focused ultrasound in localized prostate cancer. J Endourol 2001; 15:437–440; discussion 447–448.

64. Uchida T, Ohkusa H, Yamashita H, et al. Five years experience of transrectal high-intensity focused ultrasound using the Sonablate device in the treatment of localized prostate cancer. Int J Urol 2006; 13:228–233.

65. Langen KM, Jones DT. Organ motion and its management. Int J Radiat Oncol Biol Phys 2001; 50:265–278.

66. Lattanzi J, McNeely S, Hanlon A, et al. Daily CT localization for correcting portal errors in the treatment of prostate cancer. Int J Radiat Oncol Biol Phys 1998; 41:1079.

67. Lattanzi J, McNeeley S, Hanlon A, et al. Ultrasound-based stereotactic guidance of precision conformal external beam radiation therapy in clinically localized prostate cancer. Urology 2000; 55:73–78.

68. de Crevoisier R, Tucker SL, Dong L, et al. Increased risk of biochemical and local failure in patients with distended rectum on the planning CT for prostate cancer radiotherapy. Int J Radiat Oncol Biol Phys 2005; 62:965–973.

69. Teh BS, McGary JE, Dong L, et al. The use of rectal balloon during the delivery of intensity modulated radiotherapy (IMRT) for prostate cancer: more than just a prostate gland immobilization device? Cancer J 2002; 8:476–483.

70. Litzenberg D, Dawson LA, Sandler H, et al. Daily prostate targeting using implanted radiopaque markers. Int J Radiat Oncol Biol Phys 2002; 52:699–703.

71. Dehnad H, Nederveen AJ, van der Heide UA, et al. Clinical feasibility study for the use of implanted gold seeds in the prostate as reliable positioning markers during megavoltage irradiation. Radiother Oncol 2003; 67:295–302.

72. Kupelian PA, Willoughby TR, Meeks SL, et al. Intra-prostatic fiducials for localization of the prostate gland: monitoring intermarker distances during radiation therapy to test for marker stability. Int J Radiat Oncol Biol Phys 2005; 62:1291–1296.

73. Rukstalis DB, Goldknopf JL, Crowley EM, et al. Prostate cryoablation: a scientific rationale for future modifications. Urology 2002; 60:19–25.

74. Brossner C, Madersbacher S, Bayer G, et al. Comparative study of two different TRUS-guided sextant biopsy techniques in detecting prostate cancer in one biopsy session. Eur Urol 2000; 37:65–71.

75. Walz J, Graefen M, Chun FK, et al. High incidence of prostate cancer detected by saturation biopsy after previous negative biopsy series. Eur Urol 2006; 50:498–505.

76. Lattouf JB, Grubb RL III, Lee SJ, et al. Magnetic resonance imaging-directed transrectal ultrasonography-guided biopsies in patients at risk of prostate cancer. BJU Int 2007; 99:1041–1046.

77. Schlemmer HP, Merkle J, Grobholz R, et al. Can preoperative contrast-enhanced dynamic MR imaging for prostate cancer predict microvessel density in prostatectomy specimens?. Eur Radiol 14:309–317.

78. Kirkham AP, Emberton M, Allen C. How good is MRI at detecting and characterising cancer within the prostate? Eur Urol 2006; 50:1163–1174.

79. Onik G, Narayan P, Vaughan D, et al. Focal "nerve-sparing" cryosurgery for treatment of primary prostate cancer: a new approach to preserving potency. Urology 2002; 60:109–114.

80. Bahn DK, Silverman P, Lee F Sr., et al. Focal prostate cryoablation: initial results show cancer control and potency preservation. J Endourol 2006; 20:688–692.

81. Lam JS, Pisters LL, Belldegrun AS. Cryotherapy for prostate cancer. In: Wein AJ, Kavoussi LR, Novick AC, et al., eds. Campbell-Walsh Urology, Vol. 3 9th ed. Philadelphia, PA: Saunders Elsevier, 2007:3032–3052.

82. Blana A, Walter B, Rogenhofer S, et al. High-intensity focused ultrasound for the treatment of localized prostate cancer: 5-year experience. Urology 2004; 63:297–300.

83. Uchida T, Ohkusa H, Nagata Y, et al. Treatment of localized prostate cancer using high-intensity focused ultrasound. BJU Int 2006; 97:56–61.

8

The Use of Fiducial Markers for IGRT in Prostate Cancer: The Mayo Clinic Approach

BRIAN J. DAVIS, JON KRUSE, CHRISTOPHER C. GOULET, AND MICHAEL G. HERMAN

Department of Radiation Oncology, Mayo Clinic, Rochester, Minnesota, U.S.A.

INTRODUCTION

The practice of modern oncology relies in great part on imaging for screening, diagnosis, staging, therapy, and subsequent assessment. In this regard, the medical management of men with prostate cancer (CaP) does not differ. In 2007, it is estimated that nearly 219,000 men in the United States were diagnosed with CaP (1), and approximately two-thirds, or 140,000 will have CaP localized to the pelvis. Common treatment options for early-stage CaP as identified by the National Comprehensive Cancer Network (www.nccn.org) include radical prostatectomy (RRP), external beam radiation therapy (EBRT), and radioactive seed implantation, also known as permanent prostate brachytherapy (PPB). Other options exist including hormonal therapy, high-dose rate (HDR) brachytherapy, cyrotherapy, and thermal ablation. The latter two common options, EBRT and PPB, rely on ionizing radiation to eradicate the cancer and have been a mainstay in the treatment of CaP for decades. At least 40,000 men per year undergo EBRT for therapy of CaP. The efficacy of these RT options depends on accurate localization of the target and the delivery of an appropriate dose to this volume. Although many methods are widely available to improve the quality of target localization and verification, the Mayo Clinic Department of Radiation Oncology has focused primarily on the use of an electronic portal imaging device (EPID) with implanted gold markers (fiducials) for prostate localization. The main goal of this chapter is to describe our approach and experience with this method of target localization as applied to prostate image-guided radiation therapy (IGRT).

The rationale for integrating improved techniques of image guidance in RT for CaP derives from data supporting the benefits of radiation dose escalation for treatment of this disease.

One means to assess the outcome of CaP following therapy is to monitor the serum prostate-specific antigen (PSA). While controversy exists regarding the optimal means by which to interpret the PSA level following therapy, some studies have shown that conventional dose EBRT results in a poorer PSA relapse–free survival as compared to other modalities (2). However, the use of increased dose of EBRT results in comparable outcomes, but increased side effects may occur (3). Its tolerance also depends on accurate localization and the maximal exclusion of critical normal structures, also known as "organs at risk," with conformal radiation field arrangements. However, the position of the target, until recently, was typically inferred only from external reference points, such as skin markings, used to align the patient on the treatment machine. The accuracy of this alignment is monitored with periodic portal imaging of the skeletal structures of the lower pelvis. Although external reference points should be reproducibly related to skeletal structures, the use of portal imaging during EBRT delivery often reveals displacement from the intended position, which is commonly referred to as "setup variation." In CaP EBRT, several investigators demonstrated that this error in field alignment may exceed 10 mm along each of the mutually perpendicular axes of the coordinate system (4–9). However, the setup variation only partially accounts for uncertainties in the position of the target relative to the treatment beam. The position of the prostate is not fixed relative to the skin marks or the skeletal anatomy of the pelvis (5,10–13), because the state of bladder and rectal filling may result in displacement of the prostate (14–16). This organ motion adds an additional component of uncertainty, which may also exceed 10 mm, in localizing the target for treatment delivery. Both organ motion and setup variation must be taken into account in defining planning target volume (PTV) margins to adequately encompass the prostate with the intended dose (17–19). Target positional variations over a course of treatment have a number of potential sources, and their statistical descriptions as random and systematic processes have been developed to weigh their relative influences on targeting accuracy (15,16).

As stated, improved biochemical (PSA) relapse–free survival (bRFS) has been demonstrated with increased dose of EBRT (20–24). In addition, reduced rates of positive posttreatment biopsies have been observed using radiation dose escalation (22). While these improvements in outcome are observed with increased radiation dose, increased morbidity may also result when such doses are delivered.

More recently, advances in radiation dose delivery with intensity-modulated radiotherapy (IMRT) (25) and improvements in targeting with daily prostate positioning have led to apparent reduced toxicity. Consequently, National Cancer Institute (NCI)-supported multiinstitutional prospective trials using radiation dose escalation for CaP have yielded lower-than-expected toxicity rates (26–28). While the outcome for most CaPs treated with high-dose EBRT appears comparable to other common treatment modalities (2), it appears feasible that further dose escalation with EBRT is possible without an undue increase in normal tissue toxicity.

Many trials have investigated the effect of increasing dose on late rectal toxicity. Radiation Therapy Oncology Group (RTOG) 9406 escalated the dose with three-dimensional conformal EBRT using five different dose levels: 68.4, 73.8, 79.2, 74, and 78 Gy. At every dose level analyzed thus far, the grade 3 or greater gastrointestinal or genitourinary toxicities have been significantly reduced when compared to the historical controls of RTOG 7506

and RTOG 7706, which used conventional radiation rather than three-dimensional conformal radiation (26–28). At the 79.2-Gy dose level, there were no acute grade 3 or greater toxicities (29,30). The late grade 3 toxicities for the rectum and bladder were 0.6% and 1.8%, respectively, with no grade 4 or 5 toxicities reported. In the phase III randomized trial of 70 Gy versus 78 Gy from MD Anderson Cancer Center, the late grade 3 rectal toxicity was 1% in the 70-Gy arm compared to 7% in the 78-Gy arm. However, the radiation was delivered to a conventional four-field box [11×11 cm^2 anteroposteriorly (AP) and 11×9 cm^2 laterally] for the first 46 Gy followed by a slight field reduction (9×9 cm^2 in both the AP and lateral dimensions) to 70 Gy. Only after 70 Gy was the six-field three-dimensional conformal boost added to achieve the final dose of 78 Gy. Over the last several years, IMRT has been shown to further decrease the rectal toxicity over three-dimensional conformal radiation for localized CaP. A recent report of IMRT treatments from Memorial Sloan Kettering shows only 0.5% grade 3 late rectal and bladder toxicity at doses up to 8640 cGy (26). The use of IMRT also showed a decrease in the grade 2 late toxicities compared to three-dimensional conventional radiation performed at the same institution (3). Given this level of rectal toxicity, further dose escalation is likely feasible, especially if localization techniques are refined to allow tighter margins.

A 2005 study by de Creviosier et al. (31) examined the rectal cross-sectional area on patient's treatment plans, and found a significant correlation between rectal distension and poor biochemical control. The likely explanation is that for patients with a distended rectum at simulation, the internal position of the prostate did not represent its average position over the course of treatment. A systematic displacement of the target tissue was introduced for these patients, leading to a poor outcome. This study emphasized the value of image guidance in the treatment of CaP.

THE MAYO CLINIC TECHNIQUE FOR PROSTATE IGRT

Between 2001 and 2002, a phase I trial was conducted in the Department of Radiation Oncology at the Mayo Clinic using an IGRT procedure to identify intraprostatic gold markers and correct daily variations in target position during external beam radiotherapy for CaP (32). Other centers have also developed this technique, which has become commonplace. An early feasibility study by Balter et al. described the use of implanted markers to track prostate movement over the course of routine radiotherapy in 1995. Investigators at the University of California, San Francisco, recently described their five-year experience using implanted markers for prostate radiotherapy. In the approach used at our institution, pretherapy electronic portal images (EPIs) are acquired with a small portion of the therapeutic 6-megavolt (6-MV) dose from an orthogonal pair of treatment fields. The position of the intraprostatic gold markers on the EPIs are aligned with that on the treatment planning digitally reconstructed radiographs derived from axial computed tomography (CT) images. If the initial three-dimensional target displacement (3DI) exceeds 5 mm or rotations exceed 3°, the beam is realigned before the remainder of the dose is delivered. A custom spreadsheet is used to calculate three-dimensional translations from the deviations measured in each of the two portal images. If the action thresholds are exceeded, the spreadsheet supplies couch coordinates to correct the prostate position. At the end of each fraction, the data in the spreadsheet are saved to a database, which can show deviations and corrective actions taken for each patient over the course of treatment. This database is examined after the first five treatment fractions, and any systematic errors are identified and corrected before imaging for the rest of the treatment course.

In the initial clinical study of 20 patients, field-only EPIs were acquired for all fields and offline analysis was performed to determine the final three-dimensional target placement (3DF). Twenty patients completed protocol-specified treatment, and it was determined that all markers were identified on 99.6% of the pretherapy EPIs. Overall, 53% of treatment fractions were realigned. The mean 3DI was 5.6 mm in all patients (range 3.7–9.3), and the mean 3DF was 2.8 mm (range 1.6–4.0), which was statistically significant ($p < 0.001$). Rotational corrections were made on 15% of treatments. Mean treatment duration was 1.4 minutes greater for protocol patients than for similar patients in whom localization was not performed. This study demonstrated that frequent field misalignment occurs when external fiducial marks are used for patient alignment as opposed to using implanted markers. Misalignments can be readily and rapidly identified and corrected with an EPID-based online correction procedure that integrates commercially available equipment and software.

At the Mayo Clinic, gold fiducial markers are implanted via the transperineal approach with 18-gauge needles using local anesthetic only. Prior to the procedure, patients are requested to discontinue anticoagulants for several days, although bleeding is very minimal and, on occasion, patients who have been on continuous aspirin therapy undergo the procedure without having discontinued its use. Patients are placed in the dorsal lithotomy position and a stabilization device is used to maintain probe position. Those experienced with this marker placement will typically perform the needle insertion "free-hand" without the assistance of a template. Prior to needle placement, a local anesthetic is introduced into the perineum and gradually introduced to the level of the prostate before fiducial marker placement is undertaken. Two needles are typically used to implant four markers, two markers through each needle. The markers are placed in a staggered manner so that no overlap occurs on the AP or lateral images. Ideally, the markers are positioned so that they are maximally displaced from one another but are not too close (<5 mm) to the prostate periphery in order to limit the possibility of migration. From 2002 through mid-2007, over 500 patients have undergone this procedure of marker placement and daily prostate localization at our institution.

In Figure 1, the image on the left is a digitally reconstructed radiograph from the CT scan used to plan the radiation treatment. Four gold interstitial fiducial markers are readily apparent in the middle image. The images on the right show the corresponding portal images and treatment field overlay to those in the image on the far left. In blue, the field pattern produced by the multileaf collimation is evident with the small objects enclosed in pink corresponding to the fiducial markers. The object in green is the prostate as determined by the initial CT scan of the prostate. The second image on the right shows the field after it was shifted so that the prostate was

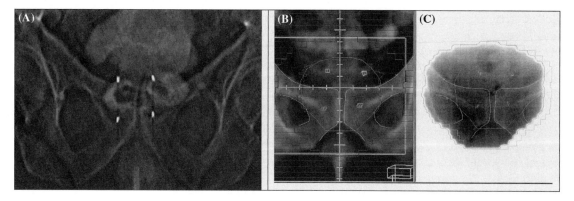

Figure 1 (**A**) Axial scout view (A-P) of pelvis with 4 implanted fiducial markers, (**B**) Digitally-reconstructed radiograph (DRR) of simulation film, (**C**) corresponding electronic portal image showing fiducial markers.

centered in the treatment beam as intended. The field is initially aligned via external tattoos on the patient. Note also that the prostate position as determined by the implanted fiducial markers has shifted relative to the bony anatomy.

OPTIMIZING IGRT IMPLEMENTATION IN PROSTATE CANCER: IGRT QUALITY CONTROL

Quality assurance (QA) of EPID-based prostate localization starts with QA of the EPID itself. Specific QA protocols will vary with EPID hardware and clinical utilization, but general prescriptions for EPID QA can be found in the literature (33), and are meant to generally ensure patient safety, image quality, and localization accuracy. At the Mayo Clinic, the EPID panels are mounted on movable robotic arms and collision sensors on the panels are tested daily to ensure that the patient will not be harmed if struck by the device. The other patient safety concern with EPID localization is excess radiation dose from imaging procedures. A pair of megavoltage portal images may deliver 6 to 8 cGy to the patient per treatment fraction—a dose that can be appreciable with a typically large number of fractions for prostate treatments. At our institution, the portal images are acquired through shaped ports, which limit the exposure to the PTV plus a 1-cm margin. The patient's treatment plan includes a pair of four-monitor unit imaging fields to be delivered at each treatment session. The dose from the imaging fields is calculated initially and is considered when the influences for the remaining five IMRT fields are optimized. In this way, the dose from the localization procedure is reflected in the treatment plan.

EPID image quality is assessed every day as part of routine linac warm-up, and the imaging panels' dark-field and flood-field corrections are calibrated every month by Physics staff.

Localization accuracy is guaranteed through a number of procedures and consistency checks. The first element of the localization process is for the EPID system to report the position of the gold markers in the portal images, relative to their prescribed locations. Some of the EPIDs at Mayo (Varian Portal Vision v. 7.3) use a gradient search algorithm to detect the radiation field edge of the portal image and compare this to the prescribed field shape, as defined on the reference digitally reconstructed radiograph (DRR). The location of isocenter is known on the DRR, and so comparison of the detected and prescribed field shapes enables the EPID software to find the isocenter on the portal image. The detection and alignment of the radiation field edges is crucial for accurate localization of the patient, and it is verified graphically by therapists on every portal image before the location of the fiducial markers is recorded. On some newer EPID systems (Varian 4D Treatment Console), the robotic support arm reports the location of isocenter

relative to the imaging panel, and this information is used in localizing the markers. On these machines, the accuracy of the arm calibration is tested daily at multiple gantry angles by placing a physical graticule tray on the head of the machine and comparing the image of the central BB to the central axis of the beam, as reported by the EPID system. The most critical and robust aspect of the IGRT QA process is physician review of images acquired during treatment. EPID images can be acquired with the therapeutic fields, showing the positions of the markers during the actual treatment. In the case of IMRT treatments, the EPID panel will integrate charge continuously through the field delivery and present a single image representing the entire field delivery. Fiducial markers are visible in these integrated images, and physicians review these images after each treatment but before the following session to verify that the prostate is positioned properly during the actual treatment. This review process serves as a comprehensive check on all other components of the localization process, and can be used to assess other processes such as intrafraction motion.

CLINICAL OUTCOME WITH INTRAPROSTATIC FIDUCIALS AND EPID

One research effort has focused on the estimation of limits of dose escalation using IMRT and precise prostate targeting (35). As described previously, recent reports of dose escalation for CaP indicate minimal toxicity using established dose constraints on normal adjacent structures. The completed multiinstitutional protocol, RTOG 94-06, enrolled 1084 patients and did not find the maximum tolerable dose (MTD). This result suggests that further dose escalation is possible before the MTD is found. In support of this concept, Zelefsky et al. (3) continued dose escalation for treatment of CaP to 8640 cGy with IMRT.

At our institution, initial investigations addressed the limits of dose escalation using five-field intensity-modulated radiotherapy (5FIMRT) as a function of PTV margins. CT data was obtained from 18 patients with localized CaP treated with 5FIMRT between September 2003 and February 2005. All patients gave permission for use of their medical records in accordance with the Mayo Clinic's institutional review board and Minnesota statutes. Patient characteristics are provided in Table 1. The beam angles employed include those described by Burman et al. and used routinely in our clinical practice and elsewhere: posterior, posterior right and left oblique (P75R, P75L), and anterior right and left oblique (A45R, A45L). The PTV of all patients in the study received 75.6 Gy delivered in 42 fractions.

Each patient was treated with interstitial fiducial markers in place and using daily electronic portal

Table 1 Patient Characteristics and Treatment Details for Simulation Study Examining the Limits of Dose Escalation for Treatment of Prostate Cancer

Patient characteristics		
Age (yr)	Avg: 70	Range: 57–80
Anterior/posterior separation (cm)	Avg: 23.5	Range: 12.1–34.1
Lateral separation (cm)	Avg: 37.0	Range: 31.1–44.8
Tumor characteristics		
T stage	T1c	12/18 (67%)
	T2a	5/18 (28%)
	T2b	1/18 (6%)
Gleason score	3 + 3	14/18 (78%)
	3 + 4	2/18 (11%)
	4 + 3	2/18 (11%)
PSA	Avg: 6.1	Range: 2.4–13.0
Low risk		10/18 (56%)
Intermediate risk		8/18 (44%)
Treatment details		
Dose = 75.6 Gy		18/18 (100%)
Interstitial Fiducial Markers		18/18 (100%)
Five field IMRT		18/18 (100%)
Prostate volume on CT (cc)	Avg: 56	Range: 32–103
Rectal volume on CT (cc)	Avg: 97	Range: 62–132

Table 2 Dose Constraints [RTOG Protocol P-0126 (www.rtog. org)].

	<15%	<25%	<35%	<50%
Bladder	V80	V75	V70	V65
Rectum	V75	V70	V65	V60
PTV	<2% less than the prescription dose <2% greater than 107% of the prescription dose			
CTV	0% less than the prescription dose			

imaging (EPI). All targets were positioned prior to treatment so that the net three-dimensional displacement of the target was less than 5 mm. The prostate to PTV margin was routinely selected as 7.5 mm uniformly around the prostate except posteriorly where it was limited to 5 mm. The prostate, rectum, and bladder were segmented by the treating radiation oncologist in a manner consistent with the specifications for contouring these structures on RTOG protocols. The clinical target volume (CTV) was defined as the prostate. For each patient, uniform 10-, 5-, and 3-mm three-dimensional expansions of the prostate were used to generate the PTV. These definitions of CTV, PTV, and others are nomenclature used in radiation treatment planning and are described in several reports by the International Commission of Radiologic Units (ICRU). Identical 6-MV 5FIMRT beam arrangements were used for every plan. The same beam orientations as described above were employed. Plans were optimized in the Eclipse Planning System (Varian Medical Systems, Palo Alto, California, U.S., version 7.2) in a manner such that the dose constraints as outlined in RTOG dose escalation protocol P0126 for the rectum, bladder, PTV, and CTV and as listed in Table 2 were maintained (www.rtog.org). Hot spots greater than 107% of the prescription were not allowed in the rectum or bladder. In addition, no point outside the PTV, except those immediately adjacent to

the PTV, was allowed to receive a calculated dose above the prescription dose. All plans used 6-MV beams, in accordance with the current institutional treatment policy. Equal priorities were assigned to the rectal V75, and the minimum and maximum PTV constraints for every plan. Additional constraints, at the same priority level, were added in the minority of plans, and only when the constraint could not otherwise be met. Iterative optimizations, adding additional 180-cGy fractions, were performed until one or more of these constraints could no longer be met. The highest dose that met all the constraints was defined as the maximum achievable dose. The relationship between maximum achievable dose and PTV margin, prostate volume, and PTV overlap with the rectum was examined.

Results of Simulation Analysis

The maximum achievable dose is limited by the rectal V75 dose constraint in 61% of cases. The other limiting constraints include the bladder V80 (19%), PTV coverage (19%), lateral subcutaneous hot spots in the P75 beams (11%), rectal V70 (4%), rectal V65 (2%), and bladder V75 (2%). Nine of the 54 plans had two criteria that were primarily responsible for limiting the dose. PTV margins of 10, 5, and 3 mm yield a mean maximum achievable dose of 83.0 Gy (range 73.8–108.0 Gy), 113.1 Gy (range 90.0–151.2 Gy), and 135.9 Gy (range 102.6–189.0 Gy), respectively. All comparisons of the maximum achievable dose between margin groups are statistically significant with one-sided p values <0.001 (paired t test). Prostate volumes of 30 to 50 cc ($n = 8$) compared with those of 50 to 70 cc ($n = 7$) and 70 to 105 cc ($n = 3$) show an inverse correlation with maximum achievable dose (Fig. 2B). Smaller prostates yield significantly higher maximum achievable dose for PTV margins of 3 and 5 mm ($p < 0.05$). For plans with 10-mm margins, prostates 30 to 50 cc yield a significantly larger maximum achievable dose than those 70 to 105 cc ($p = 0.009$). However, there is no significant difference between any of the other comparisons of prostate size with maximum achievable dose for the 10-mm margin groups.

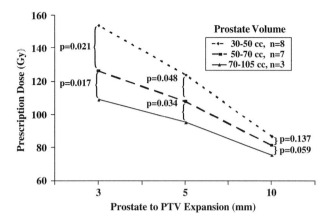

Figure 2 The estimated maximum prescription dose to the prostate using dose constraints from the protocol RTOG P-0126 as a function of treatment margin for three different cohorts of prostate size.

Decreasing the prostate to PTV margin size significantly decreases the PTV overlap with the rectum (one-sided $p < 0.001$ between all margin comparisons). The MAD shows an inverse correlation with the component of PTV volume overlapping the rectum. The linear correlation coefficient is 0.72. However, the comparison between these two variables shows a better logarithmic relationship. The correlation coefficient between the logarithm of the volume of PTV overlapping the rectum and the maximum achievable dose is 0.87 (Fig. 2). Maximum achievable dose declines from 150 to 100 Gy with 0 to 5 cc of overlap, and thereafter drops slowly to 75 Gy with 5 to 20 cc of overlap. By decreasing the PTV margin while maintaining identical dose constraints, doses significantly greater than those currently prescribed for treatment of localized CaP appear feasible. In other words, this simulation study shows that the more accurate the treatment delivery and the narrower the margin placed around the prostate, the higher the radiation dose that may be delivered.

The RTOG protocol P0126 specifies a CTV-to-PTV margin of 5 to 10 mm. However, the use of increasingly accurate target localization methods may permit smaller margins, such as 3 mm. Recently, Schallenkamp et al. in a Mayo study show that using interstitial fiducial markers and daily EPI allow margins of 2.7, 2.9, and 2.8 mm in the superoinferior (SI), AP, and right-left (RL) axes. The one-dimensional margins were defined so that 95% of patients would receive a minimum of 95% of the prescribed dose to the CTV, assuming that institutional systematic error is zero. On this protocol, patients were shifted only if the fiducial markers were greater than 5 mm (3D magnitude of displacement) from their expected position. This method of daily tracking is associated with a reduction in setup error by more than 2 mm. Cheung et al. also show

that by creating an individualized PTV using daily online positioning with interstitial fiducial markers and patient-specific respiratory and intrafraction prostate motion data, the average PTV margin was 3 mm in the RL and SI directions, and 4 mm in the AP direction (34). As such, the lower PTV treatment margin examined in this study is 3 mm, whereas those margins employed in RTOG P-0126 are 5 to 10 mm.

Intrafraction Motion

Many have studied the magnitude of intrafraction motion during prostate radiotherapy with implanted fiducial markers and EPI. Goulet et al. (35) at our institution studied the estimated increase in dose escalation possible by reducing treatment margins. For example, reduction of the treatment margin from 10 to 3 mm for an intermediate-sized prostate gland would theoretically allow an increase of maximum allowable dose from 90 to 128 Gy. Willoughby et al. (36) have analyzed the influence of tracking interfraction and intrafraction prostate motion with implanted fiducial markers and the margins required to assure that 90% of the patient population receives a minimum dose to the CTV of at least 95% of the nominal dose. By this methodology, CTV to PTV margins, mPTV, are given by:

$$mPTV = 2.5\,\Sigma + 0.7\sigma$$

where Σ is the sum of all of the routine setup errors and σ is the random error related to intrafraction motion.

For skin-based setup without and with inclusion of intrafraction motion, prostate treatments would have required average margins of 8.0, 7.3, and 10.0 mm and 8.2, 10.2, and 12.5 mm, about the left-right, AP, and cranial-caudal directions, respectively. Positioning by prostate markers at the start of the treatment fraction reduced these values to 1.8, 5.8, and 7.1 mm, respectively. Interbeam adjustment further reduced margins to an average of 1.4, 2.3, and 1.8 mm. Intrabeam adjustment yielded margins of 1.3, 1.5, and 1.5 mm, respectively. Consequently, the value of prostate localization and intrafraction tracking is substantial when considering the potential for dose escalation, reduced cancer recurrence rates, and reduced toxicity.

In the study by Willoughby et al. (36), 11 patients' data were analyzed. Using the technique of implanted fiducial markers at our institution, we studied the intrafraction motion of 39 patients receiving 1532 treatments of EBRT. In Figure 3A, the time requirement for the steps involved in delivering one fraction of radiation for a patient treated with implanted fiducial markers is given. From minutes 9 through 13, intrafraction motion may occur without compensating for its occurrence. The position of the

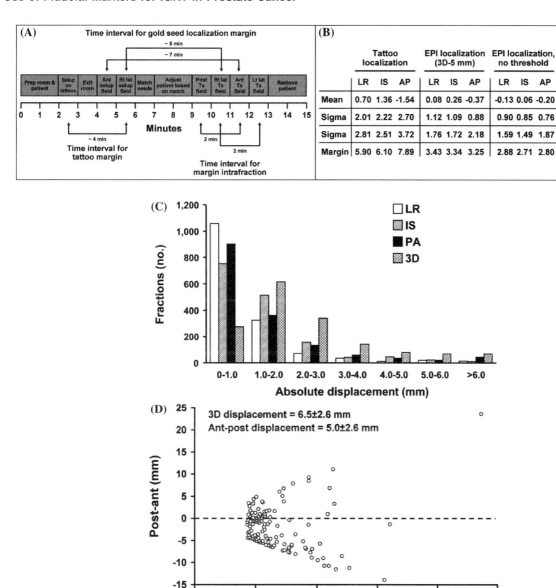

Figure 3 (**A**) Time intervals for gold seed localization during EBRT. (**B**) Localization errors based on different methods of localization. (**C**) Number of fractions versus displacements. (**D**) Worst 10% of cases, A-P versus absolute displacement. *Abbreviation*: EBRT, external beam radiation therapy. *Source*: From Ref. 37.

prostate after treatment completion is determined without determining the history of this movement. In Figure 3B, the required margin is calculated using the method of Van Herk. The first "σ" represents the systematic error and the second "σ" represents the random error. Based on using skin marks alone, it is estimated that the margin required should be from 5.9 to 7.89 mm. If localization by EPID is used and adjustments of the patient position are performed with no threshold, then the margins in all directions need to be 2.7 to 2.8 mm. Likewise, accounting for the effect of intrafraction motion by itself, required margins are 2.1 to

2.97 mm. In other words, the magnitude of the effect of intrafraction motion on required margins is essentially similar to that afforded by setting up on the prostate by itself. In the histogram of Figure 3C, the magnitude of the prostate intrafraction motion for each direction and the three-dimensional displacement is shown. From this chart, it is clear that there is a significant amount of intrafraction movement. Figure 3D shows the top 10% three-dimensional intrafraction motion, along with the corresponding posteroanterior displacement. From this graph, it is evident that intrafraction motion is a significant issue, especially in regards to the rectum, the radiation dose limiting structure, which lies posterior to the prostate. The average of the top 10% intrafraction displacement is 6.5 mm with a standard deviation of 2.6 mm; the top 10% left-right motion averages 3.3 mm with 1.9 mm standard deviation; the inferosuperior is 3.8 mm and 1.1 mm, respectively; and the posteroanterior average is 5.0 mm with a standard deviation of 2.6 mm. It is essential to develop a method that better characterizes and substantially reduces the adverse influence of intrafraction motion on CaP radiotherapy.

In this regard, current efforts to develop and test a continuous tracking device using electromagnetic transponders are worthwhile. Such a system for accurate target localization and continuous tracking has been developed by Calypso Medical, Inc. of Seattle, which will be discussed in detail in chapter 12.

Briefly, the system utilizes miniature, permanently implanted, wireless electromagnetic transponders and an array to localize them in three-dimensional space. The technical design of the system includes the use of non-ionizing electromagnetic radiation with negligible tissue interaction. The system is designed for continuous operation during EBRT and provides data at a rate up to 10 Hz. A single transponder has an accuracy less than 2 mm rms, whereas for most configurations tested, the accuracy is submillimeter when using three or more transponders. The five major components of this system include wireless transponders, a console, an array, a tracking station, and infrared cameras. The transponders are wireless, self-contained, and do not require an internal power supply. The transponders are encapsulated in biocompatible glass and are designed for permanent implantation or surface placement. The array incorporates an electromagnetic source to temporarily excite transponders at 300 to 500 kHz and induce resonant response signals. Sensors in the array measure transponder signals used to determine the positions in three-dimensional space relative to the array. Transponder signals are time-multiplexed so that different resonant frequencies may be tracked independently. The array is registered to the isocenter of the linear accelerator through infrared cameras and optical targets mounted on the array. The user interface displays localization and tracking data inside and outside the radiation treatment room.

Current Practice at Mayo Clinic

The prostate IGRT protocol has evolved over six years of implementation at Mayo Clinic. In the initial phase I study in 2001, the patients were treated with a three-dimensional conformal four-field box technique. The four fields were planned, and then additional anterior and right lateral fields were added to the plan for imaging. Monitor units were

Table 3 IGRT Protocols at the Mayo Clinic

	Original protocol	Present protocol
Imaging fields	Anterior + Right Lateral	Anterior + 60° oblique
Action threshold (3D translation)	5 mm	4 mm
Action threshold (rotation)	3°	None
Treatment fields	4 Field box	5 Field IMRT
CTV to PTV margin	7.5 mm; 5 mm posterior	7.5 mm; 5 mm posterior

transferred from the anterior and lateral treatment fields to their respective EPID fields. We found that the patient's femurs could occasionally obscure the fiducial markers in a lateral image, so the imaging view has been replaced by a 60° anterior oblique. The two EPID fields are planned for four monitor units each, and then five IMRT fields are planned to deliver the remainder of the prescribed dose. In addition to translational motion, the prostate is often observed to rotate in the AP direction, about the left-right axis. This rotation was measured in the original protocol, and the rotation of the target was matched by rotating the collimator angle of the lateral treatment fields. No straightforward correction exists for oblique IMRT treatment fields, so rotational motions of the prostate are no longer considered. The action level for translational correction has been reduced from 5 to 4 mm, although the CTV-to-PTV margins remain at 7.5 mm in all directions, with the exception of a 5-mm posterior margin. Changes in the IGRT protocol are summarized in Table 3.

SUMMARY OF PERTINENT CONCLUSIONS

- Dose escalation in CaP leads to improvement in biochemical control and a reduction in positive biopsies following CaP radiotherapy.
- In order to achieve increased dose escalation without a concomitant increase in toxicity, IGRT is essential.
- Our approach is to use implanted fiducial markers and daily EPI to achieve routine localization well within 5 mm of the intended positioning.
- Reduced margins may further allow substantially increased dose escalation based on a theoretical study presented in this chapter.
- Our measurements indicate that intrafraction prostate motion is more than 6 mm during approximately 10% of fractions.
- Tracking of the prostate during treatment may facilitate more accurate treatment achieved by the use of implanted electromagnetic beacons.

ACKNOWLEDGMENTS

The authors would like to thank Drs. Chris Beltran and Thomas M. Pisansky for their collaboration on projects and publications related to this chapter.

REFERENCES

1. American Cancer Society. Cancer Facts and Figures 2007. Atlanta: American Cancer Society, 2007.
2. Kupelian PA, Potters L, Khuntia D, et al. Radical prostatectomy, external beam radiotherapy <72 Gy, external beam radiotherapy > or =72 Gy, permanent seed implantation, or combined seeds/external beam radiotherapy for stage T1-T2 prostate cancer. Int J Radiat Oncol Biol Phys 2004; 58(1):25–33.
3. Zelefsky MJ, Fuks Z, Hunt M, et al. High dose radiation delivered by intensity modulated conformal radiotherapy improves the outcome of localized prostate cancer. J Urol 2001; 166(3):876–881.
4. el-Gayed AA, Bel A, Vijlbrief R, et al. Time trend of patient setup deviations during pelvic irradiation using electronic portal imaging. Radiother Oncol 1993; 26: 162–171.
5. Vigneault E, Pouliot J, Laverdiere J, et al. Electronic portal imaging device detection of radioopaque markers for the evaluation of prostate position during megavoltage irradiation: a clinical study. Int J Radiat Oncol Biol Phys 1997; 37:205–212.
6. Greer PB, Jose CC, Matthews JH. Set-up variation of patients treated with radiotherapy to the prostate measured with an electronic portal imaging device. Australas Radiol 1998; 42:207–212.
7. Tinger A, Michalski JM, Cheng A, et al. A critical evaluation of the planning target volume for 3-D conformal radiotherapy of prostate cancer. Int J Radiat Oncol Biol Phys 1998; 42:213–221.
8. Stryker JA, Shafer J, Beatty RE. Assessment of accuracy of daily set-ups in prostate radiotherapy using electronic imaging. Br J Radiol 1999; 72:579–583.
9. Zelefsky MJ, Crean D, Mageras GS, et al. Quantification and predictors of prostate position variability in 50 patients evaluated with multiple CT scans during conformal radiotherapy. Radiother Oncol 1999; 50:225–234.
10. Balter JM, Sandler HM, Lam K, et al. Measurement of prostate movement over the course of routine radiotherapy using implanted markers. Int J Radiat Oncol Biol Phys 1995; 31:113–118.
11. Dawson LA, Mah K, Franssen E, et al. Target position variability throughout prostate radiotherapy. Int J Radiat Oncol Biol Phys 1998; 42:1155–1161.
12. Stroom JC, Koper PC, Korevaar GA, et al. Internal organ motion in prostate cancer patients treated in prone and supine treatment position. Radiother Oncol 1999; 51: 237–248.
13. Langen KM, Jones DT. Organ motion and its management. Int J Radiat Oncol Biol Phys 2001; 50:265–278.
14. Roeske JC, Forman JD, Mesina CF, et al. Evaluation of changes in the size and location of the prostate, seminal vesicles, bladder, and rectum during a course of external beam radiation therapy. Int J Radiat Oncol Biol Phys 1995; 33:1321–1329.
15. van Herk M, Bruce A, Kroes AP, et al. Quantification of organ motion during conformal radiotherapy of the prostate by three dimensional image registration. Int J Radiat Oncol Biol Phys 1995; 33:1311–1320.
16. Beard CJ, Kijewski P, Bussiere M, et al. Analysis of prostate and seminal vesicle motion: Implications or treatment planning. Int J Radiat Oncol Biol Phys 1996; 34: 451–458.
17. International Commission on Radiation Units and Measurements. ICRU Report 62: Prescribing, Recording and Reporting Photon Beam Therapy (Supplement to ICRU Report 50). Bethesda, MD, 1999.
18. Bijhold J, Lebesque JV, Hart AA, et al. Maximizing setup accuracy using portal images as applied to a conformal boost technique for prostatic cancer. Radiother Oncol 1992; 24:261–271.
19. Bel A, Vos PH, Rodrigus PT, et al. High-precision prostate cancer irradiation by clinical application of an offline patient setup verification procedure, using portal imaging. Int J Radiat Oncol Biol Phys 1996; 35:321–332.
20. Pollack A, Zagars GK, Starkschall G, et al. Prostate cancer radiation dose response: results of the M.D. Anderson phase III randomized trial. Int J Radiat Oncol Biol Phys 2002; 53:1097–1105.
21. Zietman AL, Desilvio M, Slater JD, et al. A randomized trial comparing conventional dose (70.2 GyE) and high-dose (79.2 GyE) conformal radiation in early stage adenocarcinoma of the prostate: results of an interim analysis of PROG 95-09. Int J Radiat Oncol Biol Phys 2004; 60:S131–S132.
22. Zelefsky MJ, Chan H, Fuks Z, et al. Correlation of long-term biochemical outcome with post-treatment biopsy results for patients treated with 3-dimensional conformal radiotherapy for prostate cancer. Int J Radiat Oncol Biol Phys 2004; 60:S170.
23. Michalski JM, Purdy JA, Winter K, et al. Preliminary report of toxicity following 3D radiation therapy for prostate cancer on 3DOG/RTOG 9406. Int J Radiat Oncol Biol Phys 2000; 46:391–402.
24. Ryu JK, Winter K, Michalski JM, et al. Interim report of toxicity from 3D conformal radiation therapy (3D-CRT) for prostate cancer on 3DOG/RTOG 9406, level III (79.2 Gy). Int J Radiat Oncol Biol Phys 2002; 54:1036–1046.
25. Michalski JM, Winter K, Purdy JA, et al. Toxicity after three-dimensional radiotherapy for prostate cancer with RTOG 9406 dose level IV. Int J Radiat Oncol Biol Phys 2004; 58:735–742.
26. Zelefsky MJ, Fuks Z, Hunt M, et al. High-dose intensity modulated radiation therapy for prostate cancer: early toxicity and biochemical outcome in 772 patients. Int J Radiat Oncol Biol Phys 2002; 53:1111–1116.
27. Zelefsky MJ, Cowen D, Fuks Z, et al. Long term tolerance of high dose three-dimensional conformal radiotherapy in patients with localized prostate carcinoma. Cancer 1999; 85:2460–2468.

28. Schallenkamp JM, Herman MG, Kruse JJ, et al. Prostate position relative to pelvic bony anatomy base on intraprostatic gold markers and electronic portal imaging. Int J Radiat Oncol Biol Phys 2005; 63(3):800–811.

29. Michalski JM, Winter K, Purdy JA, et al. Trade-off to low-grade toxicity with conformal radiation therapy for prostate cancer on Radiation Therapy Oncology Group 9406. Semin Radiat Oncol 2002; 12:75–80.

30. Michalski JM, Winter K, Purdy JA, et al. Preliminary evaluation of low-grade toxicity with conformal radiation therapy for prostate cancer on RTOG 9406 dose levels I and II. Int J Radiat Oncol Biol Phys 2003; 56: 192–198.

31. de Crevoisier R, Tucker SL, Dong L, et al. Increased risk of biochemical and local failure in patients with distended rectum on the planning CT for prostate cancer radiotherapy. Int J Radiat Oncol Biol Phys 2005; 62:965–973.

32. Herman MG, Pisansky TM, Kruse JJ, et al. Technical aspects of daily on-line positioning of the prostate for three-dimensional conformal radiotherapy using an electronic portal imaging device. Int J Radiat Oncol Biol Phys 2003; 57(4):1131–1140.

33. Herman MG, Balter JM, Jaffray DA, et al. Clinical use of electronic portal imaging: report of AAPM Radiation Therapy Committee Task Group 58. Med Phys 2001; 28:712–737.

34. Cheung R, Tucker SL, Ye JS, et al. Characterization of rectal normal tissue complication probability after highdose external beam radiotherapy for prostate cancer. Int J Radiat Oncol Biol Phys 2004; 58:1513–1519.

35. Goulet CC, Herman MG, Hillman DW, et al. Estimated limits of dose escalation for localized prostate cancer using intensity modulated radiotherapy, varied planning target volume margins and established dose constraints: correlation with prostate size and target volume overlap with the rectum. Int J Radiat Oncol Biol Phys 2005; 63(suppl 1):S209.

36. Willoughby TR, Kupelian PA, Pouliot J, et al. Target localization and real-time tracking using the Calypso 4D localization system in patients with localized prostate cancer. Int J Radiat Oncol Biol Phys 2006; 65(2):528–534.

37. Beltran C, Herman MG, Davis BJ, et al. Planning Target Margin Calculations for Prostate Radiotherapy Based on Intrafraction and Interfraction Motion Using Four Localization Methods. Int J Radiat Oncol Biol Phys 2008; 70(1): 289–295.

9

IGRT in Prostate Cancer: Method and Application of Cone-Beam Computed Tomography

DAVID A. JAFFRAY

Radiation Medicine Program, Princess Margaret Hospital/University Health Network, Departments of Radiation Oncology and Medical Biophysics, University of Toronto, Toronto, Ontario, Canada

INTRODUCTION

The past 10 years has seen radiation therapy of the prostate gland evolve from a simple technique–based approach that relied on bony anatomy (1) and perturbations from the "four-field brick" to a modality that is informed from image sets derived from a variety of different imaging systems. These images are capable of illustrating the gland and its internal structures, differentiating disease from normal tissues, and demonstrating the presence of organ motion. As the design phase of prostate radiation therapy continues to advance, there is a need for parallel advancements in the methods used to verify that these planned dose distributions are effected within the patient. Recent developments in detector technology, computational horsepower, and the data-handling systems have permitted the development of volumetric imaging on the radiation therapy treatment unit using cone-beam computed tomography (CBCT) methods. These are highly integrated solutions that permit in-room imaging, alignment, and adjustment of the patient position prior to treatment.

ACHIEVING PRECISION AND ACCURACY IN RADIATION THERAPY FOR PROSTATE CANCER

The large number of sensitive adjacent structures (rectum, bladder, penile bulb, femoral heads), their complex spatial interrelationship, the mobility and distention of the rectum/colon, and the gradual filling of the bladder make the conformal treatment of the prostate gland challenging. In this context, the objective of maintaining the prescribed dose to the prostate gland [gross tumor volume (GTV) and clinical target volume (CTV)] is a complex tradeoff of competing dose-volume constraints where the fundamental limits on the dose gradients in photon beams and the presence of geometric uncertainties are in competition. These uncertainties are made complex by the fact that the structures can move and change shape both relative to bony anatomy and each other (2–6). Imaging methods such as portal imaging or radiographic imaging allow localization of bony anatomy or implanted fiducials (7–13), but do not permit characterization of the changes in shape and relative position of the gland and surrounding normal tissues (14). The use of markers in the gland provides a significant improvement in gland-targeting accuracy and precision over bony anatomy. However, further advances in imaging are desired to allow visualization of these structures directly, thereby eliminating the need for marker placement, allowing patient-specific dose accumulation, and possibly leading to subprostatic boost, and adaptive methods to further reduce the planning target volume (PTV) margins employed in the design of the treatment plan.

CBCT IMAGING

Advances in large-area electronics has led to the development of two-dimensional radiographic detectors based upon amorphous silicon technology (15). The resulting radiographic receptors employ radiation-sensitive phosphors or scintillators on large (up to 41 cm × 41 cm) arrays, free of distortion and reasonably efficient (>60%) at collecting X-rays and converting the X-ray shadow into a digital format. Such detectors make it possible to achieve coverage of a large field of view (FOV) with resolutions that are less than 1 mm. The use of area detectors to generate volumetric computed tomography images was pioneered in the field of single-photon emission computed tomography (SPECT). In this approach, it is necessary to collect projection data from multiple directions around the object of interest. The same is necessary in CBCT, wherein multiple (300–600) projections are acquired over a range of angles (∼180–360) about the patient (16,17). A sufficiently fast and effective reconstruction algorithm for reconstructing this type of data was reported by Feldkamp et al. in 1984 (18). The adaptation of the flat-panel detector to medical linear accelerators was already underway to allow better megavoltage portal imaging quality (19). These systems can now be used to generate CBCT data directly (20). Alternatively, an additional kV X-rays tube can be integrated with the accelerator, and a kV detector is employed opposite for collection of the multiple radiographs (21,22).

Currently, there are a number of commercial systems available in the market (Fig. 1). The Elekta Synergy™ System (23), Varian On-Board Imager™ (24), and Siemens Artiste™ offer kV-based CBCT integrated into the treatment unit. Siemens is the only company offering a megavoltage (MV) CBCT system (MVision™) (20). There are numerous subtleties in the operation of these systems that determine the relative merits. Factors to be considered include size of the FOV, the speed of acquisition and reconstruction, the use of correction schemes to improve imaging performance, their support for radiographic/fluoroscopic modes, the level of integration with the treatment unit, software tools, remote couch control, and connectivity to the electronic treatment record. Given that these systems have relatively recently reached the market, there continues to be significant technical advancement and ongoing development of modes of clinical use.

CBCT SYSTEMS AND ISSUES

Image Quality

The images generated by the kV CBCT systems have many features that make them attractive for image-guided radiation therapy (IGRT) of the prostate. These include

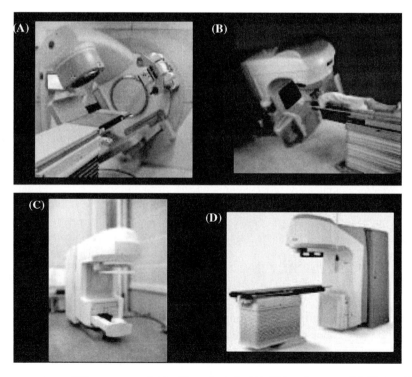

Figure 1 There are four cone-beam CT systems available. These include (**A**) Elekta Synergy, (**B**) Varian Trilogy, and (**C**) Siemens Artiste offering kV cone-beam CT. Siemens also offers the MVision adaptation to their accelerator for megavoltage cone-beam CT (**D**).

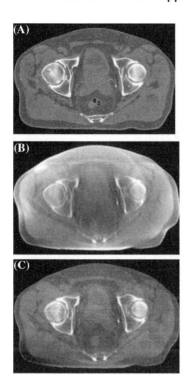

Figure 2 The quality of cone-beam CT images is influenced by the presence of X-rays scatter, detector nonlinearity, and lag. (**A**) Axial slice from a conventional CT scan of the prostate. (**B**) Cone-beam CT image acquired at ∼3 cGy. (**C**) The same image as **B** with a postprocessing correction applied to the projection data to suppress the influence of scatter.

detection of soft tissue contrast, large FOV, remarkably high spatial resolution, and relatively low imaging doses. The soft tissue contrast demonstrated with current systems is not at the level of conventional CT systems. The presence of X-rays scatter and detector lag in the CBCT systems induces significant shading artifacts such as cupping or streaks (Fig. 2B). These features do not significantly reduce the spatial resolution, as a result, very detailed images can be generated with these systems (21). Such a characteristic can be useful when considering the need to detect and localize implanted fiducials, or in the case of brachytherapy, distinguish and localize nearly 100 such seeds (25). However, the shading artifacts negatively affect the ability of these systems to produce accurate CT numbers, and therefore, accurate electron density estimation. While not critical for image guidance, it does prevent planning directly on the CBCT images unless these densities are manually assigned.

While early attempts at MV CBCT produced images of limited quality (22,26), the utilization of amorphous silicon detectors has advanced the method significantly. The quality of the images produced with these systems has many of the features outlined above for the kV systems (Fig. 3). While the fundamental limitations on noise per unit imaging dose will limit soft tissue visualization, the use of the MV beam should reduce the magnitude of scatter (27,28) and may mitigate some of the artifacts arising from detector nonlinearities and beam-hardening effects. The reduction in these effects may offset some of the fundamental noise constraints associated with the use of the megavoltage-range X-rays.

Currently, the CBCT approach requires approximately 40 to 120 seconds to generate an image. This time constraint is due in part to the maximum gantry rotation rate allowed in these systems (1 rpm). The reconstruction process assumes a static object over the course of acquisition, and given these long acquisition times, it is highly likely that some motion will occur. In terms of image quality for prostate imaging, the most disruptive artifacts arise from the motion of gas in the rectum and colon. The low density of gas makes it a high-contrast material, which can generate streak artifacts in the images if it is mobile. Efforts to reduce the presence of gas have been identified as a method of improving image quality and the utility of the images (29,30).

Integration with the Medical Linear Accelerator

The generation of a CBCT image is an important feature of the imaging system, however, it is of equal importance that these images be easily acquired with the patient

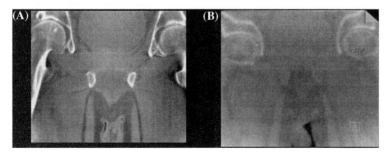

Figure 3 Cone-beam CT images of the prostate and surrounding anatomy generated using (**A**) kV cone-beam CT (Elekta XVI) and (**B**) MV cone-beam CT (Siemens MVision). These are generated with comparable imaging doses.

positioned for treatment. This requires that the imaging systems be well integrated with the medical linear accelerator. The need for rapid acquisition and seamless registration is clear; however, the central issues are geometric precision and accuracy in detection and correction.

Accuracy and Precision

The adaptation of CBCT systems to the medical linear accelerator initially raised concerns regarding the geometric integrity of the systems, both in terms of CBCT image quality and the registration of the resulting volumes to the coordinate system of the treatment unit. However, studies are demonstrating that these systems can be reliably calibrated and are capable of maintaining calibration over long time intervals (24,31). These studies suggest that the intrinsic accuracy and precision are sub-mm for unambiguous targeting tasks (e.g., Lutz-type BB phantoms) (32). These results have been verified in patient studies involving markers by comparing the alignment results of CBCT images to those produced by portal imaging methods (33). Overall, the geometric precision and accuracy of these systems is proving to be excellent with monitoring through a suitable quality assurance program (34).

Image-Guidance System

In addition to the geometric performance, there are several additional features that need to be present if volumetric targeting is to be achieved. These include the ability to overlay reference grayscale images and reference structures of interest. Automated tools to first detect bony anatomy and then identify soft tissue target offsets are an excellent way to bound allowable corrections during the online guidance procedure. The use of this approach can be used to limit displacements relative to bone in excess of some limit (e.g., 20 mm) and avoid alignment to the wrong structures. The use of subregions or "clip-boxes" to improve the registration to local structures is a valuable addition to these systems. This can be taken further with the use of automated prostate-specific localization methods (29). Once a registration has been performed, a correction must be derived by either adjusting the patient position or altering the machine parameters. For nonrotational couch corrections, any detected rotation in the registration must be accommodated in the translations. This requires the identification of a reference point at which it is desired that the rotation-induced residual error is minimized (35). The appropriate couch correction can then be transferred to the treatment unit for automated adjustment of the couch. Overall, these systems are becoming highly integrated, such that, the time required for CBCT online imaging and correction is equivalent to the time required for conventional online portal imaging based approaches (Princess Margaret Hospital, Internal Study).

Dosimetry

The use of CBCT in the guidance of prostate therapy results in a dose penalty that needs consideration. In the context of kV CBCT, these doses are distinct from the therapy dose. The energy of the kV beam is typically ~ 120 kilovolt peak (kVp) and as a result, the biological effect of the dose deposited during imaging is not easily interpreted in the context of the tumor control and normal tissue toxicity. However, this does not indicate that imaging doses should not be documented and minimized. Recent publications have reported on the imaging doses associated with kV CBCT (36–38) and the AAPM Task Group No. 75 describes the dose from a variety of radiographic image-guidance systems (39). Chow et al. have recently published a report describing the combined dose from kV CBCT imaging and therapy for a typical course of prostate treatment using daily online imaging and soft tissue guidance (40). The doses were calculated using Monte Carlo methods and accumulated. The differential dose to the bone and soft tissue structures is evident, however, these doses remain low relative to the dose from the therapy beam. Currently, imaging doses delivered for prostate gland visualization in kV CBCT of the prostate is approximately 3 cGy at isocenter per scan. It should be noted that these "quoted doses" are dependent on many variables (energy, FOV, offset geometry, use of bow-tie filter) and published quantities are no substitute for measurements that correspond to the specific technique.

USE OF CBCT FOR IMAGE-GUIDED RADIATION THERAPY OF THE PROSTATE

Online Guidance Models

The online guidance approach involves detecting and (if necessary) correcting the relative position of the prostate and treatment isocenter on a fraction-by-fraction basis. Such a method requires that all the elements of the process are highly streamlined and sufficient performance is achieved in the imaging to allow accurate and precise estimation of the gland. At the Princess Margaret Hospital, online IGRT of the prostate using CBCT has been employed in patients with and without implanted fiducial markers in the gland. This is based upon observer studies of online alignment of IGRT of the prostate with the Elekta Synergy system (33). These studies compared the appropriate couch correction for 16 prostate patients imaged and treated on the CBCT-equipped system. These corrections were derived from either gland-template (i.e., soft tissue) alignment or marker-marker alignment. The soft tissue–determined corrections did not agree precisely with that determined from the markers, however, the two systems demonstrated excellent agreement in their mean shifts for any patient. The discrepancy between marker and soft tissue results was consistent with the degree of interobserver variations found in a parallel study. Based on these results, the use of CBCT for targeting RT of the prostate is now a consideration. The agreement in mean position between the marker and soft tissue results suggests that both methods are equally good at reducing the systematic errors, which is the dominant source of the margin in these cases. It should be noted that the use of soft tissue alignment at the treatment unit opens the potential for introduction of systematic errors of another variety— systematic differences in the interpretation of the gland outline in the grayscale images. This can be resolved by the physician (that specified the gland) and the therapist (that align each day) reviewing the initial alignments to assure consistency between the GTV and target structures in the CBCT image.

The use of MV CBCT for online guidance of prostate RT has not been reported in the literature, however, it is quite reasonable to pursue this if fiducials are employed. The high contrast of these objects would allow precise and accurate localization at low doses. Soft tissue targeting may require unacceptably high imaging doses. The inclusion of these doses in the planning process may permit this to be pursued, provided the imaging dose is appropriately accommodated (41). Further developments in lower-energy beams using low–atomic number targets may also serve to further reduce the dose required for soft tissue localization.

At this point, the use of markers continues for targeting the prostate gland. The significant adoption of this approach since the development of online electronic portal imaging devices has produced a clinical practice that is well equipped to switch to soft tissue targeting. It is not clear how long this approach will persist, but it is likely to transition as image quality in CBCT continues to improve. The development of hypofractionated regimens will also drive the use of soft tissue targeting where visualization of the gland and normal tissues may be of interest for each fraction. Clearly, this will increase the time required to assess the images and may alter the workflow and delegation issues.

Off-Line Guidance Models

The Beaumont Approach (42,43) is an alternative and mature approach that readily adopts CBCT for off-line image guidance. In the original embodiment of this approach, the systematic and random characteristics of prostate position and shape are captured through repeat CT scans in the first week of therapy. This approach has now been adapted to employ CBCT as the source of data (44). In the recent report, the advantages of extending the adaptive process to include online components are described. The Netherlands Cancer Institute has recently reported on their adaptive approach using CBCT (30). An average PTV reduction of 29% was achieved with the volume of the rectum that received >65 Gy reduced by 19% on average. These processes require high-quality CBCT images for segmentation of the structures of interest (prostate, rectal wall), as opposed to isocenter alignment and localization employed in a simple online approach. Overall, the quality of the images produced with these types of systems make these approaches feasible (45). The growing interest in hypofractionated schedules will place additional pressure on adopting an online strategy. This does not mean that the principles of adaptation will not be employed to deal with the issue of intrafraction motion (46).

Hybrid Models

The distinction between online and off-line approaches is somewhat arbitrary. The magnitude and frequency of variations in gland and rectal wall configuration that can occur over the course of therapy suggest that a hybrid approach may be beneficial. Such approaches have been proposed in the past (47). Figure 4 presents a process for which the original CBCT-equipped treatment unit was designed. This process separated the translational, rotational, and deformational elements of the prostate movements to be managed by three different methods: (*i*) the online couch correction was used to adjust displacements of the prostate apex, (*ii*) multiple prestored plans were indexed to accommodate the presence of rotations, and (*iii*) an ongoing accumulation of the "database of fractions" allowed patient-specific adaptation of deformation to be fed back into an off-line process of replanning. While this approach is still beyond the technical capacity of any commercial radiation therapy management system, all the subcomponents are now available. One example of the advancements that are at the forefront of this effort has been reported by Smitsman et al. (29). In their investigations, registration success rates in excess of 80% were achieved provided rectal gas was managed through an appropriate diet. Another example is taken from the same group. Rijkhorst et al. describe an alternative approach to correct for prostate rotations employing collimator and gantry angle rotations (48).

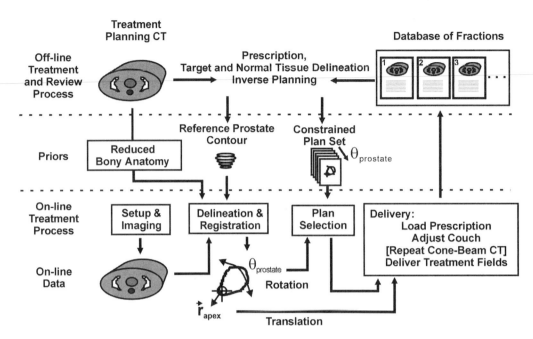

Figure 4 Flow chart for a proposed high-precision image-guidance system. The off-line planning process and preparation of priors produce reference contours and a constrained plan set. In the online process, the prostate is rapidly delineated and registered from a CBCT image, and the prostate rotation and translation determine the selected plan and couch adjustment, respectively. An optional repeat CBCT image acquired immediately prior to and/or after delivery would provide the most accurate representation of the treatment. Image data are stored in a database for off-line review of prostate and rectal doses and re-evaluation of the predefined plan set. *Abbreviation*: CBCT, cone-beam computed tomography.

Other Issues

The ability for soft tissue visualization can also impact the approach taken in planning and image guidance. Two areas of interest that have not been employed with CBCT image guidance include rectal avoidance and subprostatic boost. Literature on these concepts have been presented for the tomotherapy paradigm (49) and marker-based approaches (50). It is highly likely that these approaches will be pursued using CBCT methods. Another example of novel applications of this technology is in the targeting of postprostatectomy patients (51). In this context, the visualization of surrounding normal tissues is more relevant for image guidance. Showater and Valicenti evaluated some 176 CBCT study sets revealing that rectal and bladder borders were reliably identified in 94% of the image sets. These results are encouraging and support the application of CBCT methods in the management of prostate cancer.

An important and concerning development associated with the introduction of soft tissue imaging in the clinical setting is in the need for retraining and skill development. Broad use of CBCT will result in the radiation therapists at the treatment units dealing with an order of magnitude more volumetric with imaging data than their counterparts in the planning process (dosimetrists, planners). These images are open to interpretation and skills need to be developed to properly evaluate these images and maximize their benefit to the patient.

SUMMARY OF PERTINENT CONCLUSIONS

- The development of more volumetric with imaging data in prostate radiation therapy is maturing at a remarkable rate.
- In the past five years, we have seen a rapid transition from bone-based alignment to online markers, and now to soft tissue targeting.
- The broad deployment of CBCT technology assures that this trend will continue at a rapid pace.
- The inherent challenge of treating the prostate gland in its surrounding radiosensitive milieu makes the application of these technologies sensible and appropriate.
- Further improvements in image quality will make this a simple and broadly practiced method for assuring precise and accurate targeting in prostate radiation therapy.

REFERENCES

1. Pilepich MV, Prasad SC, Perez CA. Computed tomography in definitive radiotherapy of prostatic carcinoma, part 2: definition of target volume. Int J Radiat Oncol Biol Phys 1982; 8(2):235–239.
2. Beard CJ, Kijewski P, BussiŠre M, et al. Analysis of prostate and seminal vesicle motion: implications for treatment planning. Int J Radiat Oncol Biol Phys 1996; 34:451.
3. Crook JM, Raymond Y, Salhani D, et al. Prostate motion during standard radiotherapy as assessed by fiducial markers. Radiother Oncol 1995; 37(1):35–42.
4. Ghilezan MJ, Jaffray DA, Siewerdsen JH, et al. Prostate gland motion assessed with cine-magnetic resonance imaging (cine-MRI). Int J Radiat Oncol Biol Phys 2005; 62(2): 406–417.
5. Huang E, Dong L, Chandra A, et al. Intrafraction prostate motion during IMRT for prostate cancer. Int J Radiat Oncol Biol Phys 2002; 53(2):261–268.
6. Langen KM, Jones DT. Organ motion and its management. Int J Radiat Oncol Biol Phys 2001; 50(1):265–278.
7. Balter JM, Kwok LL, Sandler HM, et al. Automated localization of the prostate at the time of treatment using implanted radiopaque markers: technical feasibility. Int J Radiat Oncol Biol Phys 1995; 33:1281.
8. Balter JM, Lam KL, Sandler HM, et al. Automated tracking of prostate position using on-line portal imaging. Med Phys 1994; 21:951.
9. Balter JM, Sandler HM, Lam K, et al. Measurement of prostate movement over the course of routine radiotherapy using implanted markers. Int J Radiat Oncol Biol Phys 1995; 31(1):113–118.
10. Chung PW, Haycocks T, Brown T, et al. On-line aSi portal imaging of implanted fiducial markers for the reduction of interfraction error during conformal radiotherapy of prostate carcinoma. Int J Radiat Oncol Biol Phys 2004; 60(1): 329–334.
11. Gilhuijs KG, van de Ven PJ, van Herk M. Automatic three-dimensional inspection of patient setup in radiation therapy using portal images, simulator images, and computed tomography data. Med Phys 1996; 23(3):389–399.
12. Nederveen A, Lagendijk J, Hofman P. Detection of fiducial gold markers for automatic on-line megavoltage position verification using a marker extraction kernel (MEK). Int J Radiat Oncol Biol Phys 2000; 47(5):1435–1442.
13. Vigneault E, Pouliot J, Laverdiere J, et al. Electronic portal imaging device detection of radioopaque markers for the evaluation of prostate position during megavoltage irradiation: a clinical study. Int J Radiat Oncol Biol Phys 1997; 37(1):205–212.
14. Nichol AM, Brock KK, Lockwood GA, et al. A magnetic resonance imaging study of prostate deformation relative to implanted gold fiducial markers. Int J Radiat Oncol Biol Phys 2007; 67(1):48–56.
15. Antonuk LE, Boudry JM, El-Mohri Y, et al. Large area, flat-panel, amorphous silicon imagers. SPIE 1995; 2432:216.
16. Cho PS, Johnson RH, Griffin TW. Cone-beam CT for radiotherapy applications. Phys Med Biol 1995; 40(11): 1863–1883.

17. Jaffray DA, Siewerdsen JH. Cone-beam computed tomography with a flat-panel imager: initial performance characterization. Med Phys 2000; 27(6):1311–1323.
18. Feldkamp LA, Davis LC, Kress JW. Practical cone-beam algorithm. J Opt Soc Am 1984; 1:612–619.
19. Antonuk LE, Yorkston J, Huang W, et al. Megavoltage imaging with a large-area, plat-panel, amorphous silicon imager. Int J Radiat Oncol Biol Phy 1996; 36:661.
20. Pouliot J, Bani-Hashemi A, Chen J, et al. Low-dose megavoltage cone-beam CT for radiation therapy. Int J Radiat Oncol Biol Phys 2005; 61(2):552–560.
21. Jaffray DA, Siewerdsen JH, Wong JW, et al. Flat-panel cone-beam computed tomography for image-guided radiation therapy. Int J Radiat Oncol Biol Phys 2002; 53(5): 1337–1349.
22. Jaffray DA, Drake DG, Moreau M, et al. A radiographic and tomographic imaging system integrated into a medical linear accelerator for localization of bone and soft-tissue targets. Int J Radiat Oncol Biol Phys 1999; 45(3):773–789.
23. McBain CA, Henry AM, Sykes J, et al. X-ray volumetric imaging in image-guided radiotherapy: the new standard in on-treatment imaging. Int J Radiat Oncol Biol Phys 2006; 64(2):625–634.
24. Yoo S, Kim GY, Hammoud R, et al. A quality assurance program for the on-board imagers. Med Phys 2006; 33(11): 4431–4447.
25. Moseley DJ, Siewersen JH, Jaffray DA. High-contrast object localization and removal in cone-beam CT. In: SPIE. San Diego, CA, 2006.
26. Mosleh-Shirazi MA, Evans PM, Swindell W, et al. A cone-beam megavoltage CT scanner for treatment verification in conformal radiotherapy. Radiother Oncol 1998; 48(3):319–328.
27. Jaffray DA, Munro P, Fenster A, et al. X-ray scatter in megavoltage transmission radiography: physical characteristics and influence on image quality. Med Phys 1994; 21:45.
28. Siewerdsen JH, Jaffray DA. Cone-beam computed tomography with a flat-panel imager: magnitude and effects of x-ray scatter. Med Phys 2001; 28(2):220–231.
29. Smitsmans MH, de Bois J, Sonke JJ, et al. Automatic prostate localization on cone-beam CT scans for high precision image-guided radiotherapy. Int J Radiat Oncol Biol Phys 2005; 63(4):975–984.
30. Nijkamp J, Pos FJ, Nuver TT, et al. Adaptive radiotherapy for prostate cancer using kilovoltage cone-beam computed tomography: first clinical results. Int J Radiat Oncol Biol Phys 2008; 70(1):75–82 [Epub September 17, 2007].
31. Sharpe MB, Moseley DJ, Purdie TG, et al. The stability of mechanical calibration for a kV cone beam computed tomography system integrated with linear accelerator. Med Phys 2006; 33(1):136–144.
32. Yenice KM, Lovelock DM, Hunt MA, et al. CT image-guided intensity-modulated therapy for paraspinal tumors using stereotactic immobilization. Int J Radiat Oncol Biol Phys 2003; 55(3):583–593.
33. Moseley DJ, White EA, Wiltshire KL, et al. Comparison of localization performance with implanted fiducial markers and cone-beam computed tomography for on-line image-guided radiotherapy of the prostate. Int J Radiat Oncol Biol Phys 2007; 67(3):942–953.

34. Jaffray D, Bissonnette J-P, Craig, T. Modern Technology of Radiation Oncology, Volume 2 Medical Physics Publishing, Madison, Wisconsin 2005, ISBN: 9781930524255.

35. Guckenberger M, Meyer J, Wilbert J, et al. Precision of image-guided radiotherapy (IGRT) in six degrees of freedom and limitations in clinical practice. Strahlenther Onkol 2007; 183(6):307–313.

36. Islam MK, Purdie TG, Norrlinger BD, et al. Patient dose from kilovoltage cone beam computed tomography imaging in radiation therapy. Med Phys 2006; 33(6):1573–1582.

37. Amer A, Marchant T, Sykes J, et al. Imaging doses from the Elekta Synergy X-ray cone beam CT system. Br J Radiol 2007; 80(954):476–482.

38. Wen N, Guan H, Hammoud R, et al. Dose delivered from Varian's CBCT to patients receiving IMRT for prostate cancer. Phys Med Biol 2007; 52(8):2267–2276.

39. Murphy M, Balter JM, Balter S, et al. The management of imaging dose during image-guided radiotherapy: report of the AAPM Task Group 75. Med Phys 2007; 34(10):4041–4061.

40. Chow JC, Leung MKK, Norrlinger BD, Islam M, et al. Evaluation of the effect of patient dose from cone-beam computed tomography on prostate IMRT using Monte Carlo simulation. Med Phys 35(1): pp. 52–60.

41. Morin O, Gillis A, Descovich M, et al. Patient dose considerations for routine megavoltage cone-beam CT imaging. Med Phys 2007; 34(5):1819–1827.

42. Yan D, Lockman D, Brabbins D, et al. An off-line strategy for constructing a patient-specific planning target volume in adaptive treatment process for prostate cancer. Int J Radiat Oncol Biol Phys 2000; 48(1):289–302.

43. Yan D, Vicini F, Wong J, et al. Adaptive radiation therapy. Phys Med Biol 1997; 42(1):123–132.

44. Wu Q, Liang J, Yan D. Application of dose compensation in image-guided radiotherapy of prostate cancer. Phys Med Biol 2006; 51(6):1405–1419.

45. Ding GX, Duggan DM, Coffey CW, et al. A study on adaptive IMRT treatment planning using kV cone-beam CT. Radiother Oncol 2007; 85(1):116–125 [Epub August 20, 2007].

46. Litzenberg DW, Balter JM, Hadley SW, et al. Influence of intrafraction motion on margins for prostate radiotherapy. Int J Radiat Oncol Biol Phys 2006; 65(2):548–553.

47. Jaffray D, Van Herk M, Lebesque JV, et al. Image-guided radiotherapy of the prostate. In: MICCAI 2002. Utrecht, Netherlands, 2002.

48. Rijkhorst EJ, van Herk M, Lebesque JV, et al. Strategy for online correction of rotational organ motion for intensity-modulated radiotherapy of prostate cancer. Int J Radiat Oncol Biol Phys 2007; 69(5):1608–1617 [Epub October 4, 2007].

49. Mackie TR, Kapatoes J, Ruchala K, et al. Image guidance for precise conformal radiotherapy. Int J Radiat Oncol Biol Phys 2003; 56(1):89–105.

50. Nederveen AJ, Lagendijk JJ, Hofman P. Feasibility of automatic marker detection with an a-Si flat-panel imager. Phys Med Biol 2001; 46(4):1219–1230.

51. Showalter TN, Nawaz AO, Xiao Y, et al. A cone beam CT-based study for clinical target definition using pelvic anatomy during postprostatectomy radiotherapy. Int J Radiat Oncol Biol Phys 2008; 70(2):431–436.

10

IGRT in Prostate Cancer: Focus on BAT Ultrasound

JOSHUA S. SILVERMAN AND ERIC M. HORWITZ

Department of Radiation Oncology, Fox Chase Cancer Center, Philadelphia, Pennsylvania, U.S.A.

INTRODUCTION

History of Daily Image Localization at Fox Chase Cancer Center

The development of three-dimensional conformal radiation therapy (3DCRT) and its use in the treatment of prostate cancer began in the late 1980s at Fox Chase Cancer Center as Gerald Hanks and colleagues sought to more precisely deliver increasing doses of external beam radiation to the prostate while limiting the toxicities to adjacent structures. Early results were promising as biochemical control increased compared with patients treated with conventional techniques and doses as the radiation dose was increased (1). However, with these increasing control rates came increasing complications, especially in the rectum adjacent to the prostate. Initially, a lateral rectal block was added after 5600 cGy to reduce complications (2).

As more patients were treated with higher doses of radiation across the country and CT simulators and simulations became more widespread, the issue of organ motion was recognized. With this realization came the acknowledgment that to safely deliver ever higher doses of radiation, this phenomenon would need to be controlled. The development of B-mode acquisition and targeting (BAT) ultrasound emerged from the goal of obtaining an easy-to-use, reproducible, and robust method of accurately localizing the prostate and adjacent critical structures in real time prior to daily radiation treatment.

The Rationale for Image Guidance

There are several rationales for the use of daily image-guided radiation therapy (IGRT) in the management of prostate cancer. The ability to consistently and reproducibly deliver the prescribed dose of radiation to the target is the most obvious reason. Another reason is the ability to safely escalate radiation dose. The first reports illustrating this dose response appeared in 1995, and since that time, multiple single-institution prospective, retrospective, and phase III randomized prospective trials have confirmed this phenomenon in prostate cancer. These studies have consistently demonstrated an improvement in biochemical control as an increasing dose of radiation is delivered to the prostate (1,3,4). Finally, IGRT allows for the limiting of dose to adjacent critical structures and the reduction of early and late complications. Dose-volume effects have been described in the literature for both the bladder and rectum (5,6).

Because of dose-volume relations of critical structures, either conformality must be increased or the planning target volume (PTV) must be reduced when dose escalation is done, and either of these necessitates more accurate localization and verification of the target (prostate). Movement of the prostate with respect to bladder and rectal filling has been observed and characterized by several authors and similar patterns have been described (7–9). Large shifts in prostate position are associated with rectal gas pockets and can be produced from the introduction of 50 mL of contrast into the rectum (10,11). Zelefsky et al. report that rectal volume greater than 60 cm^3 and bladder volume greater than 40 cm^3 are the only independent predictors of prostate shifts greater than 3 mm (12).

THE FOX CHASE TECHNIQUE FOR ULTRASOUND-GUIDED PROSTATE IGRT

Simulation

In preparation for treatment, patients are simulated in a supine position in a cast mold of their pelvis with an ankle block. Patients are simulated with a full bladder (consuming 12–16 oz water within several hours of simulation) and empty rectum (magnesium citrate bowel preparation and, occasionally, an additional Fleet's enema). Patients are simulated using CT and MRI unless there is a contraindication to performing an MRI. A slice thickness of 3 mm is used for both scans. The scans are fused in the planning computer based on bony and soft tissue anatomy using either chamfer matching or maximization of mutual information methods. The structures outlined include the prostate, seminal vesicles, rectum (from ischial tuberosity to the sigmoid flexure), the entire bladder, and the bilateral femoral heads. The clinical tumor volume (CTV) is defined as the prostate and the proximal seminal vesicles (the first 9 mm of the seminal vesicles). The CTV is expanded by 5 to 6 mm posteriorly and 8 mm in all other directions to produce the PTV. Triangulation tattoos and the use of a cradle cast ensure efficient and reproducible daily setup and initial alignment prior to the use of BAT ultrasound daily localization. The radiation dose and targets prescribed depend on the stage of cancer (13).

Once the planning is complete and the patient is ready for treatment, the contoured images are imported into the BAT ultrasound system over a local area network (LAN). Prior to the patient entering the treatment room, the ultrasound system is moved adjacent to the treatment couch and is docked to the treatment machine collimator, and the CT- and MRI-simulation target images and isocenter are imported into the BAT system. Since 2000, intensity-modulated radiation therapy is used exclusively for all prostate cancer patients treated with external beam radiation therapy.

Daily Setup and Alignment

The BAT ultrasound system consists of a B-mode transabdominal arm attached to a precision tracking arm and connected to a computer (Fig. 1). The computer shows the real-time images from the ultrasound probe and the outlines of the image-guided contours. The BAT ultrasound

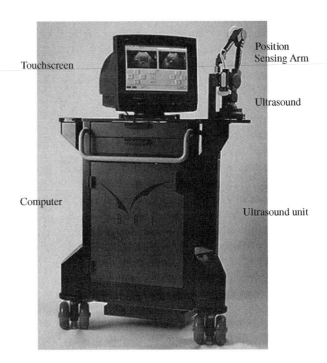

Figure 1 The BAT ultrasound equipment. The ultrasound probe is connected to a computer that enables proper alignment prior to daily treatment. *Abbreviation*: BAT, B-mode acquisition and targeting.

system uses the treatment machine isocenter as a reference point to overlay corresponding CT contours onto the ultrasound images.

Daily setup using BAT ultrasound is accomplished as follows. The patient is aligned to the simulation tattoos. Weekly portal images are used to verify that the patient's

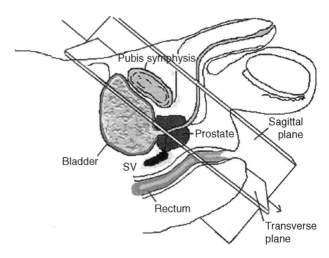

Figure 2 Ultrasound plans. The sagittal and transverse ultrasound planes commonly used for BAT ultrasound are depicted in the figure. *Abbreviation*: BAT, B-mode acquisition and targeting.

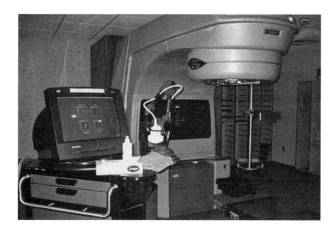

Figure 3 The BAT ultrasound in clinical practice. The ultrasound cabinet is moved adjacent to the treatment couch prior to the initiation of radiotherapy. *Abbreviation*: BAT, B-mode acquisition and targeting.

alignment corresponds to the bony anatomy of the pelvis. The patient's CT data set is chosen from a pull-down menu on the computer console and the suprapubic BAT ultrasound procedure is initiated. Typical BAT ultrasound settings are 3.5 MHz, 60% power, 80% gain, and 14-cm depth. Real-time imaging is available on the display screen. The BAT probe recognizes its three-dimensional location with respect to the machine isocenter as transverse and sagittal images are taken (Fig. 2). The BAT

probe is performed with the patient in the treatment position on the treatment couch (Fig. 3). The transverse and sagittal contours are moved by the operator using a touch-screen menu to overlay the images so that the ultrasound and contoured CT-derived images are brought into register (Fig. 4A, B) Fine (1.0 mm) and coarse (1.0 cm) adjustments can be made. The system then calculates the necessary couch shifts and displays them so that the couch can be adjusted prior to initiation of radiotherapy by the radiation therapist. If a large shift is required, the BAT ultrasound alignment is repeated to verify the accuracy of the necessary shift.

Morr et al. describes the appearance of the various anatomic structures using BAT ultrasound (14). The bladder is anechoic (dark) and prostate is of intermediate echogenicity. The bladder wall, bladder/prostate interface (difficult to determine), prostate, and rectum are hyperechoic. Often, angulation of the ultrasound probe (approximately 10°–50°) is required in the caudal direction. With BAT, the apex of the prostate is not easily seen in the sagittal image because of interference from the pubic bone. Image quality is best when scanning the widest extent of the prostate in the transverse plane and along the urethral axis in the sagittal plane (15). The probe is moved superiorly and angled inferiorly if the prostate was overshadowed by the pubic symphysis in the transverse plane. In the sagittal plane, only the base of the prostate can be fully visualized, even if the ultrasound probe is moved superiorly.

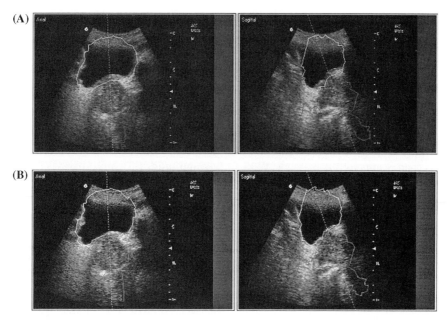

Figure 4 BAT ultrasound daily treatment alignment. The computer allows the BAT ultrasound images to be correlated with contours of the prostate, bladder, and rectum. The preshift images (**A**) illustrate the need for a shift to obtain the proper alignment (**B**). Once a shift is approved, couch shifts are given as an output and used prior to the initiation of radiotherapy. *Abbreviation*: BAT, B-mode acquisition and targeting.

Fox Chase Pilot Studies with CT and Ultrasound Guidance

At Fox Chase, early studies using image guidance in conjunction with 3DCRT utilized CT imaging (15–17). In the first study, six patients who consented to this prospective study underwent daily CT simulations to assess setup variations in portal placement and organ motion supine position. These patients underwent CT simulation with an alpha cradle immobilization, intravenous contrast, and urethrograms to determine if improved prostate localization techniques could allow for the reduction of margins around the target to facilitate dose escalation in high-risk patients while minimizing the risk of normal tissue morbidity. Patients received 46 Gy to the initial planning treatment volume (PTV1) in a four-field conformal technique with the prostate, seminal vesicles, and lymph nodes as the gross tumor volume. The prostate or prostate and seminal vesicles (GTV2) then received 56 Gy to PTV2. After five weeks of treatment (50 Gy), a second CT simulation was performed. The prostate was contoured and a new isocenter was generated with appropriate surface markers. Prostate-only treatment portals were used for the final cone down. The daily isocenter was recalculated in the anterior-posterior (A-P) and lateral dimensions and compared to the 50 Gy CT simulation isocenter. The patients were transferred to a stretcher while on the sliding board in the cast and transported to the treatment room and carefully transferred to the treatment table. The patients were then treated to the corrected isocenter. Portal films and electronic portal images were obtained for each field. Utilizing CT-CT image fusions of the daily and 50-Gy baseline CT scans, the isocenter changes were quantified to reflect the contribution of positional and absolute prostate motion relative to the bony pelvis. The maximum daily A-P shift was 7.3 mm. Motion was less than 5 mm in the remaining patients, and the overall mean magnitude change was 2.9 mm. The overall variability was quantified by a pooled standard deviation of 1.7 mm. The maximum lateral shifts were less than 3 mm for all patients. With careful attention to patient positioning, maximal portal placement error was reduced to 3 mm. On the basis of this study, the authors concluded that prostate motion after 50 Gy was significantly less than previously reported. Intrapatient and overall population variance was minimal. With daily isocenter correction of setup and organ motion errors by CT imaging, Lattanzi et al. concluded that PTV margins can be significantly reduced or eliminated (16).

The second study introduced the BAT ultrasound technology and compared results with those observed with daily CT scans to determine the precision of ultrasound localization with respect to CT scans. Thirty-five consecutive men were prospectively studied in a comparison of daily CT and ultrasound-guided localization at Fox Chase Cancer Center. Daily CT prostate localization was completed before the delivery of each final boost field. In the CT simulation suite, transabdominal ultrasound-based stereotactic localization was also performed. Sixty-nine daily CT and ultrasound prostate position shifts were recorded for 35 patients. The average directed discrepancies between the two techniques were extremely small. There were -0.09 ± 2.8 mm in the A-P axis, -0.16 ± 2.4 mm in the left-right (L-R) axis, and -0.03 ± 2.3 mm in the superior-inferior (S-I) axis. Analysis of the paired CT-ultrasound shifts revealed a high correlation between the two modalities in all three dimensions. This was the first study to demonstrate that ultrasound-directed stereotactic localization was safe and accurate compared with CT scanning in targeting the prostate for conformal external beam radiation therapy (15).

The final Fox Chase ultrasound study quantified the magnitude of the patient isocenter shift parameters encountered during clinical implementation of the BAT ultrasound-based targeting system. In this study, 54 patients underwent a second CT simulation following five weeks of 3DCRT. For each of the final cone-down treatments (2–4 fractions), patients underwent ultrasound-based stereotactic prostate localization at the treatment machine. One hundred and eighty-nine daily ultrasound prostate position shifts were recorded. The isocenter field misalignment between the baseline CT and ultrasound ranged from -26.8 to 33.8 mm in the A-P axis, -10.2 to 30.9 mm in the L-R axis, and -24.6 to 9.0 mm in the S-I axis. The corresponding directed average disagreements were -3.0 ± 8.3 mm, 1.86 ± 5.7 mm, and -2.6 ± 6.5 mm in the A-P, L-R, and S-I axes, respectively. The magnitudes of the misalignments were frequently larger than 5 mm (51%, 31%, and 35% of measurements in the A-P, L-R, and S-I axes, respectively) and occasionally larger than 10 mm (21%, 7%, and 12% of measurements in the A-P, L-R, and S-I axes, respectively). Similar to the previous study described, there was a high correlation between the ultrasound and CT modalities. This initial Fox Chase experience with the BAT system in a large cohort of prostate cancer patients revealed that substantial daily isocenter corrections were encountered in a large percentage of cases. This data suggested that daily clinical isocenter misalignments are greater than would be expected from published data on organ motion and setup variations encountered in the study setting (17,18).

The Evolving Use of BAT IGRT versus Alternative Methods

BAT ultrasound is one of the several daily localization modalities described for IGRT in prostate cancer (19–21).

Other modalities include portal images with a megavolt imager (22), daily CT using either cone-beam CT or CT-on-rails (7,8,12,16,23–25), gold seed fiducial markers (20,26–29), rectal balloons, and real-time tracking beacons (30,31).

The Use of BAT Ultrasound in Current Practice at Fox Chase Cancer Center

Since 1990, daily localization has been a mainstay of prostate cancer treatment for clinically localized prostate cancer at Fox Chase Cancer Center. Weekly electronic portal imaging has been used in conjunction with BAT ultrasound to verify accuracy of the initial patient setup to bony landmarks of the pelvis prior to ultrasound localization. More recently, gold seed fiducial markers and real-time Calypso tracking beacons have been incorporated as modalities for IGRT at Fox Chase. BAT ultrasound is typically reserved for those who cannot receive Calypso beacons, such as those with an implanted pacemaker or defibrillator and those with a body thickness greater than 23 cm that precludes beacon detection. Anticoagulation is a relative contraindication for beacon placement. BAT ultrasound cannot be used in obese men since obesity leads to poor images. Gold seed fiducial markers are used in those for whom Calypso beacons and BAT ultrasound are not appropriate.

BAT ultrasound for daily localization offers advantages that other IGRT modalities do not. Ultrasound can be used to assess the reproducibility of bladder and rectal filling. The current Fox Chase policy is to treat patients with a full bladder. BAT ultrasound provides information regarding bladder and rectal filling that other daily localization modalities do not, except for volumetric imaging methods such as cone-beam CT. Patients can be coached regarding appropriate fluid intake, and an assessment can be made of the degree of rectal filling. Fiducial markers, rectal balloons, and Calypso beacons are all invasive techniques.

OPTIMIZING IGRT IMPLEMENTATION IN PROSTATE CANCER: IGRT QUALITY CONTROL

In the era of reducing dosimetric margins using 3DCRT and IMRT for prostate cancer, an analysis of BAT ultrasound is critical in determining errors associated with organ motion. Attempts at establishing adequate margins must account for inter- and intrafraction variation. The following discussion includes the various quantitative and qualitative analysis of couch shifts determined by BAT ultrasound and quality control issues related to ultrasound-based daily localization.

Interfraction Daily Couch Shifts

There are numerous published single institution experiences documenting interfraction couch shifts using BAT ultrasound (Table 1) (32,33). Couch shifts are given in the A-P, S-I, and L-R axes. From a review of the data, several themes emerge. First, couch shifts tend to be greater in the A-P and S-I axes in comparison to the L-R axis. This is consistent with a model in which daily prostate motion is most affected by the degree and variability of bladder and rectal filling. This suggests that optimal dosimetric margins must not necessarily reflect uniform expansion of the prostate volume. Interfraction couch shifts approximate a Gaussian distribution in frequency-shift histograms (14,34–36). Dosimetric margins must account for interfraction variation in couch shifts (which reflect organ motion), if complete coverage of the target (prostate) is desired.

Comparison of the magnitude and variance in single institution experiences of BAT ultrasound may be confounded by differences in immobilization technique, image modalities used for contouring (CT vs. MRI vs. CT-MRI fusion), and factors affecting the degree of bladder and rectal filling (e.g., protocol for fluid intake and bowel preparation).

Table 1 Interfraction Shifts Using BAT Ultrasound in the Treatment of Prostate Cancer

Study	Number of patients	A-P mean ± SD (mm)	S-I mean ± SD (mm)	R-L mean ± SD (mm)
Lattanzi et al. (1999)	23	0.2 ± 4.6	0.0 ± 5.7	0.1 ± 3.4
Serago et al. (2002)	38	1.3 ± 4.7	1.0 ± 5.1	0.3 ± 2.5
Morr et al. (2002)	19	4.7 ± 2.7	4.2 ± 2.8	−2.6 ± 2.1
Huang et al. (2002)	20	0.4 ± 4.0	−1.5 ± 3.3	0.4 ± 2.2
Langen et al. (2003)	10	−0.7 ± 5.2	2.7 ± 4.5	1.8 ± 3.9
Trichter et al. (2003)	26	0.32 ± 0.6	0.31 ± 0.7	0.32 ± 0.5
Little et al. (2003)	35	−1.4 ± 6.4	−1.7 ± 6.4	−0.82 ± 3.2
Chandra et al. (2003)	147	−0.49 ± 1.9	0.59 ± 3.4	0.92 ± 3.2

Abbreviations: BAT, B-mode acquisition and targeting; A-P, anterior-posterior; S-I, superior-inferior; R-L, right-left.

Table 2 Comparison of BAT Ultrasound Daily Shifts with Shifts Using Other Daily Treatment Modalities in the Treatment of Prostate Cancer

Study	Number of patients	A-P mean ± SD (mm)	S-I mean ± SD (mm)	R-L mean ± SD (mm)
A. BAT ultrasound shifts compared to daily CT scan				
Lattanzi et al. (1999)	25	3 ± 1.8	4.6 ± 2.8	2.4 ± 1.8
Lattanzi et al. (2000)	35	−0.09 ± 2.8	−0.03 ± 2.3	−0.16 ± 2.4
B. BAT ultrasound shifts compared to fiducial marker shifts				
Langen et al. 2003	10	0.2 ± 3.7	2.7 ± 3.9	1.6 ± 3.1
McNair et al. (2006)	26	3.2 ± 3.2	−3.3 ± 3.5	−2.2 ± 3.7

Abbreviations: BAT, B-mode acquisition and targeting; A-P, anterior-posterior; S-I, superior-inferior; R-L, right-left.

Comparison with Other Localization Modalities

The comparison of ultrasound-based daily localization to other modalities addresses questions of the reproducibility of daily localization and the possible existence of systematic errors between treatment modalities. Studies have compared the shifts of ultrasound with daily CT imaging (Table 2A) and with fiducial markers (Table 2B). A recent study from Fox Chase examined BAT ultrasound to CT-on-rails measurements (37). Two hundred and eighteen alignments in 15 patients revealed a high level of correlation between BAT ultrasound and CT-on-rails with systematic differences of less than 1 mm and random differences of about 2 mm. A comparison between the magnitude and variation of interfraction couch shifts with ultrasound alone versus alternate modality shifts revealed that the magnitude of shifts was similar between the various daily localization techniques for IGRT.

Interuser Variability

Interuser variability has also been examined in the literature. McNair et al. report interuser differences between three observers, with the proportion of readings over 3 mm between the observers being in the range of 25% to 44% (38). The authors did not feel that there was a significant learning curve required. In this study, one of the observers was a radiologist specializing in United States, and the results did not differ in a statistically significantly different way from previous studies or from the other users in the study (38). Another study compared interuser variability between four radiation oncologists, two physicists, one radiation therapist, and one urologist who were all novices at BAT ultrasound (36). The standard deviations between ultrasound- and fiducial-based alignments of these users were comparable. Interobserver uncertainties have been characterized in other daily localization modalities, such as CT-based alignments (39). At Fox Chase, radiation therapists routinely perform ultrasound-based daily localization. Therapists are initially trained by those with more experience in BAT ultrasound.

Intrafraction Prostate Motion Studies Using BAT

BAT ultrasound localization has been performed both prior to and immediately following radiation treatment to assess intrafraction variability (Table 3). Sources of measured intrafraction motion include changes in rectal and bladder volume, patient respiration, patient motion, and intrinsic measurement errors. In one report, 20 men had pre- and post-treatment BAT images analyzed on 10 treatment days for a total of 400 BAT alignments (40). The percentage of measurements within 5 mm in the A-P, S-I, and L-R axes were 99, 99.5 and 100, respectively. No difference in shift was necessary 70% to 80% of the time (depending on the axis). Trichter et al. found that shifts of 0.2 cm or greater were only required 17%, 7%, and 10% of the time in the A-P, S-I and L-R axes, respectively (35).

The magnitude and standard error of intrafraction ultrasound shifts are smaller than interfraction shifts (Tables 1 and 3). Intrafraction variability with ultrasound localization is similar in magnitude to intrafraction variability using gold seed fiducial markers (29,35,40).

Table 3 Intrafraction Shifts Using BAT Ultrasound in the Treatment of Prostate Cancer

Study	Number of patients	A-P mean ± SD (mm)	S-I mean ± SD (mm)	R-L mean ± SD (mm)
Huang et al. (2002)	20	0.2 ± 1.3	0.1 ± 1.0	0.01 ± 0.4
Trichter et al. (2003)	26	0.0 ± 0.32	0.04 ± 0.48	0.02 ± 0.28

Abbreviations: BAT, B-mode acquisition and targeting; A-P, anterior-posterior; S-I, superior-inferior; R-L, right-left.

Reproducibility Over Time

Chandra et al. examined the temporal pattern of 3228 couch shifts over a one-year period at MD Andersen Cancer Center (34). Over time, there was a statistically significant increase in the standard deviation of couch shifts in the A-P and S-I axes, but not in the L-R axis. Although the impact of this increased variation on outcome is unclear, it seems that the radiotherapists performing the BAT measurements became less concerned about setup precision over time. Periodic quality review should be performed when using BAT ultrasound for daily localization. At Fox Chase, BAT ultrasound images are reviewed by the attending physician every day to verify the quality of the daily alignments. The importance of initial setup and alignment should be emphasized to BAT ultrasound operators.

The Effect Of Ultrasound Probe Pressure on Prostate Motion

Alterations in prostate localization resulting from ultrasound probe pressure have been examined. Precedence for ultrasound pressure perturbations of anatomic structures exists in the ophthalmology literature (41). McGahan et al. used a specially designed pelvic phantom with a water-filled balloon representing the bladder and rectum and a central, encapsulated sphere representing the prostate to measure organ motion with differing amounts of probe pressure (42). With increasing amounts of pressure, the sphere moved approximately 1 cm, a quantity greater than the variation of interfraction couch shifts from BAT ultrasound (Table 1). The authors recommend minimizing ultrasound pressure to prevent large errors in ultrasound-based daily localization. BAT ultrasound operators should use ample ultrasound gel to guarantee good contact between the probe and skin and reduce the pressure needed to obtain high-quality images.

The effect of ultrasound probe pressure has been directly characterized in patients. Trichter and Ennis examined prostate motion in two patients with brachytherapy implants before and after BAT ultrasound (35). Based on implant seed displacement, the largest shifts observed were 0.14 cm in the S-I axis and 0.17 cm in the A-P axis in patient 1 and 0.33 cm in the S-I axis and 0.17 cm in the A-P axis in patient 2 (35). Artignan et al. observed prostate motion in ten patients with increasing ultrasound probe pressure (43). With an abdominal displacement of 1.2 cm (the amount of pressure required for a high-quality image), the average prostate displacement was 3.1 mm. Although these numbers are small, ultrasound probe pressure can result in shifts in prostate localization.

CLINICAL OUTCOME

The theoretical benefit of daily image guidance with any IGRT modality is the ability to maximize dose to the target tissue and minimize dose to surrounding critical structures by accounting for variability in organ motion. No prospective randomized trials have been performed to specifically address the role of BAT ultrasound IGRT in the management of prostate cancer. However, there is retrospective data that supports ultrasound IGRT as an effective tool to maximize target dose while minimizing toxicity to adjacent structures.

Kupelian et al. at the Cleveland Clinic compared biochemical relapse-free survival (BRFS) and toxicity in short-course intensity-modulated radiotherapy (SCIM-RT) with 70 Gy in 28 fractions with 3DCRT with 78 Gy in 39 fractions (44). The SCIM-RT patients had daily localization with BAT ultrasound, whereas the 3DCRT patients did not. Although the delivery methods differed (hypofractionated IMRT vs. standard fractionated 3DCRT), the results suggest that BAT ultrasound allows for the safe delivery of high-dose radiotherapy with low levels of toxicity. Five-year BRFS was 94% versus 88% in the SCIM-RT and 3DCRT groups, respectively. Grade 2–3 rectal toxicity (early and late) was 5% in SCIM-RT (with BAT) versus 12% 3DCRT (without BAT), and grade 3 late toxicity was 2% in SCIM-RT versus 8% 3D-CRT. One would expect hypofractionated radiotherapy to result in greater toxicity. The extent of contributions from technique (IMRT vs. conformal RT) and BAT ultrasound localization cannot be quantified from the Cleveland Clinic experience. However, this data suggests that BAT ultrasound allows for reduced toxicity in dose-intensified fractionation schemes.

Use of external beam radiation fields that conform to the shape of the target improves biochemical control in prostate cancer by facilitating dose escalation through increased sparing of normal tissue. By correcting potential organ motion and setup errors, ultrasound-directed stereotactic localization is a method that may improve the accuracy and effectiveness of conformal technology.

The application of this technology to conformal techniques will allow the reduction of treatment margins in all dimensions. This should diminish treatment-related morbidity and facilitate further dose escalation and improved cancer control.

SUMMARY OF PERTINENT CONCLUSIONS

- BAT ultrasound is a noninvasive, reproducible, and time-efficient method of daily localization for IGRT in the management of prostate cancer.

- BAT ultrasound is used to align the patient's anatomy prior to treatment with contours designated from CT- or MR-simulation images and gives the necessary couch shifts.
- Interfraction variation in couch shifts from BAT ultrasound has been characterized in several single institution experiences. The magnitude and standard deviation of couch shifts between treatments is consistent with studies of prostate motion.
- The robustness and reliability of BAT ultrasound is supported by studies of intrafraction and interobserver variations in couch shifts and comparison studies against other daily localization modalities.
- Quality control over time should remain an integral part of a clinical program that uses BAT ultrasound for IGRT in the management of prostate cancer.
- While no multi-institutional, prospective, randomized trials have specifically compared treatment with and without BAT ultrasound using the same fractionation scheme for prostate cancer, a trial by Kupelian et al. and other clinical experiences support the use of BAT ultrasound to allow for dose escalation with acceptable toxicities.

REFERENCES

1. Hanks GE, Hanlon AL, Epstein B, et al. Dose response in prostate cancer with 8–12 years' follow-up. Int J Radiat Oncol Biol Phys 2002; 54(2):427–435.
2. Lee WR, Hanks GE, Hanlon AL, et al. Lateral rectal shielding reduces late rectal morbidity following high dose three-dimensional conformal radiation therapy for clinically localized prostate cancer: further evidence for a significant dose effect. Int J Radiat Oncol Biol Phys 1996; 35:251–257.
3. Pollack A, Zagars GK, Starkschall G, et al. Prostate cancer radiation dose response: results of the M.D. Anderson phase III randomized trial. Int J Radiat Oncol Biol Phys 2002; 53(5):1097–1105.
4. Zietman AL, DeSilvio M, Slater JD, et al. A randomized trial comparing conventional dose (70.2 GyE) and high-dose (79.2 GyE) conformal radiation in early stage adenocarcinoma of the prostate: results of an interim analysis of PROG 95-09. Int J Radiat Oncol Biol Phys 2004; 60:131–132.
5. Storey MR, Pollack A, Zagars G, et al. Complications from radiotherapy dose escalation in prostate cancer: preliminary results of a randomized trial. Int J Radiat Oncol Biol Phys 2000; 48:635–642.
6. Jackson A, Skwarchuk MW, Zelefsky MJ, et al. Late rectal bleeding after conformal radiotherapy of prostate cancer. II. Volume effects and dose-volume histograms. Int J Radiat Oncol Biol Phys 2001; 49(3):685–698.
7. Beard CJ, Kijewski P, Bussiere M, et al. Analysis of prostate and seminal vesicle motion: implications for treatment planning. Int J Radiat Oncol Biol Phys 1996; 34(2):451–458.
8. Zellars RC, Roberson PL, Strawderman M, et al. Prostate position late in the course of external beam therapy: patterns and predictors. Int J Radiat Oncol Biol Phys 2000; 47(3):655–660.
9. Roeske JC, Forman JD, Mesina CF, et al. Evaluation of changes in the size and location of the prostate, seminal vesicles, bladder, and rectum during a course of external beam radiation therapy. Int J Radiat Oncol Biol Phys 1995; 33(5):1321–1329.
10. Ten Haken RK, Forman JD, Heimburger DK, et al. Treatment planning issues related to prostate movement in response to differential filling of the rectum and bladder. Int J Radiat Oncol Biol Phys 1991; 20(6):1317–1324.
11. Stroom JC, Kroonwijk M, Pasma KL, et al. Detection of internal organ movement in prostate cancer patients using portal images. Med Phys 2000; 27(3):452–461.
12. Zelefsky MJ, Crean D, Mageras GS, et al. Quantification and predictors of prostate position variability in 50 patients evaluated with multiple CT scans during conformal radiotherapy. Radiother Oncol 1999; 50(2):225–234.
13. Eade TN, Hanlon AL, Horwitz EM, et al. What dose of external-beam radiation is high enough for prostate cancer? Int J Radiat Oncol Biol Phys 2007; 68(3):682–689.
14. Morr J, DiPetrillo T, Tsai JS, et al. Implementation and utility of a daily ultrasound-based localization system with intensity-modulated radiotherapy for prostate cancer. Int J Radiat Oncol Biol Phys 2002; 53(5):1124–1129.
15. Lattanzi JP, McNeeley S, Pinover WH, et al. A comparison of daily CT localization to a daily ultrasound-based system in prostate cancer. Int J Radiat Oncol Biol Phys 1999; 43:719–725.
16. Lattanzi J, McNeely S, Hanlon A, et al. Daily CT localization for correcting portal errors in the treatment of prostate cancer. Int J Radiat Oncol Biol Phys 1998; 41(5):1079–1086.
17. Lattanzi J, McNeeley S, Hanlon A, et al. Ultrasound-based stereotactic guidance of precision conformal external beam radiation therapy in clinically localized prostate cancer. Urology 2000; 55(1):73–78.
18. Lattanzi J, McNeeley S, Donnelly S, et al. Ultrasound-based stereotactic guidance in prostate cancer—quantification of organ motion and set-up errors in external beam radiation therapy. Comput Aided Surg 2000; 5(4):289–295.
19. Litzenberg D, Dawson LA, Sandler H, et al. Daily prostate targeting using implanted radiopaque markers. Int J Radiat Oncol Biol Phys 2002; 52(3):699–703.
20. Crook JM, Raymond Y, Salhani D, et al. Prostate motion during standard radiotherapy as assessed by fiducial markers. Radiother Oncol 1995; 37(1):35–42.
21. Soete G, Verellen D, Michielsen D, et al. Clinical use of stereoscopic X-ray positioning of patients treated with conformal radiotherapy for prostate cancer. Int J Radiat Oncol Biol Phys 2002; 54(3):948–952.
22. Groh BA, Siewerdsen JH, Drake DG, et al. A performance comparison of flat-panel imager-based MV and kV cone-beam CT. Med Phys 2002; 29(6):967–975.

23. Antolak JA, Rosen II, Childress CH, et al. Prostate target volume variations during a course of radiotherapy. Int J Radiat Oncol Biol Phys 1998; 42(3):661–672.

24. Melian E, Mageras GS, Fuks Z, et al. Variation in prostate position quantitation and implications for three-dimensional conformal treatment planning. Int J Radiat Oncol Biol Phys 1997; 38(1):73–81.

25. Roach M III, Faillace-Akazawa P, Malfatti C. Prostate volumes and organ movement defined by serial computerized tomographic scans during three-dimensional conformal radiotherapy. Radiat Oncol Investig 1997; 5(4): 187–194.

26. Balter JM, Lam KL, Sandler HM, et al. Automated localization of the prostate at the time of treatment using implanted radiopaque markers: technical feasibility. Int J Radiat Oncol Biol Phys 1995; 33(5):1281–1286.

27. Sandler HM, Bree RL, McLaughlin PW, et al. Localization of the prostatic apex for radiation therapy using implanted markers. Int J Radiat Oncol Biol Phys 1993; 27(4):915–919.

28. Vigneault E, Pouliot J, Laverdiere J, et al. Electronic portal imaging device detection of radioopaque markers for the evaluation of prostate position during megavoltage irradiation: a clinical study. Int J Radiat Oncol Biol Phys 1997; 37(1):205–212.

29. Shimizu S, Shirato H, Kitamura K, et al. Use of an implanted marker and real-time tracking of the marker for the positioning of prostate and bladder cancers. Int J Radiat Oncol Biol Phys 2000; 48(5):1591–1597.

30. Kupelian P, Willoughby T, Mahadevan A, et al. Multiinstitutional clinical experience with the Calypso System in localization and continuous, real-time monitoring of the prostate gland during external radiotherapy. Int J Radiat Oncol Biol Phys 2007; 67(4):1088–1098.

31. Willoughby TR, Kupelian PA, Pouliot J, et al. Target localization and real-time tracking using the Calypso 4D localization system in patients with localized prostate cancer. Int J Radiat Oncol Biol Phys 2006; 65(2):528–534.

32. Serago CF, Chungbin SJ, Buskirk SJ, et al. Initial experience with ultrasound localization for positioning prostate cancer patients for external beam radiotherapy. Int J Radiat Oncol Biol Phys 2002; 53(5):1130–1138.

33. Little DJ, Dong L, Levy LB, et al. Use of portal images and BAT ultrasonography to measure setup error and organ motion for prostate IMRT: implications for treatment margins. Int J Radiat Oncol Biol Phys 2003; 56(5): 1218–1224.

34. Chandra A, Dong L, Huang E, et al. Experience of ultrasound-based daily prostate localization. Int J Radiat Oncol Biol Phys 2003; 56(2):436–447.

35. Trichter F, Ennis RD. Prostate localization using transabdominal ultrasound imaging. Int J Radiat Oncol Biol Phys 2003; 56(5):1225–1233.

36. Langen KM, Pouliot J, Anezinos C, et al. Evaluation of ultrasound-based prostate localization for image-guided radiotherapy. Int J Radiat Oncol Biol Phys 2003; 57(3): 635–644.

37. Feigenberg SJ, Paskalev K, McNeeley S, et al. Comparing computed tomography localization with daily ultrasound during image-guided radiation therapy for the treatment of prostate cancer: a prospective evaluation. J Appl Clin Med Phys 2007; 8(3):2268.

38. McNair HA, Mangar SA, Coffey J, et al. A comparison of CT- and ultrasound-based imaging to localize the prostate for external beam radiotherapy. Int J Radiat Oncol Biol Phys 2006; 65(3):678–687.

39. Jaffray DA, Drake DG, Moreau M, et al. A radiographic and tomographic imaging system integrated into a medical linear accelerator for localization of bone and soft-tissue targets. Int J Radiat Oncol Biol Phys 1999; 45(3): 773–789.

40. Huang E, Dong L, Chandra A, et al. Intrafraction prostate motion during IMRT for prostate cancer. Int J Radiat Oncol Biol Phys 2002; 53(2):261–268.

41. Shammas HJ. A comparison of immersion and contact techniques for axial length measurement. J Am Intraocul Implant Soc 1984; 10(4):444–447.

42. McGahan JP, Ryu J, Fogata M. Ultrasound probe pressure as a source of error in prostate localization for external beam radiotherapy. Int J Radiat Oncol Biol Phys 2004; 60(3): 788–793.

43. Artignan X, Smitsmans MH, Lebesque JV, et al. Online ultrasound image guidance for radiotherapy of prostate cancer: impact of image acquisition on prostate displacement. Int J Radiat Oncol Biol Phys 2004; 59(2):595–601.

44. Kupelian PA, Reddy CA, Carlson TP, et al. Preliminary observations on biochemical relapse-free survival rates after short-course intensity-modulated radiotherapy (70 Gy at 2.5 Gy/fraction) for localized prostate cancer. Int J Radiat Oncol Biol Phys 2002; 53(4):904–912.

11

Image-Guided Radiation Therapy in Prostate Cancer: William Beaumont Experience

MICHEL GHILEZAN, DI YAN, AND ALVARO MARTINEZ

Department of Radiation Oncology, William Beaumont Hospital Cancer Center, Royal Oak, Michigan, U.S.A.

INTRODUCTION

During the 1980s, significant advances occurred in the planning process of radiation therapy. Three-dimensional (3D) planning was developed and introduced in the clinic as an effort to improve the treatment efficacy. In the early nineties, at William Beaumont Hospital, we started working on the development of (*i*) a system for imaging the "target" before delivery of radiation treatment to obtain a high-quality "image of the day" with soft tissues details versus bony anatomy details, as commonly produced by portal imaging devices and (*ii*) a process for adapting the beam aperture to correct the individual's daily geometrical and temporal variations. The success of 3D conformal and of intensity-modulated radiation therapy (IMRT) relies on the accurate delivery of radiation dose. Unfortunately, patient and organ treatment position variation inevitably exists. Errors in patient positioning, intertreatment and intratreatment variation of organ position, and uncertainty in target localization result in variation of the dose delivered. While it is difficult, if not impossible, to completely eliminate all sources of variation clearly, all efforts must be made to minimize their effects whenever possible.

A major source of treatment uncertainty is the variability in the daily setup of the patient. The common practice to minimize setup error is by evaluating port film weekly, which is helpful but insufficient (1). The use of immobilization devices is also common and should, in theory, enhance the reproducibility of daily patient setup. However, studies of their effectiveness for the patient treated on the thoracic and abdominal regions have produced variable results and are dissatisfying (2–5).

Two new approaches to compensate for or reduce the magnitude of treatment setup error are being developed. The first incorporates generic setup error, characterized from measurements made of the patient population, into the initial treatment planning (6–9). The variability of the dose distribution due to setup error is presented to the clinician so that compromises can be made prior to the initiation of treatment. In the second approach, decision rules for setup adjustment are implemented to reduce the magnitude of setup error and to minimize the frequency of patient repositioning (10–15). The decision rule approach requires more frequent portal imaging and complements the use of electronic portal imaging devices (EPIDs). However, the setup adjustment is not based on treatment planning information, and the potential changes in the dose delivered to the individual patient are not considered. More importantly, both approaches employ average values derived from population study as criteria for plan evaluation or setup adjustment. With "population-averaged" parameters, the opportunities to optimize the treatment for the individual patient are not exploited.

ADAPTIVE RADIATION THERAPY: BASIC PRINCIPLES, PROCESS IMPLEMENTATION, AND WORK FLOW

Optimal treatment delivery is best made on an individual patient basis. Such assertion can be supported by the following analysis of measured setup error of a group of individual patients and that of the patient population.

When a sequence of daily portal images have been acquired for the individual patient, setup error can be characterized in terms of the mean, m_i, and the standard deviation, σ_i, of the daily setup error. The former represents the "systematic error" and the latter the "random error" of the treatment setup. From a two-dimensional (2D) portal image, these parameters can be characterized on each of two coordinate directions. For example, for an anterior-to-posterior (AP) treatment, the setup error would be measured along the lateral (LAT) and superior-to-inferior (SI) directions. If the analysis were performed for a group of individual patients for a specific treatment site, one could further calculate a mean, M (m_i), and standard deviation, $\sigma(\sigma_i)$, of the systematic setup errors for these patients. Similarly, M (m_i) and $\sigma(\sigma_i)$ can be calculated to represent the root-mean-square and standard deviation of random setup errors for these patients.

When only a few portal images are available for each patient, as in the case with weekly port film exposure, it becomes necessary to pool the setup measurements of each individual patient into a larger data sample for analysis. The setup error of the patient populations for a specific treatment site can then also be characterized on each of two coordinate axes by the mean, M_p, and the standard deviation, σ_p. It has been shown that the population mean, M_p, is exactly equal to M (m_i), the mean systematic setup error for all individual patients. However, the population standard deviation of the setup error, σ_p is equal to $[M^2(\sigma_i) + \sigma^2(m_i)]^{1/2}$. It includes not only the contribution from the root-mean-square of the random setup error of the individual patient, but also the standard deviation, or variability, of the systematic setup error of each patient. The latter once detected, in theory, can be eliminated. It follows then that σ_p gives a conservative overestimation of setup error of the individual. When it is used to design a margin for setup variability, as in the case with port film data, σ_p is larger than necessary for the individual patient, provided that both systematic and random setup errors could be predicted, and the systematic error could be corrected during the course of treatment.

The above analysis shows that a major deficiency in the approach to compensate for setup error "is the lack of incorporation of individual patient uncertainties and variability." Setup error of an individual patient could be either overcompensated or undercompensated in the initial treatment plan. As a result, outcome analyses from clinical trials of 3D conformal therapy, IMRT, and dose escalation may not achieve the true potential in terms of increasing local control and decreasing toxicity. It should not be assumed that every patient would be a suitable candidate for dose escalation. A patient whose treatment exhibits a highly reproducible setup and target position might be one such candidate. Conversely, a patient with large position variation might be more suitable for conservative management (15). Unfortunately, much of the patient-specific variation is not known until after initiation of treatment. Therefore, we have introduced in the mid 1990s a new approach, named adaptive radiation therapy (ART), to minimize the deleterious effects of setup variation, organ motion, and deformation on each individual patient (15–17). A retrospective study was used to demonstrate the feasibility of the ART process. In the study, treatment plan of the individual patient was adaptively modified part way through the treatment based on the time course of setup variation predicted from portal measurements made of the earlier treatment fractions (17). By taking the advantage of a computer-controlled multileaf collimator (MLC), a second improved treatment plan was calculated and implemented by adjusting the treatment field shape and prescription dose, simultaneously (18). The ART process is outlined as follows: (*i*) The patient's initial 3D treatment plan is first optimized and delivered using MLC. (*ii*) Daily setup error is measured using an EPID and characterized early on during the treatment course. (*iii*) The treatment plan is evaluated incorporating the characterized setup error to decide if and what modification is necessary. (*iv*) The treatment plan is modified accordingly for the remaining treatments by reshaping the MLC field and adjusting the prescription dose (16,17). Results from our first ART study indicate that much could be gained with the patient specific ART approach to improve setup accuracy (17). Our simulated treatments of 30 patients with the ART showed that about one-third of the patients could have their prescription doses escalated by as much as 15%. The maximum cumulative dose reduction in the clinical target volume (CTV), as percentage of prescribed dose, due to internal target motion and organ deformation captured by serial CT measurements is shown in Figure 1. The first five CT scans were sufficient to predict the maximum cumulative dose reduction in the CTV. Equally important, we showed that up to 20% of the patients would not be qualified for a higher dose escalation because of the large position variation (19). Clinical protocols, which escalate dose with a concomitant generic reduction of the setup margin, might not produce the desirable proof of the efficacy of high dose 3D conformal therapy including IMRT plans. A more effective approach to implement high-dose conformal therapy would be to start off an individual patient with a simpler treatment strategy, which would then be modified in accordance to

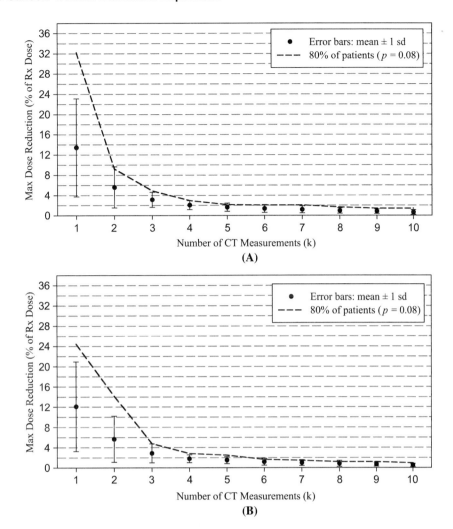

Figure 1 The maximum cumulative dose reduction in the CTV, as percentage of prescribed dose, due to internal target motion. The calculations are based on a 3D conformal four-field box treatment. The CTV is considered, alternately, as the prostate and seminal vesicles (**A**), and the prostate only (**B**). The error bars indicate the mean dose reduction and one standard deviation thereof for a population of 30 patients. The dashed lines indicate the bound on the dose reduction achieved for 80% of patients ($p = 0.08$). *Abbreviation*: CTV, clinical target volume.

the characteristics of the treatment variation measured during the early phase of the treatment course. The systematic and random setup errors of the treatment after adjustment were compared with those prior to the adjustment. The residual systematic error after adjustment was used to evaluate the accuracy and reliability of the ART process. Furthermore, the difference between the random setup errors before and after adjustment was used as a measure of the stability of the ART process. Recently at the American Society for Therapeutic Radiology and Oncology (ASTRO) meeting, we presented the quality control results of image-guided adaptive radiotherapy (IGART) from 1999 to 2006 for prostate cancer in 1017 patients with clinically treated T1-3 tumors. Only 96 patients or 9.4% of patients required a second modification of the MLC configuration including 63 corrections of

the residual systematic error in one single direction. In addition, only 5 of 1017 patients required readjustment of the target margins due to a larger random setup error (20).

Finally, patient-specific setup margins were calculated to demonstrate the potential advantages of the ART process in pursuing treatment dose escalation. Treatment setup margins for each patient were determined when a confident prediction was achieved. The setup margins were calculated by adding the predicted systematic error to twice the predicted random setup error for each coordinate direction of the treatment field if no adjustment was applied, or if an adjustment was applied, by adding 1 mm (tolerance of the prediction for the systematic error) to twice the predicted random setup error. Implementation of the ART process requires a new clinical infrastructure in which the clinical treatment procedures such as treatment planning, treatment verification, treatment evaluation, and treatment adjustment are not performed as independent tasks. Instead, a closed-loop treatment process will be used to apply the patient-specific information measured during the treatment course to reevaluate and to reoptimize the treatment plan. An optimal way to implement this feedback process integrates new technologies such as a 3D treatment planning system, an online imaging device, and MLC through information and control network. With the ART process, the physician could potentially act as a central controller to manipulate a patient's treatment using a computer network.

Modification of the treatment field shape using MLC makes the ART process possible to correct for the systematic error and to compensate for the random setup error by only reshaping the MLC once. Most importantly, reshaping the treatment fields allows one to compensate for any target shape change due to a distortion of the patient position or internal organ motion. Moreover, adjusting the MLC field allows accurate adjustment as small as 0.2 mm, minimizes the possibility of "unsettling" the patient, and reduces the workload of the therapists. However, although reshaping the treatment field alone can be used to compensate for the target shape change on the beam's eye view plane due to 3D out-of-plane rotation, it may not be acceptable when a specific setup of conformal therapy has to be precisely kept to avoid a critical adjacent organ. In this case, adjustments in the ART may also need to include the gantry or treatment couch rotation. On each of the first four days of treatment, a CT scan encompassing the entire bladder to below the ischium is obtained, and the daily CTV is contoured to assess treatment target motion. In addition, a daily portal image for each treatment field is taken using an EPID, and daily setup error is measured. The patient-specific data of daily target motion and setup error are exported to a prediction model to form the confidence limited planning target volume (cl-PTV). Then, the individual treatment plan is modified to deliver the prescribed dose to the cl-PTV by either continuing the four-field treatment or using IMRT for the remaining treatment (18,19).

To summarize, ART is a treatment process (Fig. 2), which adapts the treatment plan to patient-specific geometrical and temporal variations. Each patient initially undergoes a conventional CT simulation followed by 3D planning. A generic, but transitory PTV is constructed defined as the CTV plus a 1 cm uniform margin automatically expanded in 3D. A standard four-field conformal treatment plan with adequate beam aperture is designed to ensure that the generic PTV is covered by the prescription dose. Daily megavoltage image (MVI) portal and CT images are acquired with each of the first four days treatments without contrast. These images, documenting daily field placement and spatial organ positions, are used

as treatment feedback and are entered into a prediction model to estimate the systematic variation in daily patient setup and target motion. By taking into consideration the subsequent treatment delivery system (CRT or IMRT), the cl-PTV is constructed, subject to a predefined targeting dose tolerance, on the basis of the random variation of internal target motion and setup error obtained from the treatment images (18). Using the cl-PTV, a new treatment plan is then generated, and a prescription dose is selected based on the constraints for dose-limiting structures in the protocol, currently the rectal wall and bladder, as captured from the initial planning CT images. The subsequent treatment modality in the new treatment plan could be either a CRT or IMRT. IMRT is selected if the prescription dose could be increased by at least 5% when compared with CRT while meeting the same normal tissue constraint limits. The new beam apertures, which included adjustments for the predicted systematic variation, are transferred to the treatment machine and applied for the remaining treatments. Our protocol also includes weekly CT scans on all ART patients for quality assurance purposes (20).

DOSE ESCALATION USING THE ART PROCESS

We performed a prospective study to determine if the ART process improved the capability of dose escalation. For each patient, two conformal four-field plans were created, with respect to the generic PTV (CTV + 1 cm) and the cl-PTV, respectively. The corresponding prescription doses were selected on the basis of the dose-volume constraints on the rectal wall and bladder manifested on the initial planning image. In addition, inverse planning was also performed with both the generic and cl-PTV, respectively, for the first 30 patients treated with the ART process. The minimum and maximum doses in the PTV (the objective function) were adjusted so that the maximum prescription dose was obtained within the given constraints and the dose heterogeneity (15%) limitation in the PTV. The following constraints had to be met:

> No more than 5% of the rectal wall volume receives a dose greater than 75.6 Gy,
> No more than 30% of rectal wall volume receives a dose greater than 72 Gy,
> No more than 40% of rectal wall volume receives a dose greater than 65 Gy,
> No more than 50% of bladder volume receives a dose greater than 75.6 Gy,
> Maximum dose in the bladder is less than or equal to 80 Gy, and
> A dose inhomogeneity in the PTV of less than or equal to 10% of the prescription dose for conventional conformal treatment and less than or equal to 15% for IMRT treatment.

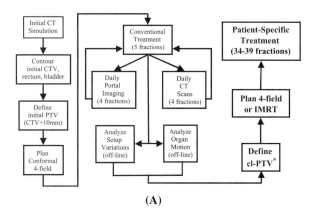

(A)

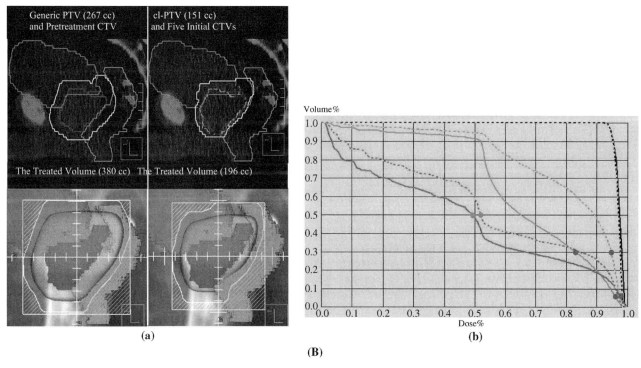

(B)

Figure 2 (**A**) Flow chart depicting the ART process. The process performs off-line analysis of the setup error and organ motion occurring during the first five days of treatment. These characterizations are used to predict variations over the remaining fractions, and the cl-PTV is designed to provide dosimetric coverage of the nonsystematic components of these variations. Systematic components are removed via commensurate block aperture shifts during replanning. (**B**) Illustration of (a) the generic PTV (*left*) and cl-PTV (*right*) of a single patient on the sagital CT image, and the corresponding treated volume (*gray shade*) on the beam eye view DRR; (b) the corresponding DVHs of PTV (black), rectal wall (*dark gray*) and bladder (*light gray*) for the generic PTV (*dashed curves*) or cl-PTV (*solid curves*). The solid dots on the curves indicate the dose/volume constraints. *Abbreviations*: ART, adaptive radiation therapy; cl-PTV, confidence limited planning target volume; DRR, digitally reconstructed radiography; DVH, dose-volume histograms.

After completing treatment and reviewing the acute toxicity of the first 40 patients, these restrictions were extended to:

No more than 5% of the rectal wall volume receives a dose greater than 82 Gy,

No more than 30% of rectal wall volume receives a dose greater than 75.6 Gy,

No more than 50% of bladder volume receives a dose greater than 75.6 Gy,

Maximum dose in the bladder is less than or equal to 85 Gy, and

A dose inhomogeneity in the PTV of less than or equal to 10% of the prescription dose for conventional conformal treatment and less than or equal to 15% for IMRT treatment.

We analyzed factors predictive of rectal toxicity and Vargas et al. published (21) on the first 331 consecutively treated patients with image-guided off-line correction with adaptive high-dose radiotherapy (IGART). The chronic rectal toxicity grade ≥ 2 risk was 9%, 18%, and 25% for the rectal wall V70 <15%, 25% to 40%, and >40%, respectively. In addition, the volume of rectum and/or rectal wall irradiated to greater than or equal to 50% was also a strong predictor of rectal damage. The use of androgen deprivation was not found predictive. We were the first ones to publish that patients experiencing acute rectal toxicity are more likely to experience chronic toxicity (21).

In a subsequent publication also from Beaumont, Vargas et al. (22) reported on prostate cancer patients treated with IGART and the use of dose-volume constraints to achieve rectal isotoxicity. High doses (79.2 Gy) to the prostate were safely delivered by our IGART process. Under the rectal dose-volume histograms (DVH) constraints for the dose-level selection, the risk of chronic rectal toxicity is similar among patients treated to different dose levels. Therefore, rectal chronic toxicity rates reflect the dose-volume cutoff used and are independent of the actual dose level (22).

More recently, Harsolia et al. (23) from Beaumont published the chronic genitourinary (GU) toxicity observed on these 331 consecutively treated patients with IGART. They were clinically stage II to stage III prostate cancer patients and were assessed using the National Cancer Institute Common Toxicity Criteria 2.0. The three-year rates of grade ≥ 2 and grade 3 chronic urinary toxicity were 17% and 3.6%, respectively. Acute urinary toxicity and bladder wall dose-volume end points are strong predictors for the development of subsequent chronic urinary toxicity. We recommend to limit the bladder wall V30 to less than 30 cc and V82 to less than 7 cc (23).

In general, the prescription dose was 92% to 93% of the isocenter dose. Figure 2A depicts the beam aperture and treated volume for both the generic PTV and the cl-PTV of a single patient with conformal four-field plans. The corresponding DVH for the target (PTVs) and normal organs, as well as the dose/volume constraints are illustrated in Figure 2B. In addition, for the first 30 patients, the potential for target miss and normal tissue overtreatment in the conventional treatment process was also evaluated by comparing the conventional generic PTV to the cl-PTV. The first prospective dose-escalation study using the ART process demonstrated that the prescription dose level for the majority of the patients could be increased up to 10% (mean 5%) or 1.8 to 7.2 Gy (mean 3.6 Gy) when compared to the conventional treatment process. That level could be further increased to 5% to 15% (mean 7.5%) or 3.2 to 10.8 Gy (mean 5.4 Gy), when the IMRT delivery was combined with the ART process. In that case, a minimum cl-PTV dose of 81 Gy [i.e., 86.7 Gy at the International Committee on Radiation Units and Measurements (ICRU) isocenter] could be prescribed to at least 50% of the patients. In contrast, there was no clear advantage on the dose escalation when the generic PTV (CTV + 1 cm margin) was applied for the IMRT treatment, except when deliberately blocking the rectal wall within the PTV (19). Our study indicated that at least 10% of patients could have potential deficiency of their treatment volumes, when treated in the conventional treatment process. In that process, a generic PTV has to be designed with a predefined confidence level regarding the patient/organ geometric uncertainty, and this confidence level has been commonly selected to be 90%. We expanded the study, and Wloch et al. (20) presented at the 2007 ASTRO meeting in Los Angeles the result on 263 patients treated with IGART who had six or more CT scans during the course of treatment during 1999 and 2003. Only 12 of 263 patients or 4.6% has a portion of their seminal vesicle missed with a range of 2 to 22 mm and average of 6.1 mm. Equally low, 5 of 263 patients or 1.9% had a portion of their prostate missed with a range of 2 to 9 mm and average of 6.3 mm. The dosimetric effect on missing dose to the PTV was assessed in these eight patients. In three patients it was less than 1%, in three patients less than 2.0%, in one patient 3.8%, and in the remaining patient 7.3% of the prescribed dose (20).

DEVELOPMENT OF THE CONE-BEAM-BASED IGART AT WILLIAM BEAUMONT HOSPITAL

Even though in 90% of the patients the prescription dose could be increased safely, the treatment quality of a small group of patients (5–10%) cannot be assured in spite of application of ART with or without IMRT. The ART process identifies this group of patients for which the dose should not be escalated above conventional levels, due to the large variations in CTV position observed during the treatment course. Special treatment intervention such as daily-based image guidance was felt as being needed in this group of patients. The identification of these patients is paramount to keep complication rates low, and thus improve the therapeutic ratio when very high doses are to be delivered. Therefore, our research efforts focused on including the position distribution of rectum/bladder in the off-line planning optimization and ultimately on real-time, online-based image guidance, where the daily target and normal organs in each patient are assessed immediately prior to treatment. Dose reconstruction and planning optimization are then performed online, based on target and normal tissue positions obtained over time. The desire to further reduce the planning target margins around the CTV has emphasized the treatment-related uncertainties such as, daily positioning and setup errors, interfraction organ motion, and intrafraction organ motion. Minimizing treatment-related uncertainties has become the intense focus of research in the recent years. Capitalizing on a series of technological innovations such as the development of amorphous-silicon flat-panel imagers, the creation of high-speed cone-beam computed tomography (CBCT) reconstruction hardware along with the realization of computer-controlled medical linear accelerators, the construction of online CBCT imaging system for IGART has been developed in our institution (25–27,40). Online image guidance should minimize some of the uncertainties related to routine radiotherapy (positioning and setup errors and interfraction organ motion). Based on our institutional experience with high-dose rate brachytherapy in prostate cancer which appear to indicate a low α/β for prostate tumors, IGRT is expected to be used in a hypofractionation regimen with higher doses per fraction and consequently, longer treatment times. As a prerequisite for the translation of the cone-beam image-guidance system into clinical use for the treatment of prostate cancer, we studied intrafraction prostate motion using serial cine-MR over about 50 minutes in patients in supine radiation treatment position. We showed that the motion of the prostate and seminal vesicles during a time frame similar to a standard treatment fraction is reduced compared to that reported in interfraction studies. The most significant predictor for intrafraction prostate motion was the status of rectal filling. A prostate displacement of less than 3 mm can be expected within 20 minutes of the initial imaging for patients with an empty rectum (28).

Using 22 image data sets from our ART prostate database, we analyzed and quantified the theoretical benefit in terms of improvement in precision and accuracy of treatment delivery and in dose increase with IGART in an ideal setting of no intrafraction motion/deformation. The conventional IMRT plan was generated on the basis of pretreatment CT, with a clinical target volume to planning target volume (CTV-to-PTV) margin of 1 cm, and the online IGART plan was created before each treatment fraction on the basis of the CT scan of the day, without CTV-to-PTV margin. The inverse planning process was similar for both conventional IMRT and online image-guided IMRT (IG-IMRT). Treatment dose for each organ of interest was quantified, including patient daily setup error and internal organ motion/deformation. We used generalized equivalent uniform dose (EUD) to compare the two approaches. The generalized EUD (percentage) of each organ of interest was scaled relative to the prescription dose at treatment isocenter for evaluation and comparison. On the basis of bladder wall and rectal wall EUD, a dose-escalation coefficient was calculated, representing the potential increment of the treatment dose achievable with online IGART as compared with conventional IMRT. The average EUDs of bladder wall and rectal wall for conventional IMRT versus online IG-IMRT were 70.1% versus 47.3%, and 79.4% versus 72.2%,

respectively. On average, a target dose increase of 13% (SD 9.7%) could be achieved with online IGART based on rectal wall EUDs and 53.3% (SD 15.3%) based on bladder wall EUDs. However, the variation (SD 9.7%) was fairly large among patients; 27% of patients had only minimal benefit (<5% of dose increment) from online IG-IMRT, and 32% had significant benefit (>15–41% of dose increment) (29).

Uncertainties in Clinical IGART Process

The IGART process reduces uncertainties in patient treatment position, but shares rest of uncertainties existing in the conventional treatment simulation, planning, and delivery. Additionally, the specific and most significant sources of uncertainties are patient image acquisition and registration, couch or MLC correction, estimation of the systematic and random position variations, treatment dose construction/evaluation, and adaptive planning modification, which will be outlined in the following sections.

Uncertainties in Treatment Position Localization

The IGART process involves frequent measurements of patient anatomical position obtained by comparing treatment images to a reference image of similar modality, i.e., the onboard CBCT image to the reference planning CT image, or the portal image to the digitally reconstructed radiography (DRR). Deformable organ registration and segmentation have been evaluated using patient image with or without inserting radio markers (30). However, the purpose of these studies was rather to validate registration methods instead of clinical QA. It would be helpful to have a deformable phantom to test registration method and verify treatment dose construction.

Uncertainties in Couch or Beam Aperture Correction

Couch position and MLC-based beam aperture adjustments have been the most common means to correct patient treatment position. However, the uncertainties associated with each correction method should be determined before a routine application in the clinic. Translational correction accuracy has been achieved within 1 mm. However, treatment position corrections using an MLC-based beam aperture shift are nontrivial due to the limited leaf width. We recently showed in a study of online image guidance and rigid body correction using MLC a maximum of 2% dose discrepancy in the target and a much higher dose discrepancy in normal tissues that could occur in both prostate and head/neck cancer treatment (31). Beam aperture correction has also been proposed and tested to compensate for target deformation (18) in conformal radiotherapy, and expanded later to IMRT (32). However, so far, the dosimetric uncertainty caused by multiple leaf segment adjustment has not been fully explored.

Uncertainties in Determining Patient Variation Parameters

A unique feature of the IGART process is the estimation of the systematic and random errors of individual treatment position. Since the estimation is performed based on limited samples of measurements, uncertainty in parameter estimation is always accompanied by statistical residuals. The systematic and random errors of treatment setup position have been systematically evaluated for prostate and head/neck cancer treatment. Following the estimation, performed at the end of the first treatment week, patient setup position has been continuously monitored for additional three to five treatment days. If the residual systematic error after the first correction in the prostate cancer treatment was 1 mm (the predetermined cutoff value) larger than the estimated value, a second correction would be performed. As we mentioned before, out of 1017 patients only 9.4% required a second correction and 0.07% a third one, which documented how robust the IGART process is (20).

Uncertainties in Treatment Dose Construction and Evaluation

At the present time, the individual patient dose tracking and feedback process is under clinical test and evaluation, instead of routine use. Treatment dose, daily as well as cumulative, in organs of interest has been constructed using volumetric image-based deformable organ registration (33). Two major factors that have been considered in the treatment or 4D dose construction are organ subvolume position displacement and variation of patient global density distribution. However, the discrepancy is commonly small (<3%) for dose evaluation in a pelvic region. Treatment dose in organs of interest can be frequently updated in the IGART process for treatment evaluation and planning modification decision. However, uncertainties in image registration and organ delineation affect directly the reliability of using the dose in treatment evaluation. Study on this aspect, therefore, needs to be systematically explored.

Uncertainties in Adaptive Planning Modification

Two typical adaptive planning methods have been explored. One is to determine patient-specific CTV-to-PTV margin (18) and then design the corresponding dose distribution. The other is to design dose distribution to compensate for patient-specific motion directly with adaptive inverse planning (34). Sources of uncertainties in the adaptive planning are very similar to those in the conventional planning reported by the Task Group 53. However, the influence could be different. The influence of organ delineation uncertainty on the accuracy of dose evaluation could be reduced because of a potential random effect in the multiple organ delineations. However, the accuracy of dose evaluation becomes more critical in the selection of the individual prescription dose. Therefore, IGART quality control should also include the selection of the most robust planning parameters, such as selecting dose/volume constraints on the relative stable portion of DVH curve for planning evaluation.

QA TESTS IN CLINICAL IGART PROCESS

Clinical development of IGART QA should aim at the most significant sources of uncertainties. QA recommendations on image acquisition, anatomical description, dose calculation, and treatment planning have been detailed in American Association of Physicists in Medicine (AAPM) Task Group Report 40 and 53. In following recommendations, we focus only on the additional QA procedures that should be applied to implement a clinical IGART process.

QA Verification for Patient Treatment Position Assessment and Correction

Staff physicists should perform integrated system test on the image localization and position correction accuracy before starting an IGART protocol to determine a baseline reference for routine monthly and daily QA tests. A therapists/image specialist performs isocenter localization tests daily for online image guided hypofractionation and monthly for offline image guidance. These tests should also be performed once when corresponding software/hardware device is updated. Staff physicists perform integrated system tests from the CT simulation to treatment delivery semiannually. A phantom with embedded radio markers can be applied for these image localization and position correction tests. In addition, phantom mounted on a motor-driven motion stage can be used for the respiratory correlated CT or CBCT imaging QA.

QA Verification for Parameter Estimation and Treatment Dose Construction

The systematic and random errors of the individual treatment position are verified in the week after the assessment by a physicist or dosimetrist and evaluated weekly by a physician during the entire course of the treatment. It is strongly recommended that one evaluates the changes in organ volume and the organ's center of mass weekly. Treatment dose to the organs of interest should be evaluated daily for hypofractionated radiotherapy and weekly for a normal fractionated treatment by a physicist. If a large dose discrepancy is observed, the corresponding treatment image and organ contours should be evaluated.

QA Verification for Treatment Evaluation and Adaptive Planning

The planning CT image should be verified to identify and eliminate the effect of contrast material and unusual events, i.e., bladder contrast and large rectal gas filling, on the dose calculation. The treatment volumetric images used in adaptive planning are verified weekly to ensure that they are appropriated for the 4D treatment dose construction. When a treatment DVH parameter is used for treatment evaluation, weekly verification is recommended to ensure that the parameter is not on the high gradient portion of the DVH curve. When patient-specific PTV is used in adaptive planning, weekly CT image verification is suggested to avoid unexpected deviation.

CLINICAL EXPERIENCE WITH IGART

In 1997 we developed and commenced clinical implementation of the ART process at William Beaumont Hospital. In 1999 we initiated an Institutional Review Board (IRB)-approved phase II prospective dose-escalation/selection trial in treating localized prostate adenocarcinoma, taking into account individual patient setup inaccuracies and internal organ motion (ART process) in the dose prescription. Hence, a patient-specific PTV was designed, along with the corresponding beam apertures. Each patient's dose prescription is selected on the basis of the dose maxima tolerable according to our specific dose-volume constraints.

Patients were eligible for this protocol if we had tissue confirmation of prostate cancer, all Gleason grades, and clinical stages (T1b-T3, NX-NO, MO). Eligibility criteria for this protocol included patients with biopsy-proven adenocarcinoma of the prostate with a clinical stage of I to III who were diagnosed within 24 weeks of enrollment. Patients with clinical or pathologic lymph node positivity were excluded from the study. For patients with a Gleason score of less than or equal to 6, a PSA less than 10, and a clinical stage T2a or less, the CTV included the prostate only (ART group I). For patients with a Gleason score greater than or equal to 7 and/or a PSA greater than or equal to 10 and/or a clinical stage greater than or equal to T2b, the CTV include the prostate and proximal 2 cm of

Table 1 Patients' Characteristics for 642 Patients

Characteristic	Median (mean)	Range
Age	73 yr	51–87
CTV	50.6 cc	18.3–214.3
Pretreatment PSA	6.7 ng/mL (9.7)	0.2–120
Gleason score	6 (6.3)	3–10
T stage	T1c	T1a–T3c
Percent biopsy cores	27%	5%–100%
Dose (minimum to PTV)	75.6 Gy	63.0–79.2
Dose (isocenter)	79.7 Gy	67.0–85.6
RT fractions	42	35–44
Follow-up	4.6 yr	0.1–7.5
PSA nadir	0.6 ng/mL	0–33.5

Abbreviations: CTV, clinical target volume; PSA, prostate-specific antigen; PTV, planning target volume; RT, radiation therapy.

seminal vesicles (ART group II). A pelvis field was never used. For the initial treatment week the PTV included the CTV plus 1 cm generic uniform margin. A total of 900 cGy (minimal prostate dose) was given in 180 cGy fractions with 18 MV photons for the first week.

All acute and chronic side effects were recorded using the Common Toxicity Criteria (CTC) version 3. The worst score seen at any time was used to score chronic toxicity.

Patient characteristics are reported in Table 1.

Before reviewing our chronic toxicity data (Tables 2–4), it is important to reiterate that using the adaptive process the PTVs are often smaller than those using standard margins of 0.5 to 1.0 cm about the CTV without compromising CTV coverage. By decreasing the treatment volume one also treats less of the normal dose limiting tissues. This potentially allows a decreased complication rate while maintaining a similar treatment dose or allows escalation of the treatment dose while maintaining similar toxicity. In our dose-escalating trial, we elected to raise the total dose while maintaining isotoxicity.

In the whole-body hyperthermia (WBH) ART trial, the rectal parameters were set so that less than or equal to 5% of the rectal wall has a dose greater than 82 Gy and less than or equal to 30% of the rectal wall has a dose greater than 75.6 Gy on the basis of the original CT set. Others have suggested that not only is the maximum rectal dose important in predicting for late toxicity, but perhaps equally important is the intermediate volume of rectum receiving lesser dose. While the trial does not impose a limit on the dose to an intermediate volume of the rectum, it has been our experience that this dose may become unacceptably high when generating IMRT plans, unless an auxiliary constraint is introduced into the optimization. The bladder constraints were set so that less than or equal to 50% of the bladder volume has a dose greater than 75.6 Gy, and the maximum allowed dose to the bladder is less than 85 Gy. The minimum prescribed dose to the

Table 2   Grade 1 Chronic Toxicity by Dose Level

Dose level (Gy)	≥70.2 to ≤72.0 (n = 109)		>72.0 to ≤75.6 (n = 301)		>75.6 to ≤79.2 (n = 232)	
Urinary incontinence (%)	8	–	5	–	11	–
Urinary retention (%)	6		5		2	–
Increased frequency/urgency (%)	–	22	–	21	–	25
Urethral stricture (%)	–	0	–	0	–	0
Hematuria (%)	2		2		6	–
Diarrhea (%)		4		5		5
Rectal pain/tenesmus (%)	4	–	7	–	7	–
Rectal bleeding (%)	–	20	–	18	–	25
Rectal ulceration (%)	–	0	–	0	–	0
Rectal fistula (%)	0	–	0	–	0	–
Proctitis (%)		4		5		2
Rectal incontinence (%)	6	–	2	–	4	–

Table 3   Grade 2 Chronic Toxicity by Dose Level

Dose level (Gy)	≥70.2– to ≤72.0 (n = 109)		>72.0 to ≤75.6 (n = 301)		>75.6 to ≤79.2 (n = 232)	
Urinary incontinence (%)	0	–	0	–	1	–
Urinary retention (%)	2	–	1	–	1	–
Increased frequency/urgency (%)	–	11	–	13	–	12
Urethral stricture (%)	–	0	–	0	–	0
Hematuria (%)	0		0		1	
Diarrhea (%)		6		2	–	2
Rectal pain/tenesmus (%)	2		0	–	1	–
Rectal bleeding (%)	–	6	–	7	–	12
Rectal ulceration (%)	–	2	–	0	–	0
Rectal fistula (%)	0	–	0	0	–	–
Proctitis (%)		8		2	6	
Rectal incontinence (%)	2	–	0	1	–	–

Table 4   Grade 3 Chronic Toxicity by Dose Level

Dose level (Gy)	≥70.2 to ≤72.0 (n = 109)		>72.0 to ≤75.6 (n = 301)		>75.6 to ≤79.2 (n = 232)	
Urinary incontinence (%)	0	–	0	–	0	–
Urinary retention (%)	4		1	–	2	–
Increased frequency/urgency (%)	–	0	–	0	–	0
Urethral stricture (%)	–	2	–	0	–	1
Hematuria (%)	3	–	0	–	0	–
Diarrhea (%)	–	0	–	0	–	0
Rectal pain/tenesmus (%)	0		0	0	–	–
Rectal bleeding (%)	–	8	1		2	–
Rectal ulceration (%)	–	0	–	0	0	–
Rectal fistula (%)	0	–	0	0	–	–
Proctitis (%)		2		0	1	–
Rectal incontinence (%)	0	–	0	–	0	–

cl-PTV ranged from 70.2 to 79.2 Gy. We want to emphasize that we are not describing central axis (CA) doses, which are generally 5% higher. Our prescription and delivered doses are specified to be the minimum dose to the patient-specific cl-PTV.

The ART acute and chronic toxicity are similar within the various dose levels used and equal or lower to those seen at other institutions that have been dose escalating (35–37). However, the prostate gland doses selected by the ART process were on the high end of the spectrum with isocentric ICRU doses being in the range of 74 to 84 Gy. This high doses may not be necessary for all patients, particularly those with low-risk features, as it has been suggested by Horwitz et al. (38), or for some with the intermediate risks factors as reported by Martinez et al. (39).

Until December 2006, we have treated at Beaumont Hospital more than 1400 patients with prostate cancer using the IGART process. To allow for a meaningful follow-up we are reporting on the initial consecutively treated 642 patients with mean follow-up of 4.6 years.

The results reported here demonstrate that the margin reduction achieved with the ART-PTV, with the corresponding improvement in accuracy and precision of dose delivery, has resulted in significant dose escalation while maintaining acceptable GU and gastrointestinal (GI) isotoxicity levels.

We compared our 3D conformal ART technique (556 patients) with the ART-IMRT technique (172 patients), and the toxicity data was presented at ASTRO 2007. The distribution of patients in group I or II was similar in both treatment cohorts. Median follow-up was 4.3 years versus 2.2 years for the three-dimensional conformal radiotherapy (3DCRT) and IMRT groups, respectively ($p < 0.01$). There were more group II patients (larger treatment fields) treated with IMRT (60%) versus 3DCRT (51%), $p < 0.01$. 3DCRT patients experienced significantly higher acute grade ≥ 2 urinary retention (7% vs. 2% for IMRT, $p = 0.03$), as well as higher acute grade ≥ 2 rectal pain/tenesmus (19% vs. 5% for IMRT, $p < 0.01$). Chronic GU and GI toxicity were generally low in both groups (Table 5). However, 17 patients (3%) in the 3DCRT group developed grade ≥ 2 chronic urinary retention versus only one patient (0.5%) in the IMRT group ($p = 0.05$). More importantly, 86 patients (16%) treated with 3DCRT developed grade ≥ 2 chronic rectal bleeding versus six patients (4%) in the IMRT group ($p < 0.01$). The median time to rectal bleeding was 1.0 year for 3DCRT versus 0.9 year for IMRT. The actuarial 1, 2, and 3 year grade ≥ 2 chronic rectal bleeding was 6%, 17%, and 18% for 3DCRT versus 3%, 3%, and 5% for IMRT, respectively ($p < 0.01$).

In terms of clinical outcome, the biochemical control using the Phoenix definition was over 90% at five years. As seen in Table 6, there are significant differences in outcome between group I (favorable-risk) and group II (intermediate/high-risk) patients, as expected. However, the five-year outcomes for group II are very encouraging.

Online Image-Guided ART-IMRT

As a natural extension of the ART process, our efforts were focused on switching from off-line image feedback to real-time image feedback where the daily target and normal organs in each patient are reassessed immediately before treatment. When required, dose reconstruction and planning optimization could be performed in real time on the basis of target and normal tissue positions obtained over the course of treatment.

An online CBCT imaging system developed as a bench-top prototype at WBH has been constructed to generate high-resolution, soft-tissue images of the patient

Table 5 Toxicity (CTC version 3) in 728 Prostate Cancer Patients Treated with A-IGRT

Treated	3DCRT (grades 2 + 3)	IMRT (grades 2 + 3)	p value
Acute			
GU frequency/urgency	34%	30%	0.29
Dysuria	5%	2%	0.15
GU incontinence	0.5%	2%	0.04
Urinary retention	7%	2%	0.03
Rectal pain/tenesmus	19%	5%	<0.01
Diarrhea	10%	8%	0.43
Chronic			
GU frequency/urgency	12%	8%	0.12
Urinary retention	3%	0.5%	0.05
Hematuria	4%	5%	0.43
Urethral stricture	1%	2%	0.10
Rectal pain/tenesmus	1%	0%	0.16
Diarrhea	3%	2%	0.51
Rectal bleeding	16%	4%	<0.01

Abbreviations: A-IGRT, adaptive image-guided radiation therapy; 3DCRT, three-dimensional conformal radiotherapy; IMRT, intensity-modulated radiation therapy; GU, genitourinary.

Table 6 ART PSA Control, 5-Year Actuarial Rates

	All patients ($n = 642$)	Group I ($n = 342$)	Group II ($n = 300$)	p value
OS	87.4%	90.3%	83.1%	0.019
CSS	97.9%	98.7%	96.8%	0.170
DFS	90.2%	93.9%	85.1%	0.001
BF	8.4%	5.1%	12.8%	0.001

Abbreviations: OS, overall survival; CSS, cause-specific survival; DFS, disease-free survival; BF, biochemical failure.

at the time of treatment for the purpose of guiding therapy and reducing geometric uncertainties in the process of radiation planning and delivery. The system includes a kilovoltage (kv) imaging unit capable of radiography, fluoroscopy, and CBCT that has been integrated with a medical linear accelerator. Kilovoltage X-rays are generated by a conventional X-ray tube mounted on a retractable arm at 90° to the treatment source. A 41 × 41 cm^2 flat-panel X-ray detector is mounted opposite the kV tube. The entire imaging system operates under computer control, with a single application providing calibration, image acquisition, processing, and CBCT reconstruction. CBCT imaging involves acquiring multiple kV radiographs as the gantry rotates through 360° of rotation. A filtered back-projection algorithm is employed to reconstruct the volumetric images (27).

To assess the potential of increasing the accuracy and precision of prostate radiotherapy delivery by using online image guidance through daily onboard CBCT scans, we designed and activated a clinical protocol with the objective of establishing IGART as a valid treatment modality in prostate cancer. Since better targeting and as a result tighter PTV margins are possible with IGART, the protocol uses a hypofractionation regimen that will shorten the total treatment time from eight and a half to four weeks, then to three weeks, two weeks, and finally to one week while delivering an equivalent minimal prostate dose of 75.6 Gy.

In the first phase, 20 patients from group I (favorable risk) and 20 patients from group II (intermediate/high risk) will be enrolled in the study and will be treated with a four-week IGART regimen. Toxicity will be evaluated at six-month interval. Target volume definition for patients in group I and II are according to our current ART protocol, i.e., prostate gland only for patients in group I and prostate plus proximal two-third of the seminal vesicles for patients in group II. If acute and late GU and GI toxicities are not in excess by more than 7% of toxicity seen with our current ART protocol, we will proceed with step 2. Twenty patients from both groups I and II will be enrolled on a three-week IGART regimen and will be followed for six months. Same toxicity criteria applied in step 1 will be used, namely, acute and late GU and GI toxicities should not exceed by more than 7% of the toxicity seen with our current ART protocol. If toxicity constraint is met, 20 patients will be enrolled on a two-week and finally 20 patients on a one-week IGART regimen. Patients will be followed for six months with the above-mentioned toxicity criteria to be met. If the recorded toxicity is greater than 7% higher than the one expected, there will be no progression to the next level.

Under local anesthesia, three Visicoil markers, 4 cm in length and 0.35 mm in diameter, are implanted into the prostate under trans-rectal ultrasound (TRUS) guidance.

Two Visicoils are placed posteriorly in each prostate lobe and the third one is placed anteriorly close to the anterior fibromuscular area. Visicoil placements are performed before the start of radiation therapy. Visicoil markers enable tracking prostate motion during treatment as well as prostate displacement between treatments. All patients undergo a pretreatment MRI that will serve as a template for precise location of prostate gland boundaries, seminal vesicles, neurovascular bundles, penile bulb, bladder, rectum, and the Visicoils.

The CTV is defined as the gross tumor volume (GTV) with a 0-mm margin for risk group I and 2 to 4 mm for risk group II patients. Planning target volume (PTV) is defined as the CTV with a 3-mm margin to compensate for variability in daily treatment setup and internal target motion due to rectal/bladder motion or other motion (respiration and muscle contractions) during treatment. Of note, this margin is significantly smaller than for the conventional 3DCRT and ART because the online correction component will account for the setup inaccuracies and interfraction organ motions.

Treatments are given five days per week. The prescription dose is 3.2 Gy prescribed to the isocenter, in 20 fractions, for a total dose of 64 Gy with a normalized total dose (NTD) of 79.4 Gy. The total number of fractions is 20, 15, 10, and 5 in the four-, three-, two-, and one-week treatment groups, respectively. For the three-, two-, and one-week treatment groups, the prescription dose is 3.9, 5.1, and 7.8 Gy per fraction, respectively. Seven-field IMRT is used with the dose prescribed at the PTV (minimum 95% coverage of prescribed dose).

Weeks of RT	4	3	2	1
Prostate, $\alpha/\beta = 4$ Gy				
Number of fractions	20	15	10	5
Dose/fraction (Gy)	3.2	3.9	5.1	7.8
Total dose (Gy)	64	58.5	51	39
NTD (Gy)	79.4	79.7	80.0	79.3
95% of NTD	75.5	75.7	76.0	75.4
Bladder, $\alpha/\beta = 2.5$ Gy				
<30% volume @ 75.6 Gy	59.4	53.6	45.9	34.5
0% volume @ 85 Gy	64.1	57.6	49.2	37.0

Before each treatment the patient undergoes a CBCT scan with images reconstructed online. This process takes approximately one to two minutes, and the imaging dose is under 3 cGy. The registration between the CT "image of the day" obtained with CBCT to the planning CT images is made automatically based on Visicoil markers. Simple positional corrections (rotations and translations) are made to ensure optimal CTV coverage. After the treatment is delivered another CBCT is obtained to verify the

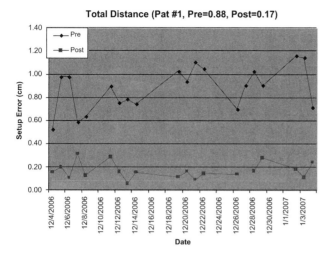

Figure 3 Pre- and postcorrection setup error using online cone-beam CT

applied online correction. There is a significant difference between the setup error before and after the CBCT-based correction as seen in Figure 3.

We have treated 12 patients so far with 64 Gy in 20 fractions over four weeks. The average time the patient is in the treatment room is 18 minutes. The maximum acute toxicity was grade 2 (increased urinary frequency) in three patients. The first four patients with a minimum follow-up of six months have grade 0 chronic GU and GI toxicity.

SUMMARY OF PERTINENT CONCLUSIONS

- A large generic PTV has been the typical way of addressing interpatient and interfraction variation in radiotherapy, which has been one of the major limiting factors for treatment improvement.
- The planning target margin can be significantly reduced by systematically managing patient-specific variation.
- However, the management of interfractional patient-specific anatomical variation requires multiple measurements of patient anatomy accomplished by different image feedbacks.
- Among them, CT image feedback, including both off-board conventional CT and ultimately onboard CBCT has been most commonly used.
- The most effective method in image feedback management of radiotherapy is the adaptive control methodology with the aim to customize each patient's treatment plan to patient-specific variation by evaluating, characterizing, and incorporating the systematic and random variations in the adaptive planning.

- On average, a target dose increase of 15% can be achieved with online IG-IMRT based on rectal wall EUDs and 48% based on bladder wall EUDs.
- Our excellent results in terms of clinical outcome and toxicity profile underline the strong clinical impact that image-guidance and the ART process have in the accuracy and precision of radiation therapy delivery.

REFERENCES

1. Valicenti RK, Michalski JM, Bosch WR, et al. Is weekly port filming adequate for verifying patient position in modern radiation therapy. Int J Radiat Oncol Biol Phys 1994; 30:431–438.
2. Hunt MA, Schultheiss TE, Desobry GE, et al. An evaluation of setup uncertainties for patients treated to pelvic sites. Int J Radiat Oncol Biol Phys 1995; 32:227–233.
3. Soffen EM, Hanks GE, Hwang CC, et al. Conformal static field therapy for low volume low grade prostate cancer with rigid immobilization. Int J Radiat Oncol Biol Phys 1990; 20:141–146.
4. Song PY, Washington M, Vaida F, et al. A comparison of four patient immobilization devices in the treatment of prostate cancer patients with three dimensional conformal radiotherapy. Int J Radiat Oncol Biol Phys 1996; 34: 213–219.
5. Verhey L. Immobilization and positioning patients for radiotherapy. Semin Radiat Oncol 1995; 5:100–114.
6. Goitein M. Calculation of the uncertainty in the dose delivered during radiation therapy. Med Phys 1985; 12 (5):608–612.
7. Kutcher GJ, Mageras GS, Leibel SA. Control, correction, and modeling of setup errors and organ motion. Semin Radiat Oncol 1995; 5(2):134–145.
8. Leong J. Implementation of random positioning error in computerized radiation treatment planning systems as a result of fractionation. Phys Med Biol 1987; 32(3): 327–334.
9. Urie MM, Goitein M, Doppke K, et al. The role of uncertainty analysis in treatment planning. Int J Radiat Oncol Biol Phys 1991; 21:91–107.
10. Bel A, Van Herk M, Bartelink H, et al. A verification procedure to improve patient setup accuracy using portal images. Radiother Oncol 1993; 29:253–260.
11. Denham JW, Dally MJ, Hunter K, et al. Objective decision-making following a portal film: the results of a pilot study. Int J Radiat Oncol Biol Phys 1993; 26:869–876.
12. Dutreix A, van der Schueren E, Leunens L. Quality control at the patient level: action or retrospective introspection. Radiother Oncol 1992; 25:146–147.
13. Shalev S, Gluhchev G. Interventional correction of patient setup using portal imaging: a comparison of decision rules. Int J Radiat Oncol Biol Phys 1995; 32(S1):216 (abstr).
14. Shalev S, Gluhchev G. When and how to correct a patient setup. In: Proceedings of the XIth International Conference on Computers in Radiation Therapy, Manchester, UK, March 20–24, 1994:274–275.

15. Yan D, Wong J, Gustafson G, et al. A new model for "accept or reject" strategies in off-line and on-line megavoltage treatment evaluation. Int J Radiat Oncol Biol Phys 1995; 31:943–952.

16. Yan D, Vicini F, Wong J, et al. Adaptive radiation therapy. Phys Med Biol 1997; 42:123–132.

17. Yan D, Wong J, Vicini F, et al. Adaptive modification of treatment planning to minimize the deleterious effects of treatment setup errors. Int J Radiat Oncol Biol Phys 1997; 38:197–206.

18. Yan D, Lockman D, Brabbins D, et al. An off-line strategy for constructing a patient-specific planning target volume in adaptive treatment process of prostate cancer. Int J Radiat Oncol Biol Phys 2000; 48:289–302.

19. Martinez A, Yan D, Brabbins D, et al. Improvement in dose escalation using the process of adaptive radiotherapy combined with 3D-conformal or intensity modulated beams for prostate cancer. Int J Radiat Oncol Biol Phys 2001; 50 (5):1226–1234.

20. Wloch J, Yan D, Brabbins D, et al. Quality control for image guided radiotherapy prostate cancer. Int J Radiat Oncol Biol Phys 2007; 69(35):520 (abstr 34).

21. Vargas C, Kestin L, Yan D, et al. Dose-volume analysis of predictors for chronic rectal toxicity following treatment of prostate cancer with adaptive image-guided radiotherapy. Int J Radiat Oncol Biol Phys 2005; 62(5):1297–1308.

22. Vargas C, Martinez AA, Yan D, et al. A phase II dose escalation study to image-guided adaptive radiotherapy for prostate cancer: use of dose constraints to achieve rectal isotoxicity. Int J Radiat Oncol Biol Phys 2005; 63(1): 141–149.

23. Harsolia A, Vargas C, Yan D, et al. Predictors for chronic urinary toxicity after the treatment for prostate cancer with adaptive 3-D conformal radiotherapy: dose-volume analysis of a phase II dose escalation study. Int J Radiat Oncol Biol Phys 2007; 69(4):1100–1109.

24. Jaffray DA, Wong JW. Exploring "target of the day" strategies for a medical linear accelerator with cone-beam CT scanning capabilities. In: Leavitt D, Starkscall G, eds. Proceedings of the XIIth International Conference on the Use of Computers in Radiation Therapy. Utah, USA: Salt Lake City, 1997:172–175.

25. Jaffray DA, Drake DG, Moreau M, et al. A radiographic and tomographic imaging system integrated into a medical linear accelerator for localization of bone and soft-tissue targets. Int J Radiat Oncol Biol Phys 1999; 45(3):773–789.

26. Jaffray DA, Siewerdsen JH. Cone-beam computed tomography with a flat-panel imager: initial performance characterization. Med Phys 2000; 27(6):1311–1323.

27. Jaffray DA, Siewerdsen JH, Wong JW, et al. Flat-panel cone-beam computed tomography for image-guided radiation therapy. Int J Radiat Oncol Biol Phys 2002; 53 (5):1337–1349.

28. Ghilezan M, Jaffray D, Siewerdsen JM, et al. 1-hour intrafraction prostate motion assessed with cine magnetic resonance imaging (cine-MRI). Int J Radiat Oncol Biol Phys 2003; 62(2):406–417.

29. Ghilezan M, Yan D, Liang J, et al. Online image-guided intensity-modulated radiotherapy for prostate cancer: how much improvement can we expect? A theoretical assessment of clinical benefits and potential dose escalation by improving precision and accuracy of radiation delivery. Int J Radiat Oncol Biol Phys 2004; 60(5):1602–1610.

30. Wu Q, Ivaldi G, Liang J, et al. Geometric and dosimetric evaluations of an online image-guided 3D conformal radiation therapy of prostate cancer. Int J Radiat Oncol Biol Phys 2006; 64:1596–1609.

31. Wu Q, Liang J, Ghilezan M, et al. A "Field to Target" (F2T) online correction technique for image guided radiation therapy. Int J Radiat Oncol Biol Phys 2006; 66(suppl): S140 (abstr).

32. Mohan R, Zhang X, Wang H, et al. Use of deformed intensity distributions for on-line modification of image-guided IMRT to account for interfractional anatomic changes. Int J Radiat Oncol Biol Phys 2005; 61:1258–1266.

33. Yan D, Lockman D. Organ/patient geometric variation in external beam radiotherapy and its effects. Med Phys 2001; 28:593–602.

34. Birkner M, Yan D, Alber M, et al. Adapting inverse planning to patient and organ geometrical variation: algorithm and implementation. Med Phys 2003; 30:2822–2831.

35. Zelefsky M, Wallner K, Ling C, et al. Comparison of the five year outcome and morbidity of 3-D conformal radiotherapy versus transperineal permanent Iodine-125 implantation for early stage prostatic cancer. J Clin Oncol 1999; 17(2):517–522.

36. Zelefsky MJ, Leibel SA, Gaudin PB, et al. Dose escalation with three-dimensional conformal radiation therapy affects the outcome in prostate cancer. Int J Radiat Oncol Biol Phys 1998; 41(3):491–500.

37. Pollack A, Zagars GK, Smith LG, et al. Preliminary results of a randomized radiotherapy dose-escalation study comparing 70 Gy with 78 Gy for prostate cancer. J Clin Oncol 2000; 18(23):3904–3911.

38. Horwitz E, Hanlon A, Pinover W, et al. Defining the optimal radiation dose with three-dimensional conformal radiation therapy for patients with non-metastatic prostate carcinoma by using recursive partitioning techniques. Cancer 2001; 92:1281–1287.

39. Martinez AA, Gonzalez J, Spencer W, et al. Conformal high dose rate brachytherapy improves biochemical control and cause specific survival in patients with prostate cancer and poor prognostic factors. J Urol 2003; 169(3):974–980.

40. Jaffray DA, Siewerdsen JH, Wong JW, et al. Flat-panel cone-beam computed tomography for image-guided radiation therapy. Int J Radiat Oncol Biol Phys 2002; 53:1337–1349.

12

IGRT in Prostate Cancer—the Calypso 4D Localization System

ARUL MAHADEVAN, KEVIN STEPHANS, AND TOUFIK DJEMIL

Cleveland Clinic Foundation, Cleveland, Ohio, U.S.A.

INTRODUCTION

Over the past decade, continuous refinement in the extent of irradiated tissue has been the focus of development in radiation oncology. The goal has been to irradiate essentially all cancerous cells and exclude surrounding normal tissue to maximize the therapeutic ratio. Advances in imaging to facilitate target delineation and enhanced treatment planning techniques like intensity-modulated treatment planning (IMRT) have led to the development of enhanced beam delivery methods like image-guided radiation therapy (IGRT). Further refinements are now largely limited by the changes in position of target, not just day to day but also during treatment. Target motion management during the course of radiation therapy (RT) has thus become a topic of heightened interest among radiation oncologists.

Tracking and adjusting to target motion during the delivery of four-dimensional radiation therapy (4D-RT) is a frontier in RT that offers substantial advantages for dose escalation and avoidance of normal tissues. 4D-RT offers the ability to record and adjust to both interfraction and intrafraction motion. It adjusts for interfraction variables such as rectal and bladder filling as well as changes in a patient's body surface or surface markers on a daily basis. Intrafraction motion is caused by breathing, bowel motility, and muscle tone. Bowel motility and gas patterns appear to be affected by rectal filling (1). Furthermore,

bladder filling and rectal motility are likely altered over the course of RT due to acute effects of treatment. Following and correcting for these changes over the course of treatment would allow for more accurate target localization, and also a better understanding of how to design margins for standard, static RT. Insufficient dose to the cancer bearing area of the prostate (2) may occur if target motion is ignored during treatment delivery. In addition, real-time organ tracking allows for the calculation of the dose actually delivered to the target accounting for any motion that was observed. Thus, dynamic dose reconstruction would allow for fine-tuning of future fractions to compensate for the influence of motion on already-delivered fractions—adaptive RT (3).

The margins established for RT often rely on "population-based margins," which attempt to ensure that at least 90% of patients receive a minimum of 95% of the prescribed planning target volume (PTV) dose (4). In any normal distribution of patients, this would cause some to be underdosed while others to be treated to a wider target than necessary. Both of these shortcomings are improved with four-dimensional radiation delivery.

Evidence mounts that increased radiation dose improves cancer outcomes. Several retrospective (5,6) and prospective randomized trials have been reported recently addressing RT dose escalation in prostate cancer (7–10). Peeters et al. (8) reported their results on a randomized phase III trial conducted in four Dutch institutions that evaluated the role of escalating the RT dose to 78 Gy from 68 Gy in 669 patients with localized prostate cancer. The five-year failure-free survival (FFS) estimate was 64% in the 78 Gy arm and 54% in the 68 Gy arm ($p = 0.01$). The Zietman et al. trial (7) reported a 19% improvement in five-year prostate-specific antigen (PSA) FFS rates (FFS of 80.4% for patients who received 79.2 Gy vs. 61.4% for those who received 70.2 Gy). This benefit to increased radiation dose was seen for higher-risk patients (44% risk reduction) as well as low-risk patients (51% risk reduction). The Pollack et al. trial (9) reported an improvement in six-year FFS of 6% (FFS of 70% for patients who received 78 Gy vs. 64% for those who received 70 Gy). There was a preferential benefit to patients with a PSA >10 µg/L who had an improvement in FFS of 19%. The PSA outcome benefit came at a cost of modest increase in genitourinary and gastrointestinal toxicity in these trials. For instance, grade 2 or higher rectal toxicity rates at six years were 12% and 26% for the 70 and 78 Gy arms, respectively ($p = 0.001$) in the Pollack trial (9). For patients in the 78 Gy arm, grade 2 or higher rectal toxicity correlated highly with the proportion of the rectum treated to greater than 70 Gy. Not only does this demonstrate the benefit of dose escalation to prostate tissue, but it also suggests significant clinical benefit to restricting rectal doses below a dose level commonly delivered to the prostate, and thus can positively influence the therapeutic ratio.

Furthermore, the α/β ratio (which describes the sensitivity of tissue to radiation fraction size) for prostate cancer is estimated to be lower (1–3 Gy) than values normally associated with most neoplasms (≥ 10 Gy) (11–13). This has led to the development of hypofractionated regimens (14) that, to date, have yielded encouraging long-term results and are being compared in randomized studies to conventionally fractionated regimens (RTOG 0415). Hypofractionated regimens thus have the advantage of addressing the potentially low α/β ratio of prostate cancer as well as improving patient convenience by reducing the number of treatment fractions required. A higher dose per fraction, however, may introduce more potential for late normal tissue effects and also increase the length of each treatment allowing more time for intrafraction motion.

Both dose escalation and hypofractionation have raised the stakes for our ability to deliver treatment accurately. There is a fine balance between increasing tumor control and limiting normal tissue toxicity. Increasing the accuracy of treatment delivery offers advantages on both fronts. In addition, the utilization of IMRT (designed to improve delivery of dose to target and minimize dose to surrounding structures) substantially increases the treatment time (15). This places further emphasis on the control of intrafraction variables.

A variety of systems can be utilized to provide information about the intrafraction motion of the prostate: transabdominal ultrasound, X-ray, CT, and cine-MRI. These systems have several disadvantages: they provide only snapshots of prostate position; they are not available during radiation delivery; most require additional ionizing radiation exposure; they are not efficient and are labor intensive; and they are subjective and operator dependant in acquisition and interpretation. Strategies such as gating afford the ability to turn the beam on and off based on target location and offer a simple solution to treating only when the target is located within the radiation beam pathway. The downside to gating is that it may increase treatment time, and in the prostate it may require manual adjustment if the target does not quickly move back into position. Hence this technology may be more applicable to cyclically moving targets (like lung or liver targets) rather than for targets moving unpredictably (like prostate). Other methods such as real-time localization based on fiducial markers may simplify the calculation of target localization and allow tracking to occur fast enough for the position of the target to be adjusted continuously during radiation delivery. One such system is the Calypso® 4D Localization System that utilizes implanted Beacon® electromagnetic transponder system (Calypso System, Calypso Medical, Seattle, Washington, U.S.) will be described in detail below.

THE CALYPSO SYSTEM

The Calypso System consists of the following components (Fig. 1).

Beacon Electromagnetic Transponders

The implantable Beacon® electromagnetic transponder measures approximately 8 mm in length and 1.85 mm in diameter and consists of a hermetically sealed biocompatible glass capsule containing a miniature passive electrical circuit made of a small ferrite core and copper coil (Fig. 2). Three transponders are implanted in specific regions in the prostate for use as fiducial markers in RT (Fig. 3). These transponders are passive and echo a signal only when excited by the nonionizing electromagnetic radiofrequency (RF) radiation generated by the system array. The response signal of each transponder is unique and is specific to that transponder. The system uses this signal to determine the location of the transponder and the location is updated at the rate of 10 Hz. Each Beacon transponder is packaged in a transfer capsule. Each capsule is color coded and labeled for prostate implantation with A for apex of the prostate, L for left base, or R for right base.

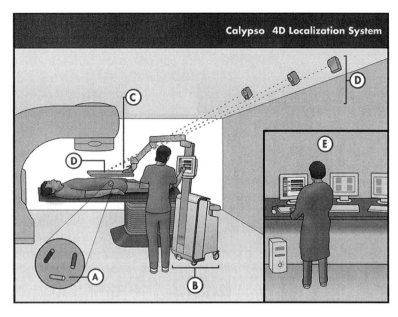

Figure 1 (**A**) Beacon® transponders; (**B**) Console; (**C**) Array; (**D**) Optical system; (**E**) Tracking station.

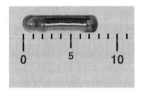

Figure 2 Calypso Beacon® transponder.

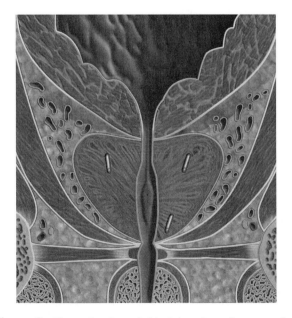

Figure 3 (*See color insert.*) Ideal location of transponders within prostate.

Implanted transponders are visible as opaque structures on kilovoltage X-ray, computed tomography (CT), and ultrasound images. Because of the low density of transponder material, their visibility on megavoltage images depends on the density of the surrounding anatomic structures. The transponders are MRI safe but will cause an image artifact around the transponder. The extent of the artifact will depend on the magnetic strength of the scanner.

4D Console

The Calypso 4D Console is a movable unit that is placed in the treatment room next to the treatment table. A mechanical arm attached to the console can be extended to allow for manual positioning of the array. It is important that the gantry can rotate freely without collision with the console or array arm. The computer on the console has a touch screen that provides objective on-screen graphics and data for QA, calibration, array positioning, and for patient localization.

Four-Dimensional Electromagnetic Array

The array is a flat panel connected to the console by means of an extendable mechanical arm. It contains components that generate and detect the nonionizing electromagnetic field used to determine the position of the target. The array is positioned over the patient during setup and is designed to be left in place during treatment. It contains circuitry that generates signals to excite the transponders and to receive the response signal of the transponders. The array also has multiple embedded optical (infrared) markers for the optical system to determine the position of the array with respect to the machine isocenter. The array is made of low density, nearly air equivalent material with peripherally positioned signal and sensor coils so that the attenuation of the megavoltage treatment beam is equivalent to between 2 and 3 mm of water (16).

Optical System

Three infrared cameras mounted permanently in the ceiling of the treatment room along with a power supply and a hub constitutes the optical system. These three cameras provide redundancy in case one of the cameras is obscured. As long as half of the optical markers are visible to two of the three cameras, the system has adequate data to continuously monitor the position of the array without compromising on accuracy.

4D Tracking Station

The 4D Tracking Station receives and interprets data from the 4D Console and the optical system, which are connected through Ethernet. Information about the target is presented to the therapist using simple, objective on-screen graphics complemented by numerical data and auditory indicators when target moves outside of the predefined limits. The tracking station is also used for system administrative functions such as user management, patient records, and daily reports.

Treatment Table Overlay

Because of the use of electromagnetic signals by the Calypso System to locate the target, the system accuracy can be affected by conductive treatment tabletops containing metal and/or other conductive materials, including carbon fiber. Therefore, a table overlay, designed to ensure that the conductive components are far enough from the transponders so that they do not interfere with localization, is needed. The tabletop overlay is a nonconductive, rigid surface and is compatible with standard treatment tables with removable inserts. It consists of a headrest, a footrest, and a central gridded part over which the treatment area of the patient is positioned.

TECHNICAL ISSUES

The 4D Electromagnetic Array consists of four source coils, which generate signals to excite the transponders, and 32 sensor coils, which detect the response signals returned by the transponders (17). The source coils generate AC electromagnetic fields in the lower end of the AM band frequency range (between 300 and 500 kHz). Prior to treatment, the relative polarity of the four source coils is selected to optimally excite each transponder at its resonant frequency. Each transponder has a unique configuration and thus is briefly excited at its distinct frequency by the nonionizing electromagnetic field generated by the source coil. These electromagnetic fields are of long wavelength (low energy) and thus do not affect treatment delivery. The resonant current amplitude in the transponder increases during signal excitation and then declines during the response period and is continuously detected by the 32 sensor coils in the array system. Several hundred repetitive response signals are averaged for each transponder to increase the signal to noise ratio. The system is able to independently track each transponder by its distinct resonant frequency. The signal from each transponder at each of the 32 coils is analyzed by the software to solve for the three-dimensional coordinates of each transponder to a measured accuracy of within 0.5 mm. The relative position of the three transponders can be used to infer the spatial position and orientation of the target.

The 4D Electromagnetic Array is designed to detect transponders placed within a $14 \times 14 \times 27$ cm^3 sensing volume determined to contain the range of common prostate positions from near to the skin surface where the array would be positioned on a retrospective review of CT scans (17). In initial phantom studies, the measured variation in transponder position readout was extremely precise at 80 mm from the source array (a typical distance for a prostate in a thin patient) with a standard deviation of 0.006, 0.01, and 0.006 mm in the x, y, and z directions, respectively (17). Reproducibility decreased with increasing distance from the array but was still submillimeter at 270 mm from the array with a standard deviation of 0.27, 0.36, and 0.48 mm in the x, y, and z directions, respectively. This introduces a physical limit to the system. Patients whose dimensions may restrict the array from being placed within 270 mm from the prostate are beyond the approved specifications of the system. No significant drifts in the location readout were observed in the phantom over a 20-minute recording period demonstrating stability compared to background electromagnetic interference beyond the time required for real-time organ motion tracking.

Dynamic accuracy for the Calypso System is defined as the static accuracy plus the effects of latency, which depend on the target motion. For a typical patient having three transponders, the latency to the tracking station screen T is less than 0.4 seconds (including all the graphics updates). Therefore, prostate moving at velocity $V = 0.5$ cm/sec (although most are slower than this) would have a latency impact of $V \times T = \sim 0.2$ cm. This is in addition to the static accuracy. Submillimeter accuracy was maintained using the dynamic phantom at speeds of up to 3 cm/s (17). The commercial system is optimized

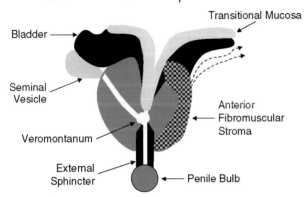

Bladder and External Sphincter Interface

Bladder

Transitional Mucosa

Seminal Vesicle

Anterior Fibromuscular Stroma

Veromontanum

External Sphincter

Penile Bulb

Figure 4.7 Prostate interface with bladder and external sphincter. Note the bladder mucosa extends to the veromontanum and the external sphincter extends to just below the veromontanum (*see page 44*).

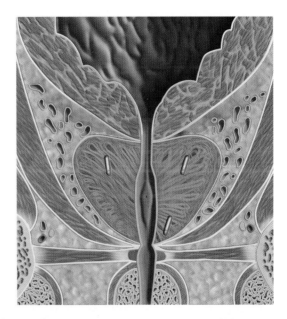

Figure 12.3 Ideal location of transponders within prostate (*see page 129*).

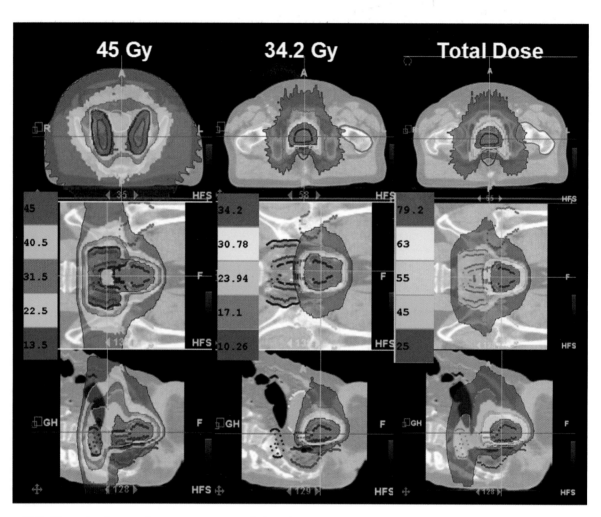

Figure 13.8 Example of a complex prostate case consisting of 45 Gy volume including lymph nodes, 34.2 Gy boost volume, and the total dose (*see page 147*).

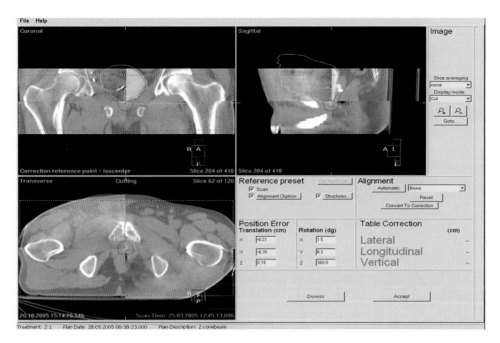

Figure 14.5 Computer monitor display for online image registration and setup error correction using cone-beam CT. Commercial software used at TJUH (Elekta AB, Sweden) (*see page 160*).

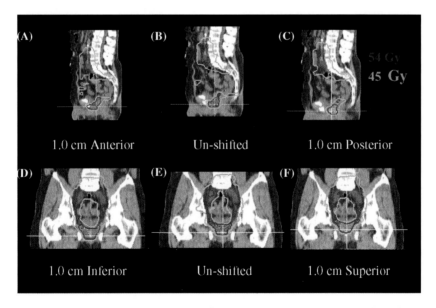

Figure 16.5 (**A–F**) The sagittal and coronal dose distributions for a patient with the prostate position shifted anteriorly (**A**), unshifted (**B** and **D**), shifted posteriorly (**C**), shifted inferiorly (**D**), and shifted superiorly (**E**). To correct for daily displacements, gold marker seeds are used to track the prostate position each day prior to each treatment. Note that the lymph nodes and prostate are always covered. To accomplish this feat, the appropriate "the plan of the day" is chosen to match position of the prostate when shown. An onboard imaging system is required to implement this approach, which we call multiple adaptive plan IMRT (MAP-IMRT) (*see page 192*).

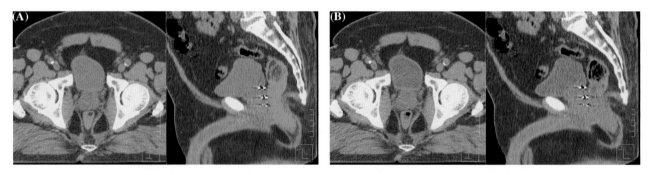

Figure 17.2 Organs at risk. (**A**) RTOG definition for rectal thickness and bladder thickness. (**B**) PROFIT definition for rectal thickness and bladder thickness (*see page 208*).

for human response times for prostate applications specifically.

CLINICAL USE OF THE CALYPSO SYSTEM
Placement of Markers

Three transponders are inserted by a radiation oncologist or a urologist transrectally or transperineally (under ultrasound guidance) using a 14-gauge introducer needle assembly, into the apical, left base, and right base regions of the prostate. The technique is similar to obtaining a prostate biopsy. Similar to gold fiducial placement, midline positioning of the transponders should be avoided to prevent loss through the urethra. Patients are prepped for implant with antibiotic prophylaxis as well as a same-day enema, and the procedure is commonly done using only local anesthesia. Implantation generally takes 10 minutes or less from the time of ultrasound probe insertion. Similar to gold fiducial placement, patients on anticoagulation or antiplatelet medications (with the exception of Aspirin) or patients unable to tolerate local anesthetics due to allergies need medical management before considering the use of this system. Patients with implanted pacemakers or other signaling medical devices should be considered with caution, as the Calypso System utilizes magnetic fields and compatibility is unknown. Patients with hip replacements or large metal implants like vascular grafts, which are in close proximity to the prostate, are contraindications to use of this system. The 4D Electromagnetic Array must be positioned over the region where the transponders are implanted and must be within 27 cm of the transponders for accurate localization and real-time tracking. In patients with a significantly large anteroposterior (AP) diameter, the Calypso System may be used for daily setup localization but not real-time tracking because of geometric constraints between the patient's upper surface, the Calypso System array, and the gantry head during full gantry rotation. In these patients, the Calypso System is moved away during radiation delivery. This situation was encountered in 6 out of 41 patients enrolled in a recent study (18).

Phantom studies have shown that target localization is accurate in the presence of either stranded or free radioactive brachytherapy seeds as well as surgical clips (19). The accuracy of real-time tracking in the presence of radioactive seeds or clips has not yet been demonstrated in patients.

Simulation

Simulation is commonly performed in the supine position as this is associated with increased patient comfort, increased ease of setup for therapists, and less intrafrac-

tion prostate position variation requiring less pretreatment adjustment when compared with prone position (20). Institutional standard immobilization devices may be used including a band around the feet, a wedge under the knees, a ring for the hands, or a Vac-Lock® bag, though no immobilization devices are required. CT simulation through the target region should be done with the smallest slice thickness available (1.0–1.5 mm), as the accuracy of array to transponder localization is submillimeter (17). Using thicker slice CT acquisition would significantly decrease the accuracy of any fiducial-based localization system for predicting prostate location as accurate fiducial coordinate identification is a critical component of the localization process. In the case of the electromagnetic transponders, the magnetic center corresponds with the radiographic center of the transponders, and a thin slice CT acquisition ensures that the radiographic centers of the transponders can be accurately identified in the CT images. The image acquisition pitch on helical CT scanners must be less than or equal to 2. The skin is marked in standard fashion (tattoos are commonly used) for initial patient setup.

Treatment Planning

Any treatment planning software can be used to identify the transponder and treatment isocenter coordinates. Automatic translation of the treatment planning coordinate reference frame (CRF) to the Calypso System CRF is supported for the Philips Pinnacle™, CMS Xio™, and Varian Eclipse™ treatment planning systems (TPS) and for any TPS that uses the IEC-61217 CRF. Coordinates of the apex, left base, and right base transponders are identified as part of the treatment planning process. When the treatment plan is complete, the transponder and isocenter positions are recorded and entered into the Calypso System.

Patient Setup

Prior to the delivery of each fraction of radiation, patients are initially set up to their marks (tattoos) from the time of simulation and aligned to the room lasers. The Calypso System array is then placed over the patient and activated to localize the position of the transponders relative to the array. The infrared cameras detect the position of the array relative to the machine isocenter. The therapist is instructed via a touch-screen PC console which shifts of the treatment couch in the AP, lateral, and craniocaudal directions are required to bring the planned prostate isocenter precisely to the machine isocenter. At this point, treatment may begin. During treatment, the array continues to localize the transponders at a frequency of 10 Hz and reports their positions outside the treatment room on a monitor at the console. The system allows for programming monitoring thresholds and when the target moves outside of the threshold, the therapist is notified visually and with an auditory alert. Predetermined action levels and protocols for corrective action may then be used to accommodate for organ motion during treatment.

CLINICAL OUTCOMES

A pilot study involving implantation of the transponders was conducted in 20 patients (21) with a prototype system and prototype transponders. This study involved the first human use of the system and evaluated the localization accuracy of this technique compared with radiographic localization. In addition, the ability to obtain real-time prostate-motion information was also evaluated in an 11-patient subset of these 20 patients (21,22). Each patient was implanted with 3 transponders and 58 of the 60 implanted transponders were usable for localization. In one patient, a single transponder was lost post-implantation (likely voided after urethral implantation), and in another patient one transponder was found to be unresponsive. A third migrated approximately 3 cm from the apex to the level of the seminal vesicles around the 4th day after implant, presumably migrating within the venous plexus, but remained suitable for localization. There were no complications from transponder placement. (Post-study processing changes improved the robustness of the transponder, and subsequent clinical studies did not encounter unresponsive transponders. In addition, the commercial system software supports localization when two of the three implanted transponders are located.)

Changes in distances between transponders (used as a proxy for transponder migration) were minimal in 15 of 20 patients by the 4th day after implantation (mean of the SD of intertransponder distance was 1.3 mm) and were stable in all patients after 14 days (21). During a mock setup session, 11 patients first underwent Calypso System localization followed by a kV radiograph and then repeat Calypso System localization. Eight minutes of real-time tracking was then done followed by a repeat of Calypso localizations and radiograph as above. Approximately 30 seconds to 1 minute elapsed between Calypso System localizations and the subsequent comparative radiograph and 10 minutes between the two radiographs. Comparison of Calypso System localization to radiograph was done to measure the reliability of the Calypso System, while comparison between the two radiograph localizations demonstrated change in prostate position over a 10-minute period. The difference in three-dimensional vector setup variation between the Calypso System and kV radiographs for these 44 comparisons was 1.5 ± 0.9 mm. Prostate motion between radiographs ranged from 0.3 to 6.6 mm, which likely accounts for some of the Calypso System to radiographic variation, given the 30 second- to 1 minute elapsing between the studies. This study demonstrated the high degree of accuracy in using the Calypso System for patient set up.

In a subsequent multiinstitutional study, 42 additional patients underwent implantation of electromagnetic transponders (18). Again, implantation was well tolerated and 125 of 126 implanted transponders remained stable and suitable for localization with one transponder being voided without discomfort (that patient later withdrew for unrelated reasons leaving 41 patients on study). One patient experienced significant pain associated with the ultrasound probe insertion and had an apical transponder placed in the prostate-rectal interface without significant associated symptoms and was able to continue with tracking. Transponder stability was again confirmed when similar comparisons between Calypso System localization to radiographs were made during 1027 treatment sessions (18). The average delay between Calypso System localization and X-rays was 152 ± 50 seconds and between the orthogonal X-rays was 18 ± 15 seconds. The average differences in lateral, longitudinal, and vertical components were -0.1 ± 0.9 mm, -0.4 ± 1.4 mm, and 0.0 ± 1.3 mm. The average vector length difference was 1.9 ± 1.2 mm and the maximum vector difference was 3.3 mm. These differences are greater than in the phantom studies (17) but likely are accounted for by prostate motion during the delay of two to three minutes from the completion of Calypso System localization to the time of filming X-rays.

Because of the closed loop system and immediate feedback given to the in-room PC console, the Calypso System is very time efficient in patient set up. Patient setup was timed during 1057 treatment sessions (18). Timing began when the patient was set up to skin marks and the Calypso System console was positioned over the patient. It ended when the therapist judged that the patient was positioned correctly (thus this included activating the Calypso System, reading the PC console instructions, and carrying out the appropriate shifts of the table). The mean setup time was 104 ± 50 seconds (less than 2 minutes). This compares favorably with other image guidance systems such as ultrasound (300 seconds) (23), kV X-rays (250 ± 113 seconds) (24), and cone-beam CT (>270 seconds) (25). In a single institution investigation, we tracked setup times for both Calypso System and an ultrasound system (Restitu[TM], Resonant Medical, Montreal, Canada) for daily treatment localization in a series of 20 consecutive patients. Eleven patients were set up with Calypso System during each treatment fraction (293 observations) and nine with ultrasound (130 observations). Therapists had prior experience with both systems. Median setup times were 1 minute to setup to tattoos and then an additional 1.6 minutes (SD 0.6 minutes) for Calypso System and 3.7 minutes (SD 1.8 minutes) for ultrasound (26). The Calypso System appears to be an efficient daily setup tool and, because of its simple interface and objective nature, can be used by therapists of all experience levels.

When the Calypso System is used for real-time tracking, the array continues to measure and report prostate position at a frequency of 10 Hz. Analyzing the tracking data over a full course of radiation therapy in 35 patients (representing 1157 treatment fractions) revealed target displacement of more than 3 mm from setup location for greater than 30 seconds in 41% of fractions and more than 5 mm for greater than 30 seconds in 15% of fractions (18). The percentage of fractions in which one particular patient experienced motion was quite variable ranging from 3% to 87% of fractions using a 3-mm cutoff and 0% to 56% using a 5-mm cutoff. If very tight margins are employed for prostate radiotherapy without continuous real-time tracking, there could be a marginal miss in a significant number of patients. The clinical significance of marginal misses deserves further study.

Graphs of prostate motion were grouped into broad categories representing typical patterns of prostate motion: Stable target at baseline, transient excursion, persistent excursion, continuous drift, high-frequency excursion, and irregular motion (Fig. 4). Stable prostates could be treated equally well with or without continuous monitoring, if one knew where the prostate was located at all times. A transient excursion would result in only slight underdosing of a proportion of the fraction delivered prior to return to baseline. Persistent excursion represents the case of most efficient use of real-time monitoring in which a single correction can restore the system to accurate treatment. Continuous drift becomes more difficult in that it may not be fixed by a single correction. However, given the anatomic constraints of the pelvis, there clearly is a limit to the extent of a continuous drift. Instead, this situation requires waiting for the prostate to settle into a new position prior to correction and is probably just a variant of persistent excursion. High-frequency excursion and erratic behavior represent cases that could be identified by real-time monitoring but would be difficult to correct for without simply increasing the margins of treatment unless the cause of motion can be determined. Of note, these could be generated by either physical patient motion on the table or motion of the patient's internal organs. Motion on the table may be correctable by an immobilization device while motion of the patient's internal organs perhaps could be corrected by medication (i.e., antispasmodics) or a physical device (rectal balloon). Other options could include motion compensation techniques like automatic table repositioning (27) or multileaf collimator (MLC) synchronization (28).

A few general observations can be made on reviewing the real-time monitoring data. First and foremost is that the motion is unpredictable, both patient to patient and, for any patient, from day to day. Secondly, the lateral shifts are minimal and appear stable over the tracking sessions. This is consistent with the prostate and pelvic anatomy. Thirdly, the longitudinal and vertical shifts typically occurred together. Finally, the prostate does not always return to baseline position after an excursion as noted in some previous cine-MRI studies (29). This underscores the clinical importance of real-time tracking as a significant portion of any long treatment fraction may miss its intended target in these circumstances.

With the knowledge of real-time prostate motion, therapeutic interventions to observed prostate motion can be implemented. These strategies could include no action—suitable for stable patterns of motion and if the margins used for treatment planning are adequate for the observed range of motion; manual gating—this can be achieved by only treating when the target is in alignment; realigning patient—this is especially needed when the pattern observed is a persistent shift and may have to be repeated in case of a continuous drift pattern.

Realignments between beams could be easily and efficiently done. Beam interruption to exercise the later options, especially in the setting of IMRT, can introduce dosimetric consequences that have to be further studied. There is sound rationale behind multiple strategies for interventions to account for intrafraction motion, and a variety of strategies have been employed to date. At the Cleveland Clinic our practice is that if a translation of 3 mm or more and lasting 30 seconds or longer occurs, we allow for completion of that individual beam but then briefly hold treatment until alignment is achieved (reposition the patient using the Calypso System, if needed) prior to the next IMRT segment.

SUMMARY OF PERTINENT CONCLUSIONS

- The Calypso System, as detailed above, represents a simple, straightforward, efficient and objective method of accurately localizing the prostate gland.
- Daily setup before initiation of RT can be performed in an efficient manner.
- Seamless transition to real-time continuous monitoring of prostate location during treatment provides valuable information to potentially prevent inadvertent geographic misses of the target.
- Setup and real-time monitoring throughout treatment delivery can be performed without exposure to additional ionizing radiation.

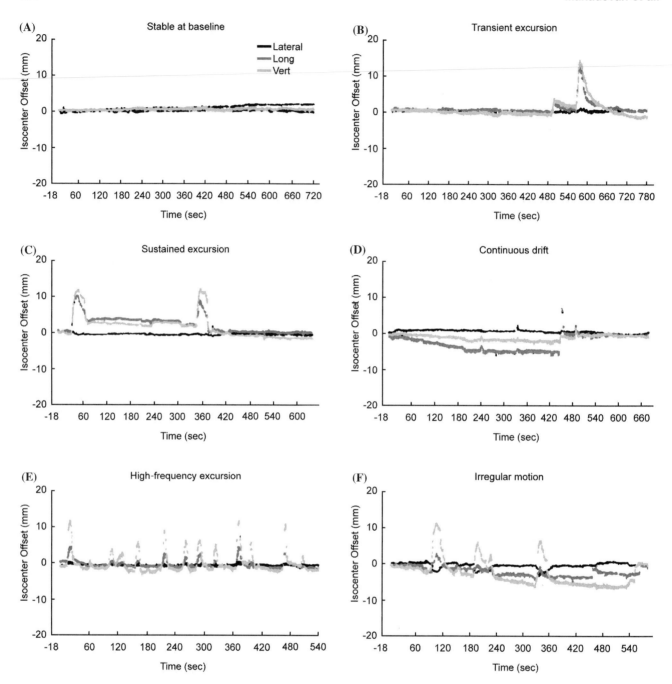

Figure 4 Patterns of prostate motion: (**A**) Stable at baseline, (**B**) transient excursion, (**C**) persistent excursion, (**D**) continuous drift, (**E**) high-frequency excursion, (**F**) irregular motion.

- Prostate motion is largely unpredictable and variable day to day and patient to patient, hence, exposes the limitations of predictive methods to account for prostate motion.
- Strategies for therapeutic intervention can be implemented on the basis of observed real-time variation in prostate location by therapists of all skill levels.

- The use of parameters for position correction due to intrafraction prostate motion provides adequate confidence to consider employing reduction in margins. This, in turn, could either decrease normal tissue toxicity at present dose levels or even allows further dose escalation without increased normal tissue toxicity.

REFERENCES

1. Ghilezan MJ, Jaffray DA, Siewerdsen JH, et al. Prostate gland motion assessed with cine-magnetic resonance imaging (cine-MRI). Int J Radiat Oncol Biol Phys 2005; 62(2): 406–417.

2. McNeal JE, Redwine EA, Freiha FS, et al. Zonal distribution of prostatic adenocarcinoma. Correlation with histologic pattern and direction of spread. Am J Surg Pathol 1988; 12(12):897–906.

3. Litzenberg DW, Hadley SW, Tyagi N, et al. Synchronized dynamic dose reconstruction. Med Phys 2007; 34(1):91–102.

4. van Herk M. Errors and margins in radiotherapy. Semin Radiat Oncol 2004; 14(1):52–64.

5. Zelefsky MJ, Fuks Z, Hunt M, et al. High-dose intensity modulated radiation therapy for prostate cancer: early toxicity and biochemical outcome in 772 patients. Int J Radiat Oncol Biol Phys 2002; 53(5):1111–1116.

6. Kupelian P, Kuban D, Thames H, et al. Improved biochemical relapse-free survival with increased external radiation doses in patients with localized prostate cancer: the combined experience of nine institutions in patients treated in 1994 and 1995. Int J Radiat Oncol Biol Phys 2005; 61(2): 415–419.

7. Zietman AL, DeSilvio ML, Slater JD, et al. Comparison of conventional-dose vs high-dose conformal radiation therapy in clinically localized adenocarcinoma of the prostate: a randomized controlled trial. JAMA 2005; 294(10): 1233–1239.

8. Peeters ST, Heemsbergen WD, Koper PC, et al. Dose-response in radiotherapy for localized prostate cancer: results of the Dutch multicenter randomized phase III trial comparing 68 Gy of radiotherapy with 78 Gy. J Clin Oncol 2006; 24(13):1990–1996.

9. Pollack A, Zagars GK, Starkschall G, et al. Prostate cancer radiation dose response: results of the M. D. Anderson phase III randomized trial. Int J Radiat Oncol Biol Phys 2002; 53(5):1097–1105.

10. Dearnaley DP, Sydes MR, Graham JD, et al. Escalated-dose versus standard-dose conformal radiotherapy in prostate cancer: first results from the MRC RT01 randomised controlled trial. Lancet Oncol 2007; 8(6):475–487.

11. Fowler J, Chappell R, Ritter M. Is alpha/beta for prostate tumors really low? Int J Radiat Oncol Biol Phys 2001; 50(4): 1021–1031.

12. Fowler JF, Ritter MA, Chappell RJ, et al. What hypofractionated protocols should be tested for prostate cancer? Int J Radiat Oncol Biol Phys 2003; 56(4):1093–1104.

13. Brenner DJ, Martinez AA, Edmundson GK, et al. Direct evidence that prostate tumors show high sensitivity to fractionation (low alpha/beta ratio), similar to late-responding normal tissue. Int J Radiat Oncol Biol Phys 2002; 52(1): 6–13.

14. Kupelian PA, Thakkar VV, Khuntia D, et al. Hypofractionated intensity-modulated radiotherapy (70 gy at 2.5 Gy per fraction) for localized prostate cancer: long-term outcomes. Int J Radiat Oncol Biol Phys 2005; 63(5):1463–1468.

15. Kry SF, Salehpour M, Followill DS, et al. The calculated risk of fatal secondary malignancies from intensity-modulated radiation therapy. Int J Radiat Oncol Biol Phys 2005; 62(4):1195–1203.

16. Pouliot J, Riley J, Werner B. Demonstration of minimal impact to radiation beam and portal image quality due to the presence of an electromagnetic array. Med Phys 2003; 30(6):1493.

17. Balter JM, Wright JN, Newell LJ, et al. Accuracy of a wireless localization system for radiotherapy. Int J Radiat Oncol Biol Phys 2005; 61(3):933–937.

18. Kupelian P, Willoughby T, Mahadevan A, et al. Multi-institutional clinical experience with the Calypso System in localization and continuous, real-time monitoring of the prostate gland during external radiotherapy. Int J Radiat Oncol Biol Phys 2007; 67(4):1088–1098.

19. Vera R, Grimm P, Zeller T, et al. Compatability of AC electromagnetic localization with brachytherapy seeds and surgical clips. Brachytherapy 2007; 6:95.

20. Bayley AJ, Catton CN, Haycocks T, et al. A randomized trial of supine vs. prone positioning in patients undergoing escalated dose conformal radiotherapy for prostate cancer. Radiother Oncol 2004; 70(1):37–44.

21. Willoughby TR, Kupelian PA, Pouliot J, et al. Target localization and real-time tracking using the Calypso 4D localization system in patients with localized prostate cancer. Int J Radiat Oncol Biol Phys 2006; 65(2):528–534.

22. Litzenberg DW, Balter JM, Hadley SW, et al. Influence of intrafraction motion on margins for prostate radiotherapy. Int J Radiat Oncol Biol Phys 2006; 65(2):548–553.

23. Chandra A, Dong L, Huang E, et al. Experience of ultrasound-based daily prostate localization. Int J Radiat Oncol Biol Phys 2003; 56(2):436–447.

24. Fox TH, Elder ES, Crocker IR, et al. Clinical implementation and efficiency of kilovoltage image-guided radiation therapy. J Am Coll Radiol 2006; 3(1):38–44.

25. Moseley DJ, White EA, Wiltshire KL, et al. Comparison of localization performance with implanted fiducial markers and cone-beam computed tomography for on-line image-guided radiotherapy of the prostate. Int J Radiat Oncol Biol Phys 2007; 67(3):942–953.

26. Warman L, Cornelli H, Mahadevan A. Online correction of setup error in prostate cancer: a comparison of an Ultrasound System and Calypso® 4D Localization System. Int J Radiat Oncol Biol Phys 2007; 69(3):S661.

27. D'Souza WD, Naqvi SA, Yu CX. Real-time intra-fraction-motion tracking using the treatment couch: a feasibility study. Phys Med Biol 2005; 50(17):4021–4033.

28. Keall PJ, Cattell H, Pokhrel D, et al. Geometric accuracy of a real-time target tracking system with dynamic multileaf collimator tracking system. Int J Radiat Oncol Biol Phys 2006; 65(5):1579–1584.

29. Mah D, Freedman G, Milestone B, et al. Measurement of intrafractional prostate motion using magnetic resonance imaging. Int J Radiat Oncol Biol Phys 2002; 54(2): 568–575.

13

Prostate Tomotherapy

RICHARD HUDES AND TIMOTHY HOLMES

St. Agnes Hospital Cancer Center, Baltimore, Maryland, U.S.A.

INTRODUCTION

Tomotherapy is a unique form of intensity-modulated radiotherapy (IMRT) based on a rotating X-ray fan beam (1–3). The term "tomotherapy" derives from *tomo*-graphic radio-*therapy*, literally meaning "slice" radiotherapy. Tomotherapy treatment delivery is conceptually similar to computed tomographic (CT) imaging where a three-dimensional image volume is acquired by helical irradiation of the patient. By analogy, a tumor volume can be helically irradiated to achieve a highly conformal three-dimensional dose distribution by modulating the intensity pattern of the incident X-ray beam profile during rotation. The intensity modulation is achieved using a fan-beam multileaf collimator (MLC) whose leaves are pneumatically driven to achieve near-instantaneous leaf transitions between open and closed states.

The Hi-ART II™ helical tomotherapy system (Tomo-Therapy Inc., Madison, Wisconsin, U.S.A.) is a dedicated image-guided IMRT radiotherapy treatment unit built on a helical CT ring gantry that incorporates a CT image detector for daily imaging of the patient prior to treatment (Fig. 1). The ring gantry design of the Hi-ART is optimal for CT scanning because it is much more mechanically stable than the C-arm type gantry used by conventional radiotherapy treatment units. Mechanical stability minimizes the potential for image artifacts due to flexing of the source-detector geometry during image acquisition. For comparison, current state-of-the-art C-arm gantry has a mechanical rotation tolerance of 1 mm whereas the Hi-ART has a tolerance of 0.1 mm similar to the Gamma-Knife and CyberKnife systems, making it suitable for stereotactic radiosurgery applications (4).

Ideally, mechanical tolerances should be less than the size of an image pixel for artifacts to be minimized without sophisticated characterization of the source-detector geometry for image reconstruction. Consistent with this requirement, Boswell et al. have confirmed that helical tomotherapy is capable of the subvoxel accuracy for phantom localization when using automatic registration of megavoltage CT (MVCT) to kilovoltage CT (kVCT) images (5). In the case of the C-arm gantry used for CT imaging, a sophisticated software model must be used to account for mechanical flexure of the source-detector geometry, and the flexure must be reproducible to minimize artifact generation.

Another major design difference between the Hi-ART II and C-arm treatment units is that the latter use a kV X-ray source oriented at 90° to the treatment beam to perform CT imaging, whereas the Hi-ART uses the same MV X-ray system to perform imaging and treatment. The difference between the two states is that the X-ray beam energy is reduced from 6 million electron volts (MeV) for treatment to 3.5 MeV for imaging in addition to a reduction in beam current resulting a very low dose of 1 to 2 cGy to the patient during imaging (6). This low dose is

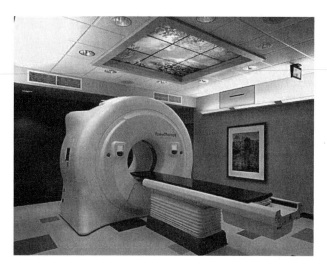

Figure 1 TomoTherapy Hi-ART II image-guided IMRT treatment unit. *Abbreviation*: IMRT, intensity-modulated radiotherapy.

also a consequence of the significantly higher penetration of the Hi-ART's MV imaging beam that results in a higher signal-to-noise ratio at the detector compared to a kV X-ray source (Fig. 2A). The increased penetration of 3.5MV X-rays reduces the likelihood of "shadow" artifacts in reconstructed images (Fig. 2B).

The Hi-ART II is designed with a high level of system integration to facilitate image-guided IMRT procedures. For example, the system is designed around a common database that is shared by the inverse treatment planning system, the MVCT imaging subsystem, the treatment delivery control system, and the record and verification subsystem.

Since the daily MVCT images can easily be accessed by the treatment planning system, they can be used to recompute an estimate of *delivered dose* to compare with the *planned dose* so that dosimetric errors can be determined and decisions can be made to adapt future treatments to compensate for these errors (7,8). A geometrical miss of the target volume constitutes the most important type of treatment error and can be caused by patient weight loss during the treatment course or internal organ shifts after the planning CT image set is acquired. The daily MVCT data is, in essence, a mathematical model of the patient that can be used for planning future treatments—a process called "adaptive radiotherapy" (9,10).

Helical tomotherapy has been successfully applied to image-guided IMRT at all body sites and target volume sizes ranging from small metastatic lesions in the brain and lung to total body irradiation with organ avoidance for bone marrow transplantation (11–20). While IMRT has wide application for curative as well as complex palliative radiotherapy, its largest caseload is for curative treatment of prostate cancer followed by head and neck and lung cancers. In all curative situations, the rationale for using CT-guided IMRT is to deliver a high tumoricidal dose (60–80 Gy) to the minimal tumor volume while simultaneously minimizing the risk of short- and long-term complications by reducing unwanted dose to adjacent critical anatomy. In the case of prostate cancer, the primary dose-limiting organ is the rectum whose anterior wall sits adjacent to the prostate. The high-dose region typically encompasses the anterior rectal wall making it the region most likely to suffer early complications in the form of tissue breakdown and bleeding. In some instances,

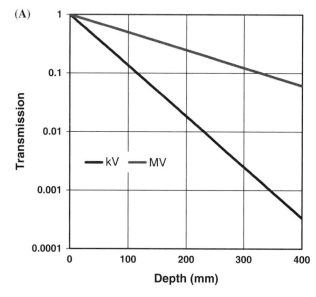

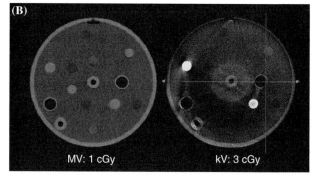

Figure 2 (**A**) Comparison of MV versus kV X-ray penetration in water. Hi-ART's megavoltage imaging beam produces a higher signal-to-noise ratio at the detector compared to a kilovoltage X-ray source. (**B**) CT images of 30 cm diameter image quality test phantom showing the "shadow" artifact produced by excessive attenuation of low energy kV X-rays compared to MV X-rays. *Abbreviations*: MV, megavoltage; kV, kilovoltage. *Source*: Courtesy of T.R. Mackie, PhD).

the bowel may also need to be considered if it is adjacent to the high-dose volume. The bladder and femoral heads are typically included in the planning process as structures to minimize unwanted dose, albeit at a lower priority than the rectum (21).

The Hi-ART II is very efficient for prostate radiotherapy where most procedures are completed within 15 to 20 minutes, with image guidance requiring less than 10 minutes and treatment delivery completed within 4 to 7 minutes, depending on the size of the target volume (22). A unique feature of the slice-based approach is that a tumor "slice" reaches full dose in one to two minutes regardless of overall treatment delivery time. This dosimetric characteristic combined with the accurate targeting of dose makes the Hi-ART II an excellent device for radiotherapy treatment of prostate cancer. In the following sections, we will discuss the features of the Hi-ART II that make it ideal for CT-guided IMRT of prostate cancer.

EQUIPMENT DESCRIPTION

The Hi-ART II uses a compact electron linear accelerator (linac) to generate X-rays for both treatment and imaging. The linac is a 30-cm long, 6 MeV, S-band (nominal 3 GHz) magnetron-powered device with a gridded gun and a solid-state modulator. An X-ray target is integrated into the body of the linac and is located 85 cm from the gantry rotation axis. Unlike conventional treatment units, the Hi-ART II does not need an X-ray flattening filter. Removal of the filter increases the X-ray output to 8 to 10 Gy/min at the gantry rotation axis, and it simplifies the treatment beam modeling and CT image reconstruction processes by providing a more monochromatic X-ray energy spectrum and reduced scatter outside the field boundary.

The treatment head has a unique "clam-shell" design that allows field widths of 5 to 50 mm (nominal). The head shielding including primary collimators was designed to limit the primary leakage to 0.01% of the primary beam, or one-tenth the limit (0.1%) used by C-arm radiotherapy treatment units. This added shielding is required since tomotherapy requires a larger number of monitor units for an IMRT treatment compared to fixed-gantry methods. Despite this, the whole-body dose from tomotherapy is lower than that from C-arm linacs, due in part to the low leakage and to the lower scatter outside the field because of the lack of a flattening filter (23–25). Additionally, Lazar et al. have estimated that the risk of developing secondary cancer from a prostate radiotherapy using tomotherapy is lower than that for fixed-gantry IMRT using a C-arm treatment unit (26).

Below the primary collimators resides the binary MLC module, consisting of 64 leaves made from 10-cm high tungsten with leakage less than 0.5%. A 13-cm thick lead counterweight is attached to the ring gantry opposite the treatment head that acts as a rotating primary barrier or beam stop. Each binary MLC leaf completely blocks a portion of the fan beam with a projected shadow of 6.25 mm (nominal) at the gantry rotation axis. The 64 leaves define a 40-cm diameter treatment field-of-view, which combined with up to 160-cm (nominal) couch travel enables very large treatment volumes to receive IMRT. Intensity modulation is achieved using pneumatic control of the binary MLC leaves by rapidly ($\sim$ 20 milliseconds) switching the open-closed state of leaves during gantry rotation. The intensity level is proportional to the time a leaf is open and there are effectively 50 intensity levels that that can be delivered.

The linac and ring gantry systems of the tomotherapy system are highly favorable for CT imaging where mechanical stability of the source-detector positions during rotation and a small source size are desirable. An additional benefit of the enclosed ring gantry is that a collision of the rotating gantry with the patient is avoided by design unlike the C-arm gantry of conventional treatment units. The tomotherapy gantry mechanical sag during rotation is approximately 0.1 mm, so no sag corrections are required in the CT reconstruction algorithm. The size of the electron beam on the target is about 1 mm so that the resolution is about 1.2 to 1.6 mm, which is comparable to a conventional CT scanner for high-contrast objects. Operating at an average dose to the patient of 1 to 2 cGy, the images produced have soft tissue contrast of 2% to 3%, which is poorer than a modern CT scanner, yet are of sufficient quality for adaptive radiotherapy processes (6). The tomotherapy unit's xenon gas detector elements have tungsten septa separating ionization cavities. In addition to the ionization collectors, the tungsten plates are embedded photon converters intercepting the MV photons and yet are thin enough to let an appreciable fraction of the electrons set in motion to deposit energy in the xenon gas. The interception of the beam by the tungsten means that the quantum efficiency of the system is about 25%, which is much more than the few percent collection efficiency of modern electronic portal imaging systems used by C-arm gantry treatment units.

Modeling the treatment delivery process requires discretization of the continuous motions of the gantry and table as well as the continuous intensities of the modulated beams. Proper sampling reduces the chance for computational aliasing that can produce "streak" or "thread" artifacts in the dose distribution (27). Consequently, each 360° gantry rotation is modeled as 51 beams spaced at 7.06° apart—a number chosen to allow a 40-cm diameter target volume to be homogeneously treated with a 2.5-cm completely blocked central avoidance structure (28). Following optimization, the intensity levels are discretized for treatment delivery, with 50 levels chosen to reduce the uncertainty in the target dose due to intensity discretization to less than 0.1%. Discretization of couch travel is determined by the pitch ratio—the ratio of the couch travel distance per rotation to the field width defined at the axis. In helical tomotherapy delivery, the pitch is usually set to be less than half to avoid threadlike dose artifacts developing near the edge of the field and becoming clinically significant (27). Given a typical pitch of 0.3 for a 25-mm field width, the table motion is modeled by offsetting adjacent beams by 0.147-mm [e.g., $(0.3 \times \times 25 \text{ mm})/51$] increments parallel to the direction of table motion.

PROSTATE TOMOTHERAPY WORKFLOW

Since the Hi-Art II design is highly integrated around a common database and software model, its workflow is efficient to carry out and is the same for all body sites. The Hi-ART II workflow can be viewed as four distinct processes: (*i*) treatment planning, (*ii*) plan verification, (*iii*) MVCT localization, and (*iv*) treatment delivery. While it is possible to carry out the full process in the same day, treatment planning and plan verification typically occur one to five days prior to the initial treatment delivery session.

IMRT Treatment Planning

The treatment planning workflow for the Hi-ART II consists of several processes that are common to most IMRT systems. A three-dimensional model of the patient is required for the planning process, so the first step is to obtain a volumetric image set of the patient in the treatment position using a CT simulator. We place the patient supine on a bean-bag positioner extending under the lower back for comfort, with their legs slightly bent using a triangular sponge under the knees, and the feet secured together with a strap to minimize knee and hip movement during the treatment procedure. Thermoplastic pelvic casts can also be used for immobilization to minimize intrafraction motion of the patient during the procedure, but they provide no useful improvement in setup accuracy in the daily image guidance, yet add to the overhead of the procedure and require storage space that may be a premium in most clinics.

The patient's CT image set is transferred to a third-party contouring software tool that supports DICOM-RT data transfers to the TomoTherapy Planning Station where

CT images are subsequently resampled from their original 512×512 pixels resolution to 256×256 pixels to reduce memory requirements.[a] Regions of interest (ROIs) are drawn for the planning target volume (PTV) and organs-at-risk (OARs) such as the bladder, rectum, femoral heads, and bowel. The TomoTherapy Planning System requires two additional nontissue structures—the couch top and the setup marks on the patient's surface. A 1-cm wide OAR "shell" is also drawn around the PTV to be used to force the high-dose region to conform to the PTV. In situations where a metal hip prosthesis is present, a nonanatomical avoidance ROI can be drawn around the prosthesis to prevent beams from passing through the implant. The TomoTherapy Planning System restricts each voxel to a single ROI; consequently, each ROI is assigned an overlap precedence ranking so that the optimization software can handle structure overlaps properly.

In the Optimization panel, the operator defines the prescription and planning parameters required by the plan optimizer. These parameters include the dose model, the dose grid resolution, helical pitch, and the beam width. Three dose models are available in increasing accuracy and computation time: (*i*) a primary ray trace model (TERMA), (*ii*) a precomputed pencil beam model (BEAMLETS), and (*iii*) a full scatter calculation (FULL SCATTER) that is performed during each cycle of the optimization. The dose model requires the selection of (*i*) the dose grid resolution (fine: 1–2 mm; normal: 2–4 mm; coarse: 4–8 mm), (*ii*) the beam width (1.0, 2.5, or 5.0 cm), and (*iii*) the helical pitch (0.1–1.0), all of which set the calculation geometry. Typical values that we use routinely for prostate treatment planning are 2.5-cm beam width, 0.25 pitch, and a modulation factor of 2.8.

The dose-volume (D-V) constraints differ depending on the type of structure. A target's set of D-V constraints define a three-point dose-volume histogram (DVH) defined by a minimum and a maximum dose limit and a third point defining where the "shoulder" falls between these limits. Only two points are defined for OARs—a maximum dose limit and a low-dose inflection point located between zero and the maximum dose limit. In addition, there are D-V penalty factors and ROI priority factors, which are used in the optimizer's objective function to compute a numerical "score" for the current plan estimate. The score allows the optimizer to determine if changes in the beam intensities produce an improvement in dose conformality. The set of D-V constraints can be saved as a class solution to be reused for future cases, if desired.

Plan optimization is performed iteratively by making changes to the incident intensity pattern for all binary

---

[a] The reason for this is that the current tomotherapy software (version 2.4) does not support creation of new contours; the newly released version 3 software provides a complete contouring toolset.

MLC leaves that intersect the target, also referred to as the *sinogram*. The name derives from the fact that each point in the target projects back to a sinusoidal path in the intensity pattern. The sinogram describes the opening and closing of the binary MLC leaves as a function of the gantry rotation angle and the translation position of the couch—it is, in effect, the operational instructions for the Hi-ART treatment delivery.

Computation time is affected by the choice of beam model and dose grid resolution. For example, if the BEAMLET model is selected then the system will initiate the computation of three-dimensional dose distributions for all binary MLC leaves that intersect the target volume, typically numbering in the thousands of beamlets. This data is computed using a multiprocessor rack consisting of 32 processors with local memory and disk storage. The results are stored locally on the processors so that they can be reused for generating an alternative plan without the need for recomputation. It takes approximately 10 to 15 minutes to compute the complete set of beamlets using the normal dose grid resolution and approximately 1.5 to 2 hours using the fine setting. At this point the optimization starts, and an iteration completes after 3 to 5 seconds, with 50 to 200 iterations needed to achieve a good plan. Alternatively, if the FULL SCATTER model is used, a single composite three-dimensional dose distribution is accurately computed during an iteration, with the computation taking about two to three minutes per iteration. The optimization can be stopped and restarted at any time to review the DVHs and dose distribution and to alter the D-V constraints, without loss of any plan data.

Once an acceptable result is achieved, the numbers of fractions are defined along with the treatment dates in the Fractionation panel. A final dose calculation is performed and corrections are applied to leaf-opening times to account for small changes in output when two adjacent leaves are opened simultaneously. Final approval of the plan requires the operator to enter their username and password, and once approved a plan cannot be changed. On plan approval, the set of daily treatments are recorded in the patient's database record.

IMRT Plan Verification

All patient treatment plans must be verified by dosimetry measurement prior to the first treatment delivery. Tomotherapy refers to this as Dosimetry Quality Assurance, or DQA. DQA is typically accomplished by using a plastic cylindrical water-equivalent phantom provided with the Hi-ART II as a surrogate for the patient. The DQA phantom supports the use of film and small volume ion chambers for performing measurements. The patient's intensity sinogram is used to compute dose in the DQA phantom for which test procedures are created. The procedures are delivered to the phantom with film and ion chambers in place. The film is developed and digitized and the information imported into the DQA analysis panel of the planning system where it is compared with the computed dose. The ion chamber measurements are converted to dose and input into the DQA analysis panel where it is compared with point data manually sampled from the three-dimensional dose distribution. The data and the comparison results are then stored in the patient's database record.

The decline in availability of automatic film processors due to increased use of digital imaging is driving the adoption of processor-less verification solutions such as radiochromic film, computed radiography, and electronic detector arrays. An example of the latter is a matrix ionization chamber having 1020 calibrated pixel ion chambers that provide a two-dimensional image of absolute dose (MatriXX, Scanditronix-Welhöfer, Germany). This device provides an electronic alternative to film, albeit at a lower spatial resolution of 7.62 mm between detector centers. Nevertheless, the example shown in Figure 3 illustrates the excellent agreement possible using this device for tomotherapy DQA. The reason for this is that the detector is being translated with the couch through the gantry at a constant speed of less than 1 mm per second while acquiring measurements at a rate of 1 sample per second. Consequently, the data samples are being acquired at less than 1 mm spacing along the direction of couch motion.

Measured and computed doses are compared by visual inspection of one-dimensional profiles and two-dimensional isodose distributions or quantified by a color wash two-dimensional γ distribution representing how well a pixel in the measured dose image agrees in magnitude and spatial position to a neighborhood of pixels in the calculated dose image (29,30). Typically, a 3-mm radius defines the neighborhood of calculated pixels used for the evaluation, and difference limits of 3% in magnitude and 3 mm in spatial position are used in computing the γ value at each pixel. A γ value of less than or equal to 1.0 indicates acceptable agreement, where value of 0.0 indicates perfect agreement. Values greater than 1.0 indicate a discrepancy that exceeds one or both limits.

MVCT Localization Imaging

The MVCT detector resolution at the axis of rotation is about 0.6 mm in the transverse direction and equal to the slice width in the longitudinal direction. The gantry rotation for MVCT imaging is 10 seconds (6 RPM) and the slice thickness is approximately 4 mm, however, a smaller slice width (i.e., 2 mm) could be used for the fine

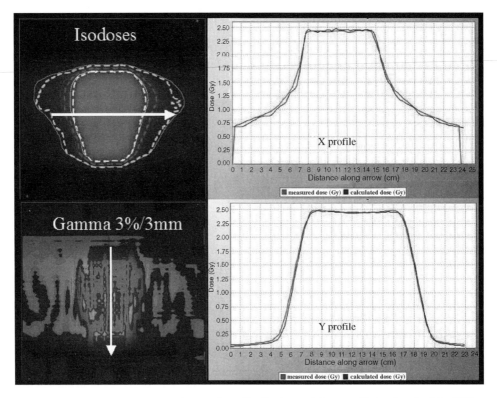

Figure 3 Tomotherapy DQA dose comparison (isodose, gamma distribution and dose profiles) using the MatriXX to measure absolute dose in a coronal plane through the center of the prostate. *Abbreviation*: DQA, dosimetry quality assurance.

resolution needed for small target volumes. The unit takes about 800 projections (or views) per rotation with two CT slices obtained per rotation. Helical pitches of 1, 1.5, and 2 are available for imaging allowing a typical tumor of 8- to 10-cm length to be imaged in as little as 2 minutes. Longer lengths of tumor and smaller pitches take more time proportionately. Image reconstruction is carried out in parallel with data acquisition, so there is little delay following acquisition for the images to be analyzed. The Hi-ART II is capable of resolving 1.2- to 1.6-mm objects near the edge of a 30-cm diameter phantom.

The X-ray energy of the verification CT is approximately 3.5 MeV. Consequently, the photons interact almost exclusively by Compton interactions so that the attenuation coefficient is linear with the electron density of the medium (31). Metal artifacts arise in conventional CT scanners because the attenuation of the metal is greatly enhanced due to the photoelectric effect. In helical CT, the beam is penetrating enough to eliminate artifacts arising from metal objects like a hip prosthesis; consequently, the verification MVCT is a more reliable CT system for patients with metal implanted appliances (32).

CT imaging is performed prior to each treatment to reduce the possibility of a geometrical miss of the target and sensitive structures. An automated comparison of verification and planning image sets is carried out immediately following image acquisition to guide the adjustment of the patient setup. The patient is assumed to be a rigid object requiring translations and rotations to bring the target anatomy and important sensitive structures into alignment with the treatment plan. The patient is positioned by aligning the patient's skin marks with lasers located outside of the bore of the unit. A sagittal representation of the patient's planning CT is shown on the operator console to aid in selecting the slices to be scanned. A verification scan is taken and reconstructed during the acquisition. The patient is then transported to the same position outside of the gantry bore while the verification image set is fused onto the planning image set, and the translation and rotation offsets are reported. Typically, the image fusion is first done automatically using a mutual information algorithm (33). Following automated registration, the patient registration can be fine-tuned manually. This allows the operator to take into account, as best as possible, the nonrigid nature of the transformation. Once the image registration is completed, the offsets also describe how the patient must be adjusted. Figure 4 is an example of a MVCT localization image registered to the planning CT using the soft-tissue anatomy of the prostate and rectum. Bone, while having less contrast than a conventional CT scan, is still clearly discernable as are the fat-muscle boundaries surrounding the prostate gland.

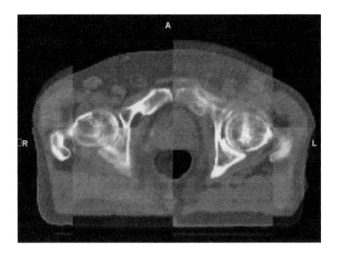

Figure 4 MVCT image registration example. The MVCT image is shown as the blue checkerboard color wash overlain on the gray scale kV planning CT. Note that the soft-tissue anatomy has been adjusted using the prostate/rectum interface, which results in a misalignment of the bony pelvis. *Abbreviations*: MVCT, megavoltage computed tomography; kV, kilovoltage.

The patient can be translated accordingly if adjustment is required. The treatment couch has automated vertical and longitudinal translations and automated gantry start angle adjustments to account for patient roll. The couch top can be manually adjusted in the lateral direction (x-direction). Yaw and pitch rotations can be accommodated using angularly calibrated immobilization/positioning aids, which are especially useful for the head and neck. Moveable CT-simulator lasers are used to verify the modified patient position.

Fully Dynamic IMRT Treatment Delivery

A Hi-ART II treatment delivery of 2.0 Gy typically takes less than 5 minutes for small target volumes like a prostate and less than 10 minutes for larger volumes that include pelvic lymph nodes and seminal vesicles. Overall treatment delivery time T is a function of target length along the axis of table motion (L), the beam width (W), the prescribed dose D, the average dose rate at the target R, and the user-defined modulation factor M defined as the ratio of the maximum leaf-open time of any leaf to the average leaf-opening time of all the nonzero values. The parameters are related by (34)

$$T = MD(L + W)/WR \sim (M/W) \times \text{constant}$$

Consequently, treatment time can be shortened by reducing the intensity modulation or by increasing the beam width in agreement with common sense.

Typically, we select a modulation factor of 2.8, with higher values not providing noticeable improvement in plan quality. On the other hand, the choice of slit width (1.0, 2.5, 5.0 cm) can alter treatment time significantly. As an example, a 7-cm prostate volume can be adequately treated with a 2.5-cm slit width in approximately 5 minutes, assuming an average dose rate at the target volume of 4 Gy/min and a modulation factor of 2.5. Yet the time would significantly increase to approximately 20 minutes if the 1-cm slit was used with the intent of achieving a more conformal dose distribution. In practice, the smaller slit does not provide much improvement in dose conformality because the effective resolution of the helical delivery in the direction of table motion is 6.25 mm when using a 2.5-cm slit with a pitch of 0.25.

Helical tomotherapy is a very efficient method to deliver a tumoricidal dose to the tumor because of the slice-based nature of the delivery. Fixed-gantry IMRT techniques used by C-arm gantry treatment units require all beam directions to be delivered before a tumor subvolume reaches full dose, hence the overall treatment time is the relevant parameter when evaluating the average dose rate at the tumor for this type of IMRT delivery. Tomotherapy delivery, on the other hand, continuously irradiates a slice of tissue so that the full dose of 1.8 to 2 Gy is reached within one to two minutes regardless of the overall length of the treatment delivery and body site. Consequently, the average dose rate at the tumor is typically 1 to 2 Gy/min, and the impact of cell repair during the delivery is minimized.

SPECIAL APPLICATION TOOLS

The availability of the CT imaging on the tomotherapy treatment unit has lead to the development of two new clinical tools based on this imaging capability. The Plan Adaptive Tool uses daily MVCT images to evaluate errors in daily treatment delivery, and it can be used to adapt future treatments to compensate for these errors. The StatRT Tool allows one use the Hi-ART II to perform the functions of CT simulation, inverse treatment planning, and treatment delivery within 10 to 15 minutes without moving the patient from the table.

Adaptive Radiotherapy: Plan Adaptive Tool

Typically, MVCT images are acquired daily for setup localization. Consequently, one has a daily model of the patient available that can be used for computing a daily estimate of delivered dose. The daily estimates can be compared with the planned dose to determine the impact of incorrect setup, changes in anatomy, or incomplete treatment delivery. Regions of unacceptable error can be automatically contoured and used to replan future treatments to compensate for these errors. This process called adaptive radiation therapy (ART) is embodied in the Plan Adaptive Tool.

The Plan Adaptive Tool has three functions: (*i*) it is used for accessing and transferring MVCT images from the patient record to the tomotherapy planner for treatment planning when anatomical changes during treatment or metal artifacts in original kVCT images warrant their use, (*ii*) it is used for computing dose using MVCT images for treatment delivery quality assurance, and (*iii*) it is used to evaluating cumulative errors in the delivered dose from which error ROIs are created and used for plan reoptimization.

A common problem faced in prostate image-guided radiation therapy (IGRT) is the presence of an implanted metal hip prosthesis that creates significant image artifacts in KVCT images used for planning and treatment setup. Tomotherapy dose computation uses CT numbers to account for tissue density. Consequently, erroneous CT numbers will cause errors in computed dose. Typically, the hip prosthesis casts a "shadow" of lower CT number in the region of the prostate. This region of lower CT number can result in significant errors exceeding 5% to 10% at the prostate. An extreme example is shown in Figure 5 where the bilateral prostheses CT artifact resulted in a 10% to 15% error in dose in the region of the prostate. It is advisable in these situations to use the Plan Adaptive Tool with a MVCT image set to determine the magnitude of the error and replan the case using the MVCT data.

Lastly, the Plan Adaptive Tool can be used for correlating acute side effects with delivered dose estimated using daily MVCT localization images. An example is shown in Figure 6 for the situation where a plan was generated for a patient with a full rectum but was treated with an empty rectum. The impact is a slightly higher local dose in the anterior rectal wall that exceeds 5%.

StatRT

StatRT is a new tool that allows the Hi-ART II to perform the functions of CT-simulation and treatment planning, in addition to treatment delivery. The intended use is for emergent palliation cases where it is desirable to efficiently simulate and treat the patient within 20 minutes and avoid moving the patient from CT simulator to treatment couch. StatRT implements a fully functional treatment planning system at the treatment unit console. Plan optimization is carried out using the FULL SCATTER model with an acceptable solution achieved in 10 to 20 iterations requiring five minutes of computation time. While this feature may not be that useful for definitive prostate treatments at normal fractionation, it may prove useful for hypofractionated prostate radiosurgery applications where it would be desirable to minimize any dose errors at the time of treatment setup.

TOMOTHERAPY IGRT QUALITY ASSURANCE

A major difference between helical tomotherapy and fixed-gantry IMRT is that the former is a fully dynamic approach where the gantry, couch, and MLC motions must be properly timed to achieve an accurate delivery. In fact, helical tomotherapy is based on the assumption of constant linac output and constant gantry rotation and couch translation speeds during imaging and delivery procedures. Conversely, in fixed-gantry IMRT, the MLC is the only system component that might move during the irradiation; hence, dynamic MLC quality assurance (QA) methods have been developed to augment the battery of classical QA tests for static treatment delivery using a C-arm linac. On the other hand, helical tomotherapy QA

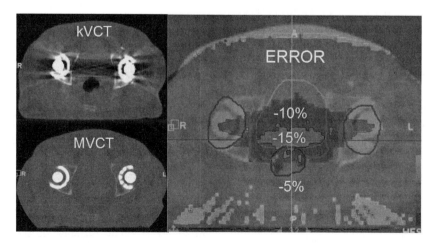

Figure 5 Bilateral hip prostheses cause significant artifacts in kVCT images used for treatment planning by overcompensating the influence. In this example dose errors of 5% to 15% occur in the region of the prostate bed. *Abbreviation*: kVCT, kilovoltage computed tomography.

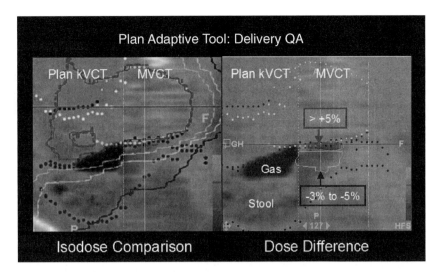

Figure 6 Pelvis midline-sagittal view showing a comparison of planned versus delivered dose where the latter was estimated using the Plan Adaptive Tool. Bowel gas and stool are present in the planning CT and absent in the MVCT localization image. The impact of this change are small hot and cold dose regions at the interface between the prostate and the rectum with the remaining region within 0% to 3% agreement. *Abbreviation*: MVCT, megavoltage computed tomography.

testing has been developed primarily with constancy of output and dynamic motions in mind (35,36).

Helical tomotherapy QA includes both static and dynamic QA tests. Examples of static QA tests are static output calibration and output readout calibration, X-ray beam alignment with the jaws and binary MLC, field size geometry, and couch offset from the setup position outside the gantry to the starting position inside the gantry. Dynamic tests include gantry rotation speed, couch speed, and MLC leaf transitions. These can be tested separately or in combination.

The approach we have developed in our clinic is to perform an imaging and treatment delivery procedure that mimics an actual patient treatment during morning warm up. This dynamic QA procedure is specially designed so that constancy of dynamic output, X-ray energy, couch-gantry speed synchronization, couch offset, movable laser calibration, MVCT localization imaging, and image quality parameters (high- and low-contrast resolutions, CT number constancy) can be evaluated in a single imaging and delivery procedure (37). Static tests are performed on a monthly basis or as necessary following a major servicing of the machine.

The main objective of a CT image-guided procedure is to reduce setup uncertainty so that smaller treatment margins can be justified and geometrical misses are minimized. It follows that some evaluation of daily setup variation should be monitored, preferably by body site. In our practice, we tabulate daily position offsets on all patients by body site for review at our monthly department QA meeting. This data is useful to evaluate if there is a dominant direction of offset, if the offsets are random or systematic, and if there are outlier patients who should be monitored more closely.

Another QA measure that is monitored is the discrepancy in DQA dosimetry measurements performed for plan verification. Two features of the DQA data are monitored: (*i*) the discrepancies in absolute dose at six points sampled in the coronal and sagittal planes and (*ii*) the spatial offsets between measured and calculated relative dose profiles extracted from the sagittal and coronal planes. Systematic discrepancies in the six-point dose samples may indicate that the output of the linac has changed from its calibrated value of 858 cGy/min or that there is an energy change in the X-ray beam. Positional shifts in the relative dose profiles may indicate that the setup lasers are out of adjustment. Hence the DQA results are monitored as a secondary indicator of dynamic performance of the Hi-ART II.

PROSTATE TOMOTHERAPY: IN THE CLINIC

Target Volume Delineation

Definitive Prostate

Typically, a kVCT simulation is performed with cystourethrogram using 3-mm thick slices and subsequent contouring of the prostate, rectum, bladder, and femoral necks (Fig. 7). For high-intermediate- or high-risk patients, the proximal 1- to 1.5-cm seminal vesicle is included and may also require an extra 2- to 3-mm margin posteriorly due to risk of extra capsular extension (38,39). For a subpopulation of high-risk patients, pelvic lymph nodes are contoured as part of the initial control target volume (CTV),

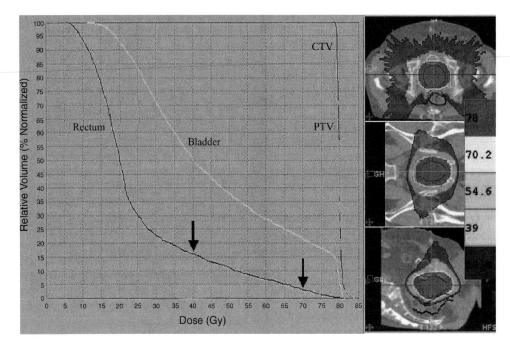

Figure 7 Example of helical tomotherapy for early stage prostate cancer. The arrows indicate two clinically relevant evaluation points on the rectum DVH. *Abbreviation*: DVH, dose-volume histogram.

as is the bowel for avoidance (Figs. 8 and 9). Occasionally, MRI fusion may be used for patients with poor kVCT imaging that leads to difficult prostate rectal interface or apex delineation. Additionally, for patients with artifacts from hip prostheses, a MVCT on the Tomotherapy unit will be used as discussed below.

In considering the PTV margin, one needs to consider setup error, interfraction motion, and intrafraction motion. Regarding interfraction movement, using kVCT localization at Fox Chase Center, Lattanzi described an error margin as low as 3 mm (35). Likewise, using a cone-beam CT, a 3-mm margin for setup errors has been reported (40). Similar results for a 3-mm margin for setup error have been found for MVCT imaging with tomotherapy (41).

Postprostatectomy

For patients' status post-prostatectomy, the simulation and contouring for patients to undergo tomotherapy are generally similar to that of other techniques described in chapter 14. The only subset that differs significantly is that with hip prostheses as discussed below.

Hip Prosthesis Artifact

A metal hip prosthesis imaged with kVCT will create significant image artifact that can deleteriously affect the ability to contour the prostate as well as the OARs

(rectum, bladder). Since the TomoTherapy Planning System uses a heterogeneity-corrected dose model, the image artifacts will create errors in the delivered dose as shown in Figure 5 for the case of bilateral hips prostheses. MRI will likewise be unable to properly image the ROIs because of the presence of metal and its distorting effects on the magnetic field of the imager. Consequently, MVCT can be acquired and used both for contouring and dose planning in this situation with the caveat that the MVCT does have increased inter- and intraobserver variability in contouring compared to kVCT (42). The MVCT with prostheses can be used for dose calculation since the artifact is minimized due to the increased penetration of the 3.5 MeV X rays used for imaging (7).

Normal Tissue Integral Dose

The integral dose equals the mean dose times the volume irradiated. Aoyama et al. (23) investigated treatment planning for prostate cancer with three-dimensional conformal radiotherapy (3DCRT), conventional linac IMRT, and helical tomotherapy. Secondary malignancy estimates showed minimal variations between these techniques. There was a benefit demonstrated for helical tomotherapy over conventional IMRT and 3DCRT for localized prostate cancer in regard to dose sparing of rectum and penile bulb without increasing normal tissue integral dose (NTID) and risk of secondary malignancy.

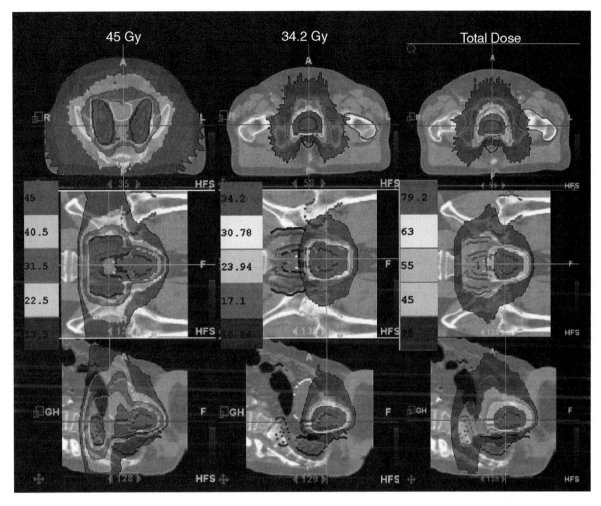

Figure 8 (*See color insert.*) Example of a complex prostate case consisting of 45 Gy volume including lymph nodes, 34.2 Gy boost volume, and the total dose.

Target Localization Technique: Daily MVCT Image Guidance

Interfraction Movement

Avoidance of geographical miss has propelled IGRT into the forefront of clinical importance for prostate cancer since there is a discrepancy between bony anatomy and prostate position for daily set up. With the TomoTherapy MVCT image guidance system, the images are acquired in the treatment position immediately prior to the treatment. The MVCT image is fused and is used for comparison with the planning kVCT for alignment prior to treatment. Alignment is made by shifts in the x, y, and z coordinates as well as a change in the roll. Automated pitch and yaw corrections are not currently addressed in the TomoTherapy Hi-Art II system.

Langen et al. (41) described three different approaches to compare the MVCT and kVCT images: (*i*) fiducial markers, (*ii*) CT anatomy, and (*iii*) kVCT contours. In studying 112 alignments from three patients, each of these approaches was analyzed compared to a reference of the center-of-mass (COM) of the three fiducial markers. Radiation therapists retrospectively registered the image sets with anatomy and contour methods. The physician registered all image sets on the basis of all three techniques. It was found that the fiducial technique was best in looking for a 3-mm difference from the reference COM. Furthermore, the fiducial and CT anatomy techniques were similar in looking for a 5-mm difference from the reference COM. It was clear that the contour-based technique was inferior than the anatomy or fiducial technique for both the radiation therapists and physician. Interestingly, there was a superiority of physician over therapist in the 3-mm threshold for anatomy compared to COM alignment, which is attributed to the physician's experience of CT image viewing (41). The authors concluded that fiducial placement is preferred, but if it is not used,

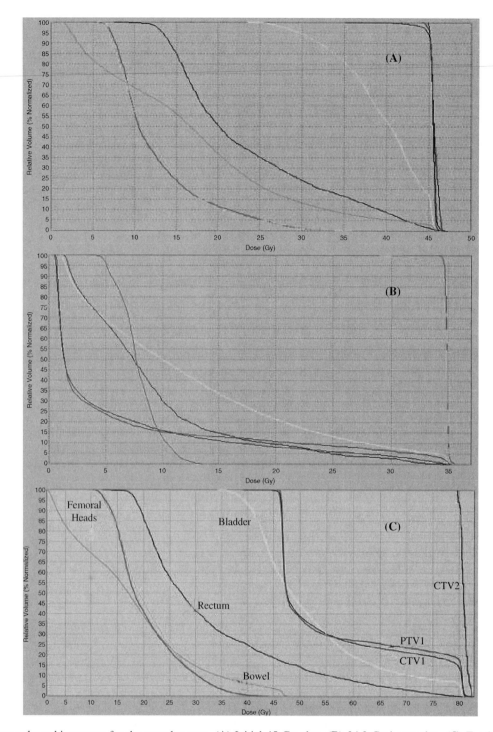

Figure 9　Dose-volume histograms for the complex case. (**A**) Initial 45 Gy plan. (**B**) 34.2 Gy boost plan. (**C**) Total dose.

then anatomy-based registration is preferred over contour-based registration because of agreement with a marker-based COM reference alignment and less interuser variability.

The use of daily image guidance results in the ability to use tighter margins compared to less than daily frequency of image guidance (43).

Intrafraction Movement

Ghilzean et al. (40) evaluated prostate motion using cine-MRI and found that a displacement of 3 mm can be expected within 20 minutes of the initial imaging for patients with an empty rectum. They found that the most significant predictor for intrafraction prostate motion is the status of rectal filling, with a full rectal state is associated with greater prostate motion. Susil et al. (40) performed an intrafraction motion study on eight prostate tomotherapy patients where they obtained MVCT following treatment to compare with the pretreatment localization scan. They found that an aggregate margin of 4 mm encompassed 95% on prostate intrafraction motion for 95% of treatment fractions examined in their study. Since tomotherapy prostate procedures can be carried out easily in a 15- to 20-minutes time slot, these results would indicate that intrafraction motion tracking is not needed for the majority of patients if they present with an empty rectum and if a minimal margin of 4 mm is used in defining the PTV. With these results in mind, typical expansion margins used for prostate tomotherapy treatment planning are 4 to 5 mm posterior and 6 to 10 mm all other directions (8,44).

The use of real-time electromagnetic tracking (Calypso 4D Localization System, Seattle, Washington, U.S.A.) is now possible, but its use is just now being studied. Litzenberg et al. (42) used this technology to study 11 patients treated with fixed-gantry IMRT, and they found that only two cases would have benefited from continuous target tracking. Langen et al. (45) found that there was a minimal dosimetric impact on a cohort of 13 prostate tomotherapy patients when the Calypso intrafraction motion data was used to calculate dose using a four-dimensional dose model and treatment margins of 4 mm posterior and 6 mm otherwise. The average percentage of treatment time that the prostate was displaced by more than 3 mm was 5%, or about 15 seconds out of a 300 seconds treatment. The random nature of day-to-day displacements reduces the cumulative impact significantly, so that in 93% of the fractions, the intrafraction motion had less than a 5% impact on the absolute dose to the PTV, and the cumulative impact on the prostate and PTV D95 was less than 1.2%. On the basis of these works, it would appear that only a very small cohort of prostate tomotherapy patients would appear to benefit from continuous target tracking.

Organ Deformation

The use of daily MVCT imaging for localization allows not only the prostate to be positioned, but also provides information regarding rectal and bladder positioning. The MVCT can be used to recalculate delivered doses. Kupelian et al. (8) have demonstrated that there is interfraction deformation of these organs that can have dosimetric consequences, particularly for the rectum. In that study of 10 prostate cancer patients treated to 78 Gy in 39 fractions, with daily MVCT images, each recontoured and recalculated dose distributions, they found the rectal deformation as the most consequential.

An example of the impact of rectal filling and deformation on the dose at the prostate rectal interface is shown in Figure 6 where local errors of 5% occur in the anterior rectal wall when a plan is generated with gas present in the bowel and subsequently used to treat with an empty rectum.

SUMMARY OF PERTINENT CONCLUSIONS

The TomoTherapy Hi-ART II is well suited for image-guided IMRT of prostate cancer for the following reasons:

- The Hi-ART II is efficient by integrating into one system the processes of treatment planning, treatment verification, MVCT image-guidance, IMRT treatment delivery, and adaptive dose recalculation.
- The Hi-ART II has mechanical accuracy similar to dedicated radiosurgery systems with an accuracy of less than 2 mm for dose localization to the target.
- MVCT image guidance only exposes the patient to approximately 1 cGy per image procedure and can avoid the need for fiducial placement.
- MVCT imaging allows imaging without artifact for patients with hip prostheses.
- Prostate margins as low as 4 mm posteriorly and 6 mm otherwise are enabled by MVCT localization.
- Fully dynamic IMRT results in maximal sparing of the rectum and bladder with homogeneous dose to the prostate.
- Fully dynamic IMRT allows quick delivery of prostate treatments, which are commonly achieved in four to seven minutes of irradiation.
- In adaptive radiotherapy, MVCT images can be used to recalculate delivered dose.
- StatRT is a new capability for real-time simulation and treatment that may prove useful for daily planning of high-dose stereotactic prostate treatments while the patient is on the treatment couch in the treatment position.

Disclosure: Timothy Holmes receives patent royalties on tomotherapy technology.

REFERENCES

1. Mackie TR, Holmes T, Swerdloff S, et al. Tomotherapy: a new concept for the delivery of dynamic conformal radiotherapy. Med Phys 2007; 20:1709–1719.
2. Mackie TR, Olivera G, Kapatoes J, et al. Helical tomotherapy. In: Palta J, Mackie TR, eds. Intensity-Modulated Radiation Therapy: The State of the Art. College Park, MD: American Association of Physicists in Medicine, 2003:247–284.
3. Mackie TR, Kapatoes J, Ruchala K, et al. Image guidance for precise conformal radiotherapy. Int J Radiat Oncol Biol Phys 2003; 56(1):89–105.

4. Holmes TW, Hu X, Dawson D, et al. Stereotactic radio-surgery using the TomoTherapy HI-ART II. Int J Radiat Oncol Biol Phys 2006; 66(3):S255.

5. Boswell S, Tome W, Jeraj R, et al. Automatic registration of megavoltage to kilovoltage CT images in helical tomotherapy: an evaluation of the setup verification process for the special case of a rigid head phantom. Med Phys 2006; 33(11):4395–4404.

6. Meeks SL, Harmon JF, Langen KM, et al. Performance characterization of megavoltage computed tomography imaging on a helical tomotherapy unit. Med Phys 2003; 32(8):2673–2681.

7. Langen KM, Meeks SL, Poole DO, et al. The use of megavoltage CT (MVCT) images for dose recomputations. Phys Med Biol 2005; 50(18):4259–4276.

8. Kupelian PA, Langen KM, Zeidan OA, et al. Daily variations in delivered doses in patients treated with radiotherapy for localized prostate cancer. Int J Radiat Oncol Biol Phys 2006; 66(3):876–882.

9. Tome WA, Jaradat HA, Nelson IA, et al. Helical tomotherapy: image guidance and adaptive dose guidance. Front Radiat Ther Oncol 2007; 40:162–178 (review).

10. Lu W, Olivera GH, Chen Q, et al. Deformable registration of the planning image (kVCT) and the daily images (MVCT) for adaptive radiation therapy. Phys Med Biol 2006; 51(17):4357–4374.

11. Schultheiss TE, Wong J, Liu A, et al. Image-guided total marrow and total lymphatic irradiation using helical tomotherapy. Int J Radiat Oncol Biol Phys 2007; 67(4):1259–1267.

12. Patel RR, Becker SJ, Das RK, et al. A dosimetric comparison of accelerated partial breast irradiation techniques: multicatheter interstitial brachytherapy, three-dimensional conformal radiotherapy, and supine versus prone helical tomotherapy. Int J Radiat Oncol Biol Phys 2007; 68(3):935–942.

13. Penagaricano JA, Yan Y, Corry P, et al. Retrospective evaluation of pediatric cranio-spinal axis irradiation plans with the Hi-ART tomotherapy system. Technol Cancer Res Treat 2007; 6(4):355–360.

14. Chen YJ, Liu A, Han C, et al. Helical tomotherapy for radiotherapy in esophageal cancer: a preferred plan with better conformal target coverage and more homogeneous dose distribution. Med Dosim 2007; 32(3):166–171.

15. Bauman G, Yartsev S, Fisher B, et al. Simultaneous infield boost with helical tomotherapy for patients with 1 to 3 brain metastases. Am J Clin Oncol 2007; 30(1):38–44.

16. Hodge W, Tome WA, Jaradat HA, et al. Feasibility report of image guided stereotactic body radiotherapy (IG-SBRT) with tomotherapy for early stage medically inoperable lung cancer using extreme hypofractionation. Acta Oncol 2006; 45(7):890–896.

17. Baisden JM, Reish AG, Sheng K, et al. Dose as a function of liver volume and planning target volume in helical tomotherapy, intensity-modulated radiation therapy-based stereotactic body radiation therapy for hepatic metastasis. Int J Radiat Oncol Biol Phys 2006; 66(2):620–625.

18. Fiorino C, Dell'Oca I, Pierelli A, et al. Significant improvement in normal tissue sparing and target coverage

for head and neck cancer by means of helical tomotherapy. Radiother Oncol 2006; 78(3):276–282.

19. Mahan SL, Ramsey CR, Scaperoth DD, et al. Evaluation of image-guided helical tomotherapy for the retreatment of spinal metastasis. Int J Radiat Oncol Biol Phys 2005; 63(5):1576–1583.

20. Orton N, Jaradat H, Welsh J, et al. Total scalp irradiation using helical tomotherapy. Med Dosim 2005; 30(3):162–168.

21. Grigorov G, Kron T, Wong E, et al. Optimization of helical tomotherapy treatment plans for prostate cancer. Phys Med Biol 2003; 48(13):1933–1943.

22. Ramsey CR, Scaperoth D, Seibert R, et al. Image-guided helical tomotherapy for localized prostate cancer: technique and initial clinical observations. J Appl Clin Med Phys 2007; 8(3):2320.

23. Aoyama H, Westerly DC, Mackie TR, et al. Integral radiation dose to normal structures with conformal external beam radiation. Int J Radiat Oncol Biol Phys 2006; 64(3):962–967.

24. Ramsey C, Seibert R, Mahan SL, et al. Out-of-field dosimetry measurements for a helical tomotherapy system. J Appl Clin Med Phys 2006; 7(3):1–11.

25. Balog J, Lucas D, DeSouza C, et al. Helical tomotherapy radiation leakage and shielding considerations. Med Phys 2005; 32(3):710–719.

26. Lazar S, Followill D, Gibbons J, et al. Risk of secondary fatal malignancies from Hi-ART Tomotherapy IMRT. Med Phys 2007; 34(6):2591.

27. Kissick MW, Fenwick J, James JA, et al. The helical tomotherapy thread effect. Med Phys 2005; 32(5):1414–1423.

28. Mackie TR, Olivera GH, Kapatoes JM, et al. Helical tomotherapy. In: Palta J, Mackie TR, eds. Intensity-Modulated Radiation Therapy: The State of the Art. College Park, MD: American Association of Physicists in Medicine, 2003:247–284.

29. Low DA, Harms WB, Mutic S, et al. A technique for the quantitative evaluation of dose distributions. Med Phys 1998; 25(5):656–661.

30. Low DA, Dempsey JF. Evaluation of the gamma dose distribution comparison method. Med Phys 2003; 30(9):2455–2464.

31. Jeraj R, Mackie TR, Balog J, et al. Radiation characteristics of helical tomotherapy. Med Phys 2004; 31(2):396–404.

32. Chen C, Meadows J, Bichay T. Improvement in IMRT dose calculation accuracy with megavoltage CT imaging in the presence of high Z materials. Med Phys 2007; 34(6):2459.

33. Ruchala KJ, Olivera GH, Kapatoes JM. Limited-data image registration for radiotherapy positioning and verification. Int J Radiat Oncol Biol Phys 2002; 54:592–605.

34. Mackie TR, Hughes J, Olivera GH, et al. The delivery time for helical tomotherapy. In: The XIVth International Conference on the Use of Computers in Radiation Therapy. 2004:750–752.

35. Fenwick JD, Tomo WA, Jaradat HA, et al. Quality assurance of a helical tomotherapy unit. Phys Med Biol 2004; 49(13):2933–2953.

36. Balog J, Olivera G, Kapatoes J. Clinical helical tomotherapy commissioning dosimetry. Med Phys 2003; 30(12):3097–3106.

37. Balog J, Holmes T, Vaden R. Helical tomotherapy dynamic quality assurance. Med Phys 2006; 33(10):3939–3950.
38. Kestin LL, Goldstein NS, Vicini FA, et al. Treatment of prostate cancer with radiotherapy: should the entire seminal vesicles be included in the clinical target volume? Int J Radiat Oncol Biol Phys 2002; 54(3):686–697.
39. Chao KK, Goldstein NS, Yan D, et al. Clinicopathologic analysis of extracapsular extension in prostate cancer: should the clinical target volume be expanded posterolaterally to account for microscopic extension? Int J Radiat Oncol Biol Phys 2006; 65(4):999–1007.
40. Letourneau D, Martinez AA, Lockman D, et al. Assessment of residual error for online cone-beam CT-guided treatment of prostate cancer patients. Int J Radiat Oncol Biol Phys 2005; 62(4):1239–1246.
41. Langen KM, Zhang Y, Andrews RD, et al. Initial experience with megavoltage CT guidance for daily prostate alignments. Int J Radiat Oncol Biol Phys 2005; 62(5):1517–1524.
42. Susil RC, Teslow TN, McNutt TR, et al. Characterization of intrafraction prostate deformation and displacement via twice daily MVCT imaging. Int J Radiat Oncol Biol Phys 2007; 69(3):S645–S646.
43. Meeks S, Kupelian PA, Lee C, et al. Does image guidance need to be performed daily in the treatment of localized prostate cancers? Implications on treatment margins. Int J Radiat Oncol Biol Phys 2007; 69(3):S82–S83.
44. Ramsey CR, Scaperoth D, Seibert R, et al. Image-guided helical tomotherapy for localized prostate cancer: technique and initial clinical observations. J Appl Clin Med Phys 2007; 8(3):37–51.
45. Langen KM, Kupelian P, Willoughby T, et al. Intra-fraction prostate motion: dosimetric impact on delivered doses. Int J Radiat Oncol Biol Phys 2007; 69(3):S336–S337.
46. Lattanzi J, McNeeley S, Hanlon A, et al. Daily CT localization for correcting portal errors in the treatment of prostate cancer. Int J Radiat Oncol Biol Phys 1998; 41(5):1079–1086.
47. Song WY, Chui B, Bauman GS, et al. Prostate contouring uncertainty in megavoltage computed tomography images acquired with a helical tomotherapy unit during image-guided radiation therapy. Int J Radiat Oncol Biol Phys 2006; 65(2):595–607.
48. Ghilezean MJ, Jaffray DA, Shetty A, et al. Prostate gland motion assessed with cine-magnetic resonance imaging (cine-MRI). Int J Radiat Oncol Biol Phys 2005; 62(2):406–417.
49. Litzenberg DW, Balter JM, Hadley SW, et al. Influence of intraprostatic motion on margins for prostate radiotherapy. Int J Radiat Oncol Biol Phys 2006; 65(2):548–553.

14

Image Guidance in Postprostatectomy Radiation Therapy

TIMOTHY N. SHOWALTER AND RICHARD K. VALICENTI

Department of Radiation Oncology, Kimmel Cancer Center, Thomas Jefferson University, Philadelphia, Pennsylvania, U.S.A.

INTRODUCTION

Salvage or adjuvant radiotherapy after radical prostatectomy (RP) has been shown to improve biochemical control for appropriately selected patients, with an acceptable level of toxicity. Enhancement in the outcome will depend on our ability to assure the safe delivery of high radiation therapy (RT) doses (>64 Gy). Image-guided radiation therapy (IGRT) is now widely used in the primary treatment of prostate cancer and proving beneficial in the postprostatectomy setting. This new development is mainly due to improved target localization techniques and the better characterization of the prostatic fossa (PF) clinical target volume (CTV). In this chapter, essential data are summarized regarding PF-CTV delineation, planning volume definition, and target localization methods for postprostatectomy IGRT.

The Role of Postprostatectomy Radiation Therapy

RP is an effective treatment for localized prostate cancer (1), but about 35% of patients exhibit biochemical failure as defined by durable rise in prostate-specific antigen (PSA) (2,3). In a series of nearly 2000 men undergoing RP at Johns Hopkins University Hospital, 15% developed a rise in PSA at a follow-up time of 15 years. Roughly a

third of those patients with biochemical failure displayed distant metastases during the study period (4), but it is presumed that the remaining two-thirds of patients with biochemical failure exhibited local recurrence. For such patients with delayed rise in PSA, salvage RT may be offered to provide local control and prevent subsequent distant dissemination (5).

Biochemical failure rates are higher after RP for patients with adverse pathologic features, such as positive surgical margins, seminal vesicle invasion (SVI), or extracapsular extension (ECE) (6). Adjuvant postoperative RT has demonstrated a biochemical disease-free survival benefit compared with historical controls in retrospective series (7–11) as well as in three randomized, prospective trials (12–14). For patients with adverse pathologic factors, adjuvant RT decreased the rate of biochemical failure by 48% and 40% in the randomized trials conducted by the Southwest Oncology Group (SWOG) and the European Organization for Research and Treatment of Cancer (EORTC), respectively (12,13). In the German study of adjuvant radiotherapy (ARO 96-02/AUO AP 09/95), which included only those patients with undetectable PSA after RP, RT provided a 21% absolute advantage in four-year freedom from biochemical progression (14). In summary, the medical evidence is compelling in favor of the routine use of adjuvant postoperative RT in appropriately selected patients (Table 1).

Table 1 Summary of Prospective Trials of Adjuvant Radiotherapy After Prostatectomy

Study	N	RT technique	RT dose (Gy)	FFBF (%)	p value
SWOG 8794 (13)	172	Conventional	60–64	65.1 (5 yr)	$p < 0.001$
	175		0	36.0 (5 yr)	
EORTC 22911 (12)	502	Conventional	60	74.0 (5 yr)	$p < 0.0001$
	503		0	52.6 (5 yr)	
ARO 96-02 (14)	108	Conventional	60	81 (4 yr)	$p < 0.0001$
	153		0	60 (4 yr)	

For patients with rising PSA, the optimal trigger point for salvage PF RT is controversial, as definitions of PSA failure after RP vary. The American Society for Therapeutic Radiology and Oncology (ASTRO) guidelines published in 1999 define biochemical failure at a PSA level of 1.5 ng/mL (15). Although the range of PSA level cut points recommended in the literature is wide (9,16–26), outcomes may be improved by instituting RT at a PSA level as low as 0.5 ng/mL (21,27).

Clinicopathologic criteria have been developed to estimate likelihood of local recurrence and appropriateness for adjuvant RT. When considering treatment for presumed local recurrence, it is important to exclude patients at significant risk of subclinical metastatic disease. Persistently detectable PSA after prostatectomy raises suspicion for possible distant metastasis, and postoperative RT should be offered only after correlating the PSA with risk of residual prostate cancer based on positive surgical margin, ECE, or SVI (5). Distant metastasis after RP may also be predicted by time to PSA failure less than 2 years, Gleason score 8 or higher, and PSA doubling time less than 10 months (4). These patients are unlikely to benefit from PF RT, and the careful selection of patients with high likelihood of local-only disease prevents the exposure of patients with metastatic prostate cancer to potential toxicity. The distinction of local residual or recurrent prostate cancer from microscopically disseminated disease is the crucial first step in the radiotherapeutic management of patients with a delayed rise in PSA after RP.

Imaging Evaluation of Postprostatectomy Failures

Given the limited value of standard imaging tests as well as clinical examination for the detection of recurrent disease after RP, the assessment of an elevated PSA after RP presents a challenge (27,28). For patient with PSA relapse after surgery, the probability of a positive bone scan or CT scan is low; rates of positive findings on bone scan are as low as 4.5% for PSA less than 10 ng/mL (28). Therefore, conventional imaging assessment with CT or bone scan is performed with a low level of

expectation for most patients in this clinical setting, and alternate approaches should be evaluated.

Magnetic Resonance Imaging

Endorectal-coil magnetic resonance imaging (eMRI) is a promising imaging modality for the detection of local recurrence after RP for patients with isolated rise in PSA. In an early study of 35 patients with clinical suspicion of PF recurrence, specificity of eMRI was 100% and sensitivity was also 100% (29). A more recent study of eMRI with 48 patients showed 95% sensitivity and 100% specificity for identifying local recurrence (30). These results, although with small patient numbers, suggest that eMRI is the preferred method for imaging PF recurrence following RP (31). Additionally, MRI-guided biopsy may be performed for the detection of recurrent disease after RP (32).

Radioimmunoscintigraphy

Functional imaging modalities have been investigated as tools for confirming local recurrence in patients with elevated PSA after RP. Radioimmunoscintigraphy (RIS) with [111]indium-capromab pendetide (ProstaScint®, Cytogen Corp., Princeton, New Jersey, U.S.) has been used for the detection of local recurrence or residual prostate tissue after RP with mixed results (33–35). In a report of 43 men with biochemical recurrence after RP, a negative [111]indium-capromab pendetide scan predicted significantly for a lower rate of biochemical progression (10% vs. 41%, $p = 0.026$) after salvage RT (36). Chance for durable biochemical control was reduced by a positive [111]indium-capromab pendetide scan outside the pelvis in a study of 23 patients (37). In contrast, Thomas et al. reported that positive [111]indium-capromab pendetide findings outside the pelvis were not predictive of biochemical control (33). It has also been purported that this test has a positive predictive value of 27% for extrapelvic disease (37), and a sensitivity of 49% for PF recurrence (38). Thus, the available data does not justify the routine use of [111]indium-capromab pendetide scans to determine the site of recurrence in patients with an isolated rise in their PSA after RP (33,39), but technical improvements such as the use of CT fusion may increase the diagnostic accuracy of this test (40).

Positron Emission Tomography

Another promising functional imaging approach is positron emission tomography (PET). PET frequently uses the tracer, 2-[^{18}F]-fluoro-2-deoxyglucose (FDG), and currently has low sensitivity for the evaluation of prostate cancer because of modest glucose consumption by these tumors and high background activity due to the proximity of the urinary tract. Local or systemic disease was detected by FDG-PET in only 31% of patients in a recent study (41). Due to the low sensitivity of FDG-PET, other PET tracers have been investigated for the detection of cancer in the prostate bed. In a retrospective report of patients with elevated PSA after surgery, ^{11}C-choline PET scans showed a true positive result in 38% of clinical local recurrences confirmed by ultrasound and/or digital rectal examination (DRE), but no positive scans were found in patients with PSA levels less than 5 ng/mL (42). Wachter and colleagues prospectively studied the use of ^{11}C-acetate PET scans fused with MRIs in the setting of post-RP biochemical failure. They found the imaging technique to be feasible, and the functional images revealed local recurrence not visible on the anatomic imaging in a handful of patients; ^{11}C-acetate PET scans affected clinical management in 28% of patients studied (43). PET studies with ^{11}C-acetate and 18F-choline successfully identify local recurrence in only about half of the cases with PSA levels less than 1 ng/mL, which is less than that reported with the use of eMRI (43,44). It has been suggested that the sensitivity of PET scans may increase with increasing PSA, suggesting a relationship between tumor burden and sensitivity (41). Currently, PET scanning has no established role in the early identification of local recurrence or residual tumor.

TARGET VOLUME DEFINITION

There is no consensus for target contouring and treatment planning for postprostatectomy RT, although the definition of CTV is often based on CT imaging data (44). Clinical investigations have revealed significant interobserver variability in defining the PF-CTV with CT, suggesting inadequate consensus and inherent uncertainty in target definition (45). It is not clear whether interobserver variability in target volume delineation for prostate cancer RT affects normal tissue toxicity in a clinically meaningful way (46), but, nonetheless, uncertainty in target definition is suboptimal and further research efforts are warranted. The PF target volume at some institutions has been determined by the prostate tumor bed, surgical clips, bladder neck, and seminal vesicle remnants. Typically, three-dimensional conformal RT (3DCRT) techniques with four to six fields have been used for postprostatectomy RT (5). In the SWOG prospective trial of adjuvant RT, 9 × 9 cm or 10 × 10 cm radiation portals were used in a four-field technique (27).

In addition to 3DCRT, intensity-modulated radiation therapy (IMRT) has been used in the postprosatectomy setting. Bastasch and colleagues delivered IMRT to a target volume defined as the prostatic fossa plus periprostatic tissues. This information was obtained from the treatment planning CT, influenced by information in the operative report and the location of surgical clips. In their study, a 5-mm margin was added to the CTV for planning purposes (47).

Most of prospective and retrospective studies provide information for RT technique, but are vague in their descriptions of the target volume. It is the goal of this section to provide insights into PF-CTV definition using both clinical and imaging data, as well as the selection of treatment margins as it applies to target localization techniques in the postprostatectomy setting.

Clinicopathologic Principles for Target Volume Definition

Principles for the design of the PF-CTV may be derived from an appreciation of the pathologic and clinical information. It is known that most local recurrences after RP occur in the caudal portion of the PF near the surgical anastamosis (48,49). DRE is 44% sensitive and 91% specific in the detection of local recurrence, while transrectal ultrasound is 76% sensitive and 67% specific (48). In a report of transrectal ultrasound examinations with biopsies for rising PSA after RP, the most common sites of local recurrence were the urethra-vesicular anastamosis (UVA) (66%), the bladder neck (16%), and posterior to the trigone (13%) (50), thus indicating the importance of including these locations in the PF-CTV.

The definition of the PF-CTV may also be based on pathologic findings and the location of surgical clips. The pathology report provides information regarding SVI, surgical margin location, and the presence and extent of ECE, and these factors should influence the CTV on an individual basis. The use of surgical clips for delineation of the PF-CTV has not been validated, so the location of the clips should be correlated with additional pathologic and anatomic data, including discussion with the urologic surgeon. A preferred approach would entail a discussion with the surgeon prior to the operation about the strategic placement of the surgical clips at the anastamosis, bladder neck, and the space posterior to the bladder adjacent to the seminal vesicle remnants.

Image-Guided Target Volume Definition

Historically, the planning CT simulation has been the primary source of volumetric imaging data for the determination of PF target volume. Although treatment planning using RIS with [111]indium-capromab pendetide may influence the identification of a clinical target when compared with the CT, (51,52), this approach is not considered standard. In this section, we will review information pertinent to anatomic and imaging considerations for optimal PF-CTV delineation.

In designing the PF-CT, alteration in pelvic relational anatomy due to the surgical procedure should be considered. Alterations of the prostate CTV by radical retropubic prostatectomy have been studied quantitatively with CT by Sanguineti and colleagues (52). Six patients were evaluated; each underwent a planning CT scan between one month and one week prior to surgery and clinical target volumes (CTV_{pre}) were contoured. One to two months after surgery, a planning CT scan was performed in the same position and target volumes (CTV_{post}) were contoured. Rectum and bladder volumes were also generated and dosimetric and volumetric analyses were performed for a standardized four-field 3DCRT plan. Postoperative CTV volumes were 30% to 50% smaller than preoperative CTV volumes, depending on whether seminal vesicles were encompassed in the volumes. The reduction in target volume size was hypothesized to be related to shifts in adjacent normal organs as such shifts may alter the anatomic boundaries of the CTV. The imaging data demonstrated that the bladder moves posteriorly and caudally after RP, but that the location of the rectum is not changed significantly due to the procedure. On average, the upper limit of CTV_{post} was more caudal than that of CTV_{pre}. The post-RP reduction in volume of CTV and alteration in bladder position favorably affected the dose-volume histograms (DVHs) for the bladder and rectum. The quantitative description of surgical alterations in target volumes and organs at risk (OARs) by Sanguineti et al. provides a framework for considering additional information regarding PF target volume delineation.

Patterns of postprostatectomy locoregional recurrence have been described by Miralbell et al. using eMRI (53). Their study, which was modeled after seminal reports that influenced RT field definition guidelines for stomach and rectal cancer (54,55), consisted of 60 consecutive patients who received salvage radiotherapy at a single institution. All patients underwent both a diagnostic eMRI and a planning CT prior to RT. The spatial coordinates of the PF tumor recurrence were transferred from the eMRI to the CT for analysis. A CTV based on the eMRI information was generated for each patient and compared with the standard, CT-based CTV designed to encompass the prostate bed. Most sites of recurrent or residual prostate tumor

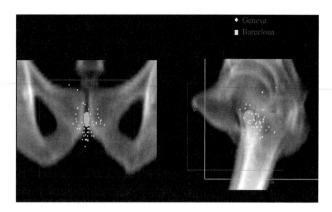

Figure 1 DRR depicting sites of local residual or recurrent disease after prostatectomy. *Source*: Ref. 53.

cells in the PF were located in the inferior and posterior aspects of the UVA. A scatter plot to show sites of local PF recurrence was produced on orthogonal digitally reconstructed radiographs (DRRs) using the spatial coordinates from the tumor recurrences visualized on eMRI (Fig. 1) (53). Ideal eMRI-based CTVs and planning target volumes (PTVs) were produced using the eMRI information and compared with the standard target volumes for a 3DCRT. In Figure 2, the Beam's eye view (BEV) image on the left depicts a left lateral field with margins around a standard PTV encompassing the PF, while the BEV on the right displays a left lateral field with a PTV produced used the investigators' recommendations. Miralbell et al. recommend a smaller, cylindrical CTV for postprostatectomy RT, including the UVA and bladder neck down to the level of the penile bulb. Their recommended CTV is generally 4-cm long and centered approximately 5 mm posterior and 3 mm inferior to the UVA (53).

The volumetric data obtained from the above studies with CT and MRI images depict the anatomic changes resultant from prostatectomy and emphasize the importance of including the caudal portion of the prostate bed in the PF-CTV.

Interfraction Organ Motion and Planning Margin

Fiorino and colleagues utilized weekly CT scans to study rectal and bladder motion during a course of postprostatectomy RT (57). The planning CT scan for each patient was coregistered with subsequent weekly CT scans obtained in the treatment position. The PF-CTV, rectum, and bladder were defined by the same observer, and variations in volumes, DVHs, and organ border position were analyzed. BEV analysis revealed a systematic anterior shift of the anterior rectal wall during RT for six of nine patients studied, with consequent worsening of the rectal DVH. The anterior rectal wall shift, which averaged 2.5 mm, was noted only within the cranial half of the

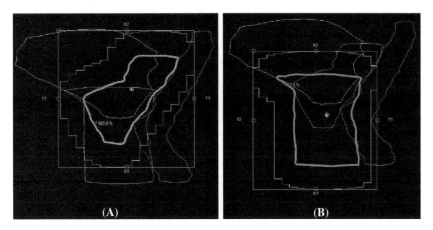

Figure 2 Beam's eye view projections showing a standard PTV with radiation portal (**A**) and the PTV proposed by authors based on sites of recurrence detected by MRI (**B**). *Source*: Ref. 53.

rectum. The anterior wall of the cranial half of the rectum also correlated with the posterior border of the PF-CTV. The region of rectal wall motion and the relationship between CTV and rectum wall are displayed in Figure 3 (57). This study characterizes interfraction pelvic organ motion in the postprostatectomy patient and shows the interrelatedness of the anterior rectal wall and the posterior PF-CTV border.

Researchers at Thomas Jefferson University Hospital (TJUH) have used cone-beam computed tomography (CBCT) images for daily setup correction and to study interfraction motion of the bladder and rectum as a method for analyzing changes in the PF during a course of RT (57). The PF was not contoured on CBCT images in the study due to reported uncertainty in postprostatectomy target delineation on helical CT (45). The rectum and bladder were readily visualized on the CBCT images, and the ability to contour the rectum with acceptable

interobserver variability has been reported (56). CBCT images obtained two to four times weekly for 10 patients in the treatment position immediately prior to RT were used to determine the interfraction motion of the posterior bladder wall and anterior rectum wall relative to the reference planning CT (CT_{ref}) and to the mean organ border position. Measurements were performed at three cranial-to-caudal levels titled "SUP," "MID," and "INF." The authors cite a prior report of correlation between PF-CTV and anterior rectum wall shifts, which was described only within the cranial half of the rectum (57). The authors also proposed CTV-to-PTV margins that were calculated with the posterior bladder wall motion and anterior rectum wall motion serving as surrogates for the movement of the anterior and posterior borders of the PF-CTV. This approach recognizes the uncertainty regarding PF definition on CT and assumes that the adjacent pelvic organs contribute to the delineation of

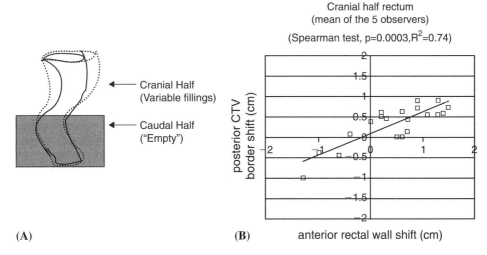

(A)   **(B)**

Figure 3 Rectal motion occurred within the cranial half of the rectum (**A**) and rectum wall motion correlated with shifts in posterior CTV border over this region (**B**). *Source*: Ref. 57.

Table 2 Organ Motion Relative to Planning CT as Observed on CBCT Images and Recommended CTV-to-PTV Margins Based on Motion of Adjacent Organ Borders

	Bladder motion (mm)			Rectal motion (mm)		
Observed motion	SUP	MID	INF	SUP	MID	INF
Relative to CT_{ref} (+ = anterior − = posterior)						
Mean	+0.1	+0.4	+1.5	−2.6	−1.6	−2.7
SD	4.4	3.7	4.0	6.0	6.3	5.8
Systematic error (Σ)	2.4	2.1	2.1	3.5	3.5	3.1
Random error (σ)	3.3	2.8	2.4	4.0	4.5	3.5
Calculated PTV margin ($2\Sigma + 0.7\sigma$)	7.1	6.2	5.9	9.8	10.2	8.6

Source: Ref. 58.

the anteroposterior (AP) target volume borders. Table 2 contains results for pelvic organ motion and for estimated CTV-to-PTV margin recommendations (58). These values may be considered when determining treatment guidelines for postprostatectomy RT.

TARGET LOCALIZATION TECHNIQUES

Image guidance during the treatment course is an important aspect of assuring precise RT delivery to the planned PF-CTV. Imaging at the time of treatment confirms the proper positioning of the target volume, allows for the correction of setup errors, and provides information regarding interfraction organ motion (59). IGRT is most likely to be beneficial when the target volume is immediately adjacent to OARs, and postprostatectomy RT dose is escalated above 64 Gy (60).

Multiple studies support the notion of radiation dose-response for RT after RP (Table 3), with RT doses of 64 Gy or higher leading to significant improvements in biochemical control (15,25,27,61,62), but potentially with an increased risk of toxicity. At TJUH, the institutional

Table 3 Summary of Published Studies Supporting Radiation Dose-Response for Treatment after Radical Prostatectomy

Study	N	RT doses (Gy)	FFBF (%)	p value
Valicenti et al. (Adjuvant − pT3) (62)	52	≥61.5	91 (3 yr)	0.01
		<61.5	57 (3 yr)	
Valicenti et al. (0.2 < PSA > 2.0) (62)	21	≥64.8	79 (3 yr)	0.02
		<64.8	33 (3 yr)	
Schild et al. (salvage) (88)	46	≥64	57 (3 yr)	0.059
		<64	17 (3 yr)	
Anscher et al. (salvage) (61)	89	>65	2.2 yr (med)	<0.001
		≤65	0	

policy is to deliver 68.4 Gy with IGRT for postprostatectomy patients. The risk of late rectal bleeding after postprostatectomy RT is reduced by restricting the amount of rectal volume receiving ≥50 Gy (63), but only by decreasing the treatment volume (64). A small treatment volume that is not localized during the course of RT delivery may lead to underdosing of the PF-CTV and a loss of treatment efficacy. To assure precise and accurate execution of the RT treatment plan, frequent examination of the online CTV during seven- to eight-week course of RT is now achievable with several IGRT techniques (65). As in the setting of primary RT for clinically localized prostate cancer, target localization methods may include the use of transabdominal ultrasound, computed tomography, or electronic portal imaging device (EPID) with fiducial markers.

Ultrasound

Chinnaiyan and colleagues reported the use of an optically guided, transabdominal ultrasound target localization system for daily positioning during postprostatectomy 3DCRT. Figure 4 shows a sample ultrasound image from their study, as well as the corresponding planning CT. The bladder neck was used as a surrogate anatomic structure for the PF, and corrective shifts were determined by the ultrasound-based position of the bladder neck. Daily localization with transabdominal 3D ultrasound was determined to be feasible in the radiation therapy clinic. In their experience, daily internal motion of the target volume for patients undergoing post-RP RT was similar in magnitude to patients with intact prostates, supporting a role for daily localization (66). Although the bladder neck was selected as an anatomic surrogate for the PF in this study, it is unclear whether this structure alone is a reliable surrogate for target localization of the PF.

Investigators from Fox Chase Cancer Center (FCCC) have described an approach for PF target localization

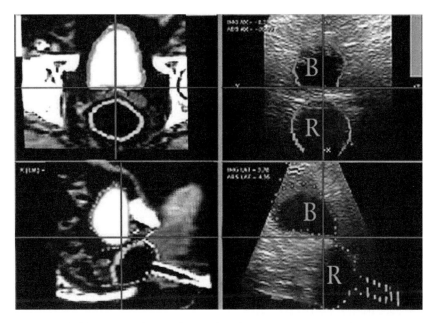

Figure 4 CT (left) and ultrasound (right) images from patient undergoing postprostatectomy IGRT with rectal balloon in place. *Source*: From Ref. 66.

using B-mode acquisition and targeting (BAT) ultrasound and CT-on-rails (67). For patients with intact prostates, the BAT ultrasound system has been demonstrated previously to be equivalent to CT for daily localization during definitive RT (68). In the FCCC study in the postprostatectomy setting, corrective shifts determined by BAT ultrasound were compared with those obtained by CT scans obtained in the treatment position prior to RT using CT-on-rails. A total of 90 pairs of CT and ultrasound images were compared for 9 patients, and the average interfraction PF target volume motions based on CT shifts were 3.0, 3.2, and 5.1 mm in the lateral, superoinferior (SI), and AP directions, respectively. Evaluation of the accuracy of BAT ultrasound localization of the PF, using CT-based localization as the standard for comparison, revealed systematic errors in alignment, potentially attributable to inherent uncertainties in postoperative target definition. The disagreement between CT and BAT ultrasound shifts was largely systematic, rather than random, and the authors noted that the discrepancies could be improved through the use of CT-based templates created using CT scans obtained during the treatment course. To resolve this discrepancy, the authors proposed a localization technique that combines information from both CT and ultrasound to provide reliable target localization (67).

Computed Tomography

Daily target localization with CT has been shown to allow reduction of PTV margins for patients receiving 3DCRT, and investigators from FCCC have recommended a 3-mm PTV margin for IGRT of the intact prostate with daily helical CT (69). Using megavoltage CT for daily target localization during postprostatectomy RT, Kupelian and colleagues reported a small average prostate motion relative to the bony anatomy. Although instances of PF motion greater than 3 mm were infrequent, the study demonstrates a discrepancy between alignments based on bony anatomy and the prostate bed (70), suggesting a potentially beneficial role for CT as daily target localization.

Kilovoltage CBCT is available for online IGRT and may improve the precision of RT (71). For patients with intact prostates, an analysis of residual setup errors using online CBCT during 3DCRT showed that a 3-mm margin would be required for patients receiving CBCT target localization (72). Furthermore, when used for online image guidance for RT of the intact prostate, CBCT has been shown to be equivalent to the technique of EPID with implanted fiducial markers, but with the added benefit of the visualization of adjacent soft tissue structures (73). Since 2005, kilovoltage CBCT has been used for online image guidance in postprostatectomy radiotherapy at TJUH and has been feasible in this capacity (58). Since online CBCT provides volumetric imaging data as well as the opportunity for setup error corrections, this can be a promising option for postprostatectomy IGRT (60). The computer monitor display shown in Figure 5 contains an example of CBCT image from TJUH used for postprostatectomy IGRT with a commercial software program (Elekta AB, Sweden).

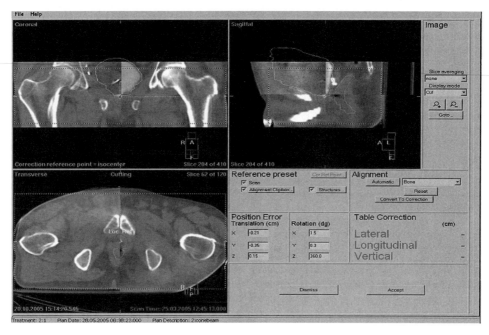

Figure 5 (*See color insert.*) Computer monitor display for online image registration and setup error correction using cone-beam CT. Commercial software used at TJUH (Elekta AB, Sweden).

Fiducials with Electronic Portal Imaging

Image-guided postprostatectomy radiotherapy has been delivered at the University of California, San Francisco (UCSF) using daily EPID with radiopaque gold markers implanted in the prostate bed (74). There is extensive experience in using this approach for daily target localization for definitive treatment of patients with intact prostates as described elsewhere in this volume (75–78). EPID with fiducial markers has also been shown to be a valuable method in postprostatectomy IGRT for the correction of interfraction motion of the prostate bed, with no significant migration of the fiducial markers during the RT course. Target positioning errors greater than 5 mm were detected in 14.1%, 38.7%, and 28.2% of RT fractions in the AP, left-right, and SI directions, respectively. Precision was improved with the use of daily target localization with EPID and implanted fiducial markers (74).

OPTIMIZING IGRT IMPLEMENTATION

IGRT has the potential to improve the quality of postprostatectomy RT through the definition of the PF target volume and the verification of the target position during the course of radiotherapy. It should be considered that the successful incorporation of complementary imaging modalities in PF target volume delineation is dependent on accurate integration of imaging modalities with optimal image registration (59). In the future, with improvements in resolution, functional imaging may become more important in treatment planning. In the mean time, CT and eMRI are the most reliable forms of volumetric anatomic imaging.

IGRT strategies for target localization have been developed with the goal of reducing geographic miss of the tumor and reducing dose to adjacent tissues, but it is important to recognize and minimize sources of inaccuracy in treatment verification. Anatomic surrogates for the PF have not been validated for target localization, and interobserver variability may limit the accuracy of targeting strategies. Although CT and ultrasound provide volumetric data that may be used to study interfraction motion and visualize adjacent normal structures, their routine use requires careful consideration and validation of protocols for image registration including the use of anatomic surrogates for the PF-CTV such as the bladder neck and posterior trigone. Daily target localization using EPID with implanted fiducial markers is appealing; the gold seed fiducials do not migrate significantly during the RT course and are readily identified (74). However, the increased information potentially available with volumetric imaging may make daily ultrasound or CT the preferred options in the future.

For patients with intact prostate glands undergoing definitive IGRT with online kilovoltage CBCT target localization, the margin required to account for residual setup errors is 3 mm. The residual error in this situation may relate to suboptimal image registration or target delineation (72). Patients undergoing postprostatectomy RT will likely require a similar margin with IGRT using daily volumetric imaging data. Studies of PF target localization using volumetric imaging have shown interfraction internal target motion errors of a magnitude similar to intact prostates (66), which supports the rationale for applying the image-guidance strategies developed for definitive RT to adjuvant or salvage RT of the PF. The correlation between late rectal bleeding and rectal DVH for patients receiving postprostatectomy RT suggests that toxicity may be reduced by efforts to shrink treatment margins with IGRT and to limit the volume of normal tissue irradiated using daily imaging. It will be difficult to quantify the benefits of IGRT over standard therapy in clinical trials using traditional metrics, but the improved precision in RT delivery should nonetheless translate into reduced toxicity and improved tumor control (60).

A potential future extension of IGRT for postoperative RT after prostatectomy may be adaptive, image-guided therapy using images obtained in the treatment position. An offline strategy, similar to the approach used for definitive prostate RT (79), may be possible for postprostatectomy RT. With CBCT images, it may be feasible to consider the anterior rectal wall and posterior bladder wall as surrogates for the AP PF borders for the purposes of offline adaptive IGRT with conformal avoidance of the adjacent normal structures (58). Further, volumetric imaging may allow online corrective strategies that adapt to patient positioning on a daily basis through conformal avoidance strategies to minimize the volume of rectum and bladder included in the radiation portals. Although there is uncertainty regarding the definition of the PF-CTV on CT, the ability to visualize the rectum and bladder on CBCT makes conformal avoidance strategies attractive.

CLINICAL OUTCOME

There are no published reports of biochemical control rates after postprostatectomy IGRT, though it is reasonable to expect improved biochemical control with IGRT due to image-guided definition of the PF-CTV and reduced risk of geographic miss with image-guided target localization. Reported biochemical outcome after postprostatectomy salvage RT varies among series, and the success of RT depends on many disease-related factors (5,80,81) and may be improved by the use of higher RT doses (15,25,62,82) or by androgen suppression in selected patients (83,84). The improvements in PSA relapse-free survival and in recurrence-free survival obtained with adjuvant RT in prospective trials were achieved with conventional RT without optimal target

localization techniques. It is anticipated that theoretical improvements in local control provided by IGRT will translate into a greater clinical benefit for postprostatectomy patients.

No data are available regarding improved normal tissue toxicity with postprostatectomy IGRT, but clinical gains are expected due to the potential to reduce the volume of irradiated normal tissue (60). Overall, current measures of toxicity show acceptable toxicities with salvage or adjuvant RT using conformal techniques. Acute toxicities from 3DCRT are tolerable and completed without interruption for 97% of patients in the EORTC 22911 trial (12). Whereas conventional RT techniques produced moderate to severe late complications in 7% to 20% of patients undergoing postprostatectomy RT, the rates of late grade II genitourinary (GU) and gastrointestinal (GI) toxicities after 3DCRT are about 5% and 9%, respectively (16). In a recent report from a large, multiinstitutional database of patients who received salvage or adjuvant RT after RP, rates of grade 2 (10%) and grade 3 (1%) late GU toxicity were low, as were rates of grade 2 (4%) and grade 3 (0.4%) late GI toxicity (85). In a prospective study, adjuvant RT was not associated with increased risk for urinary incontinence (85). Patient questionnaires have been used to study urinary and fecal continence for men treated with and without adjuvant RT after RP; although incontinence was present at a higher rate at four to eight months after RT, there was no difference in rates of incontinence at one year between those who did and did not receive RT (86).

In addition to GU and GI side effects, erectile function after adjuvant or salvage RT is important, particularly for patients who chose nerve-sparing procedures in hopes of preserving potency. It is unclear if 3DCRT adversely affects potency after RP (87). In one study, IMRT to a mean dose of 69.6 Gy after nerve-sparing prostatectomy was shown to preserve potency in all men with intact erectile function before RT (47).

Although favorable toxicity profile has been achieved with 3DCRT or IMRT, IGRT may improve upon these results through the ability to reduce RT margins and to minimize the volume of irradiated normal tissue, particularly when higher RT doses are administered.

QUALITY CONTROL

Imaging obtained prior to daily RT fractions in the treatment position provides verification data that are useful for quality assurance procedures. Interfraction organ motion or morphologic changes as a result of therapy can also be studied using these images (59). In this fashion, IGRT may improve the quality of RT through an enriched appreciation of physical variability in the target volume and surrounding normal tissues. It is incumbent upon radiation oncologists to provide data to confirm therapeutic gain from the increased precision of IGRT, but the intuitive nature of the improvements from this technology make the design of meaningful clinical trials essential (60). IGRT may improve the delivery of postprostatectomy RT in ways that are difficult to appreciate. The application of online strategies for target localization may require additional time in the clinic, (59) so changes in workflow should be documented when novel IGRT strategies are implemented. Image-guidance technologies must pass rigorous quality assurance inspection prior to implementation in the clinic. New strategies may be compared with other techniques for verification, similar to the comparison of CT to ultrasound for daily target localization for intact prostates (68).

SUMMARY OF PERTINENT CONCLUSIONS

- Postprostatectomy radiotherapy, delivered as adjuvant or salvage treatment, is supported by both retrospective data and three prospective trials (EORTC 22911, SWOG 8794, and ARO 96-02).
- Decisions to offer PF RT have been based on clinicopathologic factors, but imaging such as MRI with endorectal coil, and perhaps novel forms of functional imaging, may assist in the diagnosis of local residual or recurrent disease after prostatectomy.
- Guidelines for PF CTV definition have relied on the operative and pathology reports and the planning CT scan. More recent information obtained from CT and MRI have better characterized changes in anatomy due to prostatectomy and the tendency for disease to recur or to remain at the urethra-vesicular anastamosis and other caudal regions of the PF.
- Ultrasound, CBCT, and EPID with fiducial markers have been used as target localization strategies for postprostatectomy IGRT. All these imaging methods hold promise to improve the quality of accurate and precise RT delivery for postprostatectomy patients.
- IGRT offers the potential for improved target volume definition using complementary image modalities that may be registered to the planning CT.
- Late rectal bleeding has been correlated with rectal DVH, and the improved precision attainable with IGRT may reduce risk of clinical toxicity. Although the reported rates of toxicity are acceptable after 3DCRT after prostatectomy, the use of higher RT doses may create a more pressing need for IGRT.
- Inherent limitations of PF delineation on standard anatomic images contribute to limitations in the use of volumetric imaging techniques for daily target localization. Implementation of corrective strategies

based on daily volumetric imaging should include validation of the target localization strategy.

REFERENCES

1. Bill-Axelson A, Holmberg L, Ruutu M, et al. Radical prostatectomy versus watchful-waiting in early prostate cancer. N Engl J Med 2005; 352:1977–1984.
2. Pound CR, Partin AW, Epstein JI, et al. Prostate-specific antigen after anatomic radical retropubic prostatectomy: patterns of recurrence and cancer control. Urol Clin North Am 1997; 24:395–406.
3. Sailer SL. Radiation therapy for prostate cancer: external beam, brachytherapy, and salvage. N C Med J 2006; 67: 149–153.
4. Pound CR, Partin AW, Eisenberger MA, et al. Natural history of progression after PSA elevation following radical prostatectomy. JAMA 1999; 281:1591–1597.
5. Hayes SB, Pollack A. Parameters for treatment decisions for salvage radiation therapy. J Clin Oncol 2005; 23:8204–8211.
6. Stephenson AJ, Scardino PT, Eastham JA, et al. Postoperative nomogram predicting the 10-year probability of prostate cancer recurrence after radical prostatectomy. J Clin Oncol 2005; 23:7005–7012.
7. Valicenti RK, Gomella LG, Ismail M, et al. The efficacy of early adjuvant radiation therapy for pT3N0 prostate cancer: a matched-pair analysis. Int J Radiat Oncol Biol Phys 1999; 45:53–58.
8. Kalapurakal JA, Huang C-F, Neriamparampil MM, et al. Biochemical disease-free survival following adjuvant and salvage irradiation after radical prostatectomy. Int J Radiat Oncol Biol Phys 2002; 54:1047–1054.
9. Morris MM, Dallow KC, Zietman AL, et al. Adjuvant and salvage irradiation following radical prostatectomy for prostate cancer. Int J Radiat Oncol Biol Phys 1997; 38: 731–736.
10. Taylor N, Kelly JF, Kuban DA, et al. Adjuvant and salvage radiotherapy after radical prostatectomy for prostate cancer. Int J Radiat Oncol Biol Phys 2003; 56:755–763.
11. Vargas C, Kestin LL, Weed DW, et al. Improved biochemical outcome with adjuvant radiotherapy after radical prostatectomy for prostate cancer with poor pathologic features. Int J Radiat Oncol Biol Phys 2005; 61:714–724.
12. Bolla M, van Poppel H, Collette L, et al. Postoperative radiotherapy after radical prostatectomy: a randomised controlled trial (EORTC trial 22911). Lancet 2005; 366: 572–578.
13. Thompson IM Jr., Tangen CM, Paradelo J, et al. Adjuvant radiotherapy for pathologically advanced prostate cancer: a randomized clinical trial. JAMA 2006; 296:2329–2335.
14. Wiegel T, Bottke D, Willich N, et al. Phase III results of adjuvant radiotherapy (RT) versus "wait and see" (WS) in patients with pT3 prostate cancer following radical prostatectomy (RP) (ARO 96-02/AUO AP 09/95). J Clin Oncol, 2005 ASCO Annual Meeting Proceedings, Vol. 23, 2005:4513.
15. Panel ASfTRaOC. Consensus statements on radiation therapy of prostate cancer: guidelines for prostate rebiopsy after radiation and for radiation therapy with rising

prostate-specific antigen levels after radical prostatectomy. J Clin Oncol 1999; 17:1155–1163.

16. Zelefsky MJ, Aschkenasy E, Kelsen S, et al. Tolerance and early outcome results of postprostatectomy three-dimensional conformal radiotherapy. Int J Radiat Oncol Biol Phys 1997; 39:327–333.

17. Song DY, Thompson TL, Ramakrishnan V, et al. Salvage radiotherapy for rising or persistent PSA after radical prostatectomy. Urology 2002; 60:281–287.

18. Amling CL, Bergstralh EJ, Blute ML, et al. Defining prostate specific antigen progression after radical prostatectomy: what is the most appropriate cut point? J Urol 2001; 165:1146–1151.

19. Chawla AK, Thakral HK, Zietman AL, et al. Salvage radiotherapy after radical prostatectomy for prostate adenocarcinoma: analysis of efficacy and prognostic factors. Urology 2002; 59:726–731.

20. Duchesne GM, Dowling C, Frydenberg M, et al. Outcome, morbidity, and prognostic factors in post-prostatectomy radiotherapy: an Australian multicenter study. Urology 2003; 61:179–183.

21. Freedland SJ, Sutter ME, Dorey F, et al. Defining the ideal cutpoint for determining PSA recurrence after radical prostatectomy. Urology 2003; 61:365–369.

22. Liauw SL, Webster S, Pistenmaa DA, et al. Salvage radiotherapy for biochemical failure of radical prostatectomy: a single-institution experience. Urology 2003; 61:1204–1210.

23. Nudell DM, Grossfeld GD, Weinberg VK, et al. Radiotherapy after radical prostatectomy: treatment outcomes and failure patterns. Urology 1999; 54:1049–1057.

24. Raymond JF, Vuong M, Russell KJ. Neutron beam radiotherapy for recurrent prostate cancer following radical prostatectomy. Int J Radiat Oncol Biol Phys 1998; 41:93–99.

25. Stephenson AJ, Shariat SF, Zelefsky MJ, et al. Salvage radiotherapy for recurrent prostate cancer after radical prostatectomy. JAMA 2004; 291:1325–1332.

26. Wu JJ, King SC, Montana GS, et al. The efficacy of postprostatectomy radiotherapy in patients with an isolated elevation of serum prosate-specific antigen. Int J Radiat Oncol Biol Phys 1995; 32:317–323.

27. Swanson GP, Hussey MA, Tangen CM, et al. Predominant treatment failure pattern in postprostatectomy patients is local: analysis of patterns of treatment failure in SWOG 8794. J Clin Oncol 2007; 25:2225–2229.

28. Kane CJ, Amling CL, Johnstone PAS, et al. Limited value of bone scintigraphy and computed tomography in assessing biochemical failure after radical prostatectomy. Urology 2003; 61:607–611.

29. Silverman JM, Krebs TL. MR imaging evaluation with a transrectal surface coil of local recurrence of prostatic cancer in men who have undergone radical prostatectomy. AJR 1997; 168:379–385.

30. Sella T, Schwartz LH, Swindle PW, et al. Suspected local recurrence after radical prostatectomy: endorectal coil MR imaging. Radiology 2004; 231:379–385.

31. Walsh PC. Editorial comment on suspected local recurrence after radical prostatectomy: endorectal coil MR imaging. J Urol 2005; 173:832.

32. Hricak H, Choyke PL, Eberhardt SC, et al. Imaging prostate cancer: a multidisciplinary perspective. Radiology 2007; 243:28–53.

33. Thomas CT, Bradshaw PT, Pollock BH, et al. Indium-111-capromab pendetide radioimmunoscintigraphy and prognosis for durable biochemical response to salvage radiation therapy in men after failed prostatectomy. J Clin Oncol 2003; 21:1715–1721.

34. Raj GV, Partin AW, Polascik TJ. Clinical utility of indium 111-capromab pendetide immunoscintigraphy in the detection of early, recurrent prostate carcinoma after radical prostatectomy. Cancer 2002; 94:987–996.

35. Murphy GP, Elgamal AA, Troychak MJ, et al. Follow-up ProstaScint scans verify detection of occult soft-tissue recurrence after failure of primary prostate cancer therapy. Prostate 2000; 42:315–317.

36. Proano JM, Sodee B, Resnick MI, et al. The impact of a negative [111]indium-capromab pendetide scan before salvage radiotherapy. J Urol 2006; 175:1668–1672.

37. Kahn D, Williams RD, Haseman MK, et al. Radioimmuno-scintigraphy with In-111-labeled capromab pendetide predicts prostate cancer response to salvage radiotherapy after failed radical prostatectomy. J Clin Oncol 1998; 16: 284–289.

38. Nagda SN, Mohideen N, Lo SS, et al. Long-term follow-up of ^{111}In-capromab pendetide (Prostascint) scan as pretreatment assessment in patients who undergo salvage radiotherapy for rising prostate-specific antigen after radical prostatectomy for prostate cancer. Int J Radiat Oncol Biol Phys 2007; 67:834–840.

39. Wilkinson S, Chodak G. The role of [111]indium -capromab pendetide imaging for assessing biochemical failure after radical prostatectomy. J Urol 2004; 172:133–136.

40. Schettino CJ, Kramer EL, Noz ME, et al. Impact of fusion of indium-111 capromab pendetide volume data sets with those from MRI or CT in patients with recurrent prostate cancer. AJR 2004; 183:519–524.

41. Schoder H, Hermann K, Gonen M, et al. 2-[^{18}F]Fluoro-2-deoxyglucose positron emission tomography for the detection of disease in patients with prostate-specific antigen relapse after radical prostatectomy. Clin Cancer Res 2005; 11:4761–4769.

42. de Jong IJ, Pruim J, Elsinga PH, et al. 11-C-choline positron emission tomography for the evaluation after treatment of localized prostate cancer. Eur Urol 2003; 44:32–39.

43. Wachter S, Tomek S, Kurtaran A, et al. 11C-acetate positron emission tomography imaging and image fusion with computed tomography and magnetic resonance imaging in patients with recurrent prostate cancer. J Clin Oncol 2006; 24:2513–2519.

44. Dicker AP, Sweet JW, Valicenti RK, et al. Definition of the target volume after radical prostatectomy based on CT driven image fusion technology: implications for postoperative radiation therapy. In: American Society for Therapeutic Radiation Oncology Annual Meeting. Orlando, FL, 1997.

45. Symon Z, Tsvang L, Pfeffer R, et al. Prostatic fossa boost volume definition: physician bias and the risk of planned geographical miss. In: Radiological Society of North America Annual Meeting. Chicago, IL, 2004.

46. Livsey JE, Wylie JP, Swindell R, et al. Do differences in target volume definition in prostate cancer lead to clinically relevant differences in normal tissue toxicity? Int J Radiat Oncol Biol Phys 2004; 60:1076–1081.

47. Bastasch MD, Teh BS, Mai W-Y, et al. Post-nerve sparing prostatectomy, dose-escalated intensity-modulated radiotherapy: effect on erectile function. Int J Radiat Oncol Biol Phys 2002; 54:101–106.

48. Leventis AK, Shariat SF, Slawin KM. Local recurrence after radical prostatectomy: correlation of US features with prostatic fossa biopsy findings. Radiology 2001; 219: 432–439.

49. Scattoni V, Roscigno M, Raber M, et al. Multiple vesico-urethral biopsies following radical prostatectomy: the predictive roles of TRUS, DRE, PSA and the pathological stage. Eur Urol 2003; 44:407–414.

50. Connolly JA, Shinohara K, Presti JC Jr., et al. Local recurrence after radical prostatectomy: characteristics in size, location, and relationship to prostate-specific antigen and surgical margins. Urology 1996; 47:225–231.

51. Su A, Blend MJ, Spelbring D, et al. Postprostatectomy target-normal structure overlap volume differences using computed tomography and radioimmunoscintigraphy images for radiotherapy treatment planning. Clin Nuclear Med 2006; 31:139–144.

52. Sanguineti G, Castellone P, Foppiano F, et al. Anatomic variations due to radical prostatectomy: Impact on target volume definition and dose-volume parameters of rectum and bladder. Strahlenther Onkol 2004; 180:563–72.

53. Miralbell R, Vees H, Lozano J, et al. Endorectal MRI assessment of local relapse after surgery for prostate cancer: a model to define treatment field guidelines for adjuvant radiotherapy in patients at high risk for local failure. Int J Radiat Oncol Biol Phys 2007; 67:356–361.

54. Gunderson LL, Sosin H. Areas of failure found at reoperation (second or symptomatic look) following "curative surgery" for adenocarcinoma of the rectum. Clinicopathologic correlation and implications for adjuvant therapy. Cancer 1974; 34:1278–1292.

55. Gunderson LL, Sosin H. Adenocarcinoma of the stomach: areas of failure in a re-operation series (second or symptomatic look) clinicopathologic correlations and implications for adjuvant therapy. Int J Radiat Oncol Biol Phys 1982; 8:1–11.

56. Foppiano F, Fiorino C, Frezza G, et al. The impact of contouring uncertainty on rectal 3D dose-volume data: results of a dummy run in a multicenter trial (AIROPROS01-02). Int J Radiat Oncol Biol Phys 2003; 57:573–579.

57. Fiorino C, Foppiano F, Franzone P, et al. Rectal and bladder motion during conformal radiotherapy after radical prostatectomy. Radiother Oncol 2005; 74:187–195.

58. Showalter TN, Nawaz AO, Xiao Y, et al. A cone beam CT-based study for clinical target definition using pelvic anatomy during post-prostatectomy radiotherapy. Int J Radiat Oncol Biol Phys 2008; 70:431–436.

59. Dawson LA, Sharpe MB. Image-guided radiotherapy: rationale, benefits, and limitations. Lancet Oncol 2006; 7: 848–858.

60. Dawson LA, Jaffray DA. Advances in image-guided radiation therapy. J Clin Oncol 2007; 25:938–946.

61. Anscher MS, Clough R, Dodge R. Radiotherapy for a rising prostate-specific antigen after radical prostatectomy: the first 10 years. Int J Radiat Oncol Biol Phys 2000; 48:369–375.

62. Valicenti RK, Gomella LG, Ismail M, et al. Effect of higher radiation dose on biochemical control after radical prostatectomy for pT3N0 prostate cancer. Int J Radiat Oncol Biol Phys 1998; 42:501–506.

63. Cozzarini C, Fiorino C, Ceresoli GL, et al. Significant correlation between rectal DVH and late bleeding in patients treated after radical prostatectomy with conformal or conventional radiotherapy (66.6-70.2 Gy). Int J Radiat Oncol Biol Phys 2004; 55:688–694.

64. Fiorino C, Sanguineti G, Cozzarini C, et al. Rectal dose-volume constraints in high-dose radiotherapy of localized prostate cancer. Int J Radiat Oncol Biol Phys 2003; 57:953–962.

65. Speight JL, Roach M III. Advances in the treatment of localized prostate cancer: the role of anatomic and functional imaging in men managed with radiotherapy. J Clin Oncol 2007; 25:987–995.

66. Chinnaiyan P, Tome W, Patel R, et al. 3D-Ultrasound guided radiation therapy in the post-prostatectomy setting. Technol Cancer Res Treat 2003; 2:455–458.

67. Paskalev K, Feigenberg S, Jacob R, et al. Target localization for post-prostatectomy patients using CT and ultrasound image guidance. J Appl Clin Med Phys 2005; 6: 40–49.

68. Lattanzi J, McNeeley S, Pinover W, et al. A comparison of daily CT localization to a daily ultrasound-based system in prostate cancer. Int J Radiat Oncol Biol Phys 1999; 43:719–725.

69. Lattanzi J, McNeeley S, Hanlon A, et al. Daily CT localization for correcting portal errors in the treatment of prostate cancer. Int J Radiat Oncol Biol Phys 1998; 41:1079–1086.

70. Kupelian PA, Langen KM, Willoughby TR, et al. Daily variations in the position of the prostate bed in patients with prostate cancer receiving postoperative external beam radiation therapy. Int J Radiat Oncol Biol Phys 2006; 66:593–596.

71. Oldham M, Letourneau D, Watt L, et al. Cone-beam-CT guided radiation therapy: a model for on-line application. Radiother Oncol 2005; 75:271.e1–271.e8.

72. Letourneau D, Martinez AA, Lockman D, et al. Assessment of residual error for online cone-beam CT-guided treatment for prostate cancer patients. Int J Radiat Oncol Biol Phys 2005; 62:1239–1246.

73. Moseley DJ, White EA, Wiltshire KL, et al. Comparison of localization performance with implanted fiducial markers and cone-beam computed tomography for on-line image-guided radiotherapy of the prostate. Int J Radiat Oncol Biol Phys 2007; 67:942–953.

74. Schiffner DC, Gottschalk AR, Lometti M, et al. Daily electronic portal imaging of implanted gold see fiducials in patients undergoing radiotherapy after radical prostatectomy. Int J Radiat Oncol Biol Phys 2007; 67:610–619.

75. Alasti H, Petric MP, Catton CN, et al. Portal imaging for evaluation of daily on-line setup errors and off-line organ motion during conformal irradiation of carcinoma of the prostate. Int J Radiat Oncol Biol Phys 2001; 49:869–884.

76. Wu J, Haycocks T, Alasti H, et al. Positioning errors and prostate motion during conformal prostate radiotherapy using on-line isocentre set-up verification and implanted prostate markers. Radiother Oncol 2001; 61:127–133.

77. Chung PWM, Haycocks T, Brown T, et al. On-line aSi portal imaging of implanted fiducial markers for the reduction of interfraction error during conformal radiotherapy of prostate carcinoma. Int J Radiat Oncol Biol Phys 2004; 60:329–334.

78. Vigneault E, Pouliot J, Laverdiere J, et al. Electronic portal imaging device detection of radioopaque markers for the evaluation of prostate position during megavoltage irradiation: a clinical study. Int J Radiat Oncol Biol Phys 1997; 37:205–212.

79. Yan D, Lockman D, Brabbins D, et al. An off-line strategy for constructing a patient-specific planning target volume in adaptive treatment process for prostate cancer. Int J Radiat Oncol Biol Phys 2000; 48:289–302.

80. Katz MS, Zelefsky MJ, Venkatraman ES, et al. Predictors of biochemical outcome with salvage conformal radiotherapy after radical prostatectomy for prostate cancer. J Clin Oncol 2003; 21:483–489.

81. Tsien C, Griffith KA, Sandler HM, et al. Long-term results of three-dimensional conformal adjuvant and salvage radiotherapy after radical prostatectomy. Urology 2003; 62:93–98.

82. Macdonald OK, Schild SE, Vora SA, et al. Salvage radiotherapy for palpable, locally recurrent prostate cancer after radical prostatectomy. Int J Radiat Oncol Biol Phys 2004; 58:1530–1535.

83. King CR, Presti JC Jr., Gill H, et al. Radiotherapy after radical prostatectomy: does transient androgen suppression improve outcomes? Int J Radiat Oncol Biol Phys 2004; 59:341–347.

84. Eulau SM, Tate DJ, Stamey TA, et al. Effect of combined transient androgen deprivation and irradiation following radical prostatectomy for prostatic cancer. Int J Radiat Oncol Biol Phys 1998; 41:735–740.

85. Van Cangh PJ, Richard F, Lorge F, et al. Adjuvant radiation therapy does not cause urinary incontinence after radical prostatectomy: results of a prospective randomized study. J Urol 1998; 159:164–166.

86. Hofmann T, Gaensheimer S, Buchner A, et al. An unrandomized prospective comparison of urinary continence, bowel symptoms and the need for further procedures in patients with and with no adjuvant radiation after radical prostatectomy. BJU Int 2003; 92:360–364.

87. Formenti SC, Lieskovsky G, Skinner D, et al. Update on impact of moderate dose of adjuvant radiation on urinary continence and sexual potency in prostate cancer patients treated with nerve-sparing prostatectomy. Urology 2000; 56:453–458.

88. Schild SE, Buskirk SJ, Wong WW, et al. The use of radiotherapy for patients with isolated elevation of serum prostate specific antigen following radical prostatectomy. J Urol 1996; 156:1725–1729.

15

The Use of Image Guidance in Prostate Brachytherapy

CYNTHIA MÉNARD AND JUANITA CROOK

Department of Radiation Oncology, Princess Margaret Hospital, University Health Network, University of Toronto, Toronto, Ontario, Canada

INTRODUCTION

By virtue of the exponential decline in dose intensity with distance from the source, brachytherapy for prostate cancer requires precise and accurate source placement. Gains in the therapeutic ratio are largely accomplished with careful spatial selection of target tissues for high-dose radiation exposure. While modern techniques can achieve precision in delivery, toxicity and local control both remain an issue for a subset of patients, and expanding indications are placing more demands on the modality. Recent advances in imaging and image guidance may address this challenge.

The history of prostate brachytherapy illustrates a clear benefit to image guidance (1,2). Since Pasteau's publication in 1913 (3), describing insertion of a radium capsule into the prostatic urethra to treat carcinoma of the prostate, various techniques have been employed with unsatisfactory results. In 1917, Barringer first performed transperineal brachytherapy under transrectal tactile guidance (Fig. 1) (4). Decades later, in the early 1970s, Whitmore described open retropubic implantation guided by both direct intra-operative visualization of the prostate and transrectal palpation (5). Poor long-term outcomes were attributed to freehand source placement and inadequate dosimetry. In fact, dosimetry was calculated from plain radiographs, assuming that the target tissue was accurately

encompassed by the implant (6). The advent of transrectal ultrasound (TRUS), which permitted direct visualization of needles in relation to prostatic boundaries, and the subsequent development of the Seattle technique (7) revolutionized brachytherapy for prostate cancer.

The entire prostate gland has traditionally been considered the target for prostate brachytherapy for two reasons: (*i*) prostate cancer is inherently multifocal, placing the entire gland at risk and (*ii*) direct imaging of foci of cancer within the gland has been elusive. However, in reality, the local extent of prostate cancer is neither confined nor defined by the boundaries of the prostate gland. Although modern imaging techniques are still not able to map the extent of microscopic disease, they are capable of mapping intraprostatic sites of macroscopic tumor, knowledge of which may facilitate the study of tumor biology and virulence. These images can now be integrated in prostate brachytherapy for selective modulation of dose intensity both within and adjacent to the prostate gland (8). Given high precision in delivery, image-guided prostate brachytherapy may be the ideal platform for investigating intraprostatic dose modulation.

The term "image guidance" includes both off-line and online guidance techniques. This distinction is important since off-line imaging applies to all "image-directed" techniques where imaging is performed at a separate

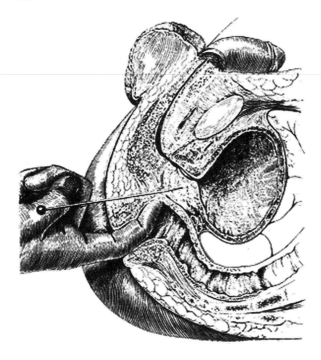

Figure 1 Transperineal brachytherapy needle placement under transrectal tactile guidance prior to the advent of image guidance. *Source*: From Ref. 4.

time from the brachytherapy procedure. In contrast "online imaging", or image guidance, is intricately integrated both temporally and spatially in the brachytherapy procedure. Furthermore, needle guidance should be distinguished from dose guidance, with needle guidance referring to the placement of brachytherapy needles or catheters, and dose guidance referring to the delivery of radiation dose. As defined by the American Brachytherapy Society (9), preplanning refers to the creation of a dose plan a few days or weeks prior to the implant procedure, while intra-operative planning includes

- Intra-operative preplanning: creation of a plan as the first step of the implant procedure

- Interactive planning: stepwise refinement of the treatment plan using computerized dose calculation derived from needle positions
- Dynamic dose calculation: constant updating of dose calculations using deposited seed or dwell positions

Since no single imaging modality embodies all the optimal characteristics for image guidance of brachytherapy for prostate cancer, multimodality guidance models will likely predominate for the foreseeable future. This chapter will place modern prostate brachytherapy techniques in the context of desired image guidance objectives, such that the promise and potential of brachytherapy can be fulfilled in the spectrum of prostate cancer treatment.

TRANSRECTAL ULTRASOUND

TRUS is considered the gold-standard image guidance modality for prostate brachytherapy. It provides good-quality images of the prostate gland boundary by using a high-frequency (5–7.5 MHz) intrarectal probe (10). The relative ease of mastering the basics of the transrectal sonograhic technique, real-time 2D feedback, and accurate volume assessment of the gland has contributed to its widespread use for image-guided brachytherapy (11). In fact, the brachytherapy community can be credited for initiating 2.5D step-TRUS image acquisition for reconstructed 3D visualization of the prostate. This technique led to the development of 3D TRUS using rotation fan scans, where overlay of sequentially acquired 2D images results in improved image quality and resolution (Fig. 3) (12). Substantial rotation (13), translation, and deformation (14) of the prostate with needle insertion highlight the value of real-time TRUS feedback during needle insertions.

One limitation of TRUS in the guidance of therapy for prostate cancer is its restricted soft tissue resolution. Conventional TRUS is neither sufficiently sensitive nor specific for visualization of intraprostatic tumor and therefore has

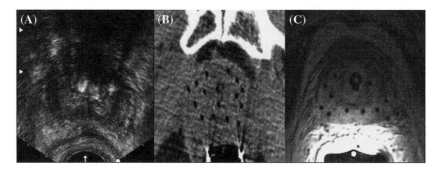

Figure 2 Images acquired after the placement of HDR brachytherapy catheters and prior to radiation delivery in one patient demonstrating the superiority of MR imaging in depicting both catheters and prostatic anatomy. (**A**) TRUS, (**B**) CT, and (**C**) MRI. *Source*: From Ref. 129.

limited use for staging purposes (8). Although prostate cancer may present as a hypoechoic area in the peripheral zone, hypoechoic features are not specific to prostate cancer and up to 40% of prostate cancers are isoechoic (10). Furthermore, implanted seeds cannot be reliably localized on TRUS (15). Seed specularity, shadowing, and tissue clutter make imaging catheters and seeds difficult using conventional ultrasound. Ongoing research in prostate ultrasound is now aimed at solving these limitations.

Color Doppler and its next generation, power Doppler technology, can show vascular profiles in tissues. Depending on the amplitude of the signal, the power Doppler image is displayed with varying hue and brightness, with color representing the total energy of the Doppler signal. Although this technology may help to reduce needle trauma to the peri-prostatic vasculature, Doppler maps cannot distinguish intraprostatic pathology, and therefore cannot guide tumor-targeted brachytherapy (16). Contrast-enhanced power Doppler TRUS has shown promise in this regard and may be useful in defining intraprostatic targets (10,11,16). Intravascular microbubble contrast agents enhance the back-scattered echo from blood flow (17) and newer bubble agents that resonate at higher frequencies may further improve the signal. 4D displays may allow for improved detection and quantification of areas of flow asymmetry (18). Further correlation with pathology is required before this technology can be incorporated in the identification of intraprostatic targets.

Ultrasound elastography, or sonoelasticity imaging, is at an early stage of development, and its potential role in image-guided brachytherapy is promising (8). Mechanical vibration is transferred to the imaging area, which contains materials of different vibration properties. The differences are detected in Doppler mode ultrasound (9). Sonoelasticity imaging may be used to detect brachytherapy catheters and seeds, and to distinguish tumor-bearing prostate tissue.

Finally, novel image-processing techniques, such as singular spectrum analysis, have shown promise preclinically in improving seed localization (19), while robotic assistance to catheter and seed segmentation and tracking may circumvent some of the limitations of TRUS (20). True interactive planning and dynamic dose calculation under TRUS guidance, will require autosegmentation of TRUS images (21,22), the subject of which is beyond the scope of this chapter.

RADIOGRAPHY AND COMPUTED TOMOGRAPHY (X RAY AND CT)

By virtue of unparalleled image resolution of implanted devices, online planar radiography has long been employed to augment TRUS in the evaluation of implant geometry and bladder wall violations. Various techniques have been proposed to objectify this integration with 3D registration of planar radiographs to TRUS images using fiducial markers attached to the ultrasound probe (23), or implanted needles (24). In this manner, images can be acquired in arbitrary positions to improve accurate mapping of seed locations relative to TRUS images. Early clinical results from the merging of fluoroscopy and TRUS to compute delivered dose intra-operatively (25), and guide placement of additional sources to underdosed areas (26) are promising.

Computed tomography (CT) essentially produces a 3D rendered image of brachytherapy catheters and seeds. Its current application lies in off-line postplanning evaluation of permanent implants, or less frequently in the treatment planning of temporary high-dose rate (HDR) brachytherapy after TRUS-guided placement of catheters and prior to dose delivery. However, the prostate is not well demarcated from surrounding structures on CT nor is intraprostatic anatomy well demonstrated (Fig. 2) (17). Compared to MR and TRUS, CT displays the largest variability and least correspondence when delineating the prostate (27,28). In general, CT defined volumes are 30% larger than those defined by TRUS (28,29). Although dynamic contrast enhanced CT can identify high-volume, poorly differentiated prostate cancers, it is unable to map intraprostatic tumor in the majority of patients (10). Attempts to improve soft-tissue delineation accuracy have resorted to the coregistration of alternative imaging modalities to CT. Some investigators have acquired postplanning CT images in the presence of a TRUS probe with subsequent registration of TRUS and CT images (30). A more common approach has been to register magnet resonance imaging (MRI) to planning CT.

Another weakness of CT in the brachytherapy scenario is the fact that artifacts from implanted material can substantially degrade CT image quality. Techniques to reduce CT metal artifacts include elegant solutions in post-processing of raw image data (31). Novel approaches have also been proposed to improve the accuracy of automatic 3D localization of seeds from CT scans, reaching sub millimeter accuracy (32,33).

There are many efforts to bring CT technology from off-line to online guidance. Fuller et al. have described a technique in which, following TRUS-guided brachytherapy, patients proceed immediately to CT for postplanning. The CT images are coregistered to TRUS images to map possible dosimetry deficiencies. If necessary, the patient is immediately re-prepped for TRUS guidance of remedial source placement (34). In order to improve efficiency, other investigators have brought diagnostic CT scanners to the brachytherapy suite, performing TRUS-guided brachytherapy on a modified CT table and thereby circumventing

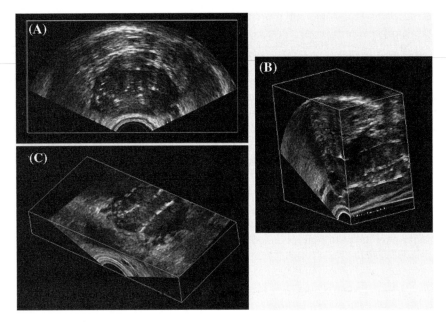

Figure 3 (**A**) A 3D TRUS prostate image post implantation sliced to visualize a transverse plane, (**B**) 3D volume sliced in the transverse and longitudinal directions, and (**C**) coronal plane. *Source*: From Ref. 130.

the need for patient transfers (35). A more cost-effective investigational solution involves using cone-beam techniques and amorphous silicon detectors in the brachytherapy suite for dual online fluoroscopic and CT guidance (Fig. 4) (9).

It is important to remember that online guidance of prostate brachytherapy using X-ray technologies risks occupational radiation exposure of health care personnel. Strategies that increase the use of X-ray in an online-guidance model must carefully consider and limit such exposures.

MAGNETIC RESONANCE IMAGING

Unlike TRUS and X-ray imaging modalities, MRI has not been widely integrated in current prostate brachytherapy guidance. Image acquisition time, complexity, space constraints, cost, and access to equipment remain as barriers to its universal adoption. However, MRI guidance of prostate brachytherapy is compelling for a number of reasons, and the subject of considerable research in both diagnostic and therapeutic communities.

First and foremost, prostate visualization is best realized with MRI, both for gland boundaries and subglandular architecture, as well as for adjacent organs at risk (9,36). For tumor-targeted dose intensification, MRI yields the highest accuracy in identifying the location and extent of both intra- and extraprostatic tumor burden. In fact, visualization of extracapsular extension on

diagnostic MRI is responsible for modification of dose plans in a substantial proportion of patients (37).

As prostate MRI acquisition techniques evolve, a combination of MR characteristics, including low T2 (38–43), rapid intravenous T1 contrast enhancement and washout (44), low diffusivity (45,46), high R2* (47–49), and high choline+creatine/citrate ratio (50–53) will create accurate maps of cancer burden. Such tumor-mapping accuracy currently requires the use of an endorectal coil, and prolonged examination times (45–60 minutes). Image voxel resolution varies depending on pulse sequence, magnetic field strength, and scan time, achieving $2 \times 0.5 \times 0.5$ mm [(T2-weighted fast spin echo (FSE)] to 5 mm^3 for (MRSI) (54,55) with modern equipment. Efforts to improve image resolution to 1 mm^3 isotropic voxels are ongoing.

MRI may also provide a window on tumor biology, virulence, and radiosensitivity. R2* maps from BOLD-MRI acquisitions (with rBV correction) have high sensitivity (95%) and reasonable specificity (70%) for defining intraprostatic tumor hypoxia, and possibly radioresistance, as defined by pimonidazole staining (49). MRSI metabolite ratios correlate with Gleason score, since prominent choline spectra correspond to increasing phospholipids cell membrane turnover in more rapidly proliferating aggressive cancers (56). Time to metabolic atrophy measured on MRSI after brachytherapy has shown promise as an early measure of response, with metabolic atrophy being seen in 95% of usable voxels in 46% of patients by 6 months and in 100% at 48 months with a mean time

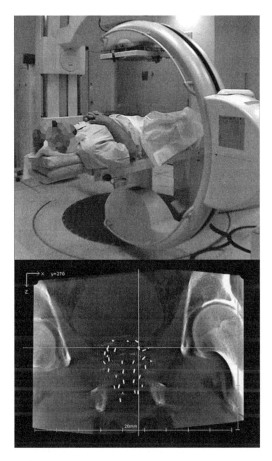

Figure 4 Cone-beam CT device (far left—Siemens Power-mobil Mobile C-arm) used for seed placement verification during a permanent seed brachytherapy procedure. Coronal CT image (*below*) shows good resolution of the seeds and surrounding soft tissue anatomy. *Source*: From Ref. 131.

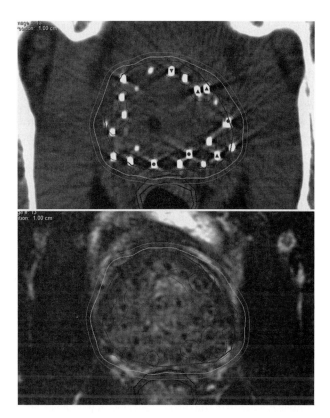

Figure 5 Fused CT (*top*) and MR (*bottom*) images from mid prostate level. Fusion is based on the seeds as fiducial markers. Both seeds and spacers leave black "holes" on MR, which therefore appear more numerous than the seeds on the CT image. However, the seed pattern on the CT is reproduced on the MR with a black void corresponding to each seed image.

to atrophy of 29 months (54). Finally, intravenous contrast kinetics may also reflect angiogenic activity in tumor-bearing regions (57). In essence, MRI guidance may bring us closer to the reality of biologically targeted brachytherapy (58).

FSE MRI provides superior visualization of brachytherapy catheters and seeds compared to TRUS, but is inferior to radiography. Brachytherapy seeds were first reported to be visible on MRI in 1997 (59,60). In phantom studies, distortion maps of different orientations of brachytherapy seeds were generated with susceptibility artifact patterns dependent on the orientation of the seeds with the main magnetic field and phase encode gradient. The highly predictable nature of these distortion patterns suggested that an automatic localization algorithm could accurately locate the implanted seeds using FSE MRI (61). This may be further enhanced using proton density weighting and IV contrast administration (62). MR elastography in a manner akin to TRUS elastography, with

vibration of interstitial needles during brachytherapy procedures, may further improve mapping of instrument geometry (63).

Off-line MRI guidance for prostate brachytherapy has focused on improving tissue delineation on postplanning CT scans. MRI-CT fusion using various image acquisition and registration techniques, has consistently demonstrated improved prostate gland delineation (Fig. 5) (64–73). The incorporation of MRI into postplanning allows assessment of dose to erectile structures, including the internal pudendal artery (74), neurovascular bundles, and penile bulb (75). Not surprisingly, performance is dependent on the details of pulse sequence acquisitions, with T2-weighted FSE techniques generally providing optimal soft tissue contrast with minimal susceptibility artifact from implanted seeds (76). However, because of the unreliability of extraprostatic source localization, postplanning based solely on MRI (77) remains problematic.

Another option involves the use of combined X-ray and MRI (XMR) interventional suites for postimplant dosimetry. XMR suites have been available for a few years and mainly applied to endovascular interventions. In such an environment, patients are transferred between the two imaging systems using a specially designed sliding table. Unlike CT/MRI image registration techniques described above, the registration process relies on a combination of calibration and tracking. All sources, including those in close clusters, are identified by two isocentric radiographs and transposed to MRI (78). By combining the highest soft tissue (MRI) and seed (X-ray) image resolution; this approach may achieve the best dosimetric accuracy in postplanning.

The off-line integration of MRI and MRSI for preplanning or intra-operative guidance by deformable registration of MR images to online 3D TRUS has also been described (79,80). An algorithm has been developed that first places the MRS positive voxel with respect to the z-axis in US/CT space. This determines the appropriate axial slice in which the MRS voxel is located. The x and y coordinates can then be determined. Using an MRS voxel size of $6.25 \times 6.25 \times 3$ mm, the reported positional accuracy was 2.2 ± 1.2 mm (80). The feasibility of this approach for brachytherapy dose intensification to intraprostatic tumor sites has been demonstrated clinically (81). However, substantial gland deformation introduces progressive registration errors through the course of a brachytherapy procedure, highlighting the need for more adaptive online MR integration.

The use of an open low-field MRI system for online-guidance of permanent seed prostate brachytherapy was first described by D'Amico et al. in 1998 (82–85). In an effort to reduce the toxicity of permanent seed brachytherapy, investigators translated the conventional transperineal ultrasound technique to an open MRI scanner architecture (85). Even at low field strength, the peripheral zone of the prostate gland could now be distinguished from the central gland and specifically targeted using custom interactive planning software (Fig. 6). Five-year results now confirm the equivalence of partial prostate brachytherapy to radical prostatectomy in biochemical disease-free survival (86). This group has also integrated off-line diagnostic MRI to online open MRI for the guidance of salvage permanent seed brachytherapy to specific subsites of recurrence visible on diagnostic MRI and MRSI (87).

For treatment planning for HDR brachytherapy, investigators at UCSF registered previous diagnostic MRI/MRSI datasets to "treatment planning" CT or MR images that were acquired after TRUS-guided insertion of brachytherapy catheters (88). Based on the diagnostic images, intraprostatic tumor sites were identified and targeted for dose escalation without exceeding tolerance for the urethra and rectum.

In order to circumvent the error associated with deformable or rigid registration of previously acquired

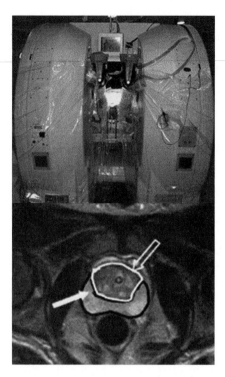

Figure 6 (*Top*) Open 0.5-T MR system for performing image-guided brachytherapy procedures. (*Below*) Prostate gland segmentation identifies peripheral zone (solid arrow) and central gland (*hollow arrow*) in interventional MR images. *Source*: From Ref. 132.

images, a technique for transperineal placement of temporary brachytherapy catheters in a 1.5 T scanner was developed (89). To access the perineum under the geometric constraint of a 60-cm diameter bore, patients were positioned in the left lateral decubitus position. Diagnostic images were acquired first, followed by the placement of brachytherapy catheters using a stereotactically registered perineal template. With the template fixed perpendicular to the rigid endorectal coil, the mean needle targeting accuracy was 2.1 mm. Once the catheters were in place, final diagnostic-quality T2-weighted images were acquired and used to plan and optimize radiation delivery (90), constraining radiation dose to the neurovascular bundle and including extracapsular extension of disease in the high-dose target volume (91).

The disadvantage of this approach is the lateral decubitus position, which is neither stable nor comfortable. Perineal access using a supine "semi-dorsal lithotomy" position on the MR table is being explored using a dedicated prostate interventional MRI table that provides ample perineal exposure. This table integrates patient immobilization devices, template hardware attachments, and can be undocked from the MR scanner for patient transport to an HDR delivery suite without disturbing the

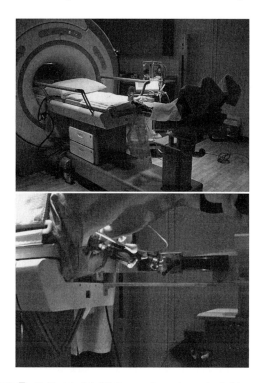

Figure 7 Cylindrical 1.5T diagnostic system adapted to prostate brachytherapy interventions using a dedicated table (Sentinelle Medical Inc., Toronto, Canada). Patient is positioned in semi-lithotomy. Dedicated table provides ample space for perineal exposure and brachytherapy devices, while undocking from the scanner to transport patients to HDR delivery suite without disrupting patient immobilization (not shown).

patient position and catheter placement (Fig. 7). Others are developing MRI-compatible robotics solving the space constraints and real-time image acquisition challenges of MRI guidance in prostate interventions (92,93).

Finally, MRI may have a role in the quality assurance of HDR delivery. Because of the dose-varying MR characteristics of exposed gel polymerization, 3D HDR dose plans can be verified using phantom polymer gel constructs (94).

NUCLEAR IMAGING (SPECT AND PET)

ProstaScint[TM] is a murine monoclonal antibody (capromab pendetide), which binds to the intracellular domain of the prostate specific membrane antigen (PSMA) and is conjugated to [111]Indium for SPECT (single-photon emission computerized tomography) imaging of prostate cancer (95). Unfortunately, problems including restricted access of the antibody to the intracellular compartment, nonspecific binding, and high blood pool activity causing a low target-to-background ratio have resulted in poor sensitivity (60%) and specificity (70%) (96) and limited clinical utility. Technical advances in SPECT imaging

resulting in superior image quality and CT registration warrant reevaluation of the role of ProstaScint in brachytherapy. Case reports (97) and mature series (98) demonstrate the feasibility of brachytherapy dose-intensification to lesions visualized on ProstaScint SPECT/CT.

Use of PET imaging for prostate cancer has been limited due to the poor sensitivity of FDG PET (99). Newer ligands, such as F18- or C11-labelled choline, and C11-labeled methionine have recently been evaluated with promising results. In a pilot study, F18-choline PET accurately discriminated positive sextants, with a sensitivity and specificity of 93% and 48%, respectively (100). This is consistent with early reports on the diagnostic accuracy of C11-choline PET (101). Pending further development and validation, these images have yet to be integrated in image guidance for prostate brachytherapy.

IMAGE GUIDANCE FOR PERMANENT LDR PROSTATE BRACHYTHERAPY

Image guidance is essential in every aspect of permanent seed prostate brachytherapy. Accurate definition of the prostate in planning of the implant, of prostate and needle position during the execution of the implant, and of prostate and seed positions in the postimplant evaluation are all vital to the success of the procedure. The current standard approach is to use TRUS for mapping of the prostate and planning of the implant, a combination of fluoroscopy and TRUS for execution of the implant, and CT for the post implant evaluation. There are some weaknesses in this standard approach, for which a variety of solutions have been developed.

Planning

When preplanning is undertaken two to three weeks prior to the procedure, the plan may not appear to "fit" when the patient is anesthetized and positioned in the operating room. With attention to the geometry of the setup including recording of probe angle and hip angles at the time of the mapping, this should be an uncommon occurrence. However, a popular solution is to perform the mapping intra-operatively as the first step in the implant procedure so that the patient only has to be set up once and there can be no alteration in prostate shape or size between mapping and implant execution.

Operative Technique

Although implants are planned with ideal coverage, with V150s and D90s within an optimal range, postplan analysis reveals that these goals can be difficult to achieve in reality. This can be attributed to either intra-operative or post-operative events.

Intra-operative Events

- Deteriorating visualization as implant progresses
- Prostate rotation 2° to needle insertion
- Seed rebound/dropping
- Prostate displacement cephalad

The quality of the TRUS images tends to deteriorate as the implant progresses due to prostate and periprostatic edema and bleeding. This can increase the uncertainty regarding needle placement with respect to the prostate contour.

Every needle insertion applies an off-axis force to the prostate, which is relatively tethered at the apex. Rotations in the coronal plane of up to 13.8° have been reported (13), resulting in seed trains that are more closely approximated at the apex but diverge at the base. This results in an area of relative under-dose at the base. Rotational displacement can be minimized by the insertion of multiple needles at a time so that centrally placed needles act as prostatic stabilizers for the more lateral needles. However, this, in turn, may cause displacement of the base in a cephalad direction. One study reported an average displacement of 1.5 cm with a range up to 3.0 cm (14). Again this will lead to significant under-dosing of the base if not recognized.

Often, if seed deposition is observed under US, seeds may appear to rebound when released because of prostatic compression, or alternatively may drop from the intended position because of placement in a cystic space or duct. Even for a preplanned implant, if such misplacements are observed, adjustments can be made in the plan to approximate the new position and determine if remedial action is required in terms of correctional seed placement.

Real-time dosimetry should allow for systematic correction of these misadventures by recalculating the dose distribution based on actual seed positions. Unfortunately most real-time intra-operative dosimetry is based on needle position rather than seed position (102). Seed visibility is inconsistent on TRUS with only 70% to 80% of the seeds being reliably identified (103). Linkage of seeds improves this situation because the inter-seed spacing is maintained. Individual seeds cannot "drop" or "rebound" as they are part of a strand, and all seed positions within the strand can thus be interpolated from any two clearly identifiable points in the strand (15).

Other efforts to improve seed localization intra-operatively and allow real-time correction include TRUS-fluoroscopy fusion (25), MR-fluoroscopy fusion, MR-TRUS fusion (79), or intra-operative CT dosimetry (35). Intra-operative dose assessment based on fluoroscopy alone has also been reported using three fluoroscopic images taken at 0°, +15°, and −15°. 3D seed coordinates can be computed and a distribution calculated in Vari-Seed. Additional seeds can be added based on deficiencies in the isodose cloud, although this method does not determine the relation of the isodose cloud to the actual prostate contour (26).

Another option to improve visibility intra-operatively is the use of single spectrum analysis, which uses eigenvalues derived from the diagonalized correlation matrix of envelope-detected radio frequency echo signals to yield a p-value indicative of the likelihood of a seed specific repetitive signal (19). This has yet to be tested in a clinical environment but accurately detects seeds implanted in animal muscle.

Postoperative Events

Another reason for discrepancy between the plan and the final dosimetry can be attributed to postoperative events including seed loss and/or migration as well as strand loss and/or migration. Migration of seeds through the blood stream to the lungs and occasionally to other organs is well recognized with loose seeds. The frequency of occurrence is 1% to 2% of seeds implanted but may affect up to 72% of patients (104–106). Vascular migration is essentially eliminated with the use of stranded preparations (107). Both seeds and strands can be lost through the urine and can migrate, usually distally, due to action of the perineal muscles (108,109). The rigidity of some newer stranding materials has led to reports of strand extrusion into the bladder and subsequent loss through the urinary tract (110). These events will not be captured by intra-operative dosimetry and may even be underappreciated when postplan imaging is performed the same day as the implant. For this reason, intra-operative dosimetry should be followed with a postplan evaluation at a later date.

Postplan Evaluation

Postplan evaluation by CT-imaging, whether performed day 1 or day 30, is not straightforward. There is a consistent discrepancy between prostate volumes as imaged by CT in comparison to TRUS or MRI, with CT volumes generally being about 30% larger (27). This discrepancy arises because the Hounsfield units of the surrounding structures (muscle, veins, bladder neck) are all very similar to those of the prostate itself. This situation is made even more difficult by the presence of metallic seeds and the resultant artifacts. Inter-observer variation in prostate contouring and postplan dosimetric evaluation has been well documented (71,73,111). For an experienced team who produces consistent technically excellent implants, the difference is minimal. Since the seeds are well placed, using their position to guide the contours will yield a result very close to the truth. For a beginner, it is perilous, fostering inappropriate confidence and leaving the operator unaware of the deficiencies in implant technique.

One solution is to use MR-CT fusion for postplans; the two sets of images can be fused with millimeter accuracy using the seeds as fiducial markers or matching through the use of mutual information (76). MR improves the soft tissue definition for contouring, while CT is used for identification of the metallic seeds (Fig. 5). Some experience with MR-CT fusion for postplans may be useful as a learning tool to give a better appreciation of the anatomy of the prostate and its surroundings (67). Another reported option is a combination of MR and X-ray, again benefiting from the enhanced soft-tissue visualization of MR for prostate contouring and using X-ray images for seed localization. This method does not have an explicit registration or fusion step but relies on system calibration and tracking (78) for stereoscopic seed localization. A method of TRUS-CT fusion (30,34) has also been developed. The TRUS probe is inserted with the patient on the CT couch and the TRUS images are recorded. The probe is then left in situ during the CT scan to serve for a registration landmark for the two image sets.

We cannot offer a recommended approach to permanent seed brachytherapy as there is not one approach that is clearly superior. Meticulous attention to detail, awareness of the various pitfalls and a consistent effort to avoid or circumvent them will inevitably lead to superior quality implants.

IMAGE GUIDANCE FOR TEMPORARY HDR PROSTATE BRACHYTHERAPY

HDR temporary implant techniques, developed in the 1990s, offer several advantages in image guidance for high precision brachytherapy. Dosimetric optimization is performed immediately following catheter placement, permitting the treatment plan to be based on the actual geometry of the implant relative to anatomical structures. A single high intensity ^{192}Ir source can be placed at any position for any length of time within each needle. These two variables (dwell position and dwell time) can be computer optimized to achieve dose distributions that conform to the target volume while limiting dose to normal structures. The treatment is subsequently delivered with an afterloading technique, and problems with source migration, inaccurate placement, and post implant edema are largely circumvented.

Image Guidance of Needles

The burden of precision in needle placement for HDR brachytherapy is considerably less than for permanent seed brachytherapy, since dwell time is such a powerful variable for dose optimization. Nonetheless, needle guidance and placement is a critical step in meeting dose-planning objectives. Experts have traditionally advocated equidistant placement of initial catheters in the periphery of the target (112). The use of online, interactive treatment planning tools and subsequent placement of additional catheters according to the estimated dosimetry has been explored and found to result in greater uniformity of treatment plans (113). Dynamic estimation of dosimetry during needle placement is feasible for TRUS-guided HDR prostate brachytherapy because it requires imaging the needles, not the individual seeds.

If the chosen target is the prostate gland, ultrasound guidance of needles with real-time image feedback is adequate. Visualization of the bladder base can be improved with fluoroscopy and cystography (112). However, the Groupe European de Curietherapie recommendations for HDR prostate brachytherapy are somewhat more refined and include

- CTV1—prostate gland,
- CTV2—peripheral zone,
- CTV3—regions infiltrated by macroscopic tumor (112).

As high-dose targets become more specific to the peripheral zone or intraprostatic burden of disease, image guidance for needle placement must evolve to meet these objectives.

TRUS guidance can be augmented by using high-resolution 3D TRUS technology, Doppler imaging, knowledge of prior biopsy results, and a finer template grid (3-mm spacing) (114). MRI for needle guidance can also be integrated in HDR brachytherapy and allows placement of needles within extraprostatic tumor (115). The use of advanced imaging for needle guidance may also reduce toxicity by avoiding needle paths through erectile structures and reducing the total number of needles (116). Given superior image resolution for mapping zonal anatomy and burden of disease, there is a need to explore further the integration of off-line or online MRI for needle guidance in HDR brachytherapy.

Image Guidance of Dose

In the modern era dose should be planned and optimized based on 3D patient anatomy rather than final implant geometry. It cannot be assumed that HDR brachytherapy catheters are ideally placed to encompass the target tissues. Anatomy-based dwell position and inverse optimization have clearly demonstrated improved dosimetry compared with more traditional catheter-based planning techniques (88,117,118). The relative merits of 3D TRUS,

CT, and MRI have already been described in the context of target delineation (Fig. 2). Precise and accurate dose planning specific to HDR brachytherapy requires that the catheter dwell positions be determined in reference to target anatomy. Although best visualized on CT and MRI, the slice thickness (2–3 mm) of CT and MRI may introduce small errors in determination of the catheter tip and first dwell position (115,119). This small uncertainty as well as uncertainties related to spatial integrity of MRI in the image-volume of interest must be measured, corrected if possible, and accounted for in dose planning (115). Planar X-ray and/or cone-beam CT may well reduce the uncertainty further in the SI dimensions.

Image Guidance of Delivery

Maintaining geometric fidelity for the delivery of HDR brachytherapy in reference to dose planning conditions is essential for accuracy. This is best accomplished by eliminating patient transfers to maintain the position of the patient and brachytherapy devices and by reducing the time interval between imaging for planning and subsequent radiation delivery. Despite these efforts, catheters can slip in the SI direction due to pelvic motion. Historically, this problem has been addressed by acquiring orthogonal radiographs of the implant catheters with reference to the contrast-filled balloon of the urethral catheter immediately prior to dose delivery (112). Integrating more advanced imaging and/or tracking methodologies during HDR delivery are desirable to ensure high-precision therapy.

IMPACT OF IMAGE GUIDANCE ON CLINICAL OUTCOMES

Disappointment with early historical results and the subsequent success of permanent seed prostate brachytherapy with the advent of TRUS and computer planning points to the impact of image guidance on clinical outcomes for prostate cancer. Improved freedom from biochemical failure (FFBF) has been demonstrated with technical maturation and the implementation of CT-based postplanning dosimetry (Fig. 8) (120). Most modern publications in this field demonstrate improved dosimetry with further advances in image guidance (26,34,35,79–81,85,88, 115,121,122). However, the relationship between dosimetry and clinical outcomes has yet to be fully defined.

There is a strong correlation of 3D dose-volume parameters with local control in prostate brachytherapy, with FFBF increasing with higher D90s (dose to 90% of the prostate) for patients with low-risk disease (123–126). It is important, however, to recognize that the accuracy of dose reporting is highly dependent on the accuracy of

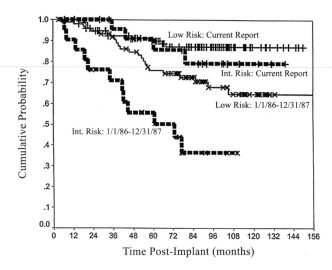

Figure 8 Comparison of freedom from prostate-specific antigen (PSA) failure by interval implanted and risk stratum. Image guidance and technical maturation with the implementation of postplanning dosimetry in 1998 may have led to improved outcomes. *Source*: From Ref. 120.

target delineation, and uncertainties in this regard may have contributed to inconsistencies in the observed dose-response relationship (71,73,111). This problem holds true for our understanding the relationship between critical organ dose and subsequent toxicity (127,128).

SUMMARY OF PERTINENT CONCLUSIONS

- Disappointment with early historical results and the subsequent success of prostate brachytherapy with the integration of TRUS imaging points to the impact and importance of image guidance.
- The entire prostate gland has traditionally been considered the target for prostate brachytherapy for two reasons (*i*) prostate cancer is inherently multifocal, placing the entire gland at risk and (*ii*) direct imaging of foci of cancer within the gland has been elusive. In reality, the local extent of prostate cancer is neither confined nor defined by the boundaries of the prostate gland.
- Modern imaging techniques, capable of mapping intraprostatic sites of macroscopic tumor, can now be integrated in prostate brachytherapy for selective modulation of dose intensity both within and adjacent to the prostate gland.
- Since no single imaging modality embodies all the optimal characteristics for image guidance of brachytherapy for prostate cancer, multimodality guidance models will likely predominate for the foreseeable future.

- The real-time 2D feedback of TRUS, the geometric integrity and brachytherapy device resolution of X-ray, and soft tissue resolution of the anatomy and biology on MRI are highly complementary.

REFERENCES

1. Rubens DJ, Yu Y, Barnes AS, et al. Image-guided brachytherapy for prostate cancer. Radiol Clin North Am 2006; 44(5):735–748, viii–ix.

2. Acher PL, Morris SL, Popert RJ, et al. Permanent prostate brachytherapy: a century of technical evolution. Prostate Cancer Prostatic Dis 2006; 9(3):215–220.

3. Pasteau O, Degrais P. De l'emploi du radium dans les cancers de la prostate. J Urol (Paris) 1913; 4:341–345.

4. Aronowitz JN. Benjamin Barringer: originator of the transperineal prostate implant. Urology 2002; 60(4):731–734.

5. Whitmore WF Jr., Hilaris B, Grabstald H. Retropubic implantation of iodine 125 in the treatment of prostatic cancer. Trans Am Assoc Genitourin Surg 1972; 64:55–57.

6. Acher PL, Dasgupta P, Popert R. Improving prostate brachytherapy by developing image guidance. BJU Int 2007; 99(2):241–243.

7. Holm HH, Juul N, Pedersen JF, et al. 125iodine seed implantation in prostatic cancer guided by transrectal ultrasonography. J Urol 1983; 130(2):283–286.

8. Carey BM. Imaging for prostate cancer. Clin Oncol (R Coll Radiol) 2005; 17(7):553–559.

9. Nag S, Ciezki JP, Cormack R, et al. Intraoperative planning and evaluation of permanent prostate brachytherapy: report of the American Brachytherapy Society. Int J Radiat Oncol Biol Phys 2001; 51(5):1422–1430.

10. Akin O, Hricak H. Imaging of prostate cancer. Radiol Clin North Am 2007; 45(1):207–222.

11. Boczko J, Messing E, Dogra V. Transrectal sonography in prostate evaluation. Radiol Clin North Am 2006; 44(5):679–687, viii.

12. Mehta SS, Azzouzi AR, Hamdy FC. Three dimensional ultrasound and prostate cancer. World J Urol 2004; 22(5):339–345.

13. Lagerburg V, Moerland MA, Lagendijk JJ, et al. Measurement of prostate rotation during insertion of needles for brachytherapy. Radiother Oncol 2005; 77(3):318–323.

14. Stone NN, Roy J, Hong S, et al. Prostate gland motion and deformation caused by needle placement during brachytherapy. Brachytherapy 2002; 1(3):154–160.

15. Xue J, Waterman F, Handler J, et al. Localization of linked 125I seeds in postimplant TRUS images for prostate brachytherapy dosimetry. Int J Radiat Oncol Biol Phys 2005; 62(3):912–919.

16. Amiel GE, Slawin KM. Newer modalities of ultrasound imaging and treatment of the prostate. Urol Clin North Am 2006; 33(3):329–337.

17. Hricak H, Choyke PL, Eberhardt SC, et al. Imaging prostate cancer: a multidisciplinary perspective. Radiology 2007; 243(1):28–53.

18. Pallwein L, Mitterberger M, Gradl J, et al. Value of contrast-enhanced ultrasound and elastography in imaging of prostate cancer. Curr Opin Urol 2007; 17(1):39–47.

19. Mamou J, Feleppa EJ. Singular spectrum analysis applied to ultrasonic detection and imaging of brachytherapy seeds. J Acoust Soc Am 2007; 121(3):1790–1801.

20. Wei Z, Ding M, Downey D, et al. Dynamic intraoperative prostate brachytherapy using 3D TRUS guidance with robot assistance. Conf Proc IEEE Eng Med Biol Soc 2005; 7(1):7429–7432.

21. Nanayakkara ND, Samarabandu J, Fenster A. Prostate segmentation by feature enhancement using domain knowledge and adaptive region based operations. Phys Med Biol 2006; 51(7):1831–1848.

22. Tutar IB, Pathak SD, Gong L, et al. Semiautomatic 3-D prostate segmentation from TRUS images using spherical harmonics. IEEE Trans Med Imaging 2006; 25(12):1645–1654.

23. Zhang M, Zaider M, Worman M, et al. On the question of 3D seed reconstruction in prostate brachytherapy: the determination of X-ray source and film locations. Phys Med Biol 2004; 49(19):N335–N445.

24. Gong L, Cho PS, Han BH, et al. Ultrasonography and fluoroscopic fusion for prostate brachytherapy dosimetry. Int J Radiat Oncol Biol Phys 2002; 54(5):1322–1330.

25. French D, Morris J, Keyes M, et al. Computing intraoperative dosimetry for prostate brachytherapy using TRUS and fluoroscopy. Acad Radiol 2005; 12(10):1262–1272.

26. Reed DR, Wallner KE, Narayanan S, et al. Intraoperative fluoroscopic dose assessment in prostate brachytherapy patients. Int J Radiat Oncol Biol Phys 2005; 63(1):301–307.

27. Smith WL, Lewis C, Bauman G, et al. Prostate volume contouring: a 3D analysis of segmentation using 3DTRUS, CT, and MR. Int J Radiat Oncol Biol Phys 2007; 67(4):1238–1247.

28. Narayana V, Roberson PL, Pu AT, et al. Impact of differences in ultrasound and computed tomography volumes on treatment planning of permanent prostate implants. Int J Radiat Oncol Biol Phys 1997; 37(5):1181–1185.

29. Kalkner KM, Kubicek G, Nilsson J, et al. Prostate volume determination: differential volume measurements comparing CT and TRUS. Radiother Oncol 2006; 81(2):179–183.

30. Steggerda M, Schneider C, van Herk M, et al. The applicability of simultaneous TRUS-CT imaging for the evaluation of prostate seed implants. Med Phys 2005; 32(7):2262–2270.

31. Takahashi Y, Mori S, Kozuka T, et al. Preliminary study of correction of original metal artifacts due to 1-125 seeds in postimplant dosimetry for prostate permanent implant brachytherapy. Radiat Med 2006; 24(2):133–138.

32. Tubic D, Beaulieu L. Sliding slice: a novel approach for high accuracy and automatic 3D localization of seeds from CT scans. Med Phys 2005; 32(1):163–174.

33. Holupka EJ, Meskell PM, Burdette EC, et al. An automatic seed finder for brachytherapy CT postplans based on the Hough transform. Med Phys 2004; 31(9):2672–2679.

34. Fuller DB, Jin H, Koziol JA, et al. CT-ultrasound fusion prostate brachytherapy: a dynamic dosimetry feedback and improvement method. A report of 54 consecutive cases. Brachytherapy 2005; 4(3):207–216.

35. Kaplan ID, Meskell P, Oldenburg NE, et al. Real-time computed tomography dosimetry during ultrasound-guided brachytherapy for prostate cancer. Brachytherapy 2006; 5(3):147–151.

36. Mayr NA, Menard C, Molloy AR, et al. Computed tomography and magnetic resonance imaging of the prostate, uterus, and cervix. In: Chao CKS, ed. Practical Essentials of Intensity Modulated Radiation Therapy. Philadelphia: Lippincott Williams & Wilkins, 2004:47–61.

37. Clarke DH, Banks SJ, Wiederhorn AR, et al. The role of endorectal coil MRI in patient selection and treatment planning for prostate seed implants. Int J Radiat Oncol Biol Phys 2002; 52(4):903–910.

38. Cheng GC, Chen MH, Whittington R, et al. Clinical utility of endorectal MRI in determining PSA outcome for patients with biopsy Gleason score 7, PSA <or = 10, and clinically localized prostate cancer. Int J Radiat Oncol Biol Phys 2003; 55(1):64–70.

39. D'Amico AV, Whittington R, Malkowicz SB, et al. Combined modality staging of prostate carcinoma and its utility in predicting pathologic stage and postoperative prostate specific antigen failure. Urology 1997; 49(3A suppl):23–30.

40. D'Amico AV, Schnall M, Whittington R, et al. Endorectal coil magnetic resonance imaging identifies locally advanced prostate cancer in select patients with clinically localized disease. Urology 1998; 51(3):449–454.

41. D'Amico AV, Whittington R, Malkowicz SB, et al. Combination of the preoperative PSA level, biopsy gleason score, percentage of positive biopsies, and MRI T-stage to predict early PSA failure in men with clinically localized prostate cancer. Urology 2000; 55(4):572–577.

42. Nguyen PL, Whittington R, Koo S, et al. Quantifying the impact of seminal vesicle invasion identified using endorectal magnetic resonance imaging on PSA outcome after radiation therapy for patients with clinically localized prostate cancer. Int J Radiat Oncol Biol Phys 2004; 59(2):400–405.

43. Poulakis V, Witzsch U, De Vries R, et al. Preoperative neural network using combined magnetic resonance imaging variables, prostate specific antigen and Gleason score to predict prostate cancer stage. J Urol 2004; 172(4 pt 1):1306–1310.

44. Ito H, Kamoi K, Yokoyama K, et al. Visualization of prostate cancer using dynamic contrast-enhanced MRI: comparison with transrectal power Doppler ultrasound. Br J Radiol 2003; 76(909):617–624.

45. Issa B. In vivo measurement of the apparent diffusion coefficient in normal and malignant prostatic tissues using echo-planar imaging. J Magn Reson Imaging 2002; 16(2):196–200.

46. Chan I, Wells W, Mulkern RV, et al. Detection of prostate cancer by integration of line-scan diffusion, T2-mapping and T2-weighted magnetic resonance imaging; a multi-channel statistical classifier. Med Phys 2003; 30(9):2390–2398.

47. Carnell D, Smith R, Taylor J, et al. Evaluation of hypoxia within human prostate carcinoma using quantified bold MRI and pimonidazole immunohistochemical mapping. Br J Cancer 2003; 88:S12.

48. Jiang L, Zhao DW, Constantinescu A, et al. Comparison of BOLD contrast and Gd-DTPA dynamic contrast-enhanced imaging in rat prostate tumor. Magn Reson Med 2004; 51(5):953–960.

49. Hoskin PJ, Carnell DM, Taylor NJ, et al. Hypoxia in prostate cancer: correlation of BOLD-MRI with pimonidazole immunohistochemistry—initial observations. Int J Radiat Oncol Biol Phys 2007; 68(4):1065–1071.

50. Kurhanewicz J, Vigneron DB, Hricak H, et al. Threedimensional H-1 MR spectroscopic imaging of the in situ human prostate with high (0.24-0.1 cm(3)) spatial resolution. Radiology 1996; 198(3):795–805.

51. Hasumi M, Suzuki K, Taketomi A, et al. The combination of multi-voxel MR spectroscopy with MR imaging improve the diagnostic accuracy for localization of prostate cancer. Anticancer Res 2003; 23(5b):4223–4227.

52. Scheidler J, Hricak H, Vigneron DB, et al. Prostate cancer: localization with three-dimensional proton MR spectroscopic imaging—clinicopathologic study. Radiology 1999; 213(2):473–480.

53. Coakley FV, Kurhanewicz J, Lu Y, et al. Prostate cancer tumor volume: measurement with endorectal MR and MR spectroscopic imaging. Radiology 2002; 223(1):91–97.

54. Pickett B, Ten Haken RK, Kurhanewicz J, et al. Time to metabolic atrophy after permanent prostate seed implantation based on magnetic resonance spectroscopic imaging. Int J Radiat Oncol Biol Phys 2004; 59(3):665–673.

55. Damyanovich A, Crook J, Jezioranski J, et al. Very high (0.05 cm3) spatial resolution three-dimensional 1H MR spectroscopic imaging of prostate pre- and post-brachytherapy. J Radiat Oncol Biol Phys 2004; 60(1 suppl):2196.

56. Hricak H. MR imaging and MR spectroscopic imaging in the pre-treatment evaluation of prostate cancer. Br J Radiol 2005; 78(Spec No 2):S103–S111.

57. Ménard C, Susil RC, Choyke P, et al. An interventional magnetic resonance imaging technique for the molecular characterization of intraprostatic dynamic contrast enhancement. Mol Imaging 2005; 4(1):63–66.

58. Ling CC, Humm J, Larson S, et al. Towards multidimensional radiotherapy (MD-CRT): biological imaging and biological conformality. Int J Radiat Oncol Biol Phys 2000; 47(3):551–560.

59. Dubois DF, Prestidge BR, Hotchkiss LA, et al. Source localization following permanent transperineal prostate interstitial brachytherapy using magnetic resonance imaging. Int J Radiat Oncol Biol Phys 1997; 39(5):1037–1041.

60. Moerland MA, Wijrdeman HK, Beersma R, et al. Evaluation of permanent I-125 prostate implants using radiography and magnetic resonance imaging. Int J Radiat Oncol Biol Phys 1997; 37(4):927–933.

61. Wachowicz K, Thomas SD, Fallone BG. Characterization of the susceptibility artifact around a prostate brachytherapy seed in MRI. Med Phys 2006; 33(12):4459–4467.

62. Bloch BN, Lenkinski RE, Helbich TH, et al. Prostate postbrachytherapy seed distribution: Comparison of

high-resolution, contrast-enhanced, T1- and T2-weighted endorectal magnetic resonance imaging versus computed tomography: initial experience. Int J Radiat Oncol Biol Phys 2007; 69(1):70–78.

63. Chan QC, Li G, Ehman RL, et al. Needle shear wave driver for magnetic resonance elastography. Magn Reson Med 2006; 55(5):1175–1179.

64. Taussky D, Austen L, Toi A, et al. Sequential evaluation of prostate edema after permanent seed prostate brachytherapy using CT-MRI fusion. Int J Radiat Oncol Biol Phys 2005; 62(4):974–980.

65. Crook J, McLean M, Yeung I, et al. MRI-CT fusion to assess postbrachytherapy prostate volume and the effects of prolonged edema on dosimetry following transperineal interstitial permanent prostate brachytherapy. Brachytherapy 2004; 3(2):55–60.

66. Vidakovic S, Jans HS, Alexander A, et al. Post-implant computed tomography-magnetic resonance prostate image registration using feature line parallelization and normalized mutual information. J Appl Clin Med Phys 2007; 8(1): 21–32.

67. Tanaka O, Hayashi S, Sakurai K, et al. Importance of the CT/MRI fusion method as a learning tool for CT-based postimplant dosimetry in prostate brachytherapy. Radiother Oncol 2006; 81(3):303–308.

68. Roberson PL, McLaughlin PW, Narayana V, et al. Use and uncertainties of mutual information for computed tomography/magnetic resonance (CT/MR) registration post permanent implant of the prostate. Med Phys 2005; 32(2):473–482.

69. Polo A, Cattani F, Vavassori A, et al. MR and CT image fusion for postimplant analysis in permanent prostate seed implants. Int J Radiat Oncol Biol Phys 2004; 60(5): 1572–1579.

70. McLaughlin PW, Narayana V, Kessler M, et al. The use of mutual information in registration of CT and MRI datasets post permanent implant. Brachytherapy 2004; 3(2):61–70.

71. Crook J, Milosevic M, Catton P, et al. Interobserver variation in postimplant computed tomography contouring affects quality assessment of prostate brachytherapy. Brachytherapy 2002; 1(2):66–73.

72. Amdur RJ, Gladstone D, Leopold KA, et al. Prostate seed implant quality assessment using MR and CT image fusion. Int J Radiat Oncol Biol Phys 1999; 43(1):67–72.

73. Dubois DF, Prestidge BR, Hotchkiss LA, et al. Intraobserver and interobserver variability of MR imaging- and CT-derived prostate volumes after transperineal interstitial permanent prostate brachytherapy. Radiology 1998; 207(3):785–789.

74. Gillan C, Kirilova A, Landon A, et al. Radiation dose to the internal pudendal arteries from permanent-seed prostate brachytherapy as determined by time-of-flight MR angiography. Int J Radiat Oncol Biol Phys 2006; 65(3): 688–693.

75. Wright JL, Newhouse JH, Laguna JL, et al. Localization of neurovascular bundles on pelvic CT and evaluation of radiation dose to structures putatively involved in erectile dysfunction after prostate brachytherapy. Int J Radiat Oncol Biol Phys 2004; 59(2):426–435.

76. McLaughlin PW, Narayana V, Drake DG, et al. Comparison of MRI pulse sequences in defining prostate volume after permanent implantation. Int J Radiat Oncol Biol Phys 2002; 54(3):703–711.

77. Tanaka O, Hayashi S, Matsuo M, et al. Comparison of MRI-based and CT/MRI fusion-based postimplant dosimetric analysis of prostate brachytherapy. Int J Radiat Oncol Biol Phys 2006; 66(2):597–602.

78. Miquel ME, Rhode KS, Acher PL, et al. Using combined x-ray and MR imaging for prostate I-125 post-implant dosimetry: phantom validation and preliminary patient work. Phys Med Biol 2006; 51(5):1129–1137.

79. Reynier C, Troccaz J, Fourneret P, et al. MRI/TRUS data fusion for prostate brachytherapy. Preliminary results. Med Phys 2004; 31(6):1568–1575.

80. Mizowaki T, Cohen GN, Fung AY, et al. Towards integrating functional imaging in the treatment of prostate cancer with radiation: the registration of the MR spectroscopy imaging to ultrasound/CT images and its implementation in treatment planning. Int J Radiat Oncol Biol Phys 2002; 54(5):1558–1564.

81. DiBiase SJ, Hosseinzadeh K, Gullapalli RP, et al. Magnetic resonance spectroscopic imaging-guided brachytherapy for localized prostate cancer. Int J Radiat Oncol Biol Phys 2002; 52(2):429–438.

82. Haker SJ, Mulkern RV, Roebuck JR, et al. Magnetic resonance-guided prostate interventions. Top Magn Reson Imaging 2005; 16(5):355–368.

83. D'Amico AV, Cormack RA, Tempany CM. MRI-guided diagnosis and treatment of prostate cancer. N Engl J Med 2001; 344(10):776–777.

84. Hurwitz MD, Cormack R, Tempany CM, et al. Three-dimensional real-time magnetic resonance-guided interstitial prostate brachytherapy optimizes radiation dose distribution resulting in a favorable acute side effect profile in patients with clinically localized prostate cancer. Tech Urol 2000; 6(2):89–94.

85. D'Amico AV, Cormack R, Tempany CM, et al. Real-time magnetic resonance image-guided interstitial brachytherapy in the treatment of select patients with clinically localized prostate cancer. Int J Radiat Oncol Biol Phys 1998; 42(3):507–515.

86. D'Amico AV, Tempany CM, Schultz D, et al. Comparing PSA outcome after radical prostatectomy or magnetic resonance imaging-guided partial prostatic irradiation in select patients with clinically localized adenocarcinoma of the prostate. Urology 2003; 62(6):1063–1067.

87. Barnes AS, Haker SJ, Mulkern RV, et al. Magnetic resonance spectroscopy-guided transperineal prostate biopsy and brachytherapy for recurrent prostate cancer. Urology 2005; 66(6):1319.

88. Pouliot J, Kim Y, Lessard E, et al. Inverse planning for HDR prostate brachytherapy used to boost dominant intra-prostatic lesions defined by magnetic resonance spectroscopy imaging. Int J Radiat Oncol Biol Phys 2004; 59(4): 1196–1207.

89. Susil RC, Camphausen K, Choyke P, et al. System for prostate brachytherapy and biopsy in a standard 1.5 T MRI scanner. Magn Reson Med 2004; 52(3):683–687.

90. Ménard C, Susil RC, Choyke P, et al. MRI-guided HDR prostate brachytherapy in standard 1.5T scanner. Int J Radiat Oncol Biol Phys 2004; 59(5):1414–1423.

91. Citrin D, Ning H, Guion P, et al. Inverse treatment planning based on MRI for HDR prostate brachytherapy. Int J Radiat Oncol Biol Phys 2005; 61:1267–1275.

92. Muntener M, Patriciu A, Petrisor D, et al. Magnetic resonance imaging compatible robotic system for fully automated brachytherapy seed placement. Urology 2006; 68(6):1313–1317.

93. Van Gellekom MP, Moerland MA, Battermann JJ, et al. MRI-guided prostate brachytherapy with single needle method—a planning study. Radiother Oncol 2004; 71(3): 327–332.

94. Kipouros P, Papagiannis P, Sakelliou L, et al. 3D dose verification in 192Ir HDR prostate monotherapy using polymer gels and MRI. Med Phys 2003; 30(8):2031–2039.

95. Jana S, Blaufox MD. Nuclear medicine studies of the prostate, testes, and bladder. Semin Nucl Med 2006; 36(1): 51–72.

96. Lange PH. PROSTASCINT scan for staging prostate cancer. Urology 2001; 57(3):402–406.

97. Sodee DB, Sodee AE, Bakale G. Synergistic value of single-photon emission computed tomography/computed tomography fusion to radioimmunoscintigraphic imaging of prostate cancer. Semin Nucl Med 2007; 37(1):17–28.

98. Ellis RJ, Zhou H, Kim EY, et al. Biochemical disease-free survival rates following definitive low-dose-rate prostate brachytherapy with dose escalation to biologic target volumes identified with SPECT/CT capromab pendetide. Brachytherapy 2007; 6(1):16–25.

99. Trabulsi EJ, Merriam WG, Gomella LG. New imaging techniques in prostate cancer. Curr Urol Rep 2006; 7(3): 175–180.

100. Kwee SA, Wei H, Sesterhenn I, et al. Localization of primary prostate cancer with dual-phase 18F-fluorocholine PET. J Nucl Med 2006; 47(2):262–269.

101. Yoshida S, Nakagomi K, Goto S, et al. 11C-choline positron emission tomography in prostate cancer: primary staging and recurrent site staging. Urol Int 2005; 74(3): 214–220.

102. Potters L, Calguaru E, Thornton KB, et al. Toward a dynamic real-time intraoperative permanent prostate brachytherapy methodology. Brachytherapy 2003; 2(3): 172–180.

103. Han BH, Wallner K, Merrick G, et al. Prostate brachytherapy seed identification on post-implant TRUS images. Med Phys 2003; 30(5):898–900.

104. Stone NN, Stock RG. Reduction of pulmonary migration of permanent interstitial sources in patients undergoing prostate brachytherapy. Urology 2005; 66(1):119–123.

105. Older RA, Synder B, Krupski TL, et al. Radioactive implant migration in patients treated for localized prostate cancer with interstitial brachytherapy. J Urol 2001; 165(5): 1590–1592.

106. Kunos CA, Resnick MI, Kinsella TJ, et al. Migration of implanted free radioactive seeds for adenocarcinoma of the prostate using a Mick applicator. Brachytherapy 2004; 3(2):71–77.

107. Al-Qaisieh B, Carey B, Ash D, et al. The use of linked seeds eliminates lung embolization following permanent seed implantation for prostate cancer. Int J Radiat Oncol Biol Phys 2004; 59(2):397–399.

108. Kaplan ID, Meskell PM, Lieberfarb M, et al. A comparison of the precision of seeds deposited as loose seeds versus suture embedded seeds: a randomized trial. Brachytherapy 2004; 3(1):7–9.

109. Fuller DB, Koziol JA, Feng AC. Prostate brachytherapy seed migration and dosimetry: analysis of stranded sources and other potential predictive factors. Brachytherapy 2004; 3(1):10–19.

110. Saibishkumar E, Yeung I, Beikiardakani A, et al. Dosimetric comparison of loose seeds and stranded seeds in I-125 permanent implant for low risk prostate cancer. Brachytherapy 2007; 6(2):pp 87–88.

111. Bice WS Jr., Prestidge BR, Grimm PD, et al. Centralized multiinstitutional postimplant analysis for interstitial prostate brachytherapy. Int J Radiat Oncol Biol Phys 1998; 41(4): 921–927.

112. Kovacs G, Potter R, Loch T, et al. GEC/ESTRO-EAU recommendations on temporary brachytherapy using stepping sources for localised prostate cancer. Radiother Oncol 2005; 74(2):137–148.

113. Edmundson GK, Yan D, Martinez AA. Intraoperative optimization of needle placement and dwell times for conformal prostate brachytherapy. Int J Radiat Oncol Biol Phys 1995; 33(5):1257–1263.

114. Kovacs G, Melchert C, Sommerauer M, et al. Intensity modulated high-dose-rate brachytherapy boost complementary to external beam radiation for intermediate- and high-risk localized prostate cancer patients—how we do it in Lubeck/Germany. Brachytherapy 2007; 6(2):142–148.

115. Citrin D, Ning H, Guion P, et al. Inverse treatment planning based on MRI for HDR prostate brachytherapy. Int J Radiat Oncol Biol Phys 2005; 61(4):1267–1275.

116. Vargas C, Ghilezan M, Hollander M, et al. A new model using number of needles and androgen deprivation to predict chronic urinary toxicity for high or low dose rate prostate brachytherapy. J Urol 2005; 174(3):882–887.

117. Yoshioka Y, Nishimura T, Kamata M, et al. Evaluation of anatomy-based dwell position and inverse optimization in high-dose-rate brachytherapy of prostate cancer: a dosimetric comparison to a conventional cylindrical dwell position, geometric optimization, and dose-point optimization. Radiother Oncol 2005; 75(3):311–317.

118. Hsu IC, Lessard E, Weinberg V, et al. Comparison of inverse planning simulated annealing and geometrical optimization for prostate high-dose-rate brachytherapy. Brachytherapy 2004; 3(3):147–152.

119. Kim Y, Hsu IC, Lessard E, et al. Dose uncertainty due to computed tomography (CT) slice thickness in CT-based high dose rate brachytherapy of the prostate cancer. Med Phys 2004; 31(9):2543–2548.

120. Grimm PD, Blasko JC, Sylvester JE, et al. 10-year biochemical (prostate-specific antigen) control of prostate cancer with (125) I brachytherapy. Int J Radiat Oncol Biol Phys 2001; 51(1):31–40.

121. D'Amico AV, Moul JW, Carroll PR, et al. Surrogate end point for prostate cancer-specific mortality after radical prostatectomy or radiation therapy. J Natl Cancer Inst 2003; 95(18):1376–1383.

122. Zelefsky MJ, Yamada Y, Cohen GN, et al. Intraoperative real-time planned conformal prostate brachytherapy: post-implantation dosimetric outcome and clinical implications. Radiother Oncol 2007; 84(2):185–189.

123. Ash D, Al-Qaisieh B, Bottomley D, et al. The correlation between D90 and outcome for I-125 seed implant monotherapy for localised prostate cancer. Radiother Oncol 2006; 79(2):185–189.

124. Nath R, Roberts K, Ng M, et al. Correlation of medical dosimetry quality indicators to the local tumor control in patients with prostate cancer treated with iodine-125 interstitial implants. Med Phys 1998; 25(12):2293–2307.

125. Stock RG, Stone NN, Tabert A, et al. A dose-response study for I-125 prostate implants. Int J Radiat Oncol Biol Phys 1998; 41(1):101–118.

126. Potters L, Morgenstern C, Calugaru E, et al. 12-year outcomes following permanent prostate brachytherapy in patients with clinically localized prostate cancer. J Urol 2005; 173(5):1562–1566.

127. DiBiase SJ, Wallner K, Tralins K, et al. Brachytherapy radiation doses to the neurovascular bundles. Int J Radiat Oncol Biol Phys 2000; 46(5):1301–1307.

128. Crook J, Potters L, Stock R, et al. Critical organ dosimetry in permanent seed prostate brachytherapy: defining the organs at risk. An American Brachytherapy Society Consensus Statement. Brachytherapy 2005; 4(3):186–194.

129. Atalar E, Menard C. MR-guided interventions for prostate cancer. Magn Reson Imaging Clin N Am 2005; 13(3):491–504.

130. Fenster A, Gardi L, Wei Z, et al. Robot-Aided and 3D TRUS-Guided Intraoperative Prostate Brachytherapy. In: Dicker AP, Merrick GS, Waterman FM, et al. eds. Basic and Advanced Techniques in Prostate Brachytherapy. Oxfordshire, UK: Taylor & Francis Group 2005; 271–283.

131. Moseley DJ, Siewerdsen JH, Jaffray DA. High-contrast detection and removal in cone-beam CT. The Physics of Medical Imaging. SPIE Proc. 5645 2005; 6(22):40–50.

132. Barnes AS, Temapny CM. Image-guided minimally invasive therapy. In: Richie JP, D'Amico, A, eds. Urologic Oncology. Philadelphia: Elsevier; 2005; pp 114–115.

16

Image-Guided Intensity-Modulated Radiotherapy for Clinically Localized Prostate Cancer: Targeting Pelvic Lymph Nodes

MACK ROACH, PING XIA, AND JEAN POULIOT

Department of Radiation Oncology, University of California, San Francisco, NCI-Designated Comprehensive Cancer Center, San Francisco, California, U.S.A.

INTRODUCTION

Why Target Lymph Nodes?

Although prophylactic irradiation of lymph nodes is a routine practice for most cancer sites, the role of prophylactic pelvic lymph node irradiation is controversial in men with localized prostate cancer. Occult lymph node involvement, despite negative imaging is a well-recognized problem in patients with cancers of the head and neck, breast, and many other solid tumors. Physicians who do not favor prophylactic pelvic radiotherapy in patients with prostate cancer tend to support their position by making the nihilistic argument that once the nodes are involved, regional therapy is of no benefit. They also argue that there is increased morbidity with pelvic nodal irradiation, and even those who favor it concede it is more time consuming and technically more challenging to treat pelvic lymph nodes (1).

There are a number of reasons prophylactic pelvic nodal irradiation should be strongly considered in men with intermediate- to high-risk prostate cancer. This chapter highlights many of these reasons and discusses technical considerations when doing so. We make the argument that there is no reason to believe prostate cancer is unique among solid tumors in terms of the need to address regional disease when present. We argue that regional disease is common, and imaging is too insensitive to detect it when present. There is a growing body of data suggesting that treatment can be effective and well tolerated when properly administered. We explain for whom we recommend prophylactic radiotherapy and how intensity-modulated image-guided radiotherapy (IGRT) is administered at the University of California San Francisco (UCSF).

How Common is Lymph Node Involvement in Men with Clinically Localized Prostate Cancer?

Lymph node involvement is more common in patients with high- to intermediate-risk disease than generally appreciated. Although commonly quoted nomograms give estimates of 2% to 38% for such patients, there are a number of reasons to believe that the true incidence is substantially underestimated. The pathological findings from the vast majority of surgical series are based on prostate patients who underwent at most a standard lymph node dissection (SLD) for what was thought to be organ confined disease. Lymph node dissections in many of these series were either limited to obrurator lymph nodes alone or inclusive of external iliac lymph nodes chains, although the internal lymph nodes are considered part of the primary lymphatic drainage. In addition, even the most aggressive node dissection surgeons tend to ignore presacral and perirectal nodes.

A limited number of surgical series reported their findings when a more extensive lymph node dissection was performed. For example, Heidenreich et al. performed extended pelvic lymphadenectomies (ELD) to assess the incidence of lymph node metastasis in 103 consecutive patients and compared their pathological findings with 100 patients undergoing an SLD (2). They noted no significant differences in age, preoperative prostate-specific antigen (PSA) or mean biopsy, and Gleason score between the patient groups. Metastases were diagnosed in 26% of those who underwent the ELD. They concluded that the use of an ELD was associated with a high rate of lymph node metastasis outside of the fields of SLD and recommended ELD in all patients with a PSA >10 ng/mL and biopsy Gleason score ≥7. According to their findings, approximately 40% of the involved nodes would have been missed by an SLD. Another series included 414 patients with a PSA level of ≤10 ng/mL and a biopsy Gleason score of ≤6 (3). According to their findings, greater than 50% of involved nodes were outside SLD nodal regions.

A series of studies conducted by Italian investigators are worthy of note (4–6). First, they constructed a nomogram on the basis of pathological data obtained from patients who had undergone an ELD. Later they demonstrated that there is a critical dependence of the likelihood of detecting positive nodes on the number of lymph nodes available for analysis. They showed that more than 10 nodes had to be sampled to have a reasonable chance of detecting involved nodes (5). In keeping with this observation, Schumacher et al. reported the finding from patients who underwent radical prostatectomy and a bilateral extended pelvic node dissection including only patients in whom 10 or more lymph nodes were removed, and who also had a preoperative PSA <10 ng/mL (7). They noted that in 73% of those with positive lymph nodes, the internal iliac chains were involved either exclusively or in combination with another area. Thus, it appears that an ELD is considerably more sensitive than an SLD. It also appears that the true incidence of lymph node involvement based on SLD is underestimated by at least 40% to 50% than when an ELD is performed (Tables 1 and 2).

Of note, however, even series based on ELD underestimate the true incidence because they largely ignore perirectal (and in some cases presacral) nodes (8,9). On the basis of limited data that is available addressing these areas, the relative risk of lymph node involvement would be 5% to 10% higher if there areas were routinely sampled. Unfortunately, even these rates are likely to underestimate the true incidence of lymph node involvement.

In addition to the problem of inadequate lymph node sampling, the rates are likely to be an additional 10% to 30% higher because of false-negative pathological evaluations and because of the lack of sensitivity of standard histopathological processing of sampling when compared with more sophisticated methods of detection (10–13). Earlier studies assumed that the "gold standard" for detecting lymph node involvement was standard cytopathological evaluation. Table 3 highlights the conclusions of selected studies demonstrating that this so-called gold standard lacks in sensitivity. Recent studies have demonstrated that more careful sectioning of the lymph nodes combined with staining for epithelial cells as well as the application of reverse transcriptase-polymerase chain reaction (RT-PCR) or PSA nRNA copy number are more sensitive methods for identifying cancer in lymph nodes that would otherwise be considered N0 (10–12).

For example, in a study conducted at the University of Southern California, immunohistochemical combined with microscopic sectioning of lymph nodes also improved the detection of lymph node involvement not recognized at initial histological examination. Using this approach, occult lymph node metastases were identified in 13% of patients with pT3N0 prostate cancer and associated with an increased risk for recurrence and death (10). Investigators from Baylor University reported that RT-PCR is also a more sensitive method than histology for detecting occult small lymph node involvement (11). They noted that 20% of patients with T3N0 disease had evidence of involvement using this assay. They used a highly sensitive and specific RT-PCR assay for human glandular kallikrein 2 (hK2) mRNA to differentially amplify splice variants of hKLK2 gene. They noted that RT-PCR/hK2 was associated with progression, failure, development of metastases, and prostate cancer–specific mortality (11). Investigators from Mt. Sinai reported a correlation between the risk of subsequent progression and the number of PSA mRNA (PSA-N) copies in pathologically N0 patients (12). Patients who were N0 by standard cytopathological evaluation but with a PSA-N ≥ 100 (17% of patients) appeared to have a substantially higher failure rate that was an independent predictor of failure than patients with a PSA-N <100 (12). Investigators from Japan performed evaluations on 2215 lymph nodes isolated from 120 patients using quantitative real-time RT-PCR and considered positive test as proof of "micrometastasis" (14). They concluded that approximately 30% of patients with clinically localized prostate cancer had "micrometastasis," the presence of which was associated with biochemical failure. Thus, it appears that approximately 13.3% to 30% of patients with pathological T3N0 disease have occult pelvic lymph node involvement.

With 40% to 50% of the involved nodes outside of the SLD areas, and an additional 5% to 10% outside of the typical ELD areas and a false-negative rate of up to 30%, it is plausible that the true estimate of lymph node involvement is as much as 65% higher than estimated

Table 1 Selected Series Assessing the Risk of Lymph Node Involvement

First author, year (reference)	Study size	Type of LND	Conclusions
Partin, 2001 (27)	$N = 5079$	Standard "staging pelvic lymphadenectomy"	Nomogram grouped patients with PSAs > 10 ng/mL, thus not useful in intermediate- to high-risk patients?
Cagiannos, 2003 (28)	$N = 5510$	"Standard" (medial inferior margin of external iliac vein down to internal iliac and obturator vessels	"… nomograms predicted most accurately when the risk of positive lymph nodes was low, roughly less than 10%. With higher risk … nomograms tended to underestimate the actual positivity"
Touijer, 2007 (41)	$N = 648$	Analysis limited to patients with Partin Table risk of >1%. LND templates of limited pelvic node dissection included the external iliac nodes, standard pelvic lymph node dissections included external iliac, obturator, and hypogastric.	Positive lymph node detection rate 7.15-fold higher for standard vs. limited pelvic lymph node dissection, with the median (mean) number of nodes retrieved was 9 (10) and 14 (15) after limited and standard pelvic lymph node dissection, respectively ($p < 0.001$).
Briganti, 2007 (5)	$N = 858$	2 to 40 nodes (median 14) were removed and examined, and 10.3% were positive. The positivity rate increased with the number of nodes removed. With 2 to 10 nodes: 5.6% positivity rate; 10–14: 8.6% positivity rate; with 15–19: 10.2% positivity rate; and 20–40: 17.6% positivity rate.	The ROC plot indicated that the removal of 28 nodes yielded a 90% ability to detect positive nodes while ≤10 or fewer nodes removed was associated with a very low probability of finding positive nodes.
Briganti, 2007 (6)	$N = 278$	The number of positive cores was 1–19 (median: 4), and the percentage of positive cores 7.1–100% (median: 37.5%).	Mean number of lymph nodes examined 17.5; 10.4% positive nodes. Nomogram based on clinical stage, PSA, and Gleason score was 79.7% accurate vs. 83% ($p < 0.001$) when percentage of positive cores added. 83.7% vs. 81%; $p < 0.001$.

Abbreviations: LND, lymph node disease; ROC, receiver operator curve.

Table 2 Examples of Estimates of Risk of Positive Nodes: Roach Equation Vs. Nomograms for Intermediate- and High-Risk Patients

First author, year (reference)	GS = 7, PSA =8, T2a	GS = 7, PSA =15, T2b	GS = 8, PSA =22, T2b	Comments
Roach, 1994 (42)	15%	20%	35%	Risk of positive nodes = (2/3) PSA + [(GS −6) × 10][a]
Partin, 2001 (27)	4%	~24%	27%	Only reports data by PSA >10 ng/mL
Cagiannos, 2003 (28)	3%	5%	10%	Standard dissection
Briganti, 2006 (43)	~17%	~22%	35%	Data based on extended lymph node dissection

[a]GS 2–4, 5, 6, 7, 8–10 (considered as 4, 5, 6, 7, and 8, respectively).
Abbreviations: GS, Gleason score; PSA, prostate-specific antigen.

Table 3 Selected Papers Highlighting More Sensitive Methods for Detecting Pelvic Lymph Node Involvement in Patients with N0 by Standard Pathological Evaluations

First author (reference)	Study design	Key findings
Shariat (11)	Archival lymph nodes tissues evaluated in 199 men with pT3N0 disease using the detection of human glandular kallikrein 2 (hK2) mRNA in men with histopathologically normal pelvic lymph nodes, removed at radical prostatectomy.	20% of patients had positive results, and on multivariable analysis models, the RT-PCR/hK2 result was associated with prostate cancer progression, development of distant metastases, and prostate cancer–specific survival.
Pagliarulo (10)	274 patients with pT3 prostate cancer treated by radical prostatectomy and bilateral lymph node dissection. 180 were staged N0, while 94 were N+. Lymph nodes from the 180 patients were evaluated for occult metastasis by immunohistochemistry. Recurrence and overall survival were compared among patients with occult tumor cells (OTN+), with patients whose lymph nodes remain negative (OLN−) and with the 94 N+ patients.	Occult tumor cells were found in 24 of 180 N0 patients (13.3%). OLN+ was associated with increased recurrence and decreased survival compared with OLN− patients. Outcome for patients with OLN+ disease was similar to that for patients with N+ disease. Immunohistochemistry can detect tumors not recognized at initial histology.
Ferrari (12)	Quantitative measures of PSA mRNA copies in N0-PLN, defined by PSA-N, and a threshold PSA-N 100 or more vs. PSA-N less than 100 copies, were assessed by continuous and categorical multivariate analyses to be independent.	4-yr biochemical failure–free survival of patients with PSA-N $\geq$ 100 vs. <100 was 55% and 77% ($p <$ 0.05). PSA-N identifies occult mets in N0-PLN. PSA-N $\geq$ 100 is an independent molecular marker for identifying patients with occult micrometastasis.
Miyake (2007) (14)	Pathological exams detected tumor cells in 29 lymph nodes from 11 patients, compared to 143 with micrometastasis using in 32 pN0 patients. In multivariate analysis only micrometastasis independently associated with PSA recurrences.	Approximately 30% of clinically localized prostate cancers shed cancer cells to the pelvic lymph nodes, and this fact may explain some of the biochemical recurrences occurring after radical prostatectomy. True incidence of lymph node involvement is 13.3–30% higher than estimated based on N0 path status.

Abbreviations: RT-PCR, real-time reverse transcriptase-PCR; PLN, pelvic lymph node.

Table 4 Conservative Estimates of the Incidence of Lymph Node Involvement in Intermediate- and High-Risk Patients with Clinically Confined Disease Vs. Hypothetical Upper Limits of Incidence[a]

PSA 6.1–10 and T stage	Gleason 3 + 4 (%)	Gleason 4 + 3 (%)	Gleason 4 + 4 (%)
T1c	2 vs. 3.3	2 vs. 3.3	3 vs. 5
T2a	3 vs. 5	5 vs. 8	5 vs. 8
T2b	6 vs. 10	8 vs. 13	8 vs. 13
T2c	10 vs. 17	13 vs. 21	13 vs. 21
PSA > 10 and T stage	Gleason 3 + 4 (%)	Gleason 4 + 3 (%)	Gleason 4 + 4 (%)
T1c	8 vs. 13	10 vs. 17	11 vs. 18
T2a	14 vs. 23	18 vs. 30	17 vs. 28
T2b	22 vs. 36	27 vs. 45	27 vs. 45
T2c	33 vs. 54	38 vs. 63	38 vs. 63

[a]Hypothetical rates are increased by 40% for lack of sensitivity associated with standard lymph node dissection, by 15% (range 10–20%) for false-negative path because of sampling errors, and by 10% for failure to sample prescral and perirectal nodes (2,8–12). Thus each nodal positivity rate was increased by 65% to come up with a hypothetical rate.
Source: From Ref. 27.

on the basis of surgical series on which nomograms have been created. Table 4 summarizes the incidence of lymph node involvement reported by Partin et al. in 2001 along with the hypothetical incidence of positive lymph nodes if the rates were 65% higher.

IMAGING AND LYMPH NODE METASTASIS FROM PROSTATE CANCER

Ideally, IGRT addressing pelvic lymph nodes should be designed using abnormalities defined using imaging modalities that establish the distribution of cancer cells in lymph nodes. Magnetic resonance imaging (MRI) provides excellent anatomical detail and soft tissue contrast but is too insensitive for routine use for the detection of nodal metastasis. Recent studies have shown that by adding lymphotropic superparamagnetic nanoparticles, the sensitivity of MRI can be improved so that lymph nodes that would have otherwise been considered normal can be identified as being involved and selectively targeted (15,16). This technology may prove useful for designing external beam radiotherapy (EBRT) fields in the future, but a lack of FDA approval in the United States has hampered the widespread adoption of this technology (16,17).

Another promising approach for identifying lymph nodes at risk for harboring microscopic metastases from prostate cancer involves combining prostate lymphoscintigraphy to identify sentinel lymph nodes (SLNs) (3). This approach involves directly transrectally applying technetium-99m nanocolloid into the prostate under ultrasonographic guidance one day before lymphadenectomy. Two hours after the injection, scintigrams were taken and the individual location of SLNs identified (3). Of note, more than half of the patients have positive lymph nodes outside the region of a standard lymph node, lending further support to the use of ELD (3).

TREATMENT OF PATIENTS WITH PELVIC LYMPH NODES: EVIDENCE OF EFFICACY

Prophylactic Irradiation for Lymph Nodes

Although there is no consensus as to the role of prophylactic pelvic lymph node irradiation in men with intermediate- to high-risk prostate cancer, two randomized trials and a number of retrospective studies have been conducted addressing this issue. The first prospective trial was conducted in the late 1970s by the Radiation Therapy Oncology Group (RTOG) 7706, and it failed to demonstrate a benefit with whole-pelvic radiotherapy (WPRT). However, this study included patients estimated to be at very low risk for lymph node involvement, and PSA data was not

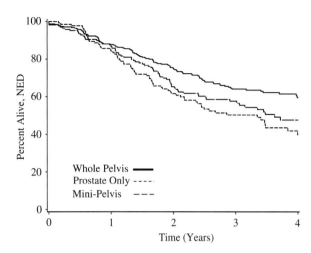

Figure 1 Taken from an analysis of patients treated on arms 1 and 2 from RTOG 9413 20. Arms 3 and 4 are excluded because they used a different timing for androgen deprivation therapy (lasted two months later). Whole pelvis (Arm 1) corresponded to a superior border placed at the L5-S1 border were compared to subsets of patients randomized to PO RT (Arm 2). Patients from Arm 2 were dichotomized as PO with a radiation field size less than the median (i.e., 10 cm × 11 cm) versus "mini pelvic" (MP) with a field size greater than or equal to the median. The "Mini-Pelvis" field was placed roughly at the bottom of the Sacral-iliac joints

available at that time (18). The largest phase III trial completed to date addressing this problem (RTOG 9413) demonstrated that patients with a risk of lymph node involvement of more than 15% might benefit from prophylactic WPRT (19). Figure 1 is taken from an analysis of patients treated on arms 1 and 2 from RTOG 9413 (20). Arms 3 and 4 are excluded because they used a different timing for androgen deprivation therapy (lasted two months later). WPRT (arm 1) corresponding to a superior border placed at the L5-S1 border was compared with subsets of patients randomized to prostate-only radiotherapy (PORT) (arm 2). Patients from arm 2 were dichotomized as PO with a radiation field size less than the median (i.e., 10 cm × 11 cm) versus those dichotomized as "mini-pelvic" (MP) with a field size greater than or equal to the median. The MP field was placed roughly at the bottom of the Sacral-iliac joints (20). Of note, the probability of progression-free survival was critically dependent on the volume of lymph nodes irradiated. In the absence of a larger, more compelling randomized trial, we believe these data suggest that this trial establishes neoadjuvant androgen deprivation therapy (NADT) and WPRT as the standard of care in patients with intermediate- to high-risk disease.

Some retrospective studies support the role of WPRT, while others do not (21–23). Investigators from UCSF observed better biochemical control rates when WPRT was administered with NADT, particularly when the risk

Table 5 Selected Papers Highlighting Benefits of Therapy Directed at Pelvic Lymph Nodes

First author (reference)	Study design	Conclusions
Seaward (21)	Retrospective analysis of patients undergoing prostate-only or whole-pelvic radiotherapy with and without hormonal therapy.	WPRT improves PFS
Roach (19)	Phase III testing whether whole-pelvic radiotherapy improves PFS	WPRT improves PFS
Spiotto (22)	Retrospective analysis of postoperative patients undergoing prostate only or WPRT with and without hormonal therapy.	WPRT improves PFS in the setting of salvage radiotherapy
Allaf (25)	Compares the outcomes of two different surgeons, each performing approximately 2000 radical prostatectomies with pelvic lymph node dissection. One surgeon tended to do extensive while the other tended to perform limited lymph node dissections.	Extended pelvic lymph node dissections may be of therapeutic value as suggested by higher biochemical control rates
Joslyn (26)	Data on all patients undergoing RP for prostate cancer obtained from the SEER Program (1988–1991). All surviving patients had a minimal follow-up of 10 yr. Of 57,764 men, 13,020 (22,5%) underwent RP. The median survival time was 127 mo. Most tumors were diagnosed as localized stage and SEER grade 2 (Gleason score 5, 6; Gleason pattern 3, moderately differentiated).	There appears to be a relationship between the number of lymph nodes removed and examined at prostatectomy for prostate cancer and the likelihood of finding lymph node metastasis and an increase in the prostate cancer–specific survival even in patients who have histologically negative lymph nodes. Patients with more than one positive lymph node had a significantly greater risk of prostate cancer–related death. Retrospective data suggest that radiotherapy and surgical resection may favorably impact outcomes in patients at risk for lymph node involvement

Abbreviations: WPRT, whole-pelvic radiotherapy; PFS, progression-free survival; RP, radical prostatectomy.

of lymph node involvement was between 15% and 35% (21,24). Investigators from Stanford noted benefits associated with WPRT in the setting of postoperative radiotherapy in patients with adverse features (22). In contrast, investigators from Fox Chase concluded that there was no benefit to the addition of NADT or WPRT to patients with a risk of nodal involvement greater than 15% (23). However, selection bias, small sample size, failure to consistently use NADT in all patients, and suboptimal field size can easily explain such findings (20). The optimal benefit of WPRT appears to require the use of NADT and WPRT with the superior border placed at the L5-S1 interspace. The point is more comprehensive coverage of lymph nodes is associated with a better outcome (20). Table 5 summarizes selected series supporting the role of prophylactic WPRT.

Evidence of Surgical Efficacy for Lymph Nodal Disease

In addition to the evidence from radiotherapy series, there is a growing body of evidence supporting a benefit for the surgical management of pelvic lymph nodes for men with prostate cancer (25,26). One study demonstrated a benefit in terms of biochemical control, while another suggested that patients who undergo a more extensive lymphadenectomy may have a reduction in prostate cancer—related deaths (25,26). Table 5 summarizes selected surgical series suggesting a therapeutic value for surgical intervention for pelvic lymph nodes.

PATIENTS SELECTION FOR WPRT

Given the fact that imaging is relatively insensitive, the selection of patients for prophylactic WPRT is usually based on assumptions about the risk of lymph node involvement as suggested by pretreatment parameters. At UCSF, patients who are at low risk (e.g., <10–15% risk of lymph node involvement) are usually treated only for the prostate. Patients with an estimated risk of lymph node involvement greater than 15% are usually offered pelvic nodal radiation with the superior border placed at the L5-S1 junction. Patients with a relative contraindication to pelvic irradiation (e.g., prior radiotherapy for seminoma and unilobar disease) are sometimes offered hemipelvic or even hemi-MP irradiation. At the other extreme, patients with imaging or pathological evidence of lymph node involvement disease are usually offered extended field irradiation that includes the common iliac with or without para-aortic node groups as well. There are a number of different methods used to estimate the risk of lymph node involvement. All patients with gross clinical T3 disease (grossly, not transrectal ultrasound, MRI, or CT) are considered at risk (>15%). For the typical patients with clinically confined disease, the most critical determinant appears to be the Gleason score ($\geq$7), followed by PSA (>10 ng/mL) and the percent positive biopsies (6,27,28). As discussed above, most nomograms are usually based on SLDs and thus are likely to underestimate the true risk of lymph node involvement, particularly if an inadequate number of nodes are taken.

RADIOTHERAPY TECHNIQUES FOR THE TREATMENT OF PELVIC LYMPH NODES

Intensity-modulated radiotherapy (IMRT) has been shown to be associated with significant clinical advantages over conventional and three-dimensional conformal radiotherapy (3DCRT) when treatment is limited to the prostate (29). There is also a growing body of data suggesting that IMRT provides even greater advantages when pelvic nodes are being irradiated. The pelvic lymph nodal regions are not adequately covered using a typical four-field arrangement designed with conventional field borders based on bony anatomy (16,30). For example, Wang-Chesebro et al. reported that the mean dose delivered by four-field box plans to 95%, 80%, and 50% of the pelvic nodal volume (defined on the basis of blood vessels with a 0.5–1.0 cm margin) were 12.7 Gy, 33.6 Gy, and 46.8 Gy, respectively. The use of conventional techniques is associated with much larger portions of the bladder and rectum being included within the high-dose portions of the radiation fields. More than 40% and 95% of the rectum and bladder volumes could receive greater than 95% of the prescription dose (typically 45 Gy). Table 4 highlights some of the most significant differences, including

inadequacy of nodal coverage, excessive small bowel and bladder doses with WPRT compared with IMRT.

TREATMENT GUIDELINES

At the UCSF, we routinely used pelvic IMRT to treat patients with intermediate- and high-risk prostate cancer. Prior to radiotherapy, three markers were implanted in the base, middle, and apex of the prostate by a urologist. Patients were simulated in supine position with an empty rectum and full bladder, and treatment planning CT scans were acquired with 3-mm slice thickness. Pelvic lymph node volumes were delineated to include obtrurator, external/internal iliac, common iliac, and presacral lymph nodes with 1- to 2-cm margins up to the vertebral level of L5-S1 and, in selected cases, perirectal nodal groups. The prostate and seminal vesicles were expanded by 2 to 3 mm for the planning tumor volume (PTV). Rectal volumes were contoured from the anus at the level of the ischial tuberosities to the sigmoid flexure. The bowel volumes (including the colon and large and small bowels) were contoured to include abdominal space. Definitive radiation for all patients consisted of a two-phase treatment course. The first portion of treatment typically utilizes 45 segments and 7 beam angles (0°, 35°, 90°, 160°, 200°, 270°, and 315°). The second cone-down portion of treatment typically utilizes 25 segments and 7 beam angles (0°, 55°, 90°, 135°, 225°, 270°, and 305°). UCSF planning objectives used as initial planning guidelines are listed in Table 6. Note that these planning objectives are used to help set computerized objectives during inverse planning; these objectives are different from final dose-volume histogram (DVH) guidelines used to evaluate treatment plans.

The first phase concurrently treated the pelvic lymph nodes and the prostate. For patients treated with external beam radiotherapy in both phases, the prescription doses to the pelvic lymph nodes and prostate (plus seminal vesicle) were 48.6 Gy/1.8 Gy and 54 Gy/2.0 Gy, concurrently (typically to the 85–91% isodose line). A typical dose distribution for WPRT in the first phase is shown in

Table 6 Typical IMRT and 3DCRT Dose Volume Comparison

Volume of interest	IMRT	WP 3DCRT	Conclusions
Lymph nodes (D95)	46 Gy	27 Gy	Lymph nodes are covered better with IMRT
Small bowel (V45Gy)	51.5 cm³	284 cm³	Small bowel is spared better with IMRT
Bladder (V40Gy)	20%	90%	Urinary bladder is spared better with IMRT

D95, dose in Gy delivered to 95% of lymph nodes; V45Gy, volume of tissue receiving 45Gy; V40Gy, percentage of bladder receiving 40Gy during whole pelvic radiotherapy.
Abbreviations: IMRT, intensity-modulated radiotherapy; WP 3DCRT, whole prostate three-dimensional conformal radiotherapy.
Source: Modified from Ref. 30.

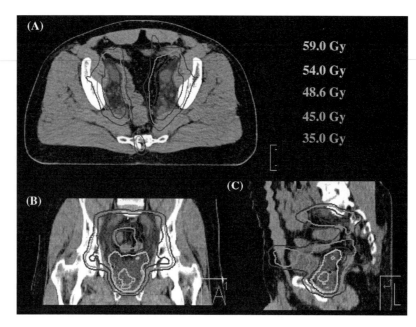

Figure 2 (A–C) A typical dose distribution for whole pelvic radiation in the first phase is used at UCSF.

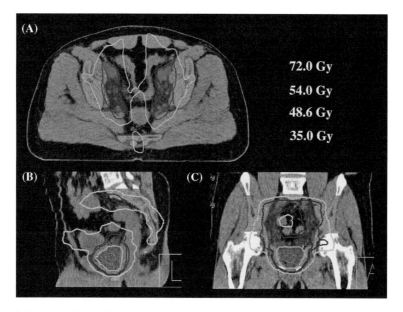

Figure 3 (A–C) A typical dose distribution for whole pelvic radiation and an IMRT boost in the second phase used at UCSF. For patients treated with external beam radiotherapy in both phases, the prescription doses to the pelvic lymph nodes and prostate (plus seminal vesicle) were 48.6 Gy/1.8 Gy and 54 Gy/2.0 Gy, concurrently (typically to the 85–91% isodose line).

Figure 2A–C. After pelvic IMRT, all patients continued the second phase of treatment to boost the prostate using either brachytherapy (prostate implant or high dose rate) or IMRT. A typical dose distribution for WPRT and an IMRT boost in the second phase is shown in Figure 3A–C. Figure 4A, B shows typical DVHs of the rectum and bladder compared with the DVHs of the same organs if

only the prostate were treated to 72 Gy. From these figures it is clear that the pelvic irradiation increased the intermediate doses to the rectum and bladder while exposing the similar amount of the rectum and bladder to the high doses.

Concurrently treating the prostate and the pelvic lymph nodes poses a technical challenge not previously

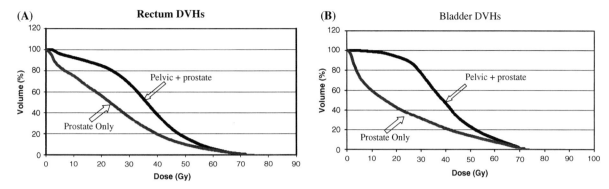

Figure 4 (**A, B**) Typical dose volume histograms of the rectum and bladder compared with the dose volume histograms of the same organs if only the prostate were treated to 72 Gy. From these figures it is clear that the pelvic irradiation increased the intermediate doses to the rectum and bladder while exposing the similar amount of the rectum and bladder to the high doses.

addressed in radiotherapy because of the independent movement of the prostate and the pelvic lymph nodes. This problem renders the conventional isocenter shifting method inadequate since prostate movement varies from a few millimeters up to 1.5 cm or more relative to the pelvic bones, while pelvic lymph nodes are relatively fixed in close proximity to vascular structures. Addressing this problem by simply adding a large planning margin to ensure adequate coverage of the target volume unavoidably results in the inclusion of normal structures in the high-dose area of the radiation fields, potentially increasing the risk of normal tissue complications. Although some investigators have concluded that this impact is of limited clinical consequence, this conclusion must be viewed with caution because it is based on fairly conservative assumptions about the magnitude of organ movement and setup errors (31).

In our experience, it is not uncommon for significant discrepancies to be associated with ignorance. We have observed several scenarios in which ignoring these discrepancies would result in rather large and clinically significant treatment errors, particularly when para-aortic irradiation is employed (see discussion below). The ideal strategy to resolve this challenge involves using online imaging and replanning on a daily basis prior to each treatment. Unfortunately, because of the extended planning time required and the potential for prostate and patient movement to occur as time is extended, online replanning is not currently a practical solution. We have developed a multiple adaptive plan IMRT (MAP-IMRT) strategy to address this issue (32). With this strategy, we created a set of IMRT plans with a series of presumed prostate positions. According to the position of the prostate detected on a daily basis, relative to the pelvic bony anatomy, an IMRT plan that is closest to "the prostate position of the day," is selected and used for treatment.

For example, we recently treated a high-risk prostate cancer patient with a "horse-shoe" abdominal kidney and adjacent lymph nodes believed to be involved with MAP-IMRT (32). The phase I plan involved concurrently treating the prostate to 54 Gy and pelvic nodes to 48.6 Gy in 27 fractions. A major dosimetric consideration for this particular patient was to minimize the dose of radiation received by the kidneys. Using the planning CT, the contour of the prostate was copied and shifted according to the eight presumed positions: 0.5 and 1.0 cm displacements along the posterior, anterior, inferior, and superior directions. These displacements were based on the established pattern of prostate movements. Subsequently, a total of nine IMRT plans were created, including the initial IMRT plan for the prostate at "the standard" unshifted position. The initial IMRT plan for the patient was created on the basis of our established planning protocol. Since the rectum and bladder are contoured in the planning CT but are not shifted with the shifted prostate, the anatomic relationships of these two organs with the shifted prostate is ignored. Therefore, the initial planning dose constraints of the rectum and bladder rendered rough approximations (Table 7). To circumvent this problem, we constructed an artificial rind structure around the shifted prostate to create a highly conformal plan, thus effectively protecting the rectum and bladder. Figures 5 and 6 show the sagittal and coronal dose distributions for a patient with the prostate position shifted 1 cm anteriorly (Fig. 5A), unshifted (Fig. 5B, D), shifted 1 cm posteriorly (Fig. 5C), shifted 1 cm inferiorly (Fig. 5D), and shifted 1 cm superiorly (Fig. 5E). To correct for daily displacements, gold marker seeds are used to track the prostate position each day prior to each treatment. Note the lymph nodes and prostate are always covered. Figure 6 shows the axial dose distributions for a patient with the prostate shifted 1 cm anteriorly (Fig. 6A), unshifted (Fig. 6B), shifted 1 cm posteriorly (Fig. 6C), shifted 1 cm inferiorly (Fig. 6D), and shifted 1 cm superiorly (Fig. 6E) using gold marker seeds to track the prostate position each day prior to each treatment. Note

Table 7 Typical Dose Constraints for Phase I Planning

Organ name	Type	Dose (cGy)	>Volume	Weight
PTV	Max. dose	5800		3
	Min. DVH	5400	95%	10
	Min dose	5200		3
PTV nodes	Max. dose	5000		3
	Min DVH	4860	95%	10
	Min. dose	4300		1
Rectum	Max. dose	5400		4
	Max. DVH	4500	7%	2
	Max. DVH	3500	30%	3
Bladder	Max dose	5400		1
	Max. DVH	4300	15%	1
Bulb	Max. dose	5400		1
	Max. DVH	3500	20%	1
Bowel	Max. dose	4860		5
	Max. DVH	4500	5%	5

Abbreviations: PTV, planning tumor volume; DVH, dose-volume histogram.

that regardless of the shift, the prostate is always well covered using "the plan of the day" to match the position of the prostate. To accomplish this feat, the appropriate plan of the day is chosen to match position of the prostate when shown. An onboard imaging system is required to implement this approach, which we call MAP-IMRT.

Onboard imaging devices are becoming widely spread and more frequently used for daily prostate alignment at a number of institutions. Several systems have been developed to provide a 3D image of the patient in treatment position moments before radiation delivery including, but not limited to, a "CT on rails" (33), a kilovoltage cone-beam CT (kVCBCT) (34), a megavoltage cone-beam CT (MVCBCT) (35), and a tomotherapy system (36). All these systems can provide a comparison of the image of the day with the planning diagnostic CT.

At UCSF, image-guided IMRT (IGRT) for targeting the pelvic nodes has been developed using the MVCBCT system Mvision™. An example of such images is shown in Figure 7A–C. Registrations on bony anatomy and on gold markers are sequentially performed to determine the setup error and the relative prostate displacement. For MVCBCT, projection images are acquired using the linear accelerator (linac) with a low dose rate 6-MV beam. The MVision system consists of a standard linac equipped with an amorphous-silicon flat panel electronic portal imaging device adapted for MeV photons. An integrated computer workspace provides automated acquisition of projection images, image reconstruction, CT to CBCT image registration, and couch shift calculation. These systems demonstrate submillimeter localization precision and sufficient soft tissue resolution to visualize structures such as the prostate (37,38). An MVCBCT acquisition is performed by rotating the linac gantry in a continuous

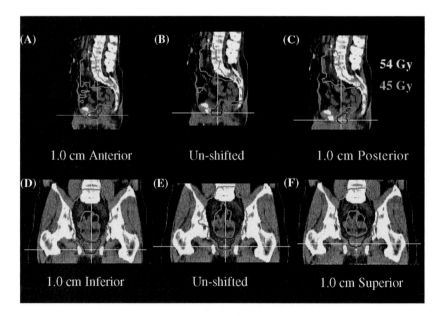

Figure 5 (**A–F**) (*See color insert.*) The sagittal and coronal dose distributions for a patient with the prostate position shifted anteriorly (**A**), unshifted (**B** and **D**), shifted posteriorly (**C**), shifted inferiorly (**D**), and shifted superiorly (**E**). To correct for daily displacements, gold marker seeds are used to track the prostate position each day prior to each treatment. Note that the lymph nodes and prostate are always covered. To accomplish this feat, the appropriate "the plan of the day" is chosen to match the position of the prostate when shown. An onboard imaging system is required to implement this approach, which we call multiple adaptive plan IMRT (MAP-IMRT).

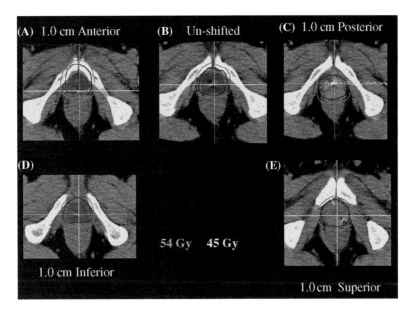

Figure 6 (**A–E**) The axial dose distributions for a patient with the prostate shifted anteriorly (**A**), unshifted (**B**), shifted posteriorly (**C**), shifted inferiorly (**D**), and shifted superiorly (**E**) using gold marker seeds to track the prostate position each day prior to each treatment. Note that regardless of the shift, the prostate is always well covered using "the plan of the day" to match the position of the prostate. An onboard imaging system is required to implement this approach, which we call multiple adaptive plan IMRT (MAP-IMRT).

200° arc. This acquisition procedure lasts for 45 seconds, and the reconstructed MVCBCT image becomes available within two minutes after the start of the acquisition. MVCBCT to CT registration can then be used to determine the proper positioning of the patient. This allows a

rapid alignment of the patient before each treatment fraction. We have found that MVCBCT acquisitions of less than 2 MU (1.7 cGy at isocenter) or 4 MU can be used for direct 3D alignment in the presence of gold seeds or with bony anatomy (Fig. 7B), respectively. Furthermore, Figure 7A–C

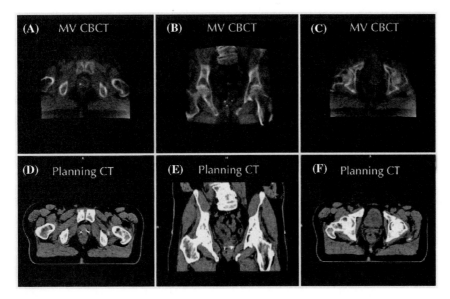

Figure 7 (**A–C**) (*top row*) Images generated at UCSF using the MVCBCT system Mvision™. The MVision system consists of a standard linac equipped with an amorphous-silicon flat panel electronic portal-imaging device adapted for MeV photons. MVCBCT projection images are acquired using the linac with a low-dose rate 6-MV beam. (**D–F**) (*lower row*) Images from the treatment planning CT. Such images are used sequentially at UCSF for implementing IGRT to target the pelvic lymph nodes during IMRT. Initially the alignment is based on bony anatomy to determine the setup error and then adjustments are made on the basis of gold markers placed in the prostate. *Abbreviations*: Linac, linear accelerator; IGRT, image-guided radiotherapy.

shows the potential of using MVCBCT to align the patient on the basis of soft tissue without the need of gold seeds. MVCBCT acquisitions of approximately 9 MU are currently required on typical pelvic patients for consistent prostate visualization without the need of gold seeds.

To implement MAP-IMRT prior to each treatment, an MVCBCT is acquired and aligned with the planning CT twice. One alignment is made with the pelvic bones and the other with the implanted markers. The couch shifts obtained from the first alignment (to the pelvic bones) is done to eliminate setup errors by shifting the treatment couch accordingly. The prostate movement of the day was obtained by the differences between two alignments. According to the detected prostate displacements, in the case described above, one of nine IMRT plans in which the prostate position was close to the prostate position of the day was chosen to treat the patient. Although online replanning may be the ideal strategy to accommodate independent movement of the prostate and pelvic lymph nodes during concurrent treatment, reoptimizing a set of IMRT plans with multiple prostate positions is proven to be clinically feasible and practical. The use of soft tissue imaging alone appears to be inadequate since there is a general consensus that registration governed by anatomy outperforms CT-contour-based registration, and that registration of implanted markers has the least interuser variability (39,40).

SUMMARY OF PERTINENT CONCLUSIONS

- The true incidence of occult pelvic lymph nodes metastasis in men with clinically localized prostate cancer appears to be substantially higher (as much as 65%) than commonly believed on the basis of the most commonly quoted nomograms.
- There is a growing body of literature that suggests that treatment of involved nodes either surgically or with NADT and EBRT improves outcomes.
- Although the optimal strategy for determining which lymph nodes are involved remains to be elucidated, general guidelines can be found in atlases of pelvic anatomy and predicted by nomograms.
- These atlases and nomograms can be used in conjunction with imaging modalities to define design treatment fields. For more selected targeting, sentinel node imaging appears to hold great promise for designing fields that are likely to encompass all of the relevant lymph nodes. When prophylactic pelvic lymph nodal radiotherapy is initiated, it appears that the more comprehensively nodes are encompassed the better the outcome.
- When patients are treated concurrently to the primary site (prostate) and pelvic lymph nodes, rules for resolving conflicting alignment issues using onboard soft tissue imaging (MV or kVCT scans) are required.
- IMRT provides clear advantages over 3DCRT when attempting to incorporate all of the nodes at risk while sparing surrounding normal tissues such as the rectum, bladder, and penile structures.
- The guidelines for selecting patients for image-guided IMRT directed at pelvic lymph nodes and the magnitude of the benefit are currently areas of active investigation by the RTOG and others.

REFERENCES

1. Ennis RD. Uncertainties regarding pelvic radiotherapy for prostate cancer. J Clin Oncol 2004; 22:2254–2255.
2. Heidenreich A, Varga Z, Von Knobloch R. Extended pelvic lymphadenectomy in patients undergoing radical prostatectomy: high incidence of lymph node metastasis. J Urol 2002; 167:1681–1686.
3. Weckermann D, Goppelt M, Dorn R, et al. Incidence of positive pelvic lymph nodes in patients with prostate cancer, a prostate-specific antigen (PSA) level of < or = 10 ng/mL and biopsy Gleason score of < or = 6, and their influence on PSA progression-free survival after radical prostatectomy. BJU Int 2006; 97:1173–1178.
4. Briganti A, Chun FK, Salonia A, et al. A nomogram for staging of exclusive nonobturator lymph node metastases in men with localized prostate cancer. Eur Urol 2007; 51:112–119; discussion 119–120.
5. Briganti A, Chun FK, Salonia A, et al. Critical assessment of ideal nodal yield at pelvic lymphadenectomy to accurately diagnose prostate cancer nodal metastasis in patients undergoing radical retropubic prostatectomy. Urology 2007; 69:147–151.
6. Briganti A, Karakiewicz PI, Chun FK, et al. Percentage of positive biopsy cores can improve the ability to predict lymph node invasion in patients undergoing radical prostatectomy and extended pelvic lymph node dissection. Eur Urol 2007; 51:1573–1581.
7. Schumacher MC, Burkhard FC, Thalmann GN, et al. Is pelvic lymph node dissection necessary in patients with a serum PSA <10 ng/ml undergoing radical prostatectomy for prostate cancer? Eur Urol 2006; 50:272–279.
8. Golimbu M, Morales P, Al-Askari S, et al. Extended pelvic lymphadenectomy for prostate cancer. J Urol 1979; 121:617–620.
9. Murray SK, Breau RH, Guha AK, et al. Spread of prostate carcinoma to the perirectal lymph node basin: analysis of 112 rectal resections over a 10-year span for primary rectal adenocarcinoma. Am J Surg Pathol 2004; 28:1154–1162.
10. Pagliarulo V, Hawes D, Brands FH, et al. Detection of occult lymph node metastases in locally advanced node-negative prostate cancer. J Clin Oncol 2006; 24: 2735–2742.
11. Shariat SF, Kattan MW, Erdamar S, et al. Detection of clinically significant, occult prostate cancer metastases in lymph nodes using a splice variant-specific rt-PCR assay

for human glandular kallikrein. J Clin Oncol 2003; 21:1223–1231.

12. Ferrari AC, Stone NN, Kurek R, et al. Molecular load of pathologically occult metastases in pelvic lymph nodes is an independent prognostic marker of biochemical failure after localized prostate cancer treatment. J Clin Oncol 2006; 24:3081–3088.

13. Miyake H, Kurahashi T, Hara I, et al. Significance of micrometastases in pelvic lymph nodes detected by real-time reverse transcriptase polymerase chain reaction in patients with clinically localized prostate cancer undergoing radical prostatectomy after neoadjuvant hormonal therapy. BJU Int 2007; 99:315–320.

14. Miyake H, Hara I, Kurahashi T, et al. Quantitative detection of micrometastases in pelvic lymph nodes in patients with clinically localized prostate cancer by real-time reverse transcriptase-PCR. Clin Cancer Res 2007; 13:1192–1197.

15. Harisinghani MG, Barentsz J, Hahn PF, et al. Noninvasive detection of clinically occult lymph-node metastases in prostate cancer. N Engl J Med 2003; 348:2491–2499.

16. Shih HA, Harisinghani M, Zietman AL, et al. Mapping of nodal disease in locally advanced prostate cancer: rethinking the clinical target volume for pelvic nodal irradiation based on vascular rather than bony anatomy. Int J Radiat Oncol Biol Phys 2005; 63:1262–1269.

17. Harisinghani MG, Saksena MA, Hahn PF, et al. Ferumoxtran-10-enhanced MR lymphangiography: does contrast-enhanced imaging alone suffice for accurate lymph node characterization? AJR Am J Roentgenol 2006; 186:144–148.

18. Asbell SO, Krall JM, Pilepich MV, et al. Elective pelvic irradiation in stage A2, B carcinoma of the prostate: Analysis of RTOG 77-06. Int J Radiat Oncol Biol Phys 1988; 15:1307–1316.

19. Roach M III, DeSilvio M, Lawton C, et al. Phase III trial comparing whole-pelvic versus prostate-only radiotherapy and neoadjuvant versus adjuvant combined androgen suppression: Radiation Therapy Oncology Group 9413. J Clin Oncol 2003; 21:1904–1911.

20. Roach M III, DeSilvio M, Valicenti R, et al. Whole pelvic, "mini-pelvic" or prostate only external beam radiotherapy field following neoadjuvant and concurrent hormonal therapy: in patients treated on RTOG 9413. Int J Radiat Oncol Bio Phys 2006; 66(3):647–653.

21. Seaward SA, Weinberg V, Lewis P, et al. Improved freedom from PSA failure with whole pelvic irradiation for high-risk prostate cancer. Int J Radiat Oncol Biol Phys 1998; 42:1055–1062.

22. Spiotto MT, Hancock SL, King CR. Radiotherapy after prostatectomy: improved biochemical relapse-free survival with whole pelvic compared with prostate bed only for high-risk patients. Int J Radiat Oncol Biol Phys 2007; 69(1):54–61.

23. Jacob R, Hanlon AL, Horwitz EM, et al. Role of prostate dose escalation in patients with greater than 15% risk of pelvic lymph node involvement. Int J Radiat Oncol Biol Phys 2005; 61:695–701.

24. Seaward SA, Weinberg V, Lewis P, et al. Identification of a high-risk clinically localized prostate cancer subgroup receiving maximum benefit from whole-pelvic irradiation. Cancer J Sci Am 1998; 4:370–377.

25. Allaf ME, Palapattu GS, Trock BJ, et al. Anatomical extent of lymph node dissection: impact on men with clinically localized prostate cancer. J Urol 2004; 172:1840–1844.

26. Joslyn SA, Konety BR. Impact of extent of lymphadenectomy on survival after radical prostatectomy for prostate cancer. Urology 2006; 68:121–125.

27. Partin AW, Mangold LA, Lamm DM, et al. Contemporary update of prostate cancer staging nomograms (Partin Tables) for the new millennium. Urology 2001; 58: 843–848.

28. Cagiannos I, Karakiewicz P, Eastham JA, et al. A preoperative nomogram identifying decreased risk of positive pelvic lymph nodes in patients with prostate cancer. J Urol 2003; 170:1798–1803.

29. Zelefsky MJ, Fuks Z, Hunt M, et al. High-dose intensity modulated radiation therapy for prostate cancer: early toxicity and biochemical outcome in 772 patients. Int J Radiat Oncol Biol Phys 2002; 53:1111–1116.

30. Wang-Chesebro A, Xia P, Coleman J, et al. Intensity-modulated radiotherapy improves lymph node coverage and dose to critical structures compared with three-dimensional conformal radiation therapy in clinically localized prostate cancer. Int J Radiat Oncol Biol Phys 2006; 66:654–662.

31. Hsu A, Pawlicki T, Luxton G, et al. A study of image-guided intensity-modulated radiotherapy with fiducials for localized prostate cancer including pelvic lymph nodes. Int J Radiat Oncol Biol Phys 2007; 68:898–902.

32. Xia P, Hwang A, Mu G, et al. Multi-adaptive-plan (MAP) IMRT to accommodate the independent movement of the prostate and pelvic-lymph nodes: a proof of principle study driven by clinical necessity. Int J Radiat Oncol Biol Phys 2007; 69(suppl 1):S724.

33. Wong JR, Cheng CW, Grimm L, et al. Clinical implementation of the world's first Primatom, a combination of CT scanner and linear accelerator, for precise tumor targeting and treatment. Med Phys 2001; 17:271–276.

34. Jaffray DA, Siewerdsen JH, Wong JW, et al. Flat-panel cone-beam computed tomography for image-guided radiation therapy. Int J Radiat Oncol Biol Phys 2002; 53: 1337–1349.

35. Pouliot J, Bani-Hashemi A, Chen J, et al. Low-dose megavoltage cone-beam CT for radiation therapy. Int J Radiat Oncol Biol Phys 2005; 61:552–560.

36. Mackie TR, Kapatoes J, Ruchala K, et al. Image guidance for precise conformal radiotherapy. Int J Radiat Oncol Biol Phys 2003; 56:89–105.

37. Morin O, Gillis A, Chen J, et al. Megavoltage cone-beam CT: system description and clinical applications. Med Dosim 2006; 31:51–61.

38. Pouliot J. Megavoltage imaging, megavoltage cone beam CT and dose-guided radiation therapy. Front Radiat Ther Oncol 2007; 40:132–142.

39. Langen KM, Zhang Y, Andrews RD, et al. Initial experience with megavoltage (MV) CT guidance for daily prostate alignments. Int J Radiat Oncol Biol Phys 2005; 62: 1517–1524.

40. Moseley DJ, White EA, Wiltshire KL, et al. Comparison of localization performance with implanted fiducial markers and cone-beam computed tomography for on-line image-guided radiotherapy of the prostate. Int J Radiat Oncol Biol Phys 2007; 67:942–953.

41. Touijer K, Rabbani F, Otero JR, et al. Standard versus limited pelvic lymph node dissection for prostate cancer in patients with a predicted probability of nodal metastasis greater than 1%. J Urol 2007; 178:120–124.

42. Roach M, Marquez C, Yuo HS, et al. Predicting the risk of lymph node involvement using the pre-treatment prostate specific antigen (PSA) and Gleason score in men with clinically localized prostate cancer. Int J Radiat Oncol Biol Phys 1994; 28:33–37.

43. Briganti A, Chun FK, Salonia A, et al. Validation of a nomogram predicting the probability of lymph node invasion based on the extent of pelvic lymphadenectomy in patients with clinically localized prostate cancer. BJU Int 2006; 98:788–793.

17

Fractionation Schemes with IGRT for Clinically Localized Prostate Cancer

HIMU LUKKA

Department of Oncology, McMaster University, Hamilton, Ontario, Canada

INTRODUCTION

The move in modern radiotherapy practice toward highly conformed, high-precision radiotherapy techniques for prostate cancer treatment has reduced treatment toxicity and has also allowed dose escalation. Dose escalation has now been shown to improve biochemical disease-free survival in the treatment of prostate cancer with radiotherapy. As a result of dose escalation, treatment courses have lengthened from six to seven weeks to eight to nine weeks. This has increased the burden on already stretched radiotherapy services, increased the cost of treatment, and placed additional social, emotional, and economic burdens on patients and their families. These problems will increase as more treatment centers acquire the technical prerequisites for dose-escalated prostatic radiotherapy and switch to longer treatment schedules. Early evidence suggests that efficacy and safety similar to that obtained with conventional fractionation schedules can be achieved with a shorter course of radiation treatment using three-dimensional conformal radiotherapy (3DCRT) and intensity-modulated radiotherapy (IMRT). If the safety and efficacy of these hypofractionated regimens are demonstrated in randomized controlled trials (RCTs), their adoption would reduce the burden of treatment for patients and their families, reduce the cost of radiotherapy treatments, and free up strained radiotherapy facilities in some jurisdictions. There are also radiobiological reasons to suggest that hypofractionated prostatic radiotherapy may result in improved efficacy while maintaining toxicity equivalent to that experienced with conventional fractionation.

This chapter will discuss (*i*) dose and fractionation issues in the treatment of prostate cancer from both radiobiological and clinical perspectives, (*ii*) normal tissue tolerance, (*iii*) evidence from recent RCTs of hypofractionated radiotherapy, (*iv*) ongoing trials that will provide additional evidence over the next few years, (*v*) indications for and contraindications to hypofractionated radiotherapy in patients with prostate cancer, and (*vi*) planning and image-guided delivery considerations particular to hypofractionated radiotherapy.

RADIOBIOLOGY

Dose and Fractionation

Traditionally, patients with prostate cancer received total doses of radiation in the range of 60 to 78 Gy, delivered in fractions of 1.8 or 2 Gy on each of five days per week over six to eight weeks. From the radiobiological perspective, these schedules may not deliver optimal radiotherapy for prostate cancer (1). General principles of radiobiology can be used to point to new schedules for investigation in clinical trials.

In very general terms, the probability of eradicating cancer cells improves with higher doses of radiation, as does the risk and severity of adverse effects. The biological effects of radiation result from the relative level of DNA damage and resultant cell kill in tumor versus normal tissues. The level of tissue-specific cell kill is dependent on a number of factors including activation of cell death pathways (e.g., apoptosis or mitotic catastrophe), cell cycle phase and resulting cell cycle arrests, and the appropriate sensing and repair of the damaged DNA. In addition to intrinsic cellular radiosensitivity, cell survival can also be modified by the tumor microenvironment and hypoxia (e.g., decreased intracellular oxygen tension leads to relative cellular radioresistance). The

radiation survival curve shows the relationship between cell survival after exposure and graded doses of radiation, which can vary among tissues. In general, the curve has an initial shallow slope (i.e., the "shoulder" region) at doses up to 4 Gy, followed by a steeper logarithmic slope at higher doses (Fig. 1A). The initial shoulder section is thought to reflect the repair of sublethal DNA damage following irradiation, and the logarithmic section reflects cell killing in the absence of repair. A linear-quadratic (LQ) model can be used to describe the cell-survival curve, so that the surviving fraction of cells S/S_0 is related to the radiation dose d as $S/S_0 = \exp(-\alpha d - \beta d^2)$. Alpha ($\alpha$) describes the initial slope of the survival curve and the nonrepairable component of DNA damage (1,2). It is the

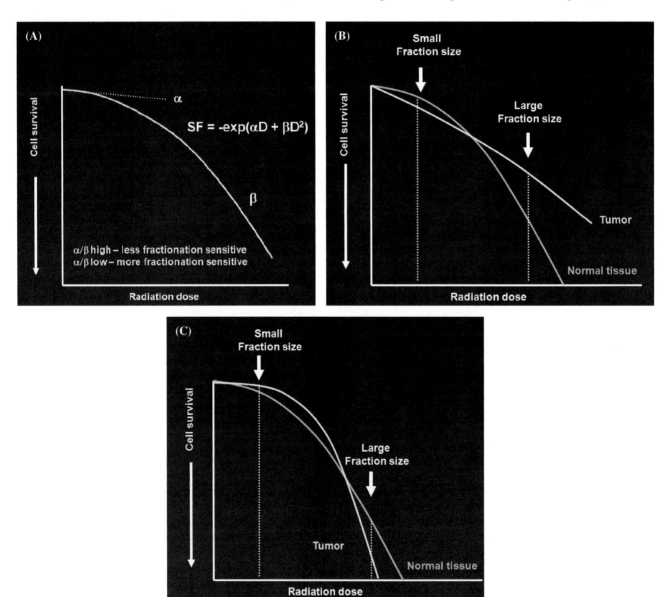

Figure 1 Cell survival versus radiation dose. (**A**) The fractionation sensitivity of a tissue is described by the α/β ratio. (**B**) If the α/β ratio for tumor greater than normal tissue. (**C**) If the α/β ratio for normal tissue greater than tumor.

most variable component among human cell types and best reflects differences in the intrinsic radiosensitivity of cells. Beta (β) describes the curvature of the survival curve and represents the transition from repairable to nonrepairable cell injury. With the linear component proportional to α and the quadratic component proportional to β, the degree to which the cell-survival curve bends from the shoulder section depends on the ratio of the coefficients alpha and beta (α/β).

While the single-fraction cell-survival curve is useful for understanding the radiobiological relationship between dose and cell survival, fractionated radiotherapy is used in clinical practice. The shoulder and linear components of the cell-survival curve are reproduced for each of these fractions. There are several reasons why fractionated radiotherapy is preferred to single fractions in the radical treatment of tumors. Fractionation capitalizes on the difference in α/β ratios between most epithelial tumors ($\alpha/\beta = 10$ Gy) and late-reacting normal tissue ($\alpha/\beta = 3$ Gy). The ratio of α to β in the LQ equation discussed above also reflects the sensitivity of tissue to radiation fraction size (3). The radiosensitivity of normal cells depends on their relative natural proliferation rate (1). Those normal tissues with slow cell proliferation rates have long cell cycle times that allow for intracellular repair between fractions. In this situation, the ratio of α to β is low. For example, in the case of bowel tissue, the ratio for late-reacting effects ranges from 2.5 to 5 and for bladder from 3 to 7 (1). In contrast, rapidly proliferating cells have little time for repair and in this scenario the α/β ratio is higher. For example, early reactions in skin can be associated with an α/β ratio of 9 to 12 and for colon it is 9 to 11 (1). In most rapidly dividing cancer cell populations, the α/β ratio is approximately 10 Gy. For these tumors, fractionated radiotherapy using fraction sizes of 1.8 to 2.0 Gy is preferred, as it produces improved tumor control while limiting normal tissue damage (Fig. 1B).

In contrast to the above scenario, there is a growing consensus that the α/β ratio for prostate cancer is low. What is actively debated is the exact α/β ratio for prostate cancer. A number of studies have suggested that the α/β ratio for prostate cancer is between 0.9 and 1.5 Gy (4–6), indicating relatively long cell cycle times, but some investigators suggest that the low values reported may be because of an artifact resulting from tumor hypoxia (7–9). This may reflect the relative proliferation within a given risk category of the prostate cancers being studied (e.g., low- vs. high-risk cancers). The evidence to support a low α/β ratio is based on basic science and clinical data. Fowler has analyzed the biochemical control rates (biochemical no evidence of disease, bNED) from published radiotherapy series and RCTs and has come to the conclusion that the α/β ratio for prostate cancer may be as low as 1.5 Gy (1). His analysis of the only hypofractio-

nation trial that has published efficacy data (10) concludes that the results would be in keeping with the α/β ratio for prostate cancer being as low as 1.0 to 1.5 Gy (1). The relatively low α/β ratio should make prostate cancer cells very sensitive to increases in fraction size or dose rate (Fig. 1C). In this setting, hypofractionated radiotherapy using a higher dose per fraction, lower total dose, and shorter overall treatment time would be more efficient at killing tumor cells than standard fractionation and should produce equivalent tumor control with reduced toxicity. Some authors suggest that, based on mathematical modeling, some higher dose per fraction hypofractionation regimens could even result in improved tumor control while maintaining the same toxicity as current high-dose 2-Gy fraction regimens (11).

Fowler et al. (11) has summarized the radiobiological implications of hypofractionation in the treatment of prostate cancer as:

> Estimates of the α/β ratio for prostate cancer are around 1.5 Gy, much lower than the typical value of 10 Gy for many other tumours. The low α/β value is comparable to, and possibly even lower than, that of surrounding late-responding normal tissue in rectal mucosa (α/β nominally 3 Gy but also likely to be in the 4–5 Gy range). This lower α/β ratio for prostate cancer than for surrounding late-responding normal tissue creates the potential for therapeutic gain.

Normal Tissue Tolerance

Radiation effects on normal tissue, which manifest clinically as adverse effects related to tissue injury, are divided into categories often labeled as acute or late (2). Adverse effects related to acute response to irradiation occur early (i.e., during or soon after radiotherapy), while those related to late response occur weeks, months, or years after completion of radiotherapy and tend to be chronic. Late adverse effects of radiotherapy can be classified as "classic" or "consequential" (12). The former are usually related to damage to slowly proliferating tissue, such as rectum or bladder. This type of late toxicity is considered a dose-limiting effect of radiotherapy. Late adverse effects may also occur as a consequence of earlier injury due to the acute effects of radiotherapy on skin and mucosa (2); these are termed "consequential." In a recent analysis of data from a radiotherapy dose-escalation study, Heemsbergen et al. investigated the link between acute and late toxicity and found that acute gastrointestinal (GI) adverse events were independent predictors of late GI adverse events in men with localized prostate cancer (12). Mild to moderate urinary, bowel, and sexual side effects are common after external beam radiotherapy for prostate cancer. Studies suggest that late bowel and bladder effects reach a plateau between 24 and 36 months after treatment (13). Although all adverse effects can impinge on patients' quality of life and many have the potential to result in serious health problems, late effects can have the added consequence of being permanent and progressive. Unlike acute effects, late effects may not heal well and may require surgical intervention.

Alteration of radiotherapy fractionation has the potential to change the pattern of adverse effects. Acute responses to radiotherapy generally occur in tissues with rapid turnover, such as GI mucosa and skin; these rapidly dividing normal tissues have an α/β ratio of approximately 10 Gy. Consequential late effects could be expected to vary with fraction size in the same way as acute adverse effects. Classic late effects are usually related to damage to slowly proliferating tissue such as rectum or bladder, which have α/β ratios of 2.5 to 5 Gy and 3 to 7 Gy, respectively. Although limited data are available for prostate cancer, a model developed for cervix cancer predicts less acute toxicity with hypofractionated regimens than for standard fractionation (14). According to this model, 60 Gy in 3 Gy fractions has less effect on acute-reacting tissue than does 78 Gy given in 2 Gy fractions. Large fractions, especially those over 2.5 Gy, are usually avoided for most tumor types because late-reacting normal tissue is generally more sensitive to large fractions than most tumor cells. In prostate cancer, however, tumor cells have an α/β ratio that is estimated to be between 0.9 and 1.5 Gy, making them sensitive to large fractions.

Thus, in theory at least, when combined with image-guided conformal or IMRT radiotherapy, hypofractionated radiotherapy has the potential to produce tumor control and late classic toxicity rates that are equivalent to conventional fractionation with less acute and consequential late toxicity. While the above discussion has summarized the radiobiological aspects of hypofractionation for prostate cancer, readers are referred to published papers and reviews for more detailed information on this subject (1,5,6,11).

EVIDENCE FROM CLINICAL TRIALS

The Role of Clinical Studies

In addition to radiobiological considerations, clinical experience and data from clinical trials can also inform choices about fraction size and total dose of radiotherapy used in clinical practice and randomized trials. Although improvement in patient survival is the definitive measure of successful cancer treatment, the long natural history of prostate cancer presents challenges to designing studies with the power to detect statistically significant improvements in overall mortality rates. For this reason, surrogate end points are often used as primary outcome variables in randomized trials in this setting. The most commonly used

of these surrogate outcomes is biochemical failure. Several definitions for biochemical failure have been described in the literature (15–17), but the American Society for Therapeutic Radiology and Oncology (ASTRO) definition has been the most widely accepted. The most recent review of the ASTRO consensus statement at a joint Radiation Therapy Oncology Group RTOG-ASTRO meeting in 2005 resulted in some changes to the definition of biochemical failure to make it generalizable to patients treated with radiotherapy plus hormonal therapy and to correct for bias in the original method for determining the date of failure used to calculate estimates of event-free survival (18). The current consensus statement recommended that the definition of prostate-specific antigen (PSA) failure be changed to PSA nadir +2; this definition is now referred to as the Phoenix definition though in the past it has been referred to as the Houston definition. The Phoenix (RTOG/ASTRO) consensus conference in 2005 also stressed the importance of adequate follow-up in clinical trials and recommended that investigators report results that reflect data from a point in time two years less than the median follow-up time. For example, when median follow-up is seven years, freedom from biochemical failure rate should be estimated at five years. Most studies reporting results to date have used the original ASTRO failure definition. It is anticipated that future studies will report outcomes on the basis of the 2005 definition of biochemical failure.

Evidence of the relative effectiveness and safety of hypofractionated radiotherapy comes from randomized trials that compare these regimens with conventional fractionation. An understanding of the evidence on total dose used for conventionally fractionated radiotherapy is important for the design and interpretation of trials comparing hypofractionated and conventional radiotherapy. The total dose and mode of delivery used for conventional radiotherapy schedules has evolved as new data emerged from randomized trials. Four randomized trials have compared conventional-dose versus high-dose conformal radiotherapy using fractions of 1.8 to 2.0 Gy (19–23). Three of four trials reported a benefit for dose-escalated radiotherapy in terms of freedom from biochemical failure based on PSA levels, but none had sufficient numbers or follow-up time to detect differences in survival. All four trials reported increased adverse effects with higher doses of radiotherapy. The trials described above used freedom from failure as their primary outcome measure. Two ongoing randomized trials, designed to detect statistically significant differences in five-year survival rate as the primary outcome, may clarify the picture on the benefits of high-dose radiotherapy in patients with localized prostate cancer (24–26). Chapter 1 includes a full discussion on the evidence and general practice guidelines for image-guided radiation treatment in prostate cancer.

Hypofractionation—Case Series

In an attempt to improve freedom from disease and survival rates, the trials described above used higher total doses of radiation with conventional fraction sizes. The net result of this approach is longer overall treatment times resulting in more trips to the treatment center by the patient and a higher burden on the radiotherapy facility. Hypofractionated radiotherapy, on the other hand, aims to achieve clinical results that are at least equivalent to conventional fractionation while shortening overall treatment time and reducing the burden on patients and treatment centers. As discussed earlier, the radiobiological data suggest that the potential exists for improved tumor control while maintaining normal tissue toxicity with hypofractionated radiotherapy using even higher dose per fraction in hypofractionated regimens.

Evidence on the clinical outcomes associated with hypofractionated radiotherapy has been evolving since the 1980s. Early reports described experiences with radiotherapy for localized prostate cancer at centers in Canada, Australia, and the United Kingdom (27–31), but three studies published since 2003 are more relevant to current practice (32–35). The largest was a retrospective case series from the Christie Hospital in the United Kingdom where 705 men with localized prostate cancer were treated with conformal radiotherapy to a dose of 50 Gy in 16 daily fractions over 22 days (fraction size 3.13 Gy) (32). The biochemical relapse-free rates in the low-, moderate-, and high-risk groups were 82%, 56%, and 39%, respectively. Grade 2 late bowel toxicity was reported in 5% of patients and grade 2 to 3 late bladder toxicity in 10% of patients. The Cleveland Clinic in the United States conducted a prospective study involving 100 men with localized prostate cancer treated to 70 Gy at 2.5 Gy/fraction (33). The five-year biochemical relapse-free survival rate was 85%, the grade 3 late rectal toxicity rate 3%, and the grade 3 late urinary toxicity rate 1%. In a prospective study at the Princess Margaret Hospital in Canada, 92 patients with prostate cancer received IMRT with a total dose of 60 Gy given as 3.0 Gy fractions over four weeks (34,35). This phase II study was designed to assess late toxicity and the feasibility of the hypofractionated regimen. At the last assessment during a median follow-up of 38 months, there was no grade 3 or 4 toxicity. Rates of grade 1/2 late adverse events were low, with 7% of patients reporting GI events and 10% reporting genitourinary (GU) events. Severe acute toxicity occurred in one patient but did not require interruption of treatment. The biochemical control rate was 97% at 14 months. In addition, high-quality evidence from a randomized trial in breast cancer, which is also postulated to have a relatively low α/β ratio, demonstrated that a 22-day course of radiotherapy using 16 fractions of 2.66 Gy produced similar rates of local recurrence–free survival to 50 Gy given in 25 fractions over 35 days, without significant increases in toxicity (36).

Hypofractionation—Randomized Trials

Evidence is available from three randomized trials that compared hypofractionated and conventionally fractionated radiotherapy regimens for localized prostate cancer (Tables 1 and 2).

A Canadian study by the Ontario Clinical Oncology Group (OCOG), published in 2005, was the first randomized trial to evaluate a fractionation schedule delivering a dose per fraction higher than 2 Gy for the treatment of localized prostate cancer (10). Between March 1995 and December 1998, 936 men with early-stage (T1 or T2) disease were randomly assigned to receive 66 Gy in 33 fractions over 45 days (long arm) or 52.5 Gy in 20 fractions of 2.625 Gy over 28 days (short arm). Patients with PSA levels ≤40 μg/L were included. They were randomized within strata on the basis of PSA level (≤ or > 15 μg/L), Gleason score (2–6 or 7–10), method of lymph node assessment (surgical or radiological), and center to enhance comparability between the long and short arms. The primary study outcome was biochemical or clinical failure (BCF), which was based on a cluster of events that included three consecutive increases in PSA, clinical evidence of local or distant failure, commencement of hormonal therapy, or death as a result of prostate cancer. The study was designed as a noninferiority trial, with statistical power to demonstrate that the treatment given in the short arm was not worse than that given in the long arm by more than 7.5% in terms of the primary outcome. The treatment planning in this study was CT-based. This study was undertaken prior to the availability of image guidance. The margin around the prostate was 1.5 cm, though posteriorly this could be reduced to 1.0 cm at the discretion of treating physician. Follow-up ranged from 4.5 to 8.3 years with a median time of 5.7 years. Kaplan-Meier estimates of BCF, based on the 1997 ASTRO definition, were 53% in the long arm and 60% in the short arm at five years [hazard ratio (HR), 1.18; 95% confidence interval (CI), 0.99–1.41], favoring conventional fractionation over hypofractionation. PSA failure accounted for 83% of BCF events. The observed difference in BCF rate (short minus long arm) was –7.0% (90% CI, –12.6% to –1.4%). Since the lower bound of the CI on this difference was lower than the predefined tolerance of –7.5%, one could not exclude the possibility that the hypofractionated regimen (short arm) was inferior to the standard regimen (long arm). Similar results were obtained when the Vancouver (17) and Houston (15) definitions for PSA failure were used. The trial did not detect statistically significant differences between treatment groups in terms of the secondary outcomes of overall

Table 1 Randomized Trials of Hypofractionated Radiotherapy in Patients with Localized Prostate Cancer

Trial	Source	Status as of latest publication	Patients	Conventional radiotherapy	Hypofractionated radiotherapy
Trial completed—results published					
OCOG (Canada)	Lukka et al., 2005 (10)	Recruitment completed, increased acute toxicity with hypofractionation; no significant differences in relapse, late toxicity, or survival	936 low, intermediate, high risk	66 Gy in 33 fractions, 2 Gy/fraction	52.5 Gy in 20 fractions, 2.62 Gy/fraction
Australian	Yeoh et al., 2006 (37,38)	Recruitment completed, increased GI toxicity in first 4 wk with hypofractionation; no significant difference in relapse and survival rates	217 low, intermediate, high risk	64 Gy in 32 fractions, 2 Gy/fraction	55 Gy in 20 fractions, 2.75 Gy/fraction
Fox Chase Cancer Center (U.S.A.)	Pollack et al., 2006 (39); clinicaltrials.gov identifier NCT00062309 (40);	Recruitment completed, follow-up ongoing, 3-mo toxicity data reported for first 100 patients: increased GI toxicity with hypofractionation	300 intermediate and high risk	76 Gy in 32 fractions, 2 Gy/fraction	70.2 Gy in 26 fractions, 2.7 Gy/fraction
Trial ongoing					
OCOG-PROFIT (Canada)	clinicaltrials.gov identifier NCT00304759 (41); Study protocol	Recruiting	1204 (target) intermediate risk	78 Gy in 39 fractions, 2 Gy/fraction[a]	60 Gy in 20 fractions, 3 Gy/fraction[a]
Institute of Cancer Research (U.K.)	clinicaltrials.gov identifier NCT00392535 (42); South et al. (43)	Recruiting	2577 low, intermediate and some high risk	74 Gy in 37 fractions, 2 Gy/fraction[a]	60 Gy in 20 fractions Or 57 Gy in 19 fractions, 3 Gy/fraction[a]
RTOG-0415 (U.S.A.)	clinicaltrials.gov identifier NCT00331773 (44); RTOG Web site (45)	Recruiting	1067 low risk	73.8 Gy in 41 fractions, 1.8 Gy/fraction[a]	70 Gy in 28 fractions, 2.5 Gy/fraction[a]

[a]Trials using three-dimensional conformal radiation treatment techniques, including intensity-modulated radiotherapy.
Abbreviations: RTOG, Radiation Therapy Oncology Group; OCOG, Ontario Clinical Oncology Group; GI, gastrointestinal.

Table 2 Published Evidence from Randomized Trials of Hypofractionated vs. Conventional Radiotherapy

Trial	Median follow-up	5-yr Kaplan-Meier estimates (hypofractionated vs. conventional RT)		Adverse effect rates (hypofractionated vs. conventional RT)	
		Biochemical-clinical relapse	Survival	Acute GI and GU toxicity (grade 3 or 4)	Late GI and GU toxicity (grade 3 or 4)
OCOG (Canada) Lukka et al., 2005 (10)	68 mo	59.95% vs. 52.95% NS[a]	87.6% vs. 85.2% NS	11.4% vs. 7.0% $P < 0.05$	3.2% vs. 3.2% NS
Australian Yeoh et al., 2006 (38)	48 mo	57.4% vs. 55.5% NS	86.4% vs. 84.1% NS	GI toxicity scores higher with hypofractionation ($P < 0.05$)	Urgency of defecation and total GU toxicity scores higher with hypofractionation ($P < 0.05$)
Fox Chase Cancer Center (U.S.A.) Pollack et al., 2006 (39)	3[b] mo	Not reported	Not reported	GI: 0% vs. 0% GU: 8% vs. 2% NS	Not reported

[a]Difference between the five-year rates for conventional and hypofractionated arms failed to meet the predefined criterion for equivalence.
[b]Preliminary results from three-month follow-up of first 100 patients.
Abbreviations: NS, difference between groups not statistically significant; RT, radiation therapy; OCGC, Ontario Clinical Oncology Group; GI, gastrointestinal; GU, genitourinary.

survival (estimated 5-year survival rates; 85.2% in the long arm and 87.6% in the short arm; HR, 0.85; 95% CI, 0.63–1.15) or positive prostate biopsy two years after radiotherapy [53.2% in the long arm vs. 51.9% in the short arm; risk difference (RD), 2.3%; 95% CI, –5.1% to 9.8%]. Patients in the long arm experienced significantly less grade 3 or 4 acute GI or GU toxicity than those in the short arm (7.0% vs. 11.4%; RD, –4.4%; 95% CI, –8.1% to –0.6%), but rates of severe late toxicity were similar (3.2% vs. 3.2%; RD, 0.0%; 95% CI, –2.4% to 2.3%). Overall, 3.2% of patients experienced grade 3 or 4 GI or GU adverse events more than five months after radiotherapy in both treatment groups, which is consistent with the α/β model for late toxicity. The small but statistically significant increase in acute toxicity with the hypofractionated regimen is consistent with a higher net rate of stem cell depletion in the rectal and bladder mucosa resulting from an increased rate of dose accumulation (13.1 Gy/wk in the short arm vs. 10 Gy/wk in the long arm).

The dose chosen for the hypofractionated regimen used in the short arm was based on data from case series published between 1982 and 1993 (27–31). The increased rate of acute toxicity observed in the short arm in the randomized trial confirms that further dose escalation would have been impossible with the treatment techniques in use during the study period. When the trial was designed in the early 1990s, a four-field technique was the standard method for delivering radiation. Current techniques such as conformal-beam radiation or IMRT together with image-guided radiation therapy (IGRT) should allow the dose per fraction to be increased to levels that could result in higher tumor-control rates (based on radiobiological considerations) while maintaining an acceptable incidence of late toxicity. Furthermore, the total dose used in the long arm in this study was low compared with current doses used in high-dose standard fractionation schedules. Thus, both the technique and dose of radiation used in this trial limit generalizability of the results to current practice.

Preliminary results from two additional randomized trials provide evidence on the adverse effects of hypofractionated radiotherapy for prostate cancer (37–40).

Yeoh et al. published two reports on an Australian randomized trial of hypofractionated radiotherapy (37,38). Median follow-up at last report was 48 months (ranging from 6 to 108 months). Two hundred and seventeen patients with localized early-stage (T1–T2) prostate cancer were randomized to receive 64 Gy in 32 fractions over 6.5 weeks (standard fractionation) or 55 Gy in 20 fractions over 4 weeks (hypofractionation). As in the OCOG trial described above, radiotherapy planning used two-dimensional computed tomography (CT) data, and treatment was delivered using a three- or four-field technique. The publication does not state if image guidance was utilized during the treatment. The primary outcome was late treatment-related toxicity. The study was designed to detect a difference between groups in the frequency of mild late toxicity of 20%. GI and GU symptoms were measured before and after one month, and then one, two, three, four, and five years consecutively after radiotherapy. Compared to conventional radiotherapy, four measures of GI toxicity (stool frequency, urgency, mucous discharge, and total GI symptom score) were significantly worse one month after starting hypofractionated radiotherapy, as were measures of the effect of GI symptoms on daily activities (38). There were no statistically significant differences in GI symptoms over the remaining follow-up, with the exception of urgency of defecation at five years, which was worse with hypofractionated radiotherapy. Hypofractionated radiotherapy was an independent predictor of increased total GI symptoms at two years (risk ratio, 1.32; 95% CI, 1.07–1.64) but not at three, four, or five years. Total GU symptom scores were worse at two and three years follow-up with hypofractionation compared to conventional fractionation, but this difference was not reflected in the effects of GU symptoms on daily activities. No statistically significant differences between treatment groups were detected for the secondary end points of biochemical ± clinical relapse (5-year estimates, 57.4% vs. 55.5% in hypofractionated and conventional arms, respectively) and overall survival (5-year estimate, 86.4% with hypofractionation vs. 84.1% with conventional fractionation).

Preliminary results are available from an American study that had higher total doses in both the conventional fractionation and hypofractionation arms than the trials described above. This trial used IMRT in both groups (39,40). Men with intermediate- or high-risk localized prostate cancer (T1b–T3c and Gleason score ≥5) were randomized to receive 76 Gy in 38 fractions (standard fractionation) or 70.2 Gy in 26 fractions (hypofractionation). Details of the planning including simulation, CTV/PTV, normal tissue delineation and constraints are described in considerable detail in the paper (39), however details of the image guidance employed is not outlined in this paper. The primary end point for the trial, biochemical failure, has not yet been analyzed, but a preliminary report on acute toxicity in the first 100 patients was published in 2006 by Pollack et al. Projected accrual is 300 patients (40). There was a significant increase in GI toxicity score during weeks 2–4 of treatment with hypofractionated IMRT compared to conventional IMRT but no differences over the remainder of the three-month follow-up period. There was no grade 3 or 4 GI toxicity, but grade 2 adverse GI effects were reported for 18% of patients in the hypofractionated arm and 8% in the control arm during radiotherapy. No statistically significant differences between groups were detected for GU toxicity.

Summary of Published Randomized Trials Using Hypofractionation

To date, one RCT has provided data on the efficacy and toxicity of moderate-dose hypofractionated radiotherapy using older (4-field) treatment techniques (10). Another study using similar doses and technique has reported toxicity data (37,38). Early results from a third study comparing higher doses of both conventional radiotherapy (76 Gy in 38 fractions) and a hypofractionated regimen (70.2 Gy in 26 fractions) suggested no difference in acute toxicity at three-months follow-up (39). These results are interesting. It is reassuring that late radiation toxicity was found to be equivalent and that the hypofractionated regimen has, in general, been found to be well tolerated.

Ongoing Trials

To evaluate the role of hypofractionated radiotherapy in the treatment of prostate cancer compared to the current standard of high-dose radiotherapy, well-designed RCTs need to be conducted evaluating hypofractionated regimens versus 76 to 78 Gy using conventional fractionation of 1.8 to 2 Gy. To enable these doses to be delivered, modern conformal and IMRT techniques need to be utilized. Three relevant ongoing randomized trials are listed in the Web site maintained by the U.S. National Institutes of Health (www.clinicaltrials.gov) (Table 1) (41,42,44). All use 3DCRT or IMRT. Doses in the standard fractionation arm range from 73.8 to 78 Gy, given in fractions of 2 Gy in two studies and 1.8 Gy in the third. Two studies use fraction sizes of 3.0 Gy in the hypofractionated arm and the third uses 2.5 Gy.

The OCOG group is conducting a randomized trial (known as "PROFIT") of hypofractionated radiotherapy (60 Gy in 20 fractions over 4 weeks) versus standard radiotherapy (78 Gy in 39 fractions over 8 weeks) in patients with intermediate-risk prostate cancer (T1–T2a, Gleason score ≤6, PSA = 10.1–20.0 ng/mL; T2b–T2c, Gleason score ≤6, PSA ≤20 ng/mL; T1–T2, Gleason score = 7, PSA ≤20 ng/mL) (41). 3DCRT or IMRT is used for both hypofractionated and standard radiotherapy. The primary outcome measure is biochemical (PSA) failure defined by the ASTRO consensus criteria. Secondary outcomes include BCF, death from cancer, toxic effects of radiotherapy, and health related quality of life. This multicenter trial started recruitment in May 2006. Total expected enrolment is 1204.

A large British trial is comparing two hypofractionated high-dose IMRT schedules (60 Gy in 20 fractions over 4 weeks and 57 Gy in 19 fractions over 3.8 weeks) with high-dose radiotherapy using conventional fractionation (74 Gy in 37 fractions over 7.5 weeks) in men with low- to high-risk-localized prostate cancer (42,43). The study population will include patients with T1b to T3a tumors, PSA ≤40 ng/mL, Gleason score <9, and estimated risk of lymph-node metastases <30% (for Gleason score <6, PSA must be ≤40 ng/mL; for Gleason score = 7, PSA must be <30 ng/mL; for Gleason score = 8, PSA must be <15 ng/mL). Primary outcomes comprise acute and late radiation–induced adverse effects, as well as recurrence of prostate cancer. Quality of life and economic impact are included among the secondary outcomes. Enrolment started in late 2002 with a target of 2577 patients to be followed for up to 15 years.

The RTOG-0415 trial started in April 2006 (44,45). One-thousand and sixty-seven men with low-risk prostate cancer (T1–T2c, Gleason score = 2–6, PSA <10 ng/mL) will be randomized to conventionally fractionated 3DCRT or IMRT (73.8 Gy in 41 fractions over 8.2 weeks) or hypofractionated 3DCRT or IMRT (70 Gy in 28 fractions over 5.6 weeks). The primary outcome is disease-free survival and secondary outcomes include biochemical recurrence, overall survival, adverse effects, quality of life, anxiety/depression, and cost utility.

These studies and other planned trials will provide evidence to help evaluate the role of hypofractionated radiotherapy in the management of localized prostate cancer. This, in turn, will help guide future research evaluating hypofractionated regimens using higher dose per fraction and even shorter regimens, as will be discussed later in this chapter.

BIOLOGICALLY EQUIVALENT DOSE

Comparisons of the biologically equivalent dose (BED) for different conventional and hypofractionated regimens is an interesting modeling exercise that aids understanding of the regimens used in clinical trials in terms of tumor control (based on a particular α/β ratio for the tumor), acute toxicity (α/β ratio of 10 Gy), and late toxicity (α/β ratio of 3 Gy) (Table 3).

While not ideal (cell proliferation is ignored, for example), the BED modeling exercise can be used as a rough comparator of the regimens used in the randomized trials discussed above. As an example, randomized trials demonstrate that bNED rates can be improved by using 78 Gy rather than 70 Gy with conventional fraction sizes of 2 Gy (12,19–23). If the α/β ratio is 1.5 Gy for prostate cancer, the BED would be 182 with a total dose of 78 Gy compared to 163 with 70 Gy. The BED for acute toxicity ($\alpha/\beta = 10$ Gy) would be expected to be 93.6 versus 84, respectively, and for late toxicity ($\alpha/\beta = 3$ Gy), 130 versus 116.7. This is supported by evidence from clinical studies, which found that rates of late rectal toxicity (grade 2 and 3) were slightly increased with higher doses of radiation.

Table 3 Biologically Equivalent Dose by α/β Ratio

Total dose (Gy)	Number of fractions	Dose/fraction (Gy)	Biologically equivalent dose (BED) assuming different α/β ratios			
			$\alpha/\beta = 1$	$\alpha/\beta = 1.5$	$\alpha/\beta = 3$ (late effects)	$\alpha/\beta = 10$ (early effects)
52.5	20	2.6	190.3	144.4	98.4	66.3
60.0	20	3.0	240.0	180.0	120.0	78.0
66.0	33	2.0	198.0	154.0	110.0	79.2
70.0	25	2.8	266.0	200.7	135.3	89.6
70.0	28	2.5	245.0	186.7	128.3	87.5
70.0	35	2.0	210.0	163.3	116.7	84.0
70.2	39	1.8	196.6	154.4	112.3	82.8
74.0	37	2.0	222.0	172.7	123.3	88.8
78.0	39	2.0	234.0	182.0	130.0	93.6

However, rates of late bladder toxicity were similar for doses of 70 and 78 Gy. The bNED rates were improved with the higher dose regimen in keeping with the increases in the BED values.

Comparison of the regimens used in the published OCOG hypofractionation trial (66 Gy/33 fractions/6.5 wk vs. 52.5 Gy/20 fractions/4 wk) would show BEDs of 154 and 144.4, respectively for tumor control, assuming an α/β ratio of 1.5 Gy (10). These BED values are consistent with the apparent "equivalence" of the two regimens in this study. The respective BED values for late toxicity would be 110 versus 98.4 and for acute toxicity, 79.2 versus 66.3. In the OCOG trial, while late toxicity rates were equivalent, acute toxicity was slightly worse with the hypofractionated regimen (grade 3 or 4 toxicity, 7% vs. 11.4%). In this case, the observed acute toxicity results are at variance with the acute toxicity BED calculations. This may, in part, be related to the radiation technique employed in the study. The observation could also arise from a higher net rate of cell depletion in the rectal and bladder mucosa resulting from an increased rate of dose accumulation.

In the ongoing OCOG-PROFIT study that randomizes patients to 78 Gy in 2 Gy fractions or 60 Gy in 3 Gy fractions, the corresponding BED values are 182 and 180 for tumor control ($\alpha/\beta = 1.5$ Gy), 130 and 120 for late toxicity ($\alpha/\beta = 3$ Gy), and 93.6 and 78 for acute toxicity ($\alpha/\beta = 10$ Gy) (41). An ongoing RTOG trial randomizes patients to 73.8 Gy in 1.80 Gy fractions or 70.0 Gy in 2.5 Gy fractions. According to the study protocol, the BED for tumor control is 162.4 versus 186.7, late toxicity 118.1 versus 128.3, and acute toxicity 87.1 versus 87.5 (45). These calculations illustrate the comparability between the hypofractionated and conventional regimens in terms of BED. The modeling exercise suggests that hypofractionated regimens have the potential to improve tumor control while maintaining late toxicity rates if the α/β ratio for prostate cancer is as low as is currently thought.

Ultimately, well-designed randomized clinical studies would need to be conducted comparing these hypofractionated regimens with conventional regimens to assess their relative efficacy and toxicity (both acute and late).

Another common method for comparing regimens is to convert the BED value to the LQ equivalent dose in 2 Gy fractions, also referred to as the normalized total dose or NTD_{2Gy}. Fowler has recently published on the comparability of hypofractionated regimens to standard 2 Gy/fraction regimens (1). Table 4 shows the comparability of hypofractionated regimens to conventionally fractionated regimens with regard to tumor control, based on equivalent late rectal toxicity. Based on this model, a regimen of 74 Gy in 37 fractions over 7.5 weeks results in a BED for late toxicity of 123.3 ($\alpha/\beta = 3$ Gy). In comparison, a regimen of 3.06 Gy in 20 fractions (total dose, 61.11 Gy) will result in a similar BED in late-responding tissue of 123.3, but the NTD_{2Gy} would be equivalent to 79.6 Gy. Fowler's calculations suggest that bNED (biochemical control) would increase from 75.5% to 84% when 74 Gy of radiotherapy (given in conventional 2 Gy fractions) is changed to a hypofractionated regimen of 61.11 Gy (in 3.06 Gy fractions). The comparability among other hypofractionated regimens, ranging from 25 fractions of 2.63 Gy to 3 fractions of 9.7 Gy, is also shown in Table 4. It needs to be emphasized that these estimates are based on modeling and must to be validated by results from well-conducted clinical trials.

INDICATIONS AND CONTRAINDICATIONS TO HYPOFRACTIONATED PROSTATE RADIOTHERAPY

Ongoing and future studies would need to confirm the role of hypofractionated radiotherapy in low-, intermediate-, and high-risk populations. If its role is proven in RCTs,

Table 4 Hypofractionated Schedules Calculated by Fowler for Constant Late Rectal Complications Assuming $\alpha/\beta = 3$ Gy

Hypofractionated schedule	Total dose (Gy)	Late rectal complications		Prostate tumor effects	
		BED_{Gy3} for $\alpha/\beta = 3$ Gy	Late rectal complications NTD_{2Gy} for $\alpha/\beta = 3$ Gy (Gy)	Calculated NTD_{2Gy} for $\alpha/\beta = 1.5$ Gy (Gy)	Estimated bNED (%)
37 F × 2.00 Gy	74.0	123.3	74.0	74.0	75.5
25 F × 2.69 Gy	65.73	123.3	74.0	78.7	82.8
20 F × 3.06 Gy	61.11	123.3	74.0	79.6	84.0
15 F × 3.69 Gy	55.33	123.3	74.0	82.0	87.3
10 F × 4.77 Gy	47.65	123.3	74.0	85.4	90.0
5 F × 7.73 Gy	36.16	123.3	74.0	90.2	94.0
3 F × 9.70 Gy	29.10	123.3	74.0	93.1	95.8

Total dose = 74 Gy × (1 + 2/3)/(1 + d/3) for the constant BED of 123.3 Gy₃.
NTD_{2Gy}, normalized total dose, the schedule using 2 Gy fractions that would give the same log cell kill. The final two columns also present the consequent prostate tumor effects, as normalized total dose (NTD_{2Gy}) assuming $\alpha/\beta = 1.5$ Gy; and the estimated five-year percentage bNED.
Abbreviations: BED, biologically equivalent dose; bNED, biochemical no evidence of disease; F, fractions; NTD, normalized total dose.
Source: From Ref. 1.

hypofractionated treatment could be considered in the ongoing treatment of these subgroups of patients.

On the basis of currently available data, it is difficult to identify specific indications or contraindications for hypofractionated radiotherapy. The inclusion criteria for entry into studies such as the PROFIT trial are broad and include any patient eligible for conventional radiotherapy to the prostate. Specific indications and contraindications for clinical practice would need to await the publication of ongoing studies. It is possible that subgroup analyses of results from ongoing trials may identify specific sets of patients who would be more optimally treated with conventional radiotherapy (as opposed to hypofractionated radiotherapy) because of better tumor control or lower toxicity. For example, in an individual patient where there is concern about bowel or bladder toxicity, it may be preferable to use conventional fractionation regimens rather than a hypofractionated regimen. Results of ongoing studies, including RCTs, are awaited. Finally, there may be selected patients who are more likely to be at risk for radiotherapy toxicity because of their inherent genetics; but further prospective studies are required to confidently predict the incidence and existence of these patients within large radiotherapy cohorts (46).

IMAGE-GUIDED PLANNING AND DELIVERY

Following publication of a randomized trial that demonstrated reduced toxicity with conformal radiotherapy compared to traditional four-field techniques, conformal techniques were adopted even when moderate doses of radiotherapy were used (47). These conformal techniques reduce dose to both rectum and bladder resulting in reduced toxicity in these organs. IMRT, which allows

further dose shaping around rectum and bladder, is now increasingly being used in clinical practice. IGRT now forms an important aspect of treatment to ensure that treatment is delivered as planned.

TECHNICAL FACTORS

Treatment Planning

Conformal radiotherapy, and particularly, IMRT techniques require careful attention be paid to definition of tumor volume and normal tissue to evaluate the dose distribution against accepted standards. These standards include definitions of maximum and minimum doses allowed within the planning target volume (PTV), as well as a set of dose-volume histogram specifications for both target and organs at risk. Examples from the RTOG and OCOG protocols defining the PTV parameters are shown in Table 5. Similarly, dose constraints on normal tissue need to be carefully evaluated with hypofractionated treatments to minimize toxicity. Studies correlating normal tissue constraints to toxicity with specific hypofractionated regimens need to be published to help confirm the safety of these regimens. Once efficacy and safety are confirmed, clinicians using such regimens need to ensure that due care and attention is paid through the planning process with regard to the PTV and clinical target volume (CTV) dosimetry, and that the doses delivered to normal tissue are within acceptable normal tissue constraints.

Two different ways of defining normal tissue have been outlined for two of the ongoing RCTs evaluating hypofractionated regimens (RTOG and OCOG) (41,44). The RTOG method is also used in other RTOG studies such as protocol 0126 (26). In the RTOG studies, the rectum is defined from the anus to the recto-sigmoid junction as a volume (including the rectal contents,

Table 5 Planning Parameters and Dose Constraints for OCOG and RTOG Trials

Dose prescription		OCOG-PROFIT		RTOG-0415	
		60 Gy in 20 (3 Gy) fractions	78 Gy in 39 (2 Gy) fractions	70 Gy in 28 (2.5 Gy) fractions	73.8 Gy in 41 (1.8) Gy fractions
CTV definition		Contoured prostate and, if applicable, seminal vesicle		Prostate and first 1 cm of seminal vesicle	
CTV dose	Minimum	60 Gy	78 Gy	70 Gy	73.8 Gy
	Maximum	64.2 Gy	83.5 Gy	–	–
PTV definition		Expansion 7 mm posteriorly (toward the rectum) and 10 mm in all other planes		5–10 mm around CTV	
PTV dose	Minimum	57 Gy	74.1 Gy	70 Gy	73.8 Gy
	Maximum	63 Gy	81.9 Gy	74.9	79
Bladder constraint	Contoured bladder wall:				
	50% to receive less than	37 Gy	53 Gy	–	–
	70% to receive less than	46 Gy	71 Gy	–	–
	Bladder volume:				
	≤15% to receive more than	–	–	79 Gy	80 Gy
	≤25% to receive more than	–	–	74 Gy	75 Gy
	≤35% to receive more than	–	–	69 Gy	70 Gy
	≤50% to receive more than	–	–	64 Gy	65 Gy
Rectum constraint	Contoured rectal wall:				
	50% to receive less than	37 Gy	53 Gy	–	–
	70% to receive less than	46 Gy	71 Gy	–	–
	Rectal volume:				
	≤15% to receive more than	–	–	74 Gy	75 Gy
	≤25% to receive more than	–	–	69 Gy	70 Gy
	≤35% to receive more than	–	–	64 Gy	65 Gy
	≤50% to receive more than	–	–	59 Gy	60 Gy
Femoral head and neck constraint	<5% to receive	>43 Gy	>53 Gy	–	–
Penile bulb constraint	Mean dose	–	–	≤51 Gy	≤52.5 Gy

Abbreviations: CTV, clinical target volume; PTV, planning target volume.
Source: From OCOG-PROFIT and RTOG-0415 protocols.

feces, and air). In the case of the bladder, the whole bladder volume is delineated (including the urine volume) in the RTOG protocols (Fig. 2A). In contrast, the OCOG-PROFIT protocol defines only the rectal wall (and not its contents) and bladder wall thickness (not urine volume) (Fig. 2B). In the OCOG-PROFIT protocol, the bowel and bladder walls are contoured 18 mm (to beam edge) beyond the most inferior and superior contoured prostate slices (or seminal vesicles when they are included in the CTV). In each protocol, the acceptable dose constraints are based on clinical experience from previous studies.

Table 5 summarizes the constraints for rectum and bladder for each of these protocols. There has not been a direct comparison of these methods of normal tissue delineation or normal tissue constraints. Both methods have advantages and disadvantages. Ultimately, it would be reasonable to expect that as long as the normal tissue delineation are adhered to and normal tissue constraints

respected, toxicity would be acceptable. The importance of ensuring this for hypofractionated regimens cannot be overemphasized. The current PTV and normal tissue constraint definitions in hypofractionated regimens are based on initial studies. The ongoing RCTs evaluating hypofractionated regimens would need to confirm the efficacy and safety of these regimens before they are routinely used in clinical practice and outside a clinical trial. Note should be made that, given that a large variety of hypofractionated regimens are potentially available for use, the efficacy and toxicity would vary by regimen. With differences in normal tissue toxicity depending on the dose per fraction and total dose, the normal tissue dose constraints will vary depending on the hypofractionated regimen used and may not be transferable to other hypofractionated regimens. It is, therefore, important that regimens and normal tissue constraints from good published hypofractionated regimens be used. Where

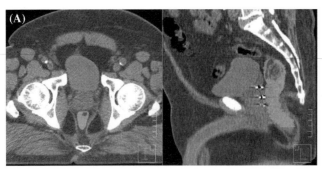 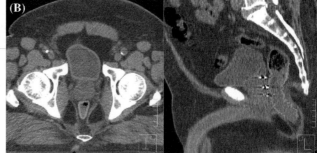

Figure 2 (*See color insert.*) Organs at risk. (**A**) RTOG definition for rectal thickness and bladder thickness. (**B**) PROFIT definition for rectal thickness and bladder thickness.

high-dose treatments are utilized, it would be extremely important to ensure that the doses within the PTV and normal tissues are in keeping with the definitions of these criteria established in protocols conducted by good clinical trial groups. With hypofractionated regimens (and higher doses per fraction), it is important to ensure that tumor and normal tissue definition and planning parameters (such as the use of convolution/superposition algorithms for heterogeneity correction, the use of appropriate margins, or the accounting of portal imaging dose) are in keeping with published and accepted data.

Treatment Delivery

High-dose prostate radiotherapy using conformal or IMRT techniques requires the monitoring of prostate position at the time of treatment delivery and adjusting the treatment parameters for accurate targeting. Several techniques are available to ensure accurate positioning for IGRT, including placement of fiducial markers, utilization of cone beam CT, and use of B-mode acquisition and targeting (BAT) system ultrasound. It is extremely important that one of these localization techniques be used as part of IGRT for prostate cancer in light of the tight margins employed to minimize the dose to normal tissue.

With hypofractionated radiotherapy, it is especially important to ensure acceptable dose distribution—particularly to normal tissue. With fewer treatments being given in hypofractionated regimens, inexact targeting of the tumor during radiotherapy for even one treatment has a larger impact on total dose delivered to the tumor than would be the case with conventional, more protracted radiotherapy involving more fractions. Suboptimal IGRT could potentially result in a higher proportion of geographic misses and consequent poorer tumor control. Conversely, the larger dose used for each treatment has the potential to produce more damage to normal tissue and thus more adverse effects to bladder and rectum, if treatment is not delivered as planned. For both these reasons, the importance of IGRT with hypofractionated regimens cannot be overemphasized.

THE FUTURE

Radiobiological principles indicate that doses per fraction beyond those employed in completed or ongoing trials warrant investigation. Fowler et al. used standard LQ modeling to determine a set of hypofractionated regimens that could be tested in randomized trials (1,11). Using data from dose-escalation studies, they developed a dose-response curve for biochemical control with bNED in intermediate-risk prostate cancer patients treated with external-beam radiotherapy alone given in conventional 2 Gy fractions. The investigators then went on to calculate the dose per fraction and total doses for regimens that would be predicted to have the same level of late toxicity as conventional radiotherapy, assuming that prostate tumors have an α/β ratio of 1.5 Gy and rectal tissue a ratio of 3 Gy (Fig. 3). The end result was a series of hypofractionated regimens that theoretically keep the rate of late complications constant while causing more damage to tumors as fraction size increases and the number of fractions decreases. Fowler et al. also considered the effect of each of the proposed hypofractionated regimens on prostate tumors by calculating the NTD, which is a measure of the total dose given in 2 Gy fractions that would give the equivalent biological effect to the hypofractionated regimen in question. For example, the effect of 60 Gy given as 20 fractions of 3 Gy corresponds to 77.1 Gy given in 2 Gy fractions. Ten fractions of 4.4 Gy should produce the same level of tumor control as 75.3 Gy given in 2 Gy fractions, but with the same late complication rate as 66 Gy in 2 Gy fractions. In the latter example, the estimated bNED would increase, in theory, from 51.6% to 77.1%. This hypothesized 25% increase in bNED could be tested against conventional radiotherapy in a randomized trial with only 72 participants in each arm. Fowler et al. warned against using treatment times of less than five weeks because of a possible risk of acute rectal toxicity, or treatments with fewer than five fractions, which might "limit the possibility of re-oxygenation or redistribution of tumor cells into more sensitive phases of cell cycles."

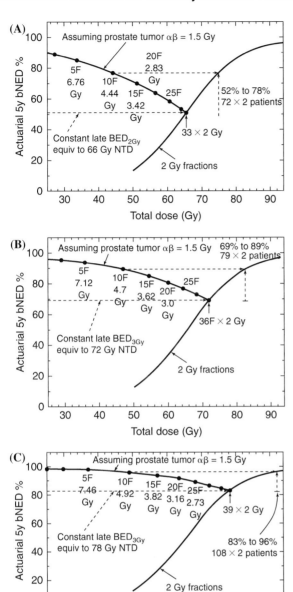

Figure 3 Estimated increase in bNED as total dose is decreased with fewer and larger fractions. Each of the three graphs shows the curve for 2 Gy rising to the right and another curve rising to the left for hypofractionated regimens with total doses calculated to keep late rectal complications constant at 66 Gy NTD$_{2Gy}$ (**A**), 72 Gy (**B**), and 78 Gy (**C**). The number of fractions and size of each fraction is noted for each point on the curve. *Abbreviations*: bNED, biochemical no evidence of disease; NTD, normalized total dose. *Source*: From Ref. 1.

Fowler's estimates show improved tumor control using some hypofractionated regimens compared to some conventional fractionation regimens, while maintaining equivalent late toxicity (1). For example, as shown in Figure 3B, there would be improved tumor control using a

regimen of either 20 fractions of 3 Gy or 10 fractions of 4.7 Gy, compared to 36 fractions of 2 Gy, while resulting in equivalent late toxicity. Other hypofractionation regimens and the impact on tumor control while maintaining the same level of late toxicity are also shown. On the basis of recent data, it would appear that 78 Gy in 2 Gy fractions is the preferred dose for intermediate-risk patients. The additional benefit, in terms of tumor control, of using hypofractionated regimens rather than conventionally fractionated treatment with a total dose of 78 Gy may not be as great as the benefit compared to lower doses such as 72 Gy in 2 Gy fractions. On the basis of Fowler's graphs, the change from 78 (2 Gy and 39 fractions) to 49.2 Gy (4.92 Gy and 10 fractions) would result in improvement in tumor control from 83% to 96%. In comparison, a change from 72 (2 Gy and 36 fractions) to 47 Gy (4.7 Gy in 10 fractions) would result in improvement in tumor control from 69% to 89%.

Current RCTs are evaluating hypofractionated regimens in the 2.5 to 3 Gy/fraction range. If these trials confirm the role of hypofractionated regimens, higher doses per fraction with fewer fractions—provided the overall treatment time is no shorter than five weeks—could be investigated. One would need to await the results of current and ongoing hypofractionated radiotherapy trials before embarking on the next generation of studies evaluating shorter, higher dose per fraction regimens. These regimens, which are based on radiobiological modeling, are interesting but would need to be carefully evaluated before they can be adopted as part of clinical practice. Phase I/II studies would be needed to confirm tolerability. If toxicity is found to be acceptable, these regimens then need to be compared with current standard treatments in well-conducted randomized trials. It is interesting to note that a phase III study has been proposed to compare 78 Gy (39 fractions of 2 Gy) to 42.7 Gy (7 fractions of 6.1 Gy in 4 weeks) (1). This regimen has a rectal-equivalent late-toxicity NTD$_{2Gy}$ of 78 Gy (assuming $\alpha/\beta = 3$ Gy), but the BED values show that the hypofractionated regimen (42.7 Gy in 7 fractions of 6.1 Gy) has a tumor-equivalent dose of 92.7 Gy in terms of NTD$_{2Gy}$ (assuming α/β ratio of 1.5 Gy for prostate cancer).

SUMMARY OF PERTINENT CONCLUSIONS

- Current high-dose treatments using 1.8 to 2 Gy fractions are more efficacious than doses used in the past and have acceptable toxicity.
- These conventional regimens may involve treatment in up to 39 fractions with associated social, emotional, and economic burdens for patients and their families. Use of these regimens has also increased the cost of treatment and increased the burden on stretched radiotherapy resources in some jurisdictions.

- Hypofractionated radiotherapy has potential advantages if found to be efficacious and to have acceptable toxicity compared to conventional radiotherapy.
- Radiobiological modeling suggests that hypofractionated prostatic radiotherapy may result in improved efficacy without increased toxicity.
- The α/β ratio for prostate cancer is likely between 0.9 and 1.5 Gy, whereas the α/β ratio is 3.0 Gy for late toxicity. This should make prostate cancer cells more sensitive to large dose fractions than to conventional fraction sizes.
- Well-designed randomized trials need to be conducted comparing hypofractionated regimens to conventionally fractionated high-dose regimens to assess their relative advantages and disadvantages.
- Early evidence suggests that efficacy and safety similar to that obtained with conventional fractionation schedules can be achieved with a shorter course of hypofractionated radiation treatment using 3DCRT and IMRT; however, the results of ongoing randomized trials are awaited.
- Ongoing and future studies need to confirm the role of hypofractionated radiotherapy in low-, intermediate-, and high-risk subgroups.
- Radiobiological principles suggest that doses per fraction beyond those employed in completed or ongoing trials warrant investigation.
- If the safety and efficacy of hypofractionated regimens are demonstrated, their adoption would reduce the burden of treatment for patients and their families, reduce the cost of radiotherapy treatments, and free up strained radiotherapy facilities in some jurisdictions.
- When hypofractionated regimens are used, conformal radiotherapy, and particularly, IMRT techniques require careful attention be paid to planning protocol: definition of tumor and organ-at-risk volumes, dose constraints, margins, method of heterogeneity corrections, dose grid resolution, and account of daily portal imaging dose.
- The normal tissue dose constraints need to be confirmed for particular hypofractionated regimens through clinical trials before use in patients off-study.
- The importance of IGRT with hypofractionated regimens cannot be overemphasized.

ACKNOWLEDGMENTS

The author wishes to thank Dr. Charles Catton, Dr. Rob Bristow, Dr. Orest Ostapiak, and Mary Johnston for assistance with the manuscript. The author also wishes to thank RTOG and OCOG (Ontario Clinical Oncology Group) for their assistance in providing details of the ongoing hypofractionation studies (0415 and PROFIT, respectively).

REFERENCES

1. Fowler JF. The radiobiology of prostate cancer including new aspects of fractionated radiotherapy. Acta Oncol 2005; 44(3):265–276.
2. Withers HR, McBride WH. Biologic basis of radiation therapy. In: Perez CA, Brady LW, eds. Principles and Practice of Radiation Oncology. 3rd ed. Philadelphia: Lippincott-Raven, 1997:79–118.
3. Hill RP, Rodemann HP, Hendry JH, et al. Normal tissue radiobiology: from the laboratory to the clinic. Int J Radiat Oncol Biol Phys 2001; 49(2):353–365.
4. Fowler J, Chappell R, Ritter M. Is alpha/beta for prostate tumors really low? Int J Radiat Oncol Biol Phys 2001; 50(4): 1021–1031.
5. Brenner DJ, Hall EJ. Fractionation and protraction for radiotherapy of prostate carcinoma. Int J Radiat Oncol Biol Phys 1999; 43(5):1095–1101.
6. Brenner DJ, Martinez AA, Edmundson GK, et al. Direct evidence that prostate tumors show high sensitivity to fractionation (low alpha/beta ratio), similar to late-responding normal tissue. Int J Radiat Oncol Biol Phys 2002; 52(1): 6–13.
7. Nahum AE, Movsas B, Horwitz EM, et al. Incorporating clinical measurements of hypoxia into tumor local control modeling of prostate cancer: implications for the alpha/beta ratio. Int J Radiat Oncol Biol Phys 2003; 57(2):391–401.
8. Orton CG. In regard: Incorporating clinical measurements of hypoxia into local tumor control modeling of prostate cancer. Int J Radiat Oncol Biol Phys 2004; 58(5):1637.
9. Nahum AE, Chapman JD. In response: Incorporating clinical measurements of hypoxia into local tumor control modeling of prostate cancer. Int J Radiat Oncol Biol Phys 2004; 58(5):1637–1639.
10. Lukka H, Hayter C, Julian JA, et al. Randomized trial comparing two fractionation schedules for patients with localized prostate cancer. J Clin Oncol 2005; 23(25):6132–6138.
11. Fowler JF, Ritter MA, Chappell RJ, et al. What hypofractionated protocols should be tested for prostate cancer? Int J Radiat Oncol Biol Phys 2003; 56(4):1093–1104.
12. Heemsbergen WD, Peeters ST, Koper PC, et al. Acute and late gastrointestinal toxicity after radiotherapy in prostate cancer patients: consequential late damage. Int J Radiat Oncol Biol Phys 2006; 66(1):3–10.
13. Zelefsky MJ, Fuks Z, Hunt M, et al. High-dose intensity modulated radiation therapy for prostate cancer: early toxicity and biochemical outcome in 772 patients. Int J Radiat Oncol Biol Phys 2002; 53(5):1111–1116.
14. Sood B, Garg M, Avadhani J, et al. Predictive value of linear-quadratic model in the treatment of cervical cancer using high-dose-rate brachytherapy. Int J Radiat Oncol Biol Phys 2002; 54(5):1377–1387.
15. American Society for Therapeutic Radiology and Oncology Consensus Panel, . Consensus Statement: guidelines for PSA following radiation therapy. Int J Radiat Oncol Biol Phys 1997; 37(5):1035–1041.
16. Pickles T, Kim-Sing C, Morris WJ, et al. Evaluation of the Houston biochemical relapse definition in men treated with prolonged neoadjuvant and adjuvant androgen ablation and

assessment of follow-up lead-time bias. Int J Radiat Oncol Biol Phys 2003; 57(1):11–18.

17. Pickles T, Duncan GG, Kim-sing C, et al. PSA relapse definitions—the Vancouver Rules show superior predictive power. Int J Radiat Oncol Biol Phys 1999; 43(3):699–700.

18. Roach M III, Hanks G, Thames H Jr., et al. Defining biochemical failure following radiotherapy with or without hormonal therapy in men with clinically localized prostate cancer: recommendations of the RTOG-ASTRO Phoenix Consensus Conference. Int J Radiat Oncol Biol Phys 2006; 65(4):965–974.

19. Pollack A, Zagars GK, Starkschall G, et al. Prostate cancer radiation dose response: results of the M. D. Anderson phase III randomized trial. Int J Radiat Oncol Biol Phys 2002; 53(5):1097–1105.

20. Zietman AL, DeSilvio ML, Slater JD, et al. Comparison of conventional-dose vs high-dose conformal radiation therapy in clinically localized adenocarcinoma of the prostate: a randomized controlled trial. JAMA 2005; 294(10):1233–1239.

21. Dearnaley DP, Hall E, Lawrence D, et al. Phase III pilot study of dose escalation using conformal radiotherapy in prostate cancer: PSA control and side effects. Br J Cancer 2005; 92(3):488–498.

22. Peeters ST, Heemsbergen WD, Koper PC, et al. Dose-response in radiotherapy for localized prostate cancer: results of the Dutch multicenter randomized phase III trial comparing 68 Gy of radiotherapy with 78 Gy. J Clin Oncol 2006; 24(13):1990–1996.

23. van der Wielen GJ, van Putten WL, Incrocci L. Sexual function after three-dimensional conformal radiotherapy for prostate cancer: results from a dose-escalation trial. Int J Radiat Oncol Biol Phys 2007; 68(2):479–484.

24. Beckendorf V, Guerif S, Le Prise E, et al. The GETUG 70 Gy vs. 80 Gy randomized trial for localized prostate cancer: feasibility and acute toxicity. Int J Radiat Oncol Biol Phys 2004; 60(4):1056–1065.

25. Available at: http://clinicaltrials.gov/ct/show/NCT00010244?order=1. Accessed March, 2008.

26. Available at: http://www.rtog.org/members/protocols/0126/p0126.pdf. Accessed March, 2008.

27. Duncan W, Warde P, Catton CN, et al. Carcinoma of the prostate: results of radical radiotherapy (1970-1985). Int J Radiat Oncol Biol Phys 1993; 26(2):203–210.

28. Preston CI, Duncan W, Kerr GR. Radical treatment of prostatic carcinoma by megavoltage X-ray therapy. Clin Radiol 1986; 37(5):473–477.

29. Kearsley JH. High-dose radiotherapy for localized prostatic cancer. An analysis of treatment results and early complications. Med J Aust 1986; 144(12):624–628.

30. Read G, Pointon RC. Retrospective study of radiotherapy in early carcinoma of the prostate. Br J Urol 1989; 63(2):191–195.

31. Jones DA, Eckert H, Smith PJ. Radical radiotherapy in the management of carcinoma of the prostate. Br J Urol 1982; 54(6):732–735.

32. Livsey JE, Cowan RA, Wylie JP, et al. Hypofractionated conformal radiotherapy in carcinoma of the prostate:

five-year outcome analysis. Int J Radiat Oncol Biol Phys 2003; 57(5):1254–1259.

33. Kupelian PA, Thakkar VV, Khuntia D, et al. Hypofractionated intensity-modulated radiotherapy (70 Gy at 2.5 Gy per fraction) for localized prostate cancer: long-term outcomes. Int J Radiat Oncol Biol Phys 2005; 63(5):1463–1468.

34. Wallace K, Haycocks T, Alasti H, et al. Hypofractionated intensity modulated radiation therapy (IMRT) for localized prostate cancer. Radiother Oncol 2003, 69 (suppl 1):S36 (abstr).

35. Martin JM, Rosewall T, Bayley A, et al. Phase II trial of hypofractionated image-guided intensity-modulated radiotherapy for localized prostate adenocarcinoma. Int J Radiat Oncol Biol Phys. 2007; 69(4):1084–1089.

36. Whelan T, MacKenzie R, Julian J, et al. Randomized trial of breast irradiation schedules after lumpectomy for women with lymph node-negative breast cancer. J Natl Cancer Inst 2002; 94(15):1143–1150.

37. Yeoh EE, Fraser RJ, McGowan RE, et al. Evidence for efficacy without increased toxicity of hypofractionated radiotherapy for prostate carcinoma: early results of a phase III randomized trial. Int J Radiat Oncol Biol Phys 2003; 55(4):943–955.

38. Yeoh EE, Holloway RH, Fraser RJ, et al. Hypofractionated versus conventionally fractionated radiation therapy for prostate carcinoma: updated results of a phase III randomized trial. Int J Radiat Oncol Biol Phys 2006; 66(4):1072–1083.

39. Pollack A, Hanlon AL, Horwitz EM, et al. Dosimetry and preliminary acute toxicity in the first 100 men treated for prostate cancer on a randomized hypofractionation dose escalation trial. Int J Radiat Oncol Biol Phys 2006; 64(2):518–526.

40. Available at: http://www.clinicaltrials.gov/ct/show/NCT00062309?order¼1. Accessed March, 2008.

41. Available at: http://www.clinicaltrials.gov/ct/show/NCT00062309?order¼1. Accessed March, 2008.

42. Available at: http://www.clinicaltrials.gov/ct/show/NCT00392535?order¼1. Accessed March, 2008.

43. South C, Naismith O, Clark C, et al. A randomised pilot study of high dose hypofractionated conformal radiotherapy in localised prostate cancer. Annual Report. Radiotherapy Physics Team (Chelsea), 2005. Available at: http://www.icr.ac.uk/research/research_sections/physics/5507.pdf. Accessed April 2007.

44. Available at: http://www.clinicaltrials.gov/ct/show/NCT00331773?order¼1. Accessed March, 2008.

45. Available at: http://www.rtog.org/members/protocols/0415/0415.pdf. Accessed March, 2008.

46. Damaraju S, Murray D, Dufour J, et al. Association of DNA repair and steroid metabolism gene polymorphisms with clinical late toxicity in patients treated with conformal radiotherapy for prostate cancer. Clin Cancer Res 2006; 12 (8):2545–2554.

47. Dearnaley DP, Khoo VS, Norman AR, et al. Comparison of radiation side-effects of conformal and conventional radiotherapy in prostate cancer: a randomised trial. Lancet 1999; 353(9149):267–272.

18

Image-Guided Proton Beam Radiation Therapy for Prostate Cancer

CARLOS E. VARGAS, JATINDER R. PALTA, DANIEL INDELICATO, AND ZUOFENG LI

Department of Radiation Oncology, University of Florida, Proton Therapy Institute, Jacksonville, Florida, U.S.A.

INTRODUCTION

Advances in technology and understanding of tumor characteristics have improved our ability to provide patients with better treatments and minimized side effects. However, these changes so far have been largely confined to realm of ionizing electromagnetic wave radiation. In this manner, radiation oncology has progressed from two-dimensional (2-D), 3-D, intensity-modulated radiation therapy (IMRT), image-guided radiation therapy (IGRT), to adaptive radiation therapy. Improved conformality is an extension of our increased ability to shape the high-dose area within the patient. We recognize, however, that our target will often vary in position, shape, or even volume during the course of therapy. Different strategies have evolved to address this problem, including image-guided radiation, consisting of daily target localization and methods of patient-specific treatment planning, so-called "adaptive radiotherapy."

Similar to conventional radiotherapy, proton therapy has to incorporate the principles of image guidance and adaptive therapy to optimize the therapeutic ratio. This is particularly true in prostate cancer, where the large interfraction positional variation makes image guidance critical.

OVERVIEW OF PROTON THERAPY AND IMAGE GUIDANCE

A comprehensive review of current proton therapy applications is beyond the scope of this chapter. However, to provide a framework of proton issues specific to prostate cancer, we will introduce some key general elements of proton therapy planning and delivery.

Proton therapy is particulate ionizing radiation. Like any charged particle, protons have a characteristic Bragg peak at the end of their ionization track. Because of their large mass (1.6726×10^{-27} kg), protons follow a relatively linear path through tissue, which allows for easier dosimetry than electrons and a predictable Bragg peak position. Basically, a proton will start depositing its energy as soon as it enters tissue but will deposit the majority of the energy at the end of its trajectory (Fig. 1). The range or the most distal penetration of the proton beam in a patient is determined by the energy of proton beam, which is continuously variable. The proton energy and spread-out Bragg peak (SOBP) are selected to cover the entire thickness of the target along the beam axis. The result is a highly homogenous dose distribution within the target as well as a sharp dose falloff beyond the target. The use of fewer beams decreases the integral dose with a

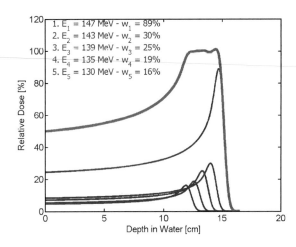

Figure 1 Diagram representing proton beam spread-out Bragg peak. *Source*: UFPTI beam data.

minimal impact on target coverage. This provides an advantage over photon therapy, where the high-dose gradient area can only be shaped with multiple beam angles, therefore increasing the low-dose volume.

Proton therapy, with its huge potential, is in its infancy. The state-of-the-art in proton therapy is to deliver proton beams that are termed as scattered proton beams. These require the fabrication of patient-specific bolus material and apertures. Even though these beams spare a significant amount of normal tissue compared with X-ray radiation therapy, they do not provide very conformal radiation dose to the tumor. Specific limitations of proton therapy are because of the differences in the creation of the high-dose gradient. For IMRT, multiple beams and segments will shape high dose to the target, relatively independent of tissues transverse. For proton therapy, each beam will create a high-dose area that will be defined by the changes in stopping power over the path of the incident proton. Thus, the target itself will help define the high-dose gradient area and changes in the tissues transverse will have a large impact on SOBP localization. For this reason, the beam angles for image-guided proton therapy must be carefully selected. For example, in prostate cancer, anterior or posterior beams, where the radiological path length may dramatically vary, are avoided. The result is treatment plans limited to lateral or lateral oblique fields. This constraint is defined by the physical properties of the particle and will not vary with proton delivery technique such as double scattering, uniform scanning, and intensity-modulated proton therapy (IMPT). The first problem can be summarized as the limitation in the beams angles that can be employed for optimal results with minimal delivery uncertainty.

The second problem is related to the smearing function. To assure target coverage, each beam plan has to be optimized to cover the target (i.e., the prostate). Each

voxel in the prostate must be expanded to a radius equivalent to the potential target motion during an image-guided approach. This information, although not used to define target size per se, is used to define the range necessary to cover distal edge of the target as the beam is realigned for each new prostate position. In other words, it represents a convex hull of all potential prostate positions encountered during treatment. The outcome is distal high-dose edge that is less conformal compared to the shape of the prostate at the time of simulation. The practical result is that improved target coverage from an image-guided approach will be limited if it is based on the initial prostate position alone.

A third problem is related to uncertainty in correlating CT numbers to the stopping power in CT-based proton treatment planning. The practical implications are that the distal and proximal margins have to be increased to provide adequate target coverage. One result is that adequate target coverage will necessarily decrease the conformality index. Another implication is that the Bragg peak cannot be stopped in front of a dose-limiting structure if it is the only beam employed or if it has a disproportional high weight among multiple beams. Thus, with improper plan design, the use of the sharp edge of the Bragg peak to limit the dose to the rectum or bladder may lead to a completely opposite result.

Currently, delivering proton therapy has been looked upon as a problem of degrading a pristine Bragg peak and pencil beam such that it becomes a clinically useful broad field. However, a narrow pencil beam, with a near mono-energetic Bragg peak, can be viewed as a single "spot" of dose, well confined in three dimensions. If it were possible to dynamically position such Bragg peaks in three dimensions throughout the target volume, then it would be possible to use this dose spot to "paint" the dose to the target as required. This is the idea behind the active scanning approach to proton therapy, which is now gaining a certain amount of popularity within the proton therapy community. With active scanning techniques, the concept of an SOBP, a central component of the passive scattering approach, is abandoned. Instead, it relies on its ability to individually place and weight spots with full flexibility, and under computer control. From the treatment planning aspect, this requires algorithms for determining the optimal weight of each Bragg peak in three dimensions.

Active scanning can be accomplished by either mechanical or magnetic means, or a combination of the two. Through computer steering, it is possible to position a Bragg peak anywhere in three dimensions within the target volume. In addition, it is also necessary to be able to individually modulate the dose delivered at each Bragg peak. As with most dynamic delivery systems, the dose at any given point is controlled by the length of time a spot dwells at each position, with the number of delivered protons being controlled by a fast monitor just before the patient. Once the desired number of monitor units has been delivered, the beam at this point is switched off using a fast magnetic deflection of the beam away from the treatment room. This fast switching off of the beam is an important aspect of the spot scanning method where the beam is switched off when the steering elements are being altered, and is only applied to the patient when all elements are stable.

We believe that we have only scratched the surface of possible technologies with protons to improve outcomes for patients. Through the development of IMPT, we should be able to deliver highly conformal radiation to the tumor while sparing the healthy normal tissue. IMPT will rival any advanced technology–based conventional radiation therapy treatment. The full potential advantage of proton therapy can be realized only if, uncertainties in the localization of the distal dose gradient region in the patient because of uncertainties in the dose calculation, biological considerations, setup and anatomical variations, and internal movement of high-density/low-density organs in the beam are minimized. Therefore, image/dose guidance, managing inter-/intraorgan motion and its effects, and minimizing residual uncertainties are essential for proton therapy. In this chapter, we describe our strategy to deal with these issues in the treatment of prostate cancer with proton beam.

RECOGNIZING RECTAL ANATOMY

Proton therapy can achieve a conformal dose distribution with one or two beam angles, but optimizing beam arrangements is crucial. For prostate cancer, we employ lateral oblique field arrangements, which provide clear access to the prostate and maximize sparing of the dose-limiting normal structures. As mentioned earlier, in the first problem, the limitation of useful beam angles and the ability to create highly conformal plans is also an oppor-

tunity. If the anatomy can be optimized for those limited angles, the doses to the normal structures can be minimal.

A rectal balloon (RB) has the theoretical advantage of distending the rectal wall and displacing it from the high-dose area anteriorly (1–5). It therefore decreases the relative volume of rectum or rectal wall radiated to intermediate and high doses. For photon therapy, it also has the relative advantage of increasing the rectal air volume and decreasing the dose at the inner rectal wall (5). Although an RB may likewise decrease the relative volume of the rectum or rectal wall radiated in proton therapy, this may provide only a small absolute advantage because of the low rectal doses being delivered. Furthermore, for proton therapy water is used in the RB to better control the proton dose distribution and decrease inhomogeneities because of the air-tissue interface. Thus, proton therapy will not necessarily have the additional advantage of decreasing the inner rectal wall dose seen with photons in the build-up region. However, water alone in the rectum may adequately distend the rectal wall during the course of proton therapy and obviate the need for an actual balloon.

We do not routinely use an RB for our prostate proton plans. As mentioned above, the absolute benefit of an RB may be clinically insignificant when low rectal doses are already achieved through highly conformal radiation. Vargas et al. reported only 9% grade 2 or higher rectal toxicity and 0.8% grade 3 toxicity if the rectal dose V70 was below 25% (6). In our study, only 17.5% of the rectum received 50 Gray Equivalent (GE) and 10.2% received 70 GE. At these V50 and V70 parameters, a respective 4.7% and 2.7% absolute benefit was observed with an RB. Furthermore, the RB will not modify the shape of the dose-volume curve; it will only shift it. As a result, the relative benefit, although similar at different dose levels (V10–V80), will be associated with a constantly decreasing real benefit (Tables 2–4).

In a detailed analysis of the topic, we found a significant benefit for the use of RB only in selected cases (Table 1 and Fig. 2). A relative improvement greater than

Table 1 Statistically Significant Dose-Volume Parameters for the Rectum ($n = 30$ scans)

	RB mean (SD) (%)	Water alone mean (SD) (%)	p value	Absolute difference (%)
Rectum V10	29.7 (7.4)	37.7 (10.3)	0.02	8.0
Rectum V20	24.6 (6.8)	31.7 (9.0)	0.02	7.1
Rectum V30	20.9 (6.0)	27.2 (8.0)	0.02	6.3
Rectum V40	17.9 (5.3)	23.3 (7.2)	0.03	5.4
Rectum V50	15.0 (4.7)	19.7 (6.2)	0.03	4.7
Rectum V60	12.2 (3.9)	16.0 (5.4)	0.04	3.8
Rectum V65	10.6 (3.9)	14.2 (5.0)	0.04	3.6
Rectum V70	8.8 (3.5)	11.5 (4.4)	0.07	2.7

Abbreviations: RB, rectal balloon; SD, standard deviation.

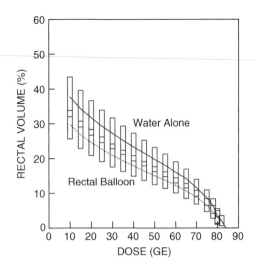

Figure 2 Line-dose graph for all rectal dose-volume parameters between V10–V82 with RB or water alone (*n* – 30). The boxes represent 95% standard error. *Abbreviation*: RB, rectal balloon.

5% at V50 was seen in 5 of 15 cases [9.2 ± 2.3% compared to 2.4 ± 1.3% for the remainder 10 cases ($p < 0.001$)]. For these same five cases, the improvement at 70 Gy persisted: 5.8 ± 2.2% compared to 1.2 ± 1.8% ($p < 0.001$). For the remaining cases, however, the difference between water alone versus an RB was less than 1% or even had a detrimental effect. Thus, patient selection is critical in realizing the role of an RB in proton radiotherapy.

We found that best predictor of an RB benefit is a sagittal view of the patient on imaging as seen in Figure 3. Specifically, we found the following three reference details to be useful in our decision: (*i*) The posterior rectal wall at the prostate level should be displaced posteriorly; (*ii*) If present, the rectal wall-prostate interface space

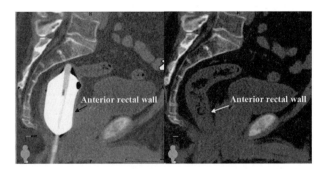

Figure 3 Sagittal projection of the planning volumetric CT-scan with RB (*left*) and with water alone (*right*). The plane between the anterior rectal wall and the prostate is lost with the RB and no posterior rectal displacement was seen. This patient did not benefit from an RB. *Abbreviation*: RB, rectal balloon.

should be preserved; and (*iii*) In intermediate- or high-risk cases, the proximal seminal vesicles should not saddle around the rectum. If all three criteria are met, the patient will likely benefit from an RB instead of water alone.

DECREASING DOSE TO NORMAL STRUCTURES

The physical and biological properties of proton therapy are desirable for many reasons (7). In addition to reducing dose to normal structures through strategic placement of the Bragg peak, protons have a biological effect similar to photons, and therefore familiar tumoricidal doses and normal tissue dose constraints can be employed (8,9). In the past, radiation doses have been limited because of the risk of chronic rectal and bladder toxicity (10–19). Proton therapy has been proposed as a means to deliver elevated doses while limiting potential toxicity to normal surrounding structures (20–25).

Cella et al. contrasted IMRT, double-scattered protons, and IMPT; however, only one case was analyzed and the IMRT and double-scattered proton plans were not actually designed for treatment purposes (26). This could have biased the IMRT plans over the double-scattered proton plan. In that study, the double-scattered proton therapy rectal dose-volume curve was superior to the IMRT plan to doses up to 60 GE or 75% of the prescribed dose; beyond this point, however, IMRT had lower doses to the rectum. For the bladder, the dose-volume curves for proton therapy and IMRT crossed over twice making interpretation difficult. Zhang et al. published the results for 10 patients treated with IMRT and created 10 companion double-scattered proton plans for retrospective analysis (27). They found that the rectal dose-volume curves favored proton therapy in the low-dose range but after a dose of 40 Gy, or 50% of the target dose, IMRT achieved a better rectal dose distribution. For the bladder dose, they found a similar proton advantage in the low-dose region (<50%) after which both curves basically overlapped. Trofimov et al. found comparable rectal dose with IMRT or proton therapy (28). Furthermore, they found lower bladder doses with IMRT at V60 and higher.

In contrast to the previous studies, we were able to demonstrate statistically significant improvements for rectal dose-volume parameters in the low-, intermediate- and high-dose areas as seen in Figure 4. This translated into a 59% improvement in the rectal mean dose over IMRT (Table 2). For the bladder, the improvement was smaller but nonetheless translated into a 35% relative decrease in the mean dose (Table 3) and curves suggested a benefit up to a dose of 65 GE (Fig. 5). The greater benefit seen in our study is likely because of the independent optimization of dose distribution, beam angle, and aperture margins for

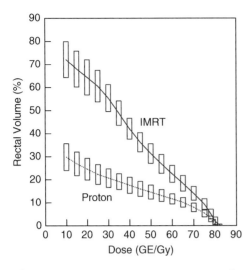

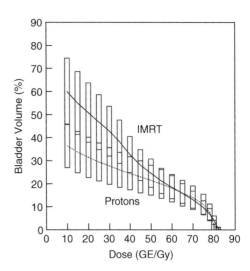

Figure 4 Combined rectal dose-volume curves for proton therapy and IMRT (*n* = 20 plans) (error box shows 95% SE). *Abbreviations*: RB, rectal balloon; IMRT, intensity-modulated radiation therapy.

Figure 5 Combined bladder dose-volume curves for proton therapy and IMRT (*n* = 20 plans) (error box shows 95% SE). *Abbreviation*: IMRT, intensity-modulated radiation therapy.

each beam combined with our compensator design. The penumbra and dose homogeneity observed in our prostate plans could also play an important role. Since our prostate technique uses lateral oblique beam arrangements, the ability to treat the target volume with small margins from planning tumor volume (PTV) to aperture (block) edge

significantly decreased our dose to surrounding dose-limiting normal structures as seen in Figure 6. Thus, for our proton plans, the distance of the 98% isodose line (IDL) to the 80% IDL was 4.4 mm for a 4.5% dose falloff per millimeter in the posterior rectal aspect compared to 5.5 mm for our IMRT plans. Although the initial dose

Table 2 Percent Volume of the Rectum Receiving Doses Between 10 GE/Gy to 80 GE/Gy and Mean Dose (*n* = 20 plans)

	Protons (SD) (%)	IMRT (SD) (%)	*p* value	Relative benefit (%)	Absolute benefit (%)
Rectum V10	29.8 (5.6)	72.1 (7.6)	<0.001	58.7	42.3
Rectum V30	20.7 (3.9)	55.4 (5.7)	<0.001	62.7	34.7
Rectum V50	14.6 (3.0)	31.3 (4.1)	<0.001	53.4	16.7
Rectum V70	7.9 (1.8)	14.0 (2.9)	<0.001	43.6	6.1
Rectum V78	2.9 (1.2)	5.0 (1.2)%	0.01	42.0	2.1
Rectum V80	0.1 (0.3)	1.8 (1.8)	0.01	94.4	1.7
Rectum mean dose	14.2 (3.7) GE	34.8 (3.0) Gy	<0.001	59.2	20.1 GE/Gy

Abbreviations: IMRT, intensity-modulated radiation therapy; SD, standard deviation.

Table 3 Percent Volume of the Bladder Receiving Doses Between 10 GE/Gy to 80 GE/Gy and Mean Dose (*n* = 20 plans)

	Protons (SD) (%)	IMRT (SD) (%)	*p* value	Relative benefit (%)	Absolute benefit (%)
Bladder V10	36.4 (13.2)	60.0 (20.1)	0.007	39.3	23.6
Bladder V20	31.4 (12.1)	50.8 (18.0)	0.01	38.2	19.4
Bladder V30	27.7 (11.1)	42.8 (15.1)	0.02	35.3	15.1
Bladder V35	26.0 (10.6)	38.2 (13.2)	0.04	31.9	12.2
Bladder mean dose	18.4 (6.2) GE	28.4 (9.4) Gy	0.01	35.2	10.0

Abbreviations: IMRT, intensity-modulated radiation therapy; SD, standard deviation.

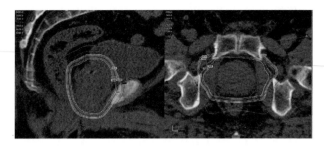

Figure 6 Sagittal (*left*) and axial (*right*) projection for the same patient as in Figure 1 including IDLs with water alone. The green line represents the 50% IDL that includes less than half the rectal circumference. *Abbreviation*: IDL, isodose line.

falloff is similar between IMRT and proton plans, the gradient beyond this region is where the advantage of proton therapy is most evident: With our proton plan, the distance between the 80% to the 20% IDL was only 7 to 9 mm in the posterior rectal aspect. This is in contrast to the >2 cm falloff seen in an optimized IMRT plan. With similar target doses of 79.2 GE at Massachusetts General Hospital (MGH) and 78 GE at out institution, the rectum V50 was 34.4% versus 31.3%, rectum V70 14.5% versus 14.0%, rectum mean dose 39.4 GE versus 33.2 GE, bladder V50 23.7% versus 25%; bladder V70 11.4% versus 14%; and bladder mean dose 29.9 GE and 28.4 GE, respectively. Overall, the doses to normal tissues for the MGH IMRT plans and our IMRT plans were similar with minor variations. Since doses to normal structures were similar for the different IMRT plans, we have concluded that the relative advantage in overall dosimetry is related to the steep gradients achieved with proton therapy.

IMAGE GUIDANCE FOR PROTON TREATMENTS

Interfraction prostate motion has been an area of major concern over the last few years in prostate cancer therapy (29–34). Large variations in daily prostate position have been described in various studies (29,30,32,34). Furthermore, studies have found a poor correlation between the location of the prostate and skin marks or bony anatomy (33,35). Ultrasound systems cannot reliably define the daily prostate position (32,33). As a result, when daily treatment setup is based on skin marks, bony anatomy, or ultrasound guidance, large margins are necessary to ensure accurate delivery of the prescribed dose (30,32,33). Several different approaches have been used in an attempt to solve the problem of prostate motion and to reduce treatment margins. Yan et al. used multiple CT scans to define prostate motion and electronic daily

images to quantify setup inaccuracies (34). They were able to derive patient-specific margins through an off-line adaptive process. PTV size was greatly reduced when compared with margin definition via class solution. A second approach, online image guidance, relies on daily information to derive the daily prostate position (30,32,33,35,36). Different approaches have been used including cone-beam CT, CT-on-rails, fiducial markers, or beacon transponders (29,30,32,33,35–39). The accuracy of these systems relies on the accuracy of the measurement and the appropriate patient translation adjustments in relation to the treatment machine isocenter. We have adopted the use of Visicoils as fiducial markers in conjunction with orthogonal X-rays. Excellent spatial resolution is possible. Fiducial displacement is minimal and thus permits a reproducible and reliable strategy for prostate positioning.

There are fundamental differences between IMRT and proton therapy treatment plans. With IMRT, the confluence of multiple beam segments arranged into five to seven beam angle directions create a high-dose area. The movement of this high-dose area will have small repercussions in the dose and shape of this high-dose area. Thus, for image guidance, few modifications are necessary when implementing an IMRT plan. For proton therapy the same is not true. First and foremost, variations in the tissues traversed by the beam path will have large repercussions in the shape and position of the proton high-dose gradient. Second, variation in the shape of the surface and relative distance changes secondary to variable external anatomy will have large impacts in the treatment plan. Thus, the plan should be modified to account for these variations, but more importantly, certain beam angles should be avoided. A proton plan should be evaluated in the light of the movements of the patients' external contours, internal organs, and prostate position. In summary, image-guided proton plans should not be evaluated on the basis of a single static target position; instead plans should be optimized and evaluated on the basis of the ability of maintaining target coverage for various different prostate positions encountered during the course of therapy.

Practical experience and plan evaluations has shown us that anterior, posterior, or lateral oblique beams more than 20° from horizontal should not be employed for double scattered, uniform scanning, or IMPT for prostate cancer unless daily cone-beam CTs can be performed and immediate range variations can be utilized. Bladder filling or rectal filling will vary from day to day modifying the radiological path length of the beam. Therefore, a particular beam can underdose the target, and more importantly, increase the dose to the rectum and bladder. Furthermore, since every radiobiology paper for proton therapy has found an increased relative biological effectiveness (RBE) at the end of the beam path, the dose-volume histogram

(DVH) advantage of a sharp distal Bragg peak falloff may be outweighed by a 10% to 30% increase in the RBE at the beam's distal margin. Another reason we generally avoid anterior and posterior beam arrangements is because the variability of the stopping power can affect the distal range for any given beam. Each beam utilized should have an additional proximal and distal margin to account for stopping power variability. Thus, a target volume that should stop at the surface of the rectum may need to extend a few millimeters into the rectum, thereby increasing the rectal dose. Furthermore, if daily prostate depth cannot be strictly maintained, the distal edge of the beam will have to take into account potential variations in prostate depth. The variability in prostate position from day to day and during each fraction will mandate that the distal margin of the beam is extended even further into the rectum.

For our institutional image-guided approach, we use a distal and proximal edge margin between 5 and 9 mm as defined by the distance between the 98% IDL and the PTV. Alternately, a general formula [(target distance $\times$ 0.018) + 2 mm] can be employed. We chose to use both the formula and IDL as a reference because we found variations in the distance to the distal edge are relatively small for our prostate patient population. However, larger variations can be seen because of bone density differences and cortical thickening across the PTV that cannot be completely characterized by a general formula for individual patients. In employing the IDL reference and the formula we can use the average calculated distance [(25 cm $\times$ 0.018) + 2 mm] and customize it for the individual patient, adding additional margin when necessary; ultimately, our minimal distal or proximal margin is 5 mm. Our calculations in water phantoms have demonstrated excellent agreement (2%) with our predicted beam profiles.

Our approach to smearing has been also based on the objectives of our image guidance approach. Smearing is an expansion of the each voxel perpendicular to the beam angle to accommodate for variation in target position and/or depth. The smearing margin was constructed based on the following formula:

$$\text{Smearing margin} = \sqrt{(\text{TM})^2 + [(\text{TD} + 2\,\text{mm}) \times 0.03]^2},$$

where TM = target motion, TD = target distance.

Our formula accounts for the TM between fractions, and to a lesser extent, intrafraction motion. The distal target position averages 25 cm with an additional 2 mm compensator thickness at the point of maximum depth. No modifications were made for setup error since with image guidance the residual setup error at our institution has been measured to be 0.3 mm (y), 0.15 mm (x), and 0.03 (z) mm. The resulting radius will be 18.8 mm. For practical purposes, the smearing margin will allow for an image-guidance approach equal to the smearing minus the residual error of the image-guided approach.

Proton radiation dose distribution relies more on tissue stopping power characteristics than IMRT. The depth of each individual Bragg peak, and therefore the resulting SOBP, depends on the energy of the beam and its interaction with tissue (40). As previously mentioned, the SOBP position will vary if changes occur in the proton stopping power of the tissues along the beam path. This raises the question of whether daily image-guided beam realignment can be safely implemented in proton therapy to account for physiological inter- and intrafraction target displacement from original simulation (41). Specifically, if the beam is realigned relative to a new target position, the beam path will likely include different bony and soft tissue structures. Changes in prostate dose with defined changes in prostate position are important in developing treatment strategies for proton therapy. For our treatments, we prescribe a minimum dose to the PTV of 74.1 GE and prescribe 78 GE to cover 95% of the PTV. Thus, the doses within the PTV are not completely homogeneous, and different clinical target volume (CTV) positions within the PTV may have different minimum doses and prescribed dose coverage.

As a result, we may face a fundamental paradox when we use image guidance for proton therapy: In attempting to deliver a more accurate radiation dose, is it possible that we compromise target coverage through realignment of proton beam positions? For the purpose of answering this question, we quantified CTV coverage for several prostate cancer patients on the basis of the initial plan compared with different target CTV locations. To fully evaluate the differences of dose distribution inside the PTV and outside the PTV, we repositioned the prostate employing unidirectional vectors of 5 and 10 mm, and multidirectional vectors of 10 mm.

Our data for alignment with motion within the PTV are shown in Table 4. With beam realignment, target coverage increased, and the entire CTV received the prescribed dose. Even without beam realignment, however, coverage greater than or equal to 99% was seen regardless of the direction of the vector of motion, when displacements were within the PTV expansion. The minimum prostate dose was decreased by a maximum of only 1.6 GE. This difference, although statistically significant, is likely not clinically relevant (Fig. 7). These findings suggest that small intrafraction motions accounted for in the PTV expansion will have negligible impact on dose delivered to the prostate with proton therapy.

Our data for alignment with motion outside the PTV is shown in Table 5. Moderate changes in coverage and minimum CTV dose were observed in the absence of

Table 4 Prostate (CTV) Coverage With and Without Image Guidance for CTV Movements Within the PTV (5 mm)

	No image guidance (SD)	Image guidance (SD)	p value
5-mm anterior			
Prostate V78 (%)	99.6% (0.5)%	100% (0.03)%	0.04
Prostate minimum dose	76.52 (1.17) GE	78.15 (0.27) GE	0.001
5-mm inferior			
Prostate V78 (%)	99.6% (0.5)%	100% (0.03)%	0.04
Prostate minimum dose	78.03 (0.34) GE	78.19 (0.23) GE	0.3
5-mm posterior			
Prostate V78 (%)	99.4% (0.8)%	100% (0.007)%	0.05
Prostate minimum dose	76.75 (1.49) GE	78.29 (0.30) GE	0.008
5-mm superior			
Prostate V78 (%)	99.9% (0.02)%	100% (0.004)%	0.2
Prostate minimum dose	78.10 (0.30) GE	78.27 (0.32) GE	0.3

Abbreviations: CTV, clinical target volume; PTV, planning tumor volume; SD, standard deviation.

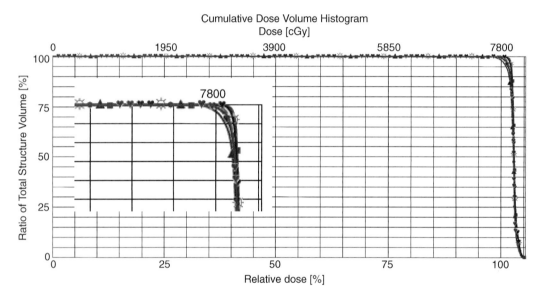

Figure 7 Dose-volume curves for 5 mm prostate shifts with (▲ ☼ ● ■) and without (♥) beam realignment. The curves for all prostate positions overlap each other, regardless of whether beam realignment was utilized.

Table 5 Prostate (CTV) Coverage With and Without Image Guidance for CTV Movements Outside the PTV (10 mm)

	No image guidance	Image guidance	p value
10-mm inferior			
Prostate V78 (%)	96.5% (1.2)%	100% (0.1)%	<0.001
Prostate minimum dose	72.47 GE (0.90) GE	78.07 GE (0.27) GE	<0.001
10-mm posterior			
Prostate V78 (%)	89.8% (3.9)%	100% (0.1)%	<0.001
Prostate minimum dose	64.75 GE (5.90) GE	78.31 GE (0.53) GE	<0.001
10 mm superior			
Prostate V78 (%)	94.4% (2.0)%	100% (0.3)%	<0.001
Prostate minimum dose	72.78 GE (0.70) GE	78.28 (0.41) GE	<0.001

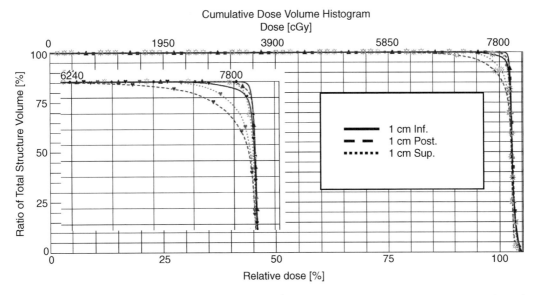

Figure 8 Dose-volume curves for 10 mm prostate shifts with (▲ ○ ●) and without (♥) beam realignment. Moderate improvements and high target coverage are seen with beam repositioning.

beam realignment. Clinically and statistically significant improvements in CTV coverage were seen with image-guided beam realignment (Fig. 8). Coverage was 99.9% or better with beam realignment, and the minimum dose to the CTV was similar to the initial plan. These findings suggest that beam realignment is necessary for target displacement greater than accounted for by the PTV expansion, but that the impact of minor changes in the length and composition of the proton beam path are likely accounted for using the smearing approach utilized in our treatment planning protocol.

Prostate displacements of 10 mm in the three axes are often seen with both inter- and intrafraction prostate motion. Our data regarding 10 mm multidirectional target displacement is seen in Table 6, which characterizes changes in dosimetry related to CTV position, with and without beam realignment. As illustrated, significant changes in mean, minimum, and maximum dose, as well as overall CTV coverage are noted without image-guided beam realignment (Fig. 9). CTV coverage improved considerably with beam realignment for most displacements.

Table 6 Prostate (CTV) Coverage With and Without Image Guidance for CTV Movements Compounding Inter- and Intrafraction Movements

	No image guidance	Image guidance	*p* value
Point A			
Prostate V78 (%)	83.56% (4.7) %	98.49% (2.8) %	<0.001
Prostate mean dose	78.48 GE (0.39) GE	79.51 GE (0.34) GE	<0.001
Prostate minimum dose	52.92 GE (4.89) GE	77.59 GE (1.27) GE	<0.001
Point B			
Prostate V78 (%)	85.57% (3.3) %	90.16% (23.5) %	<0.001
Prostate mean dose	78.66 GE (0.31) GE	79.28 GE (0.38) GE	0.002
Prostate minimum dose	54.34 GE (4.57) GE	77.15 GE (0.77) GE	<0.001
Point C			
Prostate V78 (%)	82.6% (4.2) %	99.2% (1.9) %	<0.001
Prostate mean dose	78.39 GE (0.41) GE	79.57 GE (0.29) GE	<0.001
Prostate minimum dose	52.19 GE (5.58) GE	77.54 GE (1.09) GE	<0.001
Point D			
Prostate V78 (%)	86.53% (3.9) %	97.39% (3.4)%	<0.001
Prostate mean dose	78.73 GE (0.42) GE	79.31 GE (0.36) GE	0.006
Prostate minimum dose	54.93 GE (4.47) GE	76.60 GE (0.83) GE	<0.001

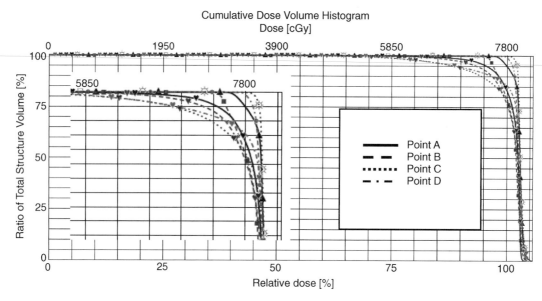

Figure 9 Dose-volume curves for 10 mm prostate shifts with (▲ ✿ ● ■) and without (♥) beam realignment. Large improvements are seen including large shifts in for the DVH curve with beam realignment. *Abbreviation*: DVH, dose-volume histogram.

Minimum CTV dose with realignment was better or equal to 77 GE (>98%) for all multidimensional shifts.

Greater benefits were documented when 10 mm changes in CTV position were made in the superior, inferior, or posterior dimension. No translations of 10 mm were performed anteriorly as they would extend the CTV unrealistically inside the symphysis pubis for all cases studied. These larger translational vectors may better characterize the potential variations in prostate position that can be encountered after the initial laser-based patient alignment for prostate cancer therapy. As seen in Table 3, without image guidance, moderate changes in CTV V78 and minimum CTV dose were observed. However, with beam realignment, we demonstrated clinically relevant and statistically significant improvements in CTV V78 and minimum CTV dose. According to multiple studies showing that changes of 8 Gy or higher will have a significant impact on prostate cancer outcomes, this cutoff was used for defining clinically relevant changes (18,21,42–46). Although large changes were seen in CTV V78 and CTV minimum dose, the maximum CTV dose and mean dose did not change substantially when compared with the initial CTV. This finding questions the utility of mean dose and maximum dose in describing changes resulting from CTV positional variation.

A difficult problem arises when we try to quantify improvements in dose distribution for motion in the vector of the proton beam direction (47). If the lateral change is because of setup error, the beam will not need to be realigned as the depth for the dose deposition will not vary and will cover the target adequately. In other words, if the prostate position changes in the beam direction in relation to the isocenter without varying its position within the pelvis, the beam will traverse a similar distance, and no variation in dose coverage location should be seen. However, if the lateral shift is within the pelvis, changes in the CTV position and variation in depth will be accompanied by corresponding changes in the proton path length. Therefore, the dose-deposition area may miss the CTV. Schallenkamp et al. described the relationship between bony anatomy and prostate motion (35). Although they found that prostate motion was independent of bony alignment (setup position) for most translational vectors, in the lateral direction setup corrections may improve target localization. Nederveen et al. also found that bony anatomy setup correction can decrease the error of the prostate position in the lateral direction by half (48). Related to this, Van Herk et al. found minimal lateral prostate motion in relation to the pelvis with cone-beam CT (0.9 mm SD) (49). Thus, although lateral prostate shifts are possible, they are mostly related to changes in position of the whole pelvic anatomy, which will not affect the proton beam depth deposition, meaning that most motion relevant to changes in dose distribution for proton prostate therapy will be described by shifts that are in the superior-inferior (SI) or anterior-posterior (AP) direction rather than the lateral direction. For this reason, it has been proposed to employ PTV margins that are dependent on the beam angle rather than anisotropic CTV expansions.

To quantify the impact of movement in the lateral direction and other potential changes resulting from inter- and intrafraction motion, we quantified CTV dose-volume variations with shifts of 10 mm in the three directions.

Although, as mentioned earlier, lateral shifts of the prostate in relation to pelvic anatomy will rarely reach 10 mm, we used this degree of displacement to mimic coverage for the potential worst-case scenario (35,48,49). For points A to D large changes in CTV V78 and minimum dose were seen. With beam realignment, we achieved clinically significant benefits in CTV V78 for all prostate positions. For points A, C, and D, CTV V78 was better or equal to 97%. Even for point B, where the CTV V78 was only improved to 90%, CTV minimum dose was 77.2 GE. In other words, although 10% of the CTV was not covered by the prescribed dose, the entire CTV did receive at least 99% of the prescribed dose.

Image guidance of daily treatment is theoretically possible with proton therapy. With appropriate target volume delineation, identification and quantification of uncertainties in treatment planning, and appropriate dose prescription, image guidance can be used to maximize the benefits of improved dose distributions achievable with proton therapy.

ACTION LEVEL THRESHOLD FOR IMAGE GUIDANCE

Accurate prostate localization for prostate cancer treatment can improve cure rates and minimize doses to dose-limiting normal structures (50–54). More reliable prostate localization will permit the delivery of higher doses to the target, and through tighter margins, reduce the normal tissue exposed to intermediate and high doses (55–58).

Target margins to account for variations in the actual prostate position have been defined for different image guidance systems (32,33,59). Serago et al. compared image guidance systems with fiducial-based megavoltage (MV) imaging (33). Since MV images are produced by the beam itself, they represent the true position of the markers in relation to the treatment axis. This method is limited by accurate representation of the crosshairs with respect to the true machine isocenter and gantry-specific isocenter variations with different beam angles (± 2 mm). Disagreements between the locations of reference fiducials have been observed between ultrasound position and MV position of 7.0 ± 4.6 mm, and kilovoltage (kV) imaging and MV position of 1.9 ± 1.5 mm. Furthermore, an additional disparity of 1.9 ± 1.2 mm has been reported between the Calypso system and kV images that theoretically should actually be added to the aforementioned MV and kV errors (60). Cone-beam CT has also shown differences between MV and CT information with linear vectors of -1.05 to 1.0 ± 0.58 to 1.29 mm (61). When evaluating an image guidance system, it is important to identify the limitations of the system in applying corrections. After image guidance, the average prostate position

variation should be close to zero and the residual difference will define the accuracy of the whole system including its systematic errors (62).

In our prostate cases, the kV images are acquired via an orthogonal pair X-ray system where one of the sources is within the nozzle, representing the beam's eye view. Images are acquired in-line with each beam prior to treatment, reducing disagreement arising from variations in gantry isocenter diameter, intrafraction error, and error in repositioning the patient. For our treatments, orthogonal pairs are acquired and single or multiple shifts based on action level threshold (ALT) of 2.5 mm in all three axes are performed as necessary.

Since our verification films are taken at the patients' final treatment position and the X-ray is directly along the beam line, no correction for couch errors or incongruence within the imaging system is necessary. Our process, therefore, has accuracy similar to a MV image for each field.

In a recent study to confirm the feasibility and performance of our prostate localization strategy, a total of 772 treatments were delivered and 3110 images acquired and analyzed employing the methods described by van Herk (63–65) and Yan et al. (66–69). Patients were treated for every fraction using image guidance and an ALT of 2.5 mm. No treatment was delivered without reaching and confirming a prostate position less than 2.5 mm from the predetermined ideal. To reach our ALT, most patients required only zero to one corrections and no patient required more than three corrections (Table 7). The high probability of a true translation (prostate in stable position) within our action level (2.5 mm) implies that the intrafraction error seen over the 3 to 4 minutes required for the correction and verification is smaller than the ALT. If the ALT was smaller than the intrafraction error for the same time period, the overall number of corrections necessary would have been higher and directly proportional to the difference. In the same study, the average error for the AP dimension (z), SI dimension (y), and right to left dimension (x) was close to 0 (Tables 8–10). The margins for each patient were very heterogeneous and ranged between 0.5 mm to 2.2 mm ($p < 0.001$).

As proposed by Van Herk, the theoretical mean error for the preparation should approach zero. Furthermore, any disagreement with zero will describe the systematic error of the approach (70). Figures 10 to 13 show the final prostate position in relation to isocenter. They illustrate positional errors for each individual patient (Figs. 10 and 12) and for all cases (Figs 11–13). The small intrafraction error found our study is in agreement with published literature based on multiple X-rays or cinefluoro. For a study involving longer treatment durations, Kotte et al. identified small intrafraction errors that did not require corrections between treated fields (71).

Table 7 Number of Corrections Needed Within Action Level Threshold of 2.5 mm for 20 Patients and All Final 772 Prostate Positions

Patient	Fractions	2.5-mm action level			
		0 corrections	1 correction	2 corrections	3 corrections
1	39	10.3	89.7	0.0	0.0
2	38	7.9	92.1	0.0	0.0
3	38	5.3	89.5	5.3	0.0
4	39	0.0	89.7	10.3	0.0
5	35	2.9	94.3	2.9	0.0
6	38	0.0	94.7	5.3	0.0
7	39	10.3	79.5	7.7	2.6
8	39	0.0	92.3	7.7	0.0
9	37	8.1	81.1	10.8	0.0
10	41	0.0	97.6	2.4	0.0
11	37	8.1	78.4	10.8	2.7
12	39	2.6	87.2	7.7	2.6
13	41	4.9	85.4	7.3	2.4
14	37	0.0	94.6	2.7	2.7
15	41	0.0	73.2	26.8	0.0
16	39	53.8	41.0	5.1	0.0
17	41	51.2	43.9	4.9	0.0
18	36	0.0	83.3	13.9	2.8
19	39	5.1	74.4	17.9	2.6
20	39	0.0	84.6	15.4	0.0
Total		8.7 (67/772)	82.1 (634/772)	8.3 (64/772)	0.9 (7/772)

Table 8 Final Prostate Position After All Corrections With Online Image Guidance for the Anterior-Posterior (z) Axis With an Action Level of 2.5 mm for 20 Patients and All 772 Final Prostate Positions

Patient	2.5-mm action level threshold			
	Mean (SD) cm	Range (cm)	Margins[a]	Margins[b]
1	0.004 (0.061)	0.330	0.0527	0.120
2	0.021 (0.063)	0.260	0.0966	0.123
3	−0.017 (0.060)	0.320	0.0845	0.118
4	−0.003 (0.071)	0.370	0.0572	0.139
5	−0.012 (0.067)	0.270	0.0769	0.131
6	−0.002 (0.072)	0.370	0.0554	0.141
7	−0.018 (0.103)	0.430	0.1171	0.202
8	−0.011 (0.104)	0.430	0.1003	0.204
9	0.015 (0.093)	0.450	0.1026	0.182
10	0.020 (0.070)	0.290	0.0990	0.137
11	−0.003 (0.134)	0.460	0.1013	0.263
12	−0.018 (0.062)	0.280	0.0884	0.122
13	0.001 (0.098)	0.440	0.0711	0.192
14	0.008 (0.078)	0.380	0.0746	0.153
15	0.019 (0.136)	0.470	0.1427	0.267
16	−0.058 (0.110)	0.470	0.2220	0.216
17	−0.028 (0.087)	0.360	0.1309	0.171
18	0.019 (0.126)	0.450	0.1357	0.247
19	0.012 (0.120)	0.450	0.1140	0.235
20	−0.005 (0.081)	0.410	0.0692	0.159
All cases	−0.003 (0.094)	0.470	0.0733	0.184

[a] $2.5\Sigma + 0.7\,\partial$.
[b] 95% of prostate positions for all cases.
Abbreviation: SD, standard deviation.

Table 9 Final Prostate Position After All Corrections With Online Image Guidance for the Superior-Inferior (y) Axis With an Action Level of 2.5 mm for 20 Patients and All 772 Final Prostate Positions

| Patient | 2.5-mm action level threshold | | | |
	Mean (SD) cm	Range (cm)	Margins[a]	Margins[b]
1	0.002 (0.052)	0.270	0.0414	0.102
2	0.029 (0.064)	0.400	0.1173	0.125
3	−0.031 (0.068)	0.320	0.1251	0.133
4	0.014 (0.052)	0.220	0.0714	0.102
5	0.015 (0.081)	0.390	0.0942	0.159
6	0.023 (0.046)	0.260	0.0897	0.090
7	0.023 (0.093)	0.430	0.1226	0.182
8	0.042 (0.058)	0.240	0.1456	0.114
9	0.041 (0.094)	0.380	0.1683	0.184
10	0.035 (0.082)	0.350	0.1449	0.161
11	0.068 (0.080)	0.420	0.2260	0.157
12	0.011 (0.036)	0.160	0.0527	0.071
13	0.032 (0.060)	0.280	0.1220	0.118
14	0.005 (0.076)	0.360	0.0657	0.149
15	0.028 (0.041)	0.230	0.0987	0.080
16	0.024 (0.075)	0.330	0.1125	0.147
17	0.040 (0.097)	0.430	0.1679	0.190
18	0.059 (0.053)	0.280	0.1846	0.104
19	0.055 (0.089)	0.360	0.1998	0.174
20	0.050 (0.064)	0.280	0.1698	0.125
All cases	0.028 (0.073)	0.430	0.1211	0.143

[a]$2.5\Sigma + 0.7\,\partial$.
[b]95% of prostate positions for all cases.
Abbreviation: SD, standard deviation.

Furthermore, Nederveen et al. have found small variations in prostate position of only 0.3 ± 0.5 mm and -0.4 ± 0.7 mm during 3 to 4 minutes employing cine-MV (72–74). Because of the short treatment times (70–80 seconds) for our prostate cancer treatments, the total time between the last verification X-ray and treatment completion is 3 to 4 minutes. In this setting, an accurate image guidance and treatment system theoretically allows very small margins.

PELVIC RADIATION AND PROTON THERAPY

Situations arise in high-risk prostate cancer where a clinician may feel compelled to irradiate the adjacent lymphatics. We compared seven-field IMRT to the pelvic lymph nodes (LNs) and prostate with a three isocenter, six-field double-scattered proton plan. Significant reductions in dose were seen for the rectum, bladder, and small bowel favoring the proton plan. Furthermore, the LN target dose of 46 GE/Gy was delivered in 23 fractions for the proton treatments while it was delivered over 39 fractions with IMRT. Although it is possible to have two plans where the LN and prostate are treated with an IMRT plan followed by a proton boost, the dose with IMRT to a

central target (i.e., prostate) will still receive a higher dose per fraction than a peripheral target (i.e., LN). As can be seen in Figures 14–16, doses to rectum, bladder, and small bowel can be decreased employing proton therapy. The improvement is larger for pelvic radiation than when treating the prostate alone. However, the integration of image guidance for pelvic radiation is not well defined. The movement of the LN vasculature in relation to the prostate and pelvic structures remains unclear.

INTENSITY-MODULATED PROTON THERAPY

Most IMPT plans seen in the literature show an advantage for IMPT over double-scattered proton therapy. Cella et al. found a substantial improvement with IMPT over proton therapy (75). However, multiple beams angles were employed including angles that used the distal falloff to decrease doses to the rectum and bladder. Since these angles cannot be used for an image-guided approach, the results are not practical in our current setting. Trofimov likewise found a small advantage with IMPT over double-scattered proton therapy (76). In this study, since the angles used for IMPT were similar to the angles employed

Table 10 Final Prostate Position After All Corrections With Online Image Guidance for the Left to Right (X) Axis With an Action Level of 2.5 mm for 20 Patients and All 772 Final Prostate Positions

| Patient | 2.5-mm Action level threshold | | | |
	Mean (SD) cm	Range (cm)	Margins[a]	Margins[b]
1	−0.017 (0.063)	0.340	0.0866	0.123
2	−0.041 (0.072)	0.260	0.1529	0.141
3	−0.033 (0.063)	0.340	0.1266	0.123
4	0.005 (0.070)	0.270	0.0615	0.137
5	−0.009 (0.049)	0.180	0.0568	0.096
6	−0.036 (0.056)	0.260	0.1292	0.110
7	0.022 (0.080)	0.410	0.1110	0.157
8	0.015 (0.071)	0.310	0.0872	0.139
9	−0.053 (0.077)	0.320	0.1864	0.151
10	0.000 (0.064)	0.320	0.0448	0.125
11	0.013 (0.066)	0.290	0.0787	0.129
12	0.004 (0.049)	0.220	0.0443	0.096
13	0.004 (0.071)	0.280	0.0597	0.139
14	0.016 (0.065)	0.230	0.0855	0.127
15	−0.028 (0.060)	0.310	0.1120	0.118
16	−0.038 (0.093)	0.370	0.1601	0.182
17	−0.058 (0.088)	0.360	0.2066	0.172
18	−0.027 (0.079)	0.370	0.1228	0.155
19	−0.023 (0.091)	0.460	0.1212	0.178
20	0.023 (0.063)	0.270	0.1016	0.123
All cases	−0.013 (0.074)	0.460	0.0843	0.145

[a] $2.5\Sigma + 0.7\,\partial$.
[b] 95% of prostate positions for all cases.
Abbreviation: SD, standard deviation.

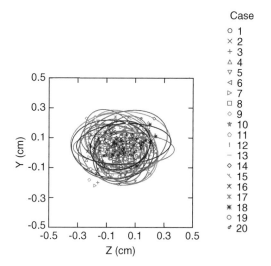

Figure 10 Final prostate positions for each case in the superior to inferior (y) and anterior to posterior (z), curves correspond to the 95% CI for each case.

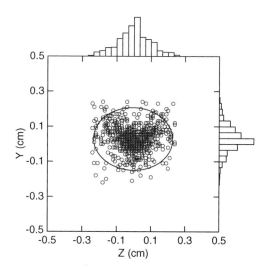

Figure 11 Final prostate positions for all cases in the superior to inferior (y) and anterior to posterior (z). Curves correspond to the 95% CI for all cases and histograms are seen in the border.

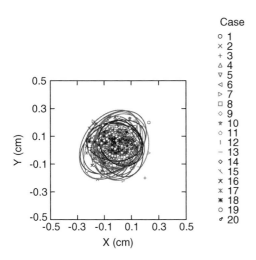

Figure 12 Final prostate positions for each case in the superior to inferior (y) and anterior to posterior (z). Curves correspond to the 95% CI for each case.

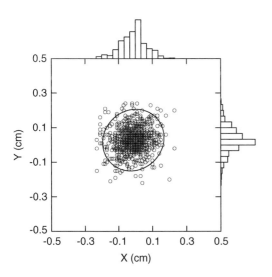

Figure 13 Final prostate positions for all cases in the superior to inferior (y) and anterior to posterior (z). Curves correspond to the 95% CI for all cases and histograms are seen in the border.

for double-scattered proton therapy, it is likely that the advantage in rectal and bladder dose was because of a sharper penumbra. Supporting this, their IMPT DVH curves are similar to the DVH curves obtained in our institution with double-scattered proton therapy. The penumbra in the lateral aspect of the beam is related to the scatter. Theoretically, an IMPT beam can achieve slightly better lateral dose profile than a double-scattered beam but the lateral penumbra is primarily governed by scatter found as the result of the depth, the composition of tissues traversed, and inherent physical characteristics of a

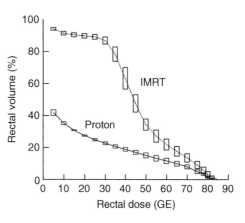

Figure 14 Mean relative rectal dose for IMRT and proton therapy. Square boxes represent the standard error. *Abbreviation*: IMRT, intensity-modulated radiation therapy.

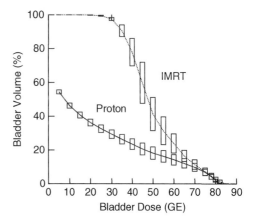

Figure 15 Mean relative bladder dose for IMRT and proton therapy. Square boxes represent the standard error. *Abbreviation*: IMRT, intensity-modulated radiation therapy.

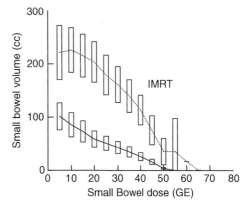

Figure 16 Mean small bowel absolute volume for IMRT and proton therapy. Square boxes represent the standard error. *Abbreviation*: IMRT, intensity-modulated radiation therapy.

particle. Thus, a well-done double-scattered plan should have a similar lateral dose profile as an IMPT plan employing similar beam arrangements. The benefit of IMPT may translate into a slightly sharper lateral falloff and a superior conformality index. If an image-guided approach and a smearing algorithm are employed with IMPT, the conformality index will be similar to a double-scattered image-guided plan for the prostate alone. However, IMPT may be superior when complex seminal vesicle shapes are encountered or the clinical situation mandates the inclusion of at-risk pelvic LNs into our target. In this case, IMPT will be superior because it allows customization of both the distal and proximal edges, rather than just the distal edge alone (as currently possible with double scattering).

SUMMARY OF PERTINENT CONCLUSIONS

- Protons' sharp distal falloff of dose is potentially a two-edged sword. On one hand, it allows the delivery of dose to the tumor while completely sparing distal tissues. On the other hand, an underestimation/overestimation of the path length for any reason could cause overshoot/undershoot of the beam with consequent complete miss of a distal portion of the tumor or irradiation of normal tissue to therapeutic doses.
- Inter-/Intrafraction motion, setup variations, bladder and rectal filling, weight loss, uncertainties in CT numbers, and stopping powers derived from approximations of dose computation models, especially in the presence of complex heterogeneities, have far more consequences in the treatment of prostate cancer with proton therapy than conventional radiation therapy.
- Understanding of the dose-deposition characteristics seen with proton therapy and the potential areas of variability of the high-dose gradient area are sources for error and opportunity with correct implementation.
- The sharp dose falloff of the lateral aspect of the beam allows lower doses to the rectum and bladder in properly designed treatment plans.
- Image guidance is possible with proton therapy. However, special considerations are necessary.
- Proton systems are highly accurate allowing for very small margins within an image-guided process.
- Complex treatment plans and beam arrangements can be optimized for the treatment of large, complex shape structures as seen for nodal pelvic proton therapy.
- The concepts explained in this chapter outline our efforts to understand potential uncertainties in our treatment preparation and execution. The problems and solutions outlined are not unique to prostate cancer but common to all nonfixed anatomy cancer

sites. These concepts can be further investigated for other treatment sites.

REFERENCES

1. Goldner G, Zimmermann F, Feldmann H, et al. 3-D conformal radiotherapy of localized prostate cancer: a subgroup analysis of rectoscopic findings prior to radiotherapy and acute/late rectal side effects. Radiother Oncol 2006; 78:36–40.
2. Goldner G, Tomicek B, Becker G, et al. Proctitis after external-beam radiotherapy for prostate cancer classified by Vienna Rectoscopy Score and correlated with EORTC/RTOG score for late rectal toxicity: results of a prospective multicenter study of 166 patients. Int J Radiat Oncol Biol Phys 2007; 67:78–83.
3. Patel RR, Orton N, Tome WA, et al. Rectal dose sparing with a balloon catheter and ultrasound localization in conformal radiation therapy for prostate cancer. Radiother Oncol 2003; 67:285–294.
4. Teh BS, McGary JE, Dong L, et al. The use of rectal balloon during the delivery of intensity modulated radiotherapy (IMRT) for prostate cancer: more than just a prostate gland immobilization device? Cancer J 2002; 8: 476–483.
5. Teh BS, Dong L, McGary JE, et al. Rectal wall sparing by dosimetric effect of rectal balloon used during intensity-modulated radiation therapy (IMRT) for prostate cancer. Med Dosim 2005; 30:25–30.
6. Vargas C, Martinez A, Kestin LL, et al. Dose-volume analysis of predictors for chronic rectal toxicity after treatment of prostate cancer with adaptive image-guided radiotherapy. Int J Radiat Oncol Biol Phys 2005; 62:1297–1308.
7. Suit H, Goldberg S, Niemierko A, et al. Proton beams to replace photon beams in radical dose treatments. Acta Oncol 2003; 42:800–808.
8. Paganetti H. Interpretation of proton relative biological effectiveness using lesion induction, lesion repair, and cellular dose distribution. Med Phys 2005; 32:2548–2556.
9. Wilkens JJ, Oelfke U. A phenomenological model for the relative biological effectiveness in therapeutic proton beams. Phys Med Biol 2004; 49:2811–2825.
10. Sohn M, Yan D, Liang J, et al. Incidence of late rectal bleeding in high-dose conformal radiotherapy of prostate cancer using equivalent uniform dose-based and dose-volume-based normal tissue complication probability models. Int J Radiat Oncol Biol Phys 2007; 67(4):1066–1073.
11. Tucker SL, Dong L, Cheung R, et al. Comparison of rectal dose-wall histogram versus dose-volume histogram for modeling the incidence of late rectal bleeding after radiotherapy. Int J Radiat Oncol Biol Phys 2004; 60:1589–1601.
12. Vargas C, Martinez A, Kestin LL, et al. Dose-volume analysis of predictors for chronic rectal toxicity after treatment of prostate cancer with adaptive image-guided radiotherapy. Int J Radiat Oncol Biol Phys 2005; 62:1297–1308.
13. Vargas C, Yan D, Kestin LL, et al. Phase II dose escalation study of image-guided adaptive radiotherapy for prostate

cancer: use of dose-volume constraints to achieve rectal isotoxicity. Int J Radiat Oncol Biol Phys 2005; 63:141–149.

14. Wachter S, Gerstner N, Goldner G, et al. Rectal sequelae after conformal radiotherapy of prostate cancer: dose-volume histograms as predictive factors. Radiother Oncol 2001; 59:65–70.

15. Cheung MR, Tucker SL, Dong L, et al. Investigation of bladder dose and volume factors influencing late urinary toxicity after external beam radiotherapy for prostate cancer. Int J Radiat Oncol Biol Phys 2007; 67(4):1059–1065.

16. Jani AB, Su A, Correa D, et al. Comparison of late gastrointestinal and genitourinary toxicity of prostate cancer patients undergoing intensity-modulated versus conventional radiotherapy using localized fields. Prostate Cancer Prostatic Dis 2007; 10(1):82–86.

17. Peeters ST, Heemsbergen WD, van Putten WL, et al. Acute and late complications after radiotherapy for prostate cancer: results of a multicenter randomized trial comparing 68 Gy to 78 Gy. Int J Radiat Oncol Biol Phys 2005; 61:1019–1034.

18. Pollack A, Zagars GK, Starkschall G, et al. Prostate cancer radiation dose response: results of the M. D. Anderson phase III randomized trial. Int J Radiat Oncol Biol Phys 2002; 53:1097–1105.

19. Michalski JM, Winter K, Purdy JA, et al. Toxicity after three-dimensional radiotherapy for prostate cancer on RTOG 9406 dose Level V. Int J Radiat Oncol Biol Phys 2005; 62:706–713.

20. Rossi CJ Jr., Slater JD, Yonemoto LT, et al. Influence of patient age on biochemical freedom from disease in patients undergoing conformal proton radiotherapy of organ-confined prostate cancer. Urology 2004; 64:729–732.

21. Shipley WU, Verhey LJ, Munzenrider JE, et al. Advanced prostate cancer: the results of a randomized comparative trial of high dose irradiation boosting with conformal protons compared with conventional dose irradiation using photons alone. Int J Radiat Oncol Biol Phys 1995; 32:3–12.

22. Slater JD, Yonemoto LT, Rossi CJ Jr., et al. Conformal proton therapy for prostate carcinoma. Int J Radiat Oncol Biol Phys 1998; 42:299–304.

23. Slater JD, Rossi CJ Jr., Yonemoto LT, et al. Conformal proton therapy for early-stage prostate cancer. Urology 1999; 53:978–984.

24. Slater JD, Rossi CJ Jr., Yonemoto LT, et al. Proton therapy for prostate cancer: the initial Loma Linda University experience. Int J Radiat Oncol Biol Phys 2004; 59:348–352.

25. Zietman AL, DeSilvio ML, Slater JD, et al. Comparison of conventional-dose vs high-dose conformal radiation therapy in clinically localized adenocarcinoma of the prostate: a randomized controlled trial. JAMA 2005; 294:1233–1239.

26. Cella L, Lomax A, Miralbell R. Potential role of intensity modulated proton beams in prostate cancer radiotherapy. Int J Radiat Oncol Biol Phys 2001; 49:217–223.

27. Zhang X, Dong L, Lee AK, et al. Effect of anatomic motion on proton therapy dose distributions in prostate cancer treatment. Int J Radiat Oncol Biol Phys 2007; 67:620–629.

28. Trofimov A, Nguyen PL, Coen JJ, et al. Radiotherapy treatment of early-stage prostate cancer with IMRT and protons: a treatment planning comparison. Int J Radiat Oncol Biol Phys 2007; 69(2):444–453.

29. Letourneau D, Martinez AA, Lockman D, et al. Assessment of residual error for online cone-beam CT-guided treatment of prostate cancer patients. Int J Radiat Oncol Biol Phys 2005; 62:1239–1246.

30. Litzenberg DW, Balter JM, Hadley SW, et al. Influence of intrafraction motion on margins for prostate radiotherapy. Int J Radiat Oncol Biol Phys 2006; 65:548–553.

31. Rudat V, Schraube P, Oetzel D, et al. Combined error of patient positioning variability and prostate motion uncertainty in 3D conformal radiotherapy of localized prostate cancer. Int J Radiat Oncol Biol Phys 1996; 35: 1027–1034.

32. Scarbrough TJ, Golden NM, Ting JY, et al. Comparison of ultrasound and implanted seed marker prostate localization methods: implications for image-guided radiotherapy. Int J Radiat Oncol Biol Phys 2006; 65:378–387.

33. Serago CF, Buskirk SJ, Igel TC, et al. Comparison of daily megavoltage electronic portal imaging or kilovoltage imaging with marker seeds to ultrasound imaging or skin marks for prostate localization and treatment positioning in patients with prostate cancer. Int J Radiat Oncol Biol Phys 2006; 65:1585–1592.

34. Yan D, Lockman D, Brabbins D, et al. An off-line strategy for constructing a patient-specific planning target volume in adaptive treatment process for prostate cancer. Int J Radiat Oncol Biol Phys 2000; 48:289–302.

35. Schallenkamp JM, Herman MG, Kruse JJ, et al. Prostate position relative to pelvic bony anatomy based on intraprostatic gold markers and electronic portal imaging. Int J Radiat Oncol Biol Phys 2005; 63:800–811.

36. de Boer HC, van Os MJ, Jansen PP, et al. Application of the No Action Level (NAL) protocol to correct for prostate motion based on electronic portal imaging of implanted markers. Int J Radiat Oncol Biol Phys 2005; 61:969–983.

37. Kupelian P, Willoughby T, Mahadevan A, et al. Multi-institutional clinical experience with the Calypso System in localization and continuous, real-time monitoring of the prostate gland during external radiotherapy. Int J Radiat Oncol Biol Phys 2007; 67:1088–1098.

38. Madsen BL, Hsi RA, Pham HT, et al. Intrafractional stability of the prostate using a stereotactic radiotherapy technique. Int J Radiat Oncol Biol Phys 2003; 57:1285–1291.

39. Serago CF, Chungbin SJ, Buskirk SJ, et al. Initial experience with ultrasound localization for positioning prostate cancer patients for external beam radiotherapy. Int J Radiat Oncol Biol Phys 2002; 53:1130–1138.

40. Ciangaru G, Polf JC, Bues M, et al. Benchmarking analytical calculations of proton doses in heterogeneous matter. Med Phys 2005; 32:3511–3523.

41. Zhang X, Dong L, Lee AK, et al. Effect of anatomic motion on proton therapy dose distributions in prostate cancer treatment. Int J Radiat Oncol Biol Phys 2007; 67:620–629.

42. Dearnaley DP, Hall E, Lawrence D, et al. Phase III pilot study of dose escalation using conformal radiotherapy in prostate cancer: PSA control and side effects. Br J Cancer 2005; 92:488–498.

43. Peeters ST, Heemsbergen WD, Koper PC, et al. Dose-response in radiotherapy for localized prostate cancer: results of the Dutch multicenter randomized phase III

trial comparing 68 Gy of radiotherapy with 78 Gy. J Clin Oncol 2006; 24:1990–1996.

44. Sathya JR, Davis IR, Julian JA, et al. Randomized trial comparing iridium implant plus external-beam radiation therapy with external-beam radiation therapy alone in node-negative locally advanced cancer of the prostate. J Clin Oncol 2005; 23:1192–1199.

45. Vargas CE, Martinez AA, Boike TP, et al. High-dose irradiation for prostate cancer via a high-dose-rate brachy-therapy boost: results of a phase I to II study. Int J Radiat Oncol Biol Phys 2006; 66:416–423.

46. Zietman AL, DeSilvio ML, Slater JD, et al. Comparison of conventional-dose vs high-dose conformal radiation therapy in clinically localized adenocarcinoma of the prostate: a randomized controlled trial. JAMA 2005; 294:1233–1239.

47. Thomas SJ. Margins for treatment planning of proton therapy. Phys Med Biol 2006; 51:1491–1501.

48. Nederveen AJ, Dehnad H, van der Heide UA, et al. Comparison of megavoltage position verification for prostate irradiation based on bony anatomy and implanted fiducials. Radiother Oncol 2003; 68:81–88.

49. Van Herk M, Bruce A, Kroes AP, et al. Quantification of organ motion during conformal radiotherapy of the prostate by three dimensional image registration. Int J Radiat Oncol Biol Phys 1995; 33:1311–1320.

50. Kupelian PA, Reddy CA, Klein EA, et al. Short-course intensity-modulated radiotherapy (70 GY at 2.5 GY per fraction) for localized prostate cancer: preliminary results on late toxicity and quality of life. Int J Radiat Oncol Biol Phys 2001; 51:988–993.

51. Kupelian PA, Thakkar VV, Khuntia D, et al. Hypofractio-nated intensity-modulated radiotherapy (70 gy at 2.5 Gy per fraction) for localized prostate cancer: long-term out-comes. Int J Radiat Oncol Biol Phys 2005; 63:1463–1468.

52. Martinez A, Vargas C, Kestin L, et al. Interim results of a phase II dose escalating trial with image guided adaptive radiotherapy for the treatment of early to high risk prostate cancer patients: improved outcome with increased EBRT doses. Int J Radiat Oncol Biol Phys 2005; 63:S305–S306.

53. Vargas C, Yan D, Kestin LL, et al. Phase II dose escalation study of image-guided adaptive radiotherapy for prostate cancer: use of dose-volume constraints to achieve rectal isotoxicity. Int J Radiat Oncol Biol Phys 2005; 63:141–149.

54. Vargas C, Martinez A, Kestin LL, et al. Dose-volume analysis of predictors for chronic rectal toxicity after treat-ment of prostate cancer with adaptive image-guided radio-therapy. Int J Radiat Oncol Biol Phys 2005; 62:1297–1308.

55. Yan D, Wong J, Vicini F, et al. Adaptive modification of treatment planning to minimize the deleterious effects of treatment setup errors. Int J Radiat Oncol Biol Phys 1997; 38:197–206.

56. Yan D, Lockman D, Brabbins D, et al. An off-line strategy for constructing a patient-specific planning target volume in adaptive treatment process for prostate cancer. Int J Radiat Oncol Biol Phys 2000; 48:289–302.

57. Kupelian PA, Langen KM, Zeidan OA, et al. Daily varia-tions in delivered doses in patients treated with radiother-apy for localized prostate cancer. Int J Radiat Oncol Biol Phys 2006; 66:876–882.

58. Zhang X, Dong L, Lee AK, et al. Effect of anatomic motion on proton therapy dose distributions in prostate cancer treatment. Int J Radiat Oncol Biol Phys 2007; 67:620–629.

59. Kupelian P, Willoughby T, Mahadevan A, et al. Multi-institutional clinical experience with the Calypso System in localization and continuous, real-time monitoring of the prostate gland during external radiotherapy. Int J Radiat Oncol Biol Phys 2007; 67:1088–1098.

60. Kupelian P, Willoughby T, Mahadevan A, et al. Multi-institutional clinical experience with the Calypso System in localization and continuous, real-time monitoring of the prostate gland during external radiotherapy. Int J Radiat Oncol Biol Phys 2007; 67:1088–1098.

61. Moseley DJ, White EA, Wiltshire KL, et al. Comparison of localization performance with implanted fiducial markers and cone-beam computed tomography for on-line image-guided radiotherapy of the prostate. Int J Radiat Oncol Biol Phys 2007; 67:942–953.

62. Yan D, Lockman D, Martinez A, et al. Computed tomog-raphy guided management of interfractional patient varia-tion. Semin Radiat Oncol 2005; 15:168–179.

63. van Herk M, Bruce A, Kroes AP, et al. Quantification of organ motion during conformal radiotherapy of the prostate by three dimensional image registration. Int J Radiat Oncol Biol Phys 1995; 33:1311–1320.

64. van Herk M, Remeijer P, Rasch C, et al. The probability of correct target dosage: dose-population histograms for deriving treatment margins in radiotherapy. Int J Radiat. Oncol. Biol. Phys. 2000; 47:1121–1135.

65. van Herk M, Remeijer P, Lebesque JV. Inclusion of geo-metric uncertainties in treatment plan evaluation. Int J Radiat Oncol Biol Phys 2002; 52:1407–1422.

66. Yan D, Wong J, Vicini F, et al. Adaptive modification of treatment planning to minimize the deleterious effects of treatment setup errors. Int J Radiat Oncol Biol Phys 1997; 38:197–206.

67. Yan D, Lockman D, Brabbins D, et al. An off-line strategy for constructing a patient-specific planning target volume in adaptive treatment process for prostate cancer. Int J Radiat Oncol Biol Phys 2000; 48:289–302.

68. Yan D, Xu B, Lockman D, et al. The influence of interpatient and intrapatient rectum variation on external beam treatment of prostate cancer. Int J Radiat Oncol Biol Phys 2001; 51:1111–1119.

69. Yan D, Lockman D, Martinez A, et al. Computed tomog-raphy guided management of interfractional patient varia-tion. Semin Radiat Oncol 2005; 15:168–179.

70. Yan D, Lockman D, Martinez A, et al. Computed tomog-raphy guided management of interfractional patient varia-tion. Semin Radiat Oncol 2005; 15:168–179.

71. Kotte AN, Hofman P, Lagendijk JJ, et al. Intrafraction motion of the prostate during external-beam radiation therapy: analysis of 427 patients with implanted fiducial markers. Int J Radiat Oncol Biol Phys 2007; 69(2):419–425.

72. Nederveen A, Lagendijk J, Hofman P. Detection of fiducial gold markers for automatic on-line megavoltage position verification using a marker extraction kernel (MEK). Int J Radiat Oncol Biol Phys 2000; 47:1435–1442.

73. Nederveen AJ, Lagendijk JJ, Hofman P. Feasibility of automatic marker detection with an a-Si flat-panel imager. Phys Med Biol 2001; 46:1219–1230.

74. Nederveen AJ, van der Heide UA, Dehnad H, et al. Measurements and clinical consequences of prostate motion during a radiotherapy fraction. Int J Radiat Oncol Biol Phys 2002; 53:206–214.

75. Cella L, Lomax A, Miralbell R. Potential role of intensity modulated proton beams in prostate cancer radiotherapy. Int J Radiat Oncol Biol Phys 2001; 49:217–223.

76. Trofimov A, Nguyen PL, Coen JJ, et al. Radiotherapy treatment of early-stage prostate cancer with IMRT and protons: a treatment planning comparison. Int J Radiat Oncol Biol Phys 2007; 69(2):444–453.

19

The Testing of Prostate IGRT in Clinical Trials

VINCENT S. KHOO

Urology Oncology Unit, Royal Marsden NHS Foundation Trust and Institute of Cancer Research, Chelsea, London, U.K.

DAVID P. DEARNALEY

Academic Department of Radiotherapy, Institute of Cancer Research and Royal Marsden NHS Foundation Trust, Sutton, Surrey, U.K.

HISTORY OF CLINICAL TRIALS FOR RADIOTHERAPY TECHNOLOGY

Testing of radiotherapy technology is as old as the field of radiation itself. However, the application of formal clinical trials in radiotherapy technology is a relatively newer activity compared with the numerous clinical studies undertaken in this arena. Part of the issue lies in the defining what is meant by testing within "clinical studies" versus "clinical trials." The term clinical study is a relatively "loose" and a general idiom that is often used to group any form of clinical or technological assessment and evaluation. It does not necessarily encompass the methodological rigors required for a formal clinical trial. Clinical studies can include a large spectrum of assessments that range from case reports to feasibility studies or retrospective reviews to prospective but noncomparative assessments. Critically, such clinical studies may be flawed by sources of data uncertainty such as systematic errors or biases and random errors. These sources of data uncertainty can severely limit the strength of the evidence produced by the study and restrict the validity of the study's outcomes.

A clinical trial should have formal methods to address and minimize these sources of systematic and random uncertainty to ensure appropriate validity of the trial results. These sources of uncertainty will be discussed in more detail in section Systematic and Random Errors in Trial Design. It is important for investigators to understand that these sources of study error can be controlled by appropriate and proper trial design but cannot be accounted for subsequently by statistical analysis alone. Thus, it is critical to have a well-designed clinical trial that addresses these issues at the outset to ensure authenticity of trial outcomes.

It is also important to consider the motivations involved in undertaking clinical research and subsequently in performing clinical trials in radiotherapy. The incentive to carry out clinical radiotherapy research is to discover appropriate evidence and to provide relevant information for the project. Good clinical research is about asking important and well-defined questions and obtaining reliable answers. This is an opportunity to assess current or new therapies, to compare and contrast different image-guided strategies, and to provide new directions in research or strategies. A clinical trial is one of the means whereby the value or effectiveness of a new radiotherapy strategy such as image-guided radiation therapy (IGRT) can be established. Clinical trials should be prospective and controlled to provide results that can be validated. It should provide evidence produced with scientific rigor to rationalize decision making rather than merely plausible reasoning to support the study's conclusions.

It is evident that there have been numerous advances made in medicine and radiation therapy without conducting formal clinical trials. This is usually possible when the treatment effects, differences, or advantages are very large, and when these treatment effects remain significant despite the potential presence of bias and uncertainty when using less than formal methods of assessment. Good examples of this in medicine include the introduction of penicillin and in radiotherapy technology, the application of cross-sectional imaging information using computed tomography (CT) for radiotherapy treatment planning. Other advances in radiotherapy technology include the replacement of cobalt-60 and betatron machines by computer-controlled linear accelerators (Linacs) and the use of multileaf collimators (MLCs). The use of CT together with Linac hardware developments, such as MLCs and electronic portal imaging devices (EPIDs), as well as the computer revolution has led to the foundation of modern radiotherapy. The next logical technological development for precision radiotherapy is the introduction of image-guided strategies.

It is evident that previous technological advances in radiotherapy have been undertaken in numerous small steps but few, if any, of these steps have been formally evaluated within randomized controlled trials to fully justify its clinical value or have been deemed to have achieved level 1 evidence as judged by modern contemporaneous criteria used in evidence-based medicine (EBM) (1). In brief, EBM is the conscientious, judicious, and explicit use of current best clinical evidence in making decisions regarding the management of patients. EBM involves integrating the best available external clinical evidence from systematic research with individual or peer group expertise and incorporates the process whereby different types of clinical evidence are categorized and ranked according to the strength of the trials/studies that are free from the various biases, which may limit their findings. In this hierarchy of evidence-based levels, level 1 is the strongest evidence level for a particular therapeutic intervention and is provided by systematic review of appropriate randomized comparative trials. There are several systems in use, and they are based on similar principles. Two common examples of EBM systems are provided from the United States (Table 1) and from the United Kingdom (Tables 2A and 2B) describing their evidence categorization (2,3).

In the history of clinical trials for radiotherapy technology, one important historical example is the use of CT in radiotherapy. It is fair to say that the integration of CT has revolutionized radiotherapy practice, but yet there have been no randomized clinical trials defining its introduction in radiotherapy. Its relative value in radiotherapy has been inferred from the many studies undertaken when CT was initially introduced in the diagnostic field. Some examples of clinical studies defining the utility of CT in both diagnostic imaging and radiotherapy practice are illustrated below and some of the limitations of these studies are discussed.

One of the earliest imaging studies of CT assessed the detection of brain metastasis by comparing the standard imaging method used at that time which was radionuclide scanning with CT (4). This clinical study reported similar diagnostic rates using radionuclide brain scanning and contrast enhanced CT. However, only just over half (53%) of the patients in this 47-patient study underwent both radionuclide scanning and CT. Obvious limitations of this study are that not all cases were imaged with both imaging modalities, the small patient cohort, and potential patient selection bias in recruitment. In this initial setting to define the utility of CT for the detection of brain metastasis, it is clear that a larger better-designed comparative study was needed. Subsequently, a National Cancer Institute (NCI) multicentre study of 2928 patients compared radionuclide brain scanning with CT, plain radiography, and angiography (5). This NCI study also evaluated the relative comparative ability to diagnose intracranial

Table 1 Evidence-Based Medicine: Levels of Evidence

Level schema	Description of U.S. Preventive Services Task Force
Level I	This would arise from evidence obtained from at least one properly designed randomized controlled trial.
Level II-1	This would arise from evidence obtained from well-designed controlled trials without randomization.
Level II-2	This would arise from evidence obtained from well-designed cohort or case-control analytic studies, preferably from more than one center or research group.
Level II-3	This would arise from evidence obtained from multiple time series with or without the intervention. Dramatic results in uncontrolled trials might also be regarded as this type of evidence.
Level III	This would arise from opinions of respected authorities, based on clinical experience, descriptive studies, or recommendations from expert based committees.

Source: From Ref. 2.

Table 2A Oxford Center for Evidence-Based Medicine Levels of Evidence (May 2001)

Level	Therapy/prevention, etiology/harm	Prognosis	Diagnosis	Differential diagnosis/ symptom prevalence study	Economic and decision analyses
1a	SR (with homogeneity[a]) of RCTs	SR (with homogeneity[a]) of inception cohort studies; CDR[b] validated in different populations	SR (with homogeneity[a]) of level 1 diagnostic studies; CDR[b] with 1b studies from different clinical centers	SR (with homogeneity[a]) of prospective cohort studies	SR (with homogeneity[a]) of level 1 economic studies
1b	Individual RCT (with narrow confidence interval[c])	Individual inception cohort study with $\geq$80% follow-up; CDR[b] validated in a single population	Validating[j] cohort study with good[h] reference standards; or CDR[b] tested within one clinical center	Prospective cohort study with good follow-up[l]	Analysis based on clinically sensible costs or alternatives; systematic review(s) of the evidence; and including multiway sensitivity analyses
1c	All or none[d]	All or none case series	Absolute SpPins and SnNouts[g]	All or none case series	Absolute better-value or worse-value analyses[i]
2a	SR (with homogeneity[a]) of cohort studies	SR (with homogeneity[a]) of either retrospective cohort studies or untreated control groups in RCTs	SR (with homogeneity[a]) of level >2 diagnostic studies	SR (with homogeneity[a]) of 2b and better studies	SR (with homogeneity[a]) of level >2 economic studies
2b	Individual cohort study (including low-quality RCT; e.g., <80% follow-up)	Retrospective cohort study or follow-up of untreated control patients in an RCT; derivation of CDR[b] or validated on split sample[f] only	Exploratory[j] cohort study with good[h] reference standards; CDR[b] after derivation, or validated only on split sample[f] or databases	Retrospective cohort study, or poor follow-up	Analysis based on clinically sensible costs or alternatives; limited review(s) of the evidence, or single studies, and including multiway sensitivity analyses
2c	"Outcomes" research; ecological studies	"Outcomes" research		Ecological studies	Audit or outcomes research
3a	SR (with homogeneity[a]) of case-control studies		SR (with homogeneity[a]) of 3b and better studies	SR (with homogeneity[a]) of 3b and better studies	SR (with homogeneity[a]) of 3b and better studies
3b	Individual case-control study		Nonconsecutive study; or without consistently applied reference standards	Nonconsecutive cohort study, or very limited population	Analysis based on limited alternatives or costs, poor quality estimates of data, but including sensitivity analyses incorporating clinically sensible variations
4	Case series (and poor quality cohort and case-control studies[e])	Case series (and poor quality prognostic cohort studies[l])	Case-control study, poor, or nonindependent reference standard	Case series or superseded reference standards	Analysis with no sensitivity analysis

(Continued)

Table 2A Oxford Center for Evidence-Based Medicine Levels of Evidence (May 2001) (*Continued*)

Level	Therapy/prevention, etiology/harm	Prognosis	Diagnosis	Differential diagnosis/ symptom prevalence study	Economic and decision analyses
5	Expert opinion without explicit critical appraisal, or based on physiology, bench research, or "first principles"	Expert opinion without explicit critical appraisal, or based on physiology, bench research or "first principles"	Expert opinion without explicit critical appraisal, or based on physiology, bench research or "first principles"	Expert opinion without explicit critical appraisal, or based on physiology, bench research or "first principles"	Expert opinion without explicit critical appraisal, or based on economic theory or "first principles"

Users can add a minus sign "−" to denote the level of that fails to provide a conclusive answer because of either a single result with a wide confidence interval (e.g., an ARR in an RCT is not statistically significant but whose confidence intervals fail to exclude clinically important benefit or harm) or a systematic review with troublesome (and statistically significant) heterogeneity. Such evidence is inconclusive, and therefore can only generate grade D recommendations.

[a]Homogeneity mean a systematic review that is free of worrisome variations (heterogeneity) in the directions and degrees of results between individual studies. Not all systematic reviews with statistically significant heterogeneity need be worrisome, and not all worrisome heterogeneity need be statistically significant. As noted above, studies displaying worrisome heterogeneity should be tagged with a "−" at the end of their designated level.

[b]Clinical decision rule. (These are algorithms or scoring systems, which lead to a prognostic estimation or a diagnostic category.)

[c]See note #2 for advice on how to understand, rate, and use trials or other studies with wide confidence intervals.

[d]Met when *all* patients died before the Rx became available, but some now survive on it; or when some patients died before the Rx became available, but *none* now die on it.

[e]Poor quality *cohort* study failed to clearly define comparison groups and/or failed to measure exposures and outcomes in the same (preferably blinded), objective way in both exposed and nonexposed individuals and/or failed to identify or appropriately control known confounders and/or failed to carry out a sufficiently long and complete follow-up of patients. Poor quality *case-control* study failed to clearly define comparison groups and/or failed to measure exposures and outcomes in the same (preferably blinded), objective way in both cases and controls and/or failed to identify or appropriately control known confounders.

[f]Split-sample validation is achieved by collecting all the information in a single tranche, then artificially dividing this into "derivation" and "validation" samples.

[g]An "Absolute SpPin" is a diagnostic finding whose *Specificity* is so high that a *Positive* result rules-*in* the diagnosis. An "Absolute SnNout" is a diagnostic finding whose *Sensitivity* is so high that a *Negative* result rules-*out* the diagnosis.

[h]*Good* reference standards are independent of the test, and applied blindly or objectively to all patients. *Poor* reference standards are haphazardly applied, but still independent of the test. Use of a nonindependent reference standard (where the "test" is included in the "reference," or where the "testing" affects the "reference") implies a level 4 study.

[i]Better-value treatments are clearly as good but cheaper, or better at the same or reduced cost. Worse-value treatments are as good and more expensive, or worse and the equally or more expensive.

[j]Validating studies test the quality of a specific diagnostic test, based on prior evidence. An exploratory study collects information and trawls the data (e.g. using a regression analysis) to find which factors are 'significant'.

[k]Poor quality prognostic cohort study is one in which sampling was biased in favor of patients who already had the target outcome, or the measurement of outcomes was accomplished in <80% of study patients, or outcomes were determined in an unblinded, nonobjective way, or there was no correction for confounding factors.

[l]Good follow-up in a differential diagnosis study is >80%, with adequate time for alternative diagnoses to emerge (e.g., 1–6 months acute, 1–5 years chronic). Produced by Bob Phillips, Chris Ball, Dave Sackett, Doug Badenoch, Sharon Straus, Brian Haynes, Martin Dawes since November 1998. *Source*: From Ref: 3.

Table 2B Evidence-Based Medicine: Recommendation Grading Based on Oxford Center for EBM

Recommendation grades	Description of Oxford Center for EBM, United Kingdom
Grade A	Consistent level 1 studies
Grade B	Consistent level 2 or 3 studies or extrapolations[a] from level 1 studies
Grade C	Level 4 studies or extrapolations[a] from level 2 or level 3 studies
Grade D	Level 5 evidence or troublingly inconsistent or inclusive studies of any level

[a]This is where data is used in a situation, which has potentially clinically important differences than the original study situation. *Abbreviation*: EBM, evidence-based medicine. *Source*: From Ref. 3.

lesions depending on the order in which CT and radionuclide scanning was performed. This study reported that CT with and without contrast enhancement was more accurate than radionuclide brain scanning and plain radiography but was as accurate as angiography in detecting brain masses. It also reported that randomizing for the imaging order was not a crucial determinant of the results and concluded that randomization for the order of imaging was not necessary (6). The important feature here is to blind the reporting of the imaging tests. It is clear that this study only evaluated diagnostic ability for metastasis detection and did not address the CT value of providing cross-sectional internal anatomy information that will not be available from radionuclide or angiographic imaging. For modern radiotherapy including stereotactic radiotherapy, cross-sectional anatomical information is vital for three-dimensional spatial localization and treatment planning.

In radiotherapy practice, the utility of CT compared with conventional methods of radiotherapy planning which used imaging with radiographic examinations, xerograms, lymphangiograms, arteriograms, air contrast studies, isotopic studies, and ultrasound was prospectively assessed in this early study (7). This study revealed that 44 of 77 (52%) of the cases had their conventional treatment changed as a result of using CT. Inadequate coverage of the target volume was noted in 32 of 77 (42%) treatment plans, and 24 of 77 (31%) cases had some portion of the target outside of the 50% isodose region. Compared with CT, it was demonstrated that planning volumes of interest (VOI) clinically estimated from plain radiographs could not accurately define tumor extent. Using an empirical predictive model, Goitein suggested that the improved tumor volume localization using CT could result in an increase in local tumor control probability by an average of 6% with the chance of five-year cancer survival increasing by an average of 3.5% (8). It is clear that CT has permitted more accurate tumor/target volume delineation and provided the foundation for precise treatment planning.

Another important issue in radiotherapy is the proper assessment of the spatial relationship of the target volume with its surrounding critical organs at risk (OAR). This assessment is needed to limit and reduce the likelihood of treatment related complications and remains a crucial aspect to maintain the therapeutic ratio in radiotherapy. Despite the lack of randomized clinical trials for the use of CT in radiotherapy treatment planning, the integration of CT in radiotherapy remains the current "standard of care" and is the basis for conformal radiotherapy (CFRT) and intensity-modulated radiotherapy (IMRT). The use of CFRT and IMRT techniques will also permit the treatment paradigm of "conformal avoidance" of OARs to be achieved once the three-dimensional treatment space is known. It has also instigated the establishment of treatment volume nomenclature from the International Commission for Radiation Units (ICRU) Reports 50 and 62 (9,10) that allow for uniformity in treatment planning and delivery as well as in consistency in reporting. In addition, the application of cross-sectional imaging is also one of the means through which IGRT is implemented.

In the clinical assessment of conformal planning technology for prostate radiotherapy, a phase III external beam radiotherapy UK clinical trial randomised prostate cancer patients to unshaped treatment fields (conventional) or shaped treatment fields (conformal) with the same dose and dose per fraction in each arm (11). In this

trial of 225 men, a significant reduction in late rectal toxicity, which is the dose limiting constraint for prostate radiotherapy, was reported for the conformal treatment arm. Level 1 evidence from this U.K. trial eventually provided the basis for its country's advisory body National Institute for heath and Clinical Excellence (NICE) to support the widespread implementation of conformal techniques for prostate radiotherapy. It is good quality evidence of this type that can influence and change national policies and lead to better outcomes for our patients.

Another example for the testing of radiotherapy technology is in the clinical application of IMRT. There is a rapidly growing and almost voluminous amount of published reports demonstrating the superiority of IMRT compared with CFRT techniques in dosimetric terms with better coverage of the nominated target volume and with substantially less dose to the adjacent OAR or critical structures. Some of these planning studies have been comparative physics evaluations but remain theoretical exercises. Many of these planning studies have been followed by numerous clinical studies undertaken in almost every tumor site ranging from the central nervous system to soft-tissue sarcomas. In particular, irradiation of the prostate gland has been extensively studied. Most of the clinical IMRT studies in prostate cancer have been either feasibility studies assessing the potential of delivering IMRT (12) or noncomparative studies assessing patient cohorts for dose escalation using IMRT (13). Most of the reported randomized controlled trials in prostate cancer are evaluating the benefits of CFRT dose escalation with conventional 1.8 to 2 Gy dose per fraction schedules (14–17) or testing the potential radiobiological advantage of hypofractionation (18,19). It is clear that these clinical trials are not testing the value of the IMRT technique itself in a comparative study.

The dosimetric assessments from these clinical studies do appear impressive for IMRT usage. Although non-randomized clinical studies may provide early evidence of the potential benefit of IMRT, the true clinical value of the IMRT technique on treatment related morbidity, local tumor control, and disease survival will need to be assessed in formal prospective and randomized clinical trials. Such randomized trials are currently being undertaken in a few clinical cancer subsites (e.g., head and neck and breast) and are easier to perform in some countries than in others for a number of reasons that include clinician bias, popular patient beliefs and local advocacy groups, and the restructuring of reimbursement for radiotherapy. This is a crucial pragmatic issue for if there is a lack of objective observer or participant equality about the treatment arms of a randomized trial, it would be difficult to initiate uptake and completion of the trial either from investigators or patients alike. Such a trial would be doomed from the outset irrespective of the appropriateness or importance of the therapeutic question under investigation. This issue has plagued randomized comparative studies of IMRT to standard treatment methods in some countries and may also limit similar studies in the assessment of IGRT for prostate cancer.

Some studies, for example the U.K. multicentre randomized control trial CHHiP of conventional or hypofractionated high-dose IMRT permit either more simple forward-planned or inverse-planned solutions (20,21). This trial will provide high quality but nonrandomized comparative data [U.S. level 2–1 evidence (Table 1) and U.K. level 2 evidence (Table 2)] relating planning and delivery techniques to dosimetry, treatment related sequela using physician, and patient-based instruments as well as disease control end points. In a similar fashion, level 2 evidence for the use of MLCs rather than low melting point alloy blocks and portal imaging rather than film verification was generated from the Medical Research Council (MRC) RT01 trial by detailed analysis of patients receiving treatment using different combinations of techniques (17,22).

There is emerging evidence that IGRT is important and relevant for prostate radiotherapy. The standard method of using a single planning CT scan to determine the three-dimensional spatial location and shape of the prostate position can lead to systematic errors in treatment planning. A consequence of such systematic errors is a loss of biochemical prostate-specific antigen (PSA) control rates in external beam prostate radiotherapy, as reported recently from retrospective analyses from two randomized studies of prostate dose escalation (23,24).

ISSUES OF CLINICAL TRIAL DESIGN FOR PROSTATE IGRT

The study components of any well-executed clinical trial for prostate IGRT will need to include close attention to trial design, IGRT method implementation and execution, quality control, collection and analysis of data, and interpretation of results. These components are summarized in Table 3. The initiation for the development of any clinical trial in prostate IGRT is to answer a relevant or important therapeutic or management question that deals with minimizing or limiting the temporal-spatial uncertainty in target volume definition, treatment delivery, or verification. This question will need to be carefully considered and refined on the basis of a careful analysis of the current standard of care in prostate radiotherapy, the known limitations in treatment delivery, the potential advantage of the image-guided technique to current radiotherapy methods, as well as a review of previous research in this area. It is important for the investigators to involve all key radiotherapy health professionals at the outset of any

clinical trial design for prostate IGRT. This group should include clinicians, physicists, radiation therapists, dosimetrists, radiotherapy nurses, and other relevant ancillary staff. It is imperative that this investigative group should critically evaluate the current evidence concerning the radiotherapeutic management of prostate radiotherapy with respect to the new image-guided strategy being investigated. In general, this should involve a review of the published literature and current ongoing clinical trials on the topic. This will provide a sound knowledge base to determine whether any preliminary studies needed to evaluate a prostate IGRT strategy is feasible and promising. This is particularly important if a comparative study to determine the value of IGRT for relevant patient outcomes is being contemplated.

Types of Clinical Trials

The type and the intention of clinical trial need to be clarified and defined at the outset. The conventional phases of clinical trials are described in Table 4. This description pertains mainly to clinical drug or biological therapy trials. The situation for radiotherapy technology is slightly different but the principles are broadly similar and can be translated over to trials in radiotherapy technology.

The initial incentive for clinical drug trials may either be an observational/case study report or laboratory evidence of anticancer activity using a particular drug agent. In radiotherapy, particularly for IGRT strategies, initial study incentive may arise from clinical observational or case studies demonstrating variations in temporal-spatial variation of the tumor target and theoretical planning or mechanical studies outlining a potential IGRT method that may deal with this uncertainty. Such studies only provide passive observational data with no control of the observed parameters and substantial inherent biases. It cannot define the appropriate patient group, the IGRT methodology may not be feasible or practical, and the impact on treatment outcomes is unknown.

A phase I drug trial would be designed to determine the appropriate drug dose for use in phase II. For clinical trials in IGRT, this could be a feasibility study to assess the methodology and practicality of the IGRT process. This could be undertaken in a manner similar to drug trials where initial cohorts of three patients are tested with the IGRT method and if successful, a further three patient cohort is tested up to a total of 9 or 12 patients. Clear and relevant thresholds or limits for the success of the process will need to be defined to either enable stoppage or continuation of the study. If the phase I or feasibility study for the IGRT method is successful, then a phase II study can be conducted whereby the IGRT method is applied to larger cohort of patients to further define its usage, safety, as well as potential effectiveness. Finally, a

Table 3 Steps in the Design of a Successful Clinical IGRT Trial

Contents	Description of the steps
Aims/goals of the trial	General • To formulate an important and relevant therapeutic or management IGRT question that can be addressed through a clinical trial Specific • To define the primary and secondary end points for the trial
Trial methods	General • To develop the study methodology and IGRT study protocol Specific • To define the patient population to be studied • To provide clear indications for patient inclusion and exclusion • To obtain informed patient consent • To define the method of radiation treatment and image guided strategy involved • To establish the process of image guidance • To address statistical consideration with respects to the power and significance levels for the study • To predetermine interim analysis for the trial with stopping or continuation rules where appropriate
Regulatory trial approval	General process • All clinical trials will need approval by the relevant authority or regulatory body for the country in which the trial is being performed • The regulatory approval process for clinical trials will differ in different countries. In general, a clinical trial will have to undergo an independent scientific review or peer review followed by approval by a research ethics committee Specific process • In the United States, this will involve the Institutional Review Board (IRB) that may be central and local • In the United Kingdom, this will involve both independent peer and ethics review. If the trial involves more than 1 center then a multicenter research ethics committee (MREC) approval is needed. Otherwise a local research ethics committees (LREC) approval will suffice
Study execution	• To ensure the logistics and mechanics for efficient and seamless execution of the study • To have adequate trained personnel for patient recruitment, assessment, and radiotherapy treatment • To have sufficient quality assured radiotherapy facilities to enable trial completion
Data collection and preparation	• To provide for complete data collection • To quality assure the collected data • To make full notes on any inconsistencies in the collection of the data • To provide for analysis of the trial data
Quality control and trial monitoring	• To ensure quality assurance for the radiotherapy and image-guided methodology. This is a particularly important aspect for any radiotherapy technology trial • To have a system in place for the reporting of any serious unexpected adverse events (SUSARS) • Data Monitoring Committee (DMC). If the trial is substantial or multicenter, then a DMC is likely to be convened. The DMC, together with the ethics committee will monitor any serious unexpected side effects and they can stop the trial at any time if there are any concerns about the welfare of the participating patients
Dissemination of results	• To present trial results to local, national, and international meetings/conferences • To submit a manuscript for peer review and publication in a recognized journal.
Other issues	• To obtain adequate funding for the conduct and completion of the clinical trial • To declare any potential conflict of interest from the investigators and minimize this issue • To provide participants with understanding of the trial rationale and design; adequate time to digest the trial information and opportunity to clarify any concerns in participation • To ensure that all investigators are appropriately trained to conduct the study according to best clinical practice

Table 4 Conventional Description for the Phases in Clinical Trials

Type of trial	Description of trial
Phase I	Dose finding studies: An experimental drug or therapy is tested for the first time in a small group of patients (20–80) to evaluate a safe dose range and identify side effects
Phase II	Safety and activity studies: The experimental drug or therapy is used in a larger cohort of patients (100–300) to see if it is effective and to further evaluate its safety
Phase III	Comparative studies: The experimental drug or therapy is given to larger groups of patients (500–3000) and compared to standard or commonly used therapies to confirm its effectiveness, monitor side effects, and collect other information on its use

Table 5 Evidence-Based Medicine: End Points

Grading schema	Description of end points (direct and indirect in descending order of strength)
A	Total mortality
B	Cause specific mortality
C	Quality of life
D	Indirect surrogates
	Disease-free survival
	Progression-free survival
	Survival or tumor response rate

clinical randomized trial can be conducted to compare the experimental or IGRT arm with the current radiotherapy standard of delivery looking at appropriate clinical end points (Table 5) such as superior local tumor control rates, reduction in the incidence of treatment related morbidity, or improved quality of life measures.

Systematic and Random Errors in Trial Design

The strength and validity of a clinical trial result is dependent on methods to control and minimize systematic and random errors. In principle, these sources of errors will be the same irrespective of the method of image guidance under investigation for prostate IGRT. They are important issues in the design for any prostate IGRT clinical trial and will be discussed below. In clinical trials, any unaccounted for bias can produce a systematically higher or lower incorrect estimate of the true treatment effect. Methods to reduce bias include the use of appropriate eligibility criteria and randomization, which will reduce the probability of selection bias in the estimation of any treatment differences arising from the clinical trial. More importantly, significant biases may arise after entry of patients into the clinical trial by (*i*) subsequent exclusion of patients after randomization; (*ii*) loss of patient data that may be due to inappropriate censoring or noncompliance; (*iii*) use of different outcome assessments for different treatment groups; and (*iv*) applying retrospective definitions or thresholds in the protocol.

Another aspect of uncertainties in clinical trials is the errors attributable to chance or random errors. In traditional terms, there are two categories of random errors. Type 1 error is a "false positive" in which there is no treatment effect or difference noted in the clinical trial but where the investigators have wrongly concluded there is. Type 1 error must be carefully considered by the trial investigators as this aspect is often under the control of the investigators when either designing the clinical trial or analyzing it. Type 1 errors can occur when multiple statistical tests are performed, especially, when examining accumulating data or during sequential interim data reviews. It can be normally controlled by selecting the appropriate level of significance to be used in the statistical tests.

Type II error is a "false negative" whereby the investigators fail to detect a treatment effect or difference when it is actually present. This type of error can be controlled by selecting the appropriate sample size for the study and relates to the power of the clinical trial. By having a large enough sample size, the clinical trial is then adequately powered to note a treatment effect of a specified size to be statistically significant when it occurs. This type of error cannot be controlled by any statistical analysis. While a small study may have power to detect a very large treatment difference, it may be unable to detect smaller or modest treatment differences, which can be still clinically relevant to clinicians. This is an extremely important issue to consider in the design of clinical trials. It would not be logical to undertake a trial when the chance of missing a clinically relevant finding is larger than the chance of finding it.

Other Trial Issues

Other issues that may arise in the conduct of any clinical trial include the motivation of its participants and addressing the trial resource issues (Table 3).

Motivation for trial participation applies to research investigators as well as to the patients themselves. This can play a subconscious but important part for both investigators and patients. It can have a negative or positive effect on the trial's success or failure. If there is a belief that the experimental prostate radiotherapy arm utilizing IGRT is superior, then investigators will not be in a position to conduct the trial while patients will be unwilling to be randomized to the standard radiotherapy arm which will be perceived to be a less effective treatment. Patient beliefs and perceptions can be greatly influenced by manufacturing advertising as well as impartial patient advocacy groups. Greater understanding for the image-guided technology and current radiotherapy standards in prostate radiotherapy are needed in these situations. Careful objective explanation of the prostate IGRT rationale and design will need to be provided by the trial investigators.

Adequate resources are needed for the initiation, development, efficient management, and timely completion of any clinical trial. This aspect is often underestimated and is particularly important when undertaking a radiotherapy technology clinical trial such as that with prostate IGRT. This involves confirmed commitment of time and finances from investigators and their staff. Infrastructure for the trial and all its individual steps remain crucial.

CURRENT CLINICAL TRIALS TESTING IMAGE-GUIDANCE TECHNOLOGY

Listings of Current Clinical Trials Testing Prostate IGRT

Although there are numerous reports of centers testing technology for IGRT in prostate radiotherapy, there are few randomized clinical trials formally testing the utility of IGRT or the impact of prostate IGRT on patient outcomes. Most published studies remain initial technology assessments or feasibility studies. A search (August, 2007) was performed of the trial databases for the NCI, National Cancer Institute of Canada (NCIC), National Cancer Research Network (NCRN), and European Organization for Research and Treatment of Cancer (EORTC) reflecting the past and current listing of prostate radiotherapy clinical trials in the United States, Canada, United Kingdom, and Europe, respectively. This search will not be a complete listing of all worldwide prostate IGRT trials but provides a relatively comprehensive review of the current state of affairs for clinical trials in prostate IGRT. There will be some overlap between these databases as some trials will be listed in several databases.

In the search undertaken of the NCI web database for clinical trials in prostate cancer, two searches were performed for active and closed trials (25). The following search filters were used: cancer type—prostate cancer; trial type—treatment and methods development; stage of cancer—stages 1 to 3; status of trial—active or closed; phase of trial—all; sponsor of trial—all, and special

category—all. This search revealed 178 active clinical trials and 219 closed clinical trials. Each of the trials listed was manually reviewed online. There was only one phase III trial listed with the aim of examining the role of IGRT from France. Although there were no web/online details for this French comparative study, details for this trial will be outlined in the next section. There are no other open or closed prostate cancer clinical trials listed on the NCI database that is expressively designed to evaluate the utility of prostate IGRT.

In the search undertaken of the Clinical Trials Group of the NCIC database (26), there are 19 clinical trials in prostate cancer listed in their website, of which 4 are open, 10 are closed, 3 are planned, and 2 have been withdrawn. Most of these listed trials are randomized phase III clinical trials, but again none are addressing the value of IGRT in prostate radiotherapy.

In the search of the NCRN clinical trial portfolio database (27), there are 32 listed prostate cancer trials of which 16 are open, 16 are closed, and 2 are planned. None of the listed trials are addressing the issue of IGRT in prostate cancer. In the search of the EORTC protocols database (28), there are 26 trial protocols listed for prostate cancer of which 2 trials are open. In the section for radiotherapy, there are 109 trials of which 11 are open, 97 are closed, and 1 is being planned. There are again no listed protocols or trials that are examining the utility of prostate IGRT.

Practical Assessment of IGRT in Prostate Cancer

Image-guided strategies and its related technology is such a new field that this term can be broadly used for every aspect in the radiotherapy management chain, as each link or step in the radiotherapy process involves some form of imaging from the definition of volumes of interest for radiotherapy treatment planning to the determination of field placement accuracy and subsequently radiotherapy margins. Thus, image guidance for prostate radiotherapy may have a different definition depending whether it is taken from the clinicians' or physicists' perspective. In this section, we will provide examples and methods of clinical trials/studies to evaluate each of these important steps.

Assessment of Target Volumes for Prostate IGRT

CT has been the standard imaging modality used to determine VOI for the prostate and seminal vesicles as well as surrounding tissue structures or OAR positions for radiotherapy treatment planning. However, CT is of no value in defining areas of cancer within the prostate gland. Magnetic resonance imaging (MRI) techniques including T2-weighted sequences, dynamic contrast–enhanced images, diffusion-weighted images, and MR spectroscopy (MRS), all hold the promise of defining significant tumor nodules within the prostate itself (29). Radiotherapy planning case studies have shown, in principle, that it is certainly possible to selectively boost regions of apparent tumor or single tumor nodules using IMRT methods with dose distributions, which are likely to maintain low toxicity profiles (30–32).

How should this prostate IGRT approach be tested? The initial and fundamental requirement is that the imaging modality to be used needs to precisely identify appropriate regions of cancer nodules within the prostate gland. To achieve this, there must be confirmation that the imaging modality used, such as MRI or MRS, correlates accurately and reliably with the histopathology. The type of study needed will be a technical evaluation using patients pre-imaged and undergoing radical prostatectomies. There can be many potential problems that will need to be overcome before clinical testing of this prostate IGRT can be appropriately undertaken.

Firstly, there needs to be accurate spatial alignment between the whole mount histopathological prostate sections and corresponding MR images. This type of procedure is not usually performed in routine practice. We have developed a customized prostate holder and slicing device specifically for the purpose of processing and orientating whole mount histopathological slices with their corresponding MR images (Fig. 1) (33). Other tissue processing issues that will need to be dealt with include the problem of tissue deformation during the slicing process and shrinkage due to fixation in formalin so that subsequent three-dimensional spatial alignment and localization of the tumor regions with the imaging remains accurate.

There are also other issues with MR imaging whereby reliability of the MR parameters will need to be defined and thresholds established to distinguish imaging criteria best associated with benign or malignant prostate tissue. Once the most promising parameters are defined, then sensitivity and specificity can be reviewed to see whether or not this imaging assessment is likely to be useful in clinical practice. For example, using dynamic contrast-enhanced MRI, our preliminary studies have suggested a very high specificity (93%) with a sensitivity of approximately 60% for prostate adenocarcinoma that increases to 73% for cancer nodules that are greater than 1 cm^3 (34).

The next appropriate set of studies would be to model this IGRT strategy of creating a deliberately heterogeneous dose distribution by escalating dose (86–90 Gy) to the cancer nodule(s) while maintaining a "standard" dose to the rest of the prostate gland. These studies can be performed on a small number of patients, in the order of 6 to 12 cases, to evaluate the distribution of intraprostatic nodule(s) locations that would be best treated using this IGRT strategy and the treatment technique. In addition, estimations of the potential tumor control probabilities (TCP) and normal tissues complication probabilities

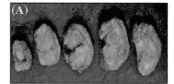
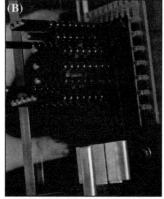
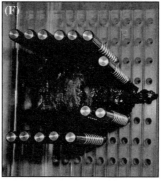
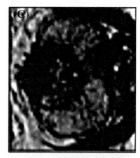
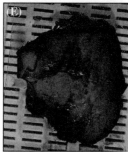
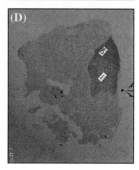

Figure 1 A study method to correlate radical prostatectomy histopathological findings with magnetic resonance imaging (MRI). (**A**) Mounting of the resected prostate gland in the same orientation as the imaging procedure. (**B**) Slicing of the mounted prostate gland. (**C**) Sliced prostate sections to correspond to the imaging slices. (**D**) An example for one of the macroscopic whole mount slides of the prostate. (**E**) Corresponding macroscopic whole prostate section. (**F**) The image section of the prostate gland using MRI.

(NTCP) can be profiled to determine the appropriate tumor boost or even to individualize boost doses for each patient.

It is evident that substantial studies of this nature are needed before clinical testing of this prostate IGRT strategy should be undertaken. For these studies outlined above, randomized trials are indeed not appropriate as these studies are designed to establish the methodology. Subsequently, following confirmation of accurate histopathological imaging correlation and the radiotherapeutic design of boost strategies with attention to four-dimensional delivery issues, feasibility studies can be initiated to determine the safety of this method and its potential impact on clinical patient outcomes.

For the example of the IGRT prostate strategy given above to treat single or multiple dominant intraprostatic nodules, this can be undertaken as a phase I/II feasibility study. Acceptable clinical parameters for both acute and late toxicity will need to be defined. It is also important to ensure that adequate follow-up time is provided to capture any untoward late side effects. In this situation, study follow-up at a minimum time of two years is often mandatory to make a preliminary assessment of late morbidity before progressing to the next stage of clinical trials. If toxicity end points are being considered, then the number of patients needed for these feasibility studies will be dependent on the nominated toxicity grades and thresholds. For example, if we wished to exclude a level of grade 2 Radiation Therapy Oncology Group (RTOG) toxicity rate at 25%, then approximately 30 patients will be needed with 90% confidence assuming that the "real" toxicity rate is 10%. A more realistic assessment would be to exclude RTOG grade 2 toxicity rates of 20% or more, and this lower threshold will now require approximately 130 patients.

In such a study, the outcomes will be strongly dependent on radiotherapy technique, planning margins used, and methods of treatment delivery and verification. In consideration of the definitive randomized trial, there is a strong argument to perform a randomized phase II type study following the feasibility studies whereby patients will be randomized between the "experimental" treatment and standard arm. Several trial comparisons may be undertaken in this regard. One clinical trial option is to randomize between the experimental boost dose and the standard dose (which may range from 74 to 78 Gy) to the whole prostate (14–17,35). Using the patient numbers quoted above, the power to detect differences between the treatment groups may be relatively weak, but the advantage of this approach is that it can act as a good pilot for the definitive randomized control trial, which will need to assess treatment efficacy.

Treatment efficacy may be considered in terms of local disease control or treatment related morbidity. In prostate cancer trials, control of biochemical PSA levels is commonly chosen as the principal end point, although there is no convincing data that this is a good proxy for clinically relevant end points such as development of metastases, use of salvage therapy (hormonal therapy), or cause-specific or overall survival. For a phase III clinical trial intending to evaluate an improvement in PSA biochemical control levels from 70% to 85%, the required number of cases for 80% power and a two-sided α value of 0.05 would be 175 per randomized arm. If a smaller improvement in biochemical PSA levels was anticipated, for example from 70% to 80%, then for 90% power and a two-sided α value of 0.05, the number needed per randomized arm would be 445 cases.

Another trial option would be to assess the utility of image-guided technology by comparing radiotherapy delivery given with or without the use of the new in-room methods of daily target guidance but with daily EPID verification in both arms as the standard. This will be discussed in more depth in the following section.

Assessment of Treatment Planning Margins, Target Tracking, and Treatment Verification

Some of the issues relevant to studies of IGRT include the determination of treatment planning margins, target tracking, and treatment verification. We have performed three small randomized control trials relating to these aspects of treatment delivery. They will be discussed to illustrate the types of methodology that can be adopted to evaluate other aspects of radiotherapy technology.

The determination of radiotherapy treatment margins for prostate radiotherapy remains a crucial issue. There have been many different methods used to assess the magnitude of prostate motion such as repeated CT scanning during radiotherapy to implanted intraprostatic markers (36,37). The aim of these methods is to rationalize the design of treatment margins for patients receiving high doses of radiation. On the basis of population statistics, margin recipes have been developed to aid the determination of treatment margins (38). However, irrespective of the margin selected, clinical relevance and potential impact on patient outcomes can only be determined through clinical trials. One example of a clinical trial assessing the appropriateness of a set of treatment margins is illustrated here. In the United Kingdom, in the mid-late nineties, most radiotherapy centers were using uniform margins around the prostate of 1.0 to 1.5 cm. The question posed was which of these treatment margins was most appropriate. In a randomized pilot study of dose escalation comparing 64 Gy versus 74 Gy (35), we added a second randomization. A 2×2 factorial design randomized patients to radiotherapy with either a 1.0-cm or 1.5-cm margin. One hundred and twenty five men were included in the study and this was enough to show a statistically significant increase in the RTOG ≥ 2 rate of late bowel toxicity (21% vs. 13%, $p = 0.005$). The biochemical PSA control rate of disease was identical between the treatment arms suggesting no loss of local tumor control using the 1-cm margin.

However, although this is the only randomized control trial at any tumor site, to our knowledge, to compare a radiotherapy margin, the evidence falls far short of proving equivalence in efficacy between the two treatment groups. To do this, adequately, a noninferiority clinical trial design would be required. If a clinical trial is aimed at determining noninferiority between the trial arms, then the number of patients needed will depend on the level of

Table 6 Allocation of Patients Numbers Needed Within Clinical Trials That Aim for Noninferiority

Difference allowed	Number per group	
	80% power	90% power
5%	1039	1439
6%	721	999
7%	530	734
8%	406	562
9%	321	444
10%	260	360

difference allowed and the confidence limits needed. Examples of this are listed in Table 6 where if a difference of 10% is allowed, the number of patients required per randomized arm for 80% and 90% power is 260 and 360 cases, respectively. However, if only a difference of 5% is allowed, then the number of patients required per randomized arm for 80% and 90% power increases to 1039 and 1439 cases, respectively. Clearly, such a trial is impractical, and the evidence from this small pilot study was sufficient to convince the U.K. investigators that the 1.0-cm margin was more appropriate. This planning margin was then used in the subsequent larger international MRC RT01 phase III trial (17).

Compared with the clinical trials described above, a "technical" trial may require considerably less patients. For example, our initial assessment of an EPID in the early 1990s evaluated 12 patients with portal imaging at the beginning and end of their treatments for hypofractionated (6 Gy/fraction) radiotherapy in prostate and bladder cancer and assessed the value of portal imaging by reimaging the patient at the end of their treatment (39). Each patient had the "order" of their treatment randomized to be either corrected on the basis of the portal image or not. This study showed that at the end of therapy in the conventionally managed treatment fractions, there was a displacement of 4.9 ± 2 mm compared with 2.1 ± 1.5 mm ($p < 0.01$) for the corrected treatments. Furthermore, the proportion of treatments delivered with a field-placement error of ≥ 5 mm decreased from 69% to 7%. This study verified the value of interventional portal imaging to improve treatment accuracy. More importantly, this study demonstrates that this format of intrapatient randomization can be used effectively to assess the value of a technical innovation in radiotherapy and has definite applications for the evaluation of IGRT in prostate cancer.

However, not all technical studies will produce the expected benefits (and desired) result. We have also undertaken a small randomized control trial evaluating the use of the "Vacfix" pelvic immobilization device (40). In this study, 30 patients were recruited and treated

radically with prostate radiotherapy. All patients were "double planned" both using our standard immobilization system (knee support and ankle stocks) or the same with the addition of a Vacfix pelvic immobilization device. In this study, a similar intrapatient randomization was used for patients being treated either with or without the Vacfix bag for weeks 1 to 3 or 4 to 6 of treatment. Neither random nor systematic errors were improved by the pelvic immobilization device. In contrast, the accuracy of treatment setup was marginally better with the standard setup technique despite the patients reporting that the use of the pelvic immobilization device was more comfortable during treatment. This is a valuable finding as many departments may have assumed that new technology will improve treatment outcomes, and this clinical trial of radiotherapy technology was salutary in showing the opposite! Accuracy, however, was very good in both groups of treatment and was deemed improved on our previous experience, which we judged to be because of the introduction of electronic portal imaging.

We are using a broadly similar clinical design to test the value of a new prostate localizing obturator called "ProSpare" (patent pending). This endorectal device containing radiopaque markers has been designed to sit comfortably within the anorectum and be self-positioned by the patient. The intention of this device is to stabilize the position of the prostate by maintaining a constant rectal volume as the device is "vented," to offer some normal tissue sparing as the anterior and posterior rectal walls are separated, as well as to provide markers for treatment localization. The accuracy of treatment will be judged by comparing fiducial markers implanted into the prostate with those within the ProSpare device. Again, patients will act as their own controls being "double planned" with and without the ProSpare device, and weeks 1 and 2 of treatment will be randomized to be either with or without the device. An initial cohort of 25 patients will assess acceptability and tolerability using an actual device tolerability rate of 85%. This will exclude a lower limit of tolerability of 50% with 90% power. This study will also allow a paired standardized difference of 0.67 mm (2-mm difference with standard deviation of 3 mm) between treatments with and without ProSpare to be detected (89% power, two-sided α 0.05 using a paired t test).

By illustration of the trial methodologies, these small detailed technical studies reveal how innovative and technical methods of treatment delivery can be tested in an appropriate fashion in small numbers of patients. However, these clinical trials do not prove that they are clinically of benefit. As outlined above, many more patients are needed to show benefits in terms of clinical efficacy of treatment albeit lower numbers may be adequate to appropriately measure benefits in terms of reduction of toxicity.

The French multicentre trial of IGRT in prostate cancer mentioned earlier has two parts (Dr. R. de Crevoisier, personal communication). The first part aims to evaluate the accuracy of conventional portal imaging for the localization of the prostate gland by also incorporating daily in-room cone-beam imaging during prostate external beam radiotherapy. This part of the study aims to recruit 80 patients. The second part of the trial randomizes 404 patients to two different frequencies of prostate position verification, which is either for daily cone beam imaging pre-treatment or for cone beam imaging during the first 3 days of treatment followed by weekly cone beam imaging. For this study, the main end point is biochemical disease-free survival with the intention of showing a 12% benefit in the five-year biochemical disease-free survival rates for the use of daily cone-beam imaging. This is calculated to require 202 patients in each arm (power = 80%, α 0.05 using 2 –sided log-rank test).

FUTURE DIRECTIONS

Current studies in prostate IGRT have been exploratory investigations assessing methodology of the IGRT process, quantifying the IGRT mechanism, or early feasibility or phase I/II studies. There are many groups that may believe it is not ethical to randomize patients into randomized control trials comparing the utility of IGRT with standard delivery methods for prostate radiotherapy whether it be for dose escalation, boost strategies, or hypofractionation regimes. However, similar to the situation that currently exists for the value of IMRT, it is clear that randomized controlled trials are the only method to truly determine the utility of IGRT procedures or strategies on patient outcomes whether it is to reduce treatment related toxicity or to improved local tumor control rates. Irrespectively of the IGRT question under trial, it is important for all radiotherapy trials to incorporate adequate and appropriate quality assurance.

Another important understanding is that while IGRT for treatment delivery may substantially reduce the magnitude of systematic error and limit random error in treatment setup and target localization, this does not necessarily mean that treatment planning margins can be zero. Random errors in treatment delivery by nature cannot be completely eliminated, and thus some form of margin for treatment uncertainty will always remain. As IGRT methods for four-dimensional treatment delivery are validated and assessed in clinical trials, attention will need to be directed to the definition of target volumes, as this will remain the main and largest source of uncertainty. This will both influence intra- and interobserver variability and can be a major concern for multicentre clinical trials.

It is also clear that sophisticated treatment planning technique such as IMRT will need to incorporate some form of IGRT so that the potential benefits for the closely shaped high-dose regions can be directed to the target volume accurately and reliably in time and space to maintain the expected patient outcomes. Again, for clinical efficacy, this can only be properly validated in comparative randomized controlled trials.

SUMMARY OF PERTINENT CONCLUSIONS

- Clinical trials in prostate IGRT need to be well designed and executed to reliably separate treatment effects from study uncertainties such as bias and random error.
- Clinical trials for prostate IGRT will need to define appropriate end points for the image-guided strategy under investigation.
- The magnitude of anticipated difference together with the confidence limit will determine the number of patients required for any clinical trial.
- Small clinical trials ($\leq$30 patients) using intrapatient randomizations can be designed to determine if new technologies improve treatment accuracy.
- Relatively small randomized controlled trials can be designed to assess if a new technique reduces treatment related side effects compared with standard treatment ($<$300 patients).
- Large randomized controlled trials are required to show equivalent efficacy of new and standard techniques ($>$1000 to 2000 patients).
- The prospective randomized comparative clinical trial in prostate IGRT will be the only method of logically confirming the true value for patient outcomes whether it is a reduction in treatment related toxicity or improvement in biochemical PSA control rates.
- The successful conduct of any clinical trial on radiation technology will need to include (*i*) the development of appropriate study protocols and technology methodology; (*ii*) the definition of suitable study end points; (*iii*) obtaining the necessary regulatory approvals; (*iv*) the provisions of suitable resources for study execution and quality assurance; (*v*) data collection and analysis; and (*vi*) dissemination of the study results.

REFERENCES

1. Evidence-Based Medicine Working Group. Evidence-based medicine. A new approach to teaching the practice of medicine. JAMA 1992; 268(17):2420–2425.
2. USPSTF. U.S. Preventive Services Task Force; Agency for Health Care Research and Quality: Evidence-based Practice Program. Available at: http://www.ahrq.gov/clinic/uspstfix.htm 2007. Accessed on July 2007.

3. Oxford U. Centre for Evidence-Based Medicine. Available at: http://www.cebm.net/index.aspx 2007. Accessed on July 2007.

4. Bardfeld PA, Passalaqua AM, Braunstein P, et al. A comparison of radionuclide scanning and computed tomography in metastatic lesions of the brain. J Comput Assist Tomogr 1977; 1(3):315–318.

5. Baker HL Jr., Houser OW, Campbell JK. National Cancer Institute study: evaluation of computed tomography in the diagnosis of intracranial neoplasms. I. Overall results. Radiology 1980; 136(1):91–96.

6. Buncher CR. National Cancer Institute study: evaluation of computed tomography in the diagnosis of intracranial neoplasms. II. Was randomization necessary? Radiology 1980; 136(3):651–655.

7. Goitein M, Wittenberg J, Mendiondo M, et al. The value of CT scanning in radiation therapy treatment planning: a prospective study. Int J Radiat Oncol Biol Phys 1979; 5(10): 1787–1798.

8. Goitein M. The utility of computed tomography in radiation therapy: an estimate of outcome. Int J Radiat Oncol Biol Phys 1979; 5(10):1799–1807.

9. ICRU-50. International Commission on Radiation Units and Measurements. ICRU Report 50: Prescribing, recording, and reporting photon beam therapy. Bethesda, MD: International Commission on Radiation Units and Measurement, 1993:3–16.

10. ICRU-62. International Commission on Radiation Units and Measurements. ICRU Report 62: Prescribing, recording, and reporting photon beam therapy. Bethesda, MD: International Commission on Radiation Units and Measurement, 1999:3–20.

11. Dearnaley DP, Khoo VS, Norman AR, et al. Comparison of radiation side-effects of conformal and conventional radiotherapy in prostate cancer: a randomised trial. Lancet 1999; 353(9149):267–272.

12. Zelefsky MJ, Fuks Z, Happersett L, et al. Clinical experience with intensity modulated radiation therapy (IMRT) in prostate cancer. Radiother Oncol 2000; 55(3):241–249.

13. Zelefsky MJ, Chan H, Hunt M, et al. Long-term outcome of high dose intensity modulated radiation therapy for patients with clinically localized prostate cancer. J Urol 2006; 176 (4 pt 1):1415–1419.

14. Pollack A, Zagars GK, Starkschall G, et al. Prostate cancer radiation dose response: results of the M. D. Anderson phase III randomized trial. Int J Radiat Oncol Biol Phys 2002; 53(5):1097–1105.

15. Peeters ST, Heemsbergen WD, van Putten WL, et al. Acute and late complications after radiotherapy for prostate cancer: results of a multicenter randomized trial comparing 68 Gy to 78 Gy. Int J Radiat Oncol Biol Phys 2005; 61(4): 1019–1034.

16. Zietman AL, DeSilvio ML, Slater JD, et al. Comparison of conventional-dose vs high-dose conformal radiation therapy in clinically localized adenocarcinoma of the prostate: a randomized controlled trial. JAMA 2005; 294(10):1233–1239.

17. Dearnaley DP, Sydes MR, Graham JD, et al. Escalated-dose versus standard-dose conformal radiotherapy in prostate cancer: first results from the MRC RT01 randomised controlled trial. Lancet Oncol 2007; 8(6):475–487.

18. Lukka H, Hayter C, Julian JA, et al. Randomized trial comparing two fractionation schedules for patients with localized prostate cancer. J Clin Oncol 2005; 23(25): 6132–6138.

19. Yeoh EE, Holloway RH, Fraser RJ, et al. Hypofractionated versus conventionally fractionated radiation therapy for prostate carcinoma: updated results of a phase III randomized trial. Int J Radiat Oncol Biol Phys 2006; 66(4):1072–1083.

20. South CP, Khoo VS, Naismith O, et al. A comparison of treatment planning techniques used in two randomised UK external beam radiotherapy trials for localised prostate cancer. Clin Oncol (R Coll Radiol) 2008; 20(1):15–21.

21. Khoo VS, Dearnaley DP. Question of dose, fractionation and technique: ingredients for testing hypofractionation in prostate cancer—the CHHiP trial. Clin Oncol (R Coll Radiol) 2008; 20(1):12–14.

22. Stanley S, Griffiths S, Sydes MR, et al. Accuracy and reproducibility of conformal radiotherapy using data from a randomised controlled trial of conformal radiotherapy in prostate cancer (MRC RT01, ISRCTN47772397). Clin Oncol 2007 (in press).

23. de Crevoisier R, Tucker SL, Dong L, et al. Increased risk of biochemical and local failure in patients with distended rectum on the planning CT for prostate cancer radiotherapy. Int J Radiat Oncol Biol Phys 2005; 62(4):965–973.

24. Heemsbergen WD, Hoogeman MS, Witte MG, et al. Increased risk of biochemical and clinical failure for prostate patients with a large rectum at radiotherapy planning: results from the Dutch trial of 68 GY versus 78 Gy. Int J Radiat Oncol Biol Phys 2007; 67(5):1418–1424.

25. NCI. Available at: http://www.cancer.gov/clinicaltrials. In: Accessed on August 2007.

26. NCIC. Available at: http://www.ctg.queensu.ca/public/Clinical_Trials/clinical_trials.html. In: Accessed on August 2007.

27. NCRN. Available at: http://www.ncrn.org.uk/portfolio/dbase.asp. In: Accessed on August 2007.

28. EORTC. Available at: http://www.eortc.be/protoc/default.htm. In: Accessed on August 2007.

29. Khoo VS, Joon DL. New developments in MRI for target volume delineation in radiotherapy. Br J Radiol 2006; 79 (Spec No 1):S2–S15 (review).

30. Pickett B, Vigneault E, Kurhanewicz J, et al. Static field intensity modulation to treat a dominant intra-prostatic lesion to 90 Gy compared to seven field 3-dimensional radiotherapy. Int J Radiat Oncol Biol Phys 1999; 44(4): 921–929.

31. Xia P, Pickett B, Vigneault E, et al. Forward or inversely planned segmental multileaf collimator IMRT and sequential tomotherapy to treat multiple dominant intraprostatic lesions of prostate cancer to 90 Gy. Int J Radiat Oncol Biol Phys 2001; 51(1):244–254.

32. Nutting CM, Corbishley CM, Sanchez-Nieto B, et al. Potential improvements in the therapeutic ratio of prostate cancer irradiation: dose escalation of pathologically identified tumour nodules using intensity modulated radiotherapy. Br J Radiol 2002; 75(890):151–161.

33. Jhavar SG, Fisher C, Jackson A, et al. Processing of radical prostatectomy specimens for correlation of data from histopathological, molecular biological, and radiological

studies: a new whole organ technique. J Clin Pathol 2005; 58(5):504–508.

34. Reinsberg SA, Moore LM, Sohaib A, et al. Methodology for the histopathologic correlation with functional MR images of the prostate by successive morphing. Proc. Intl. Soc. Mag. Reson. Med. 2004; 11(1):751.

35. Dearnaley DP, Hall E, Lawrence D, et al. Phase III pilot study of dose escalation using conformal radiotherapy in prostate cancer: PSA control and side effects. Br J Cancer 2005; 92(3):488–498.

36. Zelefsky MJ, Crean D, Mageras GS, et al. Quantification and predictors of prostate position variability in 50 patients evaluated with multiple CT scans during conformal radiotherapy. Radiother Oncol 1999; 50(2):225–234.

37. Enmark M, Korreman S, Nystrom H. IGRT of prostate cancer; is the margin reduction gained from daily IG time-dependent? Acta Oncol 2006; 45(7):907–914.

38. van Herk M, Remeijer P, Lebesque JV. Inclusion of geometric uncertainties in treatment plan evaluation. Int J Radiat Oncol Biol Phys 2002; 52(5):1407–1422.

39. Gildersleve J, Dearnaley DP, Evans PM, et al. A randomised trial of patient repositioning during radiotherapy using a megavoltage imaging system. Radiother Oncol 1994; 31(2):161–168.

40. Nutting CM, Khoo VS, Walker V, et al. A randomized study of the use of a customized immobilization system in the treatment of prostate cancer with conformal radiotherapy. Radiother Oncol 2000; 54(1):1–9.

20

Future Developments I: Online Dosimetric Verification with Fiducial Dosimeter Planning and Verification

MARK WIESMEYER, HABEEB SALEH, MARTIN MURPHY, AND MITCHELL S. ANSCHER
Department of Radiation Oncology, Virginia Commonwealth University School of Medicine, Richmond, Virginia, U.S.A.

GLORIA P. BEYER AND CHARLES W. SCARANTINO
Sicel Technologies, Morrisville, North Carolina, U.S.A.

JOANNA E. CYGLER
Department of Medical Physics, Ottawa Hospital Regional Cancer Centre, Ottawa, Ontario, Canada

INTRODUCTION

The tolerance of normal tissues limits the dose of radiation that can be delivered in the treatment of malignancy (1). Nevertheless, advances in treatment delivery technology, combined with improvements in imaging that facilitate better tumor targeting, have enabled the radiation oncologist to deliver higher doses using external beam radiation therapy than had been previously thought possible. Usually, the strategy employed to deliver high radiation doses depends on the ability to reduce the margin of normal tissue around the target that receives full-dose irradiation. In this situation, it is incumbent upon the radiation oncologist to demonstrate that the planned dose is actually being delivered to the target.

The treatment of prostate cancer with external beam radiation therapy (EBRT) is one of the few situations in oncology in which level-one evidence exists to support radiation dose escalation in selected patient populations (2). Equally compelling is the evidence of a dose-volume relationship for late toxicity in the pelvic organs surrounding the prostate, especially the rectum (2,3). Despite its location in the floor of the pelvis beneath the peritoneum, the prostate can demonstrate considerable movement between treatment fractions, and to a lesser extent, during a treatment fraction (4,5). Thus, accurate dose delivery, with narrow margins around the target, can present a technical challenge. Even more challenging can be accurate dose verification within the target. Until recently, it was not possible to measure dose in vivo, except on the skin surface and in easily accessible regions of body cavities (6), and a true in situ dose measurement, for most cancers, was impossible, since the dose measuring devices had to be removed from the body in order to be interrogated.

Currently, it is now possible, with certain limitations, to implant a dosimeter into or adjacent to a tumor and to determine the actual dose delivered to the target telemetrically throughout a course of treatment. Herein, we will review the history of in vivo dosimetry, describe the design and operation of a new in situ dose verification system, review the available animal and human data that display its capabilities, and offer practical guidelines for implementation of in situ dosimetry into routine clinical practice.

HISTORY OF IN VIVO DOSIMETRY

During the first decades of practice in radiation therapy, there were no standardized quantitative units to measure the patient's radiation exposure. Dose was typically expressed in terms of some physiological response, e.g., the "erythema dose" (7), which would have been the amount of radiation needed to induce skin reddening. The corresponding dose to internal treatment sites would then have been extrapolated from the skin dose. One common practice used to calibrate an applicator for radium therapy involved holding it to the skin of a healthy subject until a skin reaction appeared (8). This procedure established a reference exposure level for use during the therapy. Thus, early dosimetry was in vivo by definition, insofar as it measured dose to tissue directly, but more specifically, it was entrance dosimetry that required calculation and inference to estimate the dose to internal organs.

Subsequently, various film and electronic systems have replaced the skin as the radiosensitive element for entrance and exit dosimetry. A comprehensive historical survey of the large literature on this subject is beyond the scope of this chapter, but some specific examples to illustrate the various methods and their place in the development time line will be presented below.

Contemporary in vivo dosimetry methods are distinguished by the type and placement of the radiosensitive elements. The detectors can be film or discrete element sensors such as diodes and MOSFET (metal oxide semiconductor field effect transistor) sensors, or electronic detector systems such as an electronic portal imaging device (EPID). They can be placed on the skin at the point of beam entry (entrance dosimetry) or behind the patient (exit dosimetry). In these geometries, the inference of the dose at the treatment site is an extrapolation problem. Transit dosimetry measures both the entrance and exit dose. This changes the extrapolation problem into an interpolation issue, which generally is better constrained and thus will give more accurate results. Finally, placement of the sensor directly at the treatment site minimizes calculation and inference, while giving the most direct measurement.

In 1978, Hassan and Pearce (9) described a technical study of a swallowable pill containing a mercuric iodide detector and radiotransmitter that could potentially be used for in situ measurements of ionizing radiation. However, the modern era of in vivo dosimetry using external detectors began circa 1990. Initially, entrance and exit dose measurements were made with diodes and thermoluminescent detectors (TLDs) (10–12). By the mid 1990s,

commercial diode systems were available for skin dosimetry. These provided multiple diode detectors coupled to a multichannel readout unit (13).

Portal films present the opportunity to measure exit dose radiographically (14). In vivo dosimetry using EPIDs was introduced somewhat later (15,16). The MOSFET was first conceived by Lilienfeld in the 1920s (17), but its first practical realization was not until 1960 by Kahng and Atalla at Bell Labs. The major technical advances required to realize Lilienfeld's idea were the silicon planar process developed in the late 1950s by McCaldin and Hoerni and the integrated circuit developed by Kilby and Noyce. The notion of MOSFET-based dosimetry was introduced in 1978 by Holmes-Siedle in the form of a space-charge measuring device (18). Since then, MOSFETs have mostly been used to monitor radiation encountered by man-made earth-orbiting satellites. Perhaps, Thomson et al. (19), in 1984, published the earliest description of a MOSFET dosimeter that might be used in a radiation therapy setting. Subsequently, the detector was introduced into the discussion (20) as an alternative to the TLD for skin placement.

Although all of these methods are commonly called in vivo dosimetry, they still require inference of the dose at the internal tumor and critical structures from remote measurements. If one considers the more explicit form of in situ dosimetry, where one measures the dose directly at the internal sites of interest, one finds only a very small number of historical and recent examples.

An early and somewhat theatrical attempt at in situ dosimetry was motivated by the development of rotation therapy in the early 1950s. The use of rotation therapy to increase the dose to deep tumors (an early approach to three-dimensional therapy) made dose calculations significantly more complicated and greatly increased the importance of dose verification measurements at the time of treatment. To demonstrate in situ dosimetry for rotation therapy, Webb employed a professional sword swallower to insert a long rod with an ionization chamber at its tip through his esophagus into the thorax (21). The typical patient, though, would probably balk at this procedure.

Endoscopic insertion of dosimeters, however, can provide a more conventional access to some internal sites. This has motivated the development of scintillator crystals that can be passed through an endoscope while optically coupled via fiber to an external photomultiplier tube or photodiode (22). High dose rate (HDR) brachytherapy provides some opportunities for approximately in situ dosimetry by attaching dosimeters to the applicator. For example, Pai et al. (23) described use of radiochromic film taped to the outside of the applicator for cervical HDR brachytherapy. However, because of the extreme difficulty of getting dose-measuring sensors into most internal treatment sites, using external detectors has largely satisfied the measurement of in vivo dose during external beam radiotherapy.

Much of the incentive to develop in situ dosimetry has come from radioimmunotherapy (RIT), which is not amenable to the use of external detectors. In 1994, Gladstone et al. (24) described a miniature MOSFET dosimeter designed to be inserted in a 16-gauge needle and thence directly into tissue. This dosimeter was tested in mice during RIT (25). Yorke et al. (26) addressed the particular issues that arise in the use of TLDs for in situ dosimetry in RIT. TLDs are sensitive to temperature, chemical environment, time delays between exposure and readout, and other factors. In contrast to external beam (i.e., entrance) dosimetry, where the TLDs are exposed to air at room temperature and read out within 48 hours, a TLD implanted in situ for RIT is in a tissue environment at mammalian temperature for up to two weeks. Such significant differences would be expected to alter their in situ performance relative to their better-documented external characteristics. These issues were pursued further in studies by Demidecki et al. (27), which measured the effects on TLDs of prolonged immersion in in vitro media intended to simulate a tissue environment. However, these were feasibility studies that did not extend to animal or human subject testing.

Molecular imaging techniques offer promise as a means to measure dose deposition at the target site directly and noninvasively. For in situ dosimetry during proton therapy, Paans and Schippers (28) proposed in a feasibility study to use positron emission tomography (PET) imaging of the resulting proton-induced activity at the treatment site.

Finally, in 2002, Ishikawa et al. (29) patented an internal dosimetry system using small radiosensitive transponders injected directly into the tumor. The transponders included electronics to communicate dose data with a remote external receiver. This device operates, in principle, in a manner similar to a more recently developed commercially available MOSFET-based system for in situ dosimetry.

MOSFET AS A PATIENT DOSIMETER

Structure and Operation

MOSFETs are a type of transistor, and as such, they can be used to control the flow of electrical charge (current) in electronic circuits. There are two basic types of MOSFETs: n-type and p-type. The "n" in n-type and "p" in p-type refer to the fact that semiconductors such as silicon can be "doped" (i.e., trace atomic impurities can be added to pure silicon). By doping, imperfections are formed in the silicon matrix that has either a surplus of electrons (n-type) or shortage of them (p-type). A shortage

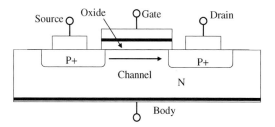

Figure 1 Cross section of a p-type MOSFET. *Abbreviation*: MOSFET, metal oxide semiconductor field effect transistor.

of electrons is often called a "hole." The doped silicon acquires the property that its electrical conductance can be modulated by an external electric field.

Transistors, in general, can be thought of as charge "faucets." Figure 1 shows the schematic of a p-type MOSFET, which shows that this analogy is reflected in the naming of some MOSFET components (e.g., source, gate, drain, channel). By convention, MOSFETs are categorized according to the doping of their source and drain or, equivalently, by the type of "channel" that is formed between source and drain. Thus, the schematic of an n-type MOSFET would be identical in structure to the p-type MOSFET shown in Figure 1, differing only in the doping of the source, drain, and substrate. Most dosimetry applications use p-type MOSFETs.

When a negative voltage with respect to the body electrode is applied to the gate of a p-type MOSFET, an electric field is produced that attracts holes from the body substrate, source, and drain to the region immediately below the oxide insulator. With a sufficient gate voltage, V_G, a sufficient number of holes may accumulate forming a channel that allows current to flow between the source and drain. The minimum voltage required allowing flow of current between the source and drain is known as threshold voltage (V_{TH}). The operation of an n-type MOSFET is precisely the same as that of a p-type, except that the activating gate voltage polarity is positive and the role of holes and electrons is reversed.

MOSFETs make suitable radiation dosimeters, because, with irradiation, the relationship between gate voltage and current flow changes in a predictable manner. They have the added features of small size, simple interface circuitry, low power during readout, and the ability to measure radiation while in a powered down (passive) state.

When a metal oxide semiconductor device is irradiated, several things occur within the insulating oxide: trapped charge builds up in the oxide, the number of interface traps increases, and the number of bulk oxide traps increases (19). Electron-hole pairs are created within the oxide insulator by the incident ionizing radiation. Electrons, having about four orders of magnitude greater mobility than holes in SiO_2 tend to move quickly toward positively biased contacts and exit the oxide layer (30). Depending on the applied electric field, some fraction of electrons and holes will recombine. Holes that escape initial recombination are relatively stable and remain near their point of generation in the oxide layer. Thus, when a p-type MOSFET is exposed to radiation, the threshold voltage magnitude increases. When MOSFET dosimeters are unbiased, their radiation sensitivity is lower, less linear, and they may exhibit less signal drift, also known as "fade."

If the change in threshold voltage due to a known radiation dose can be characterized, then the MOSFET may be used to accurately measure radiation dose. The sensitivity of MOSFET devices (*i*) increases with a positive gate bias during irradiation, which increases long-term survival of holes by decreasing electron-hole recombination, and (*ii*) increases with an increase in the thickness of the oxide layer, which promotes overall electron-hole generation.

Supporting Electronics

For any p-type MOSFET, the V_{TH} that is required to sustain a specific drain-to-source current (I_{DS}) increases with irradiation. Electronics supporting the use of these devices are designed to adjust, measure, and report the input voltage required to obtain a specific current flow. The change in V_{TH} before and after irradiation to sustain this current flow multiplied by a calibration factor yields dose for the irradiation fraction.

For an individual MOSFET detector, the relationship between V_{TH} and I_{DS} can be especially susceptible to temperature and the dose to which the detector has been exposed (other dependencies will be discussed later). Temperature changes can affect V_{TH} by as much as 4 to 5 mV/°C; exposure to high irradiation levels can affect the linearity of dose response. Dual bias dual MOSFET detector circuits were devised to limit these dependencies (31). They have the additional benefit of enabling the sensitivity of the detector to be modulated.

Figure 2 shows a dual bias dual detector circuit with two MOSFETs and their immediate supporting circuitry; they are typically fabricated on the same silicon substrate allowing the MOSFETs to be very near to each other. Because of their proximity and very small size, the MOSFETs are assumed exposed identically when irradiated. The voltage applied to the MOSFET gates is different, as implied by the circuit's name. Target drain-to-source currents may be the same or different when dosimeters are read. As with the single dosimeter discussion above, the V_{TH} is adjusted to obtain a specific

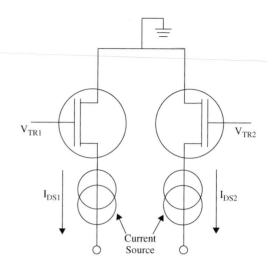

Figure 2 Readout circuitry for dual bias, dual MOSFET. *Abbreviation*: MOSFET, metal oxide semiconductor field effect transistor. *Source*: From Ref. 31.

I_{DS}. The reported dose is equal to $k(\Delta V_{TH1} - \Delta V_{TH2})$, where k is a constant of proportionality with units Gy/V.

Patient Dosimetry

The use of MOSFETS for dosimetry of EBRT is relatively recent. Thomson first proposed the idea in 1984 (19). This paper discussed the use of these devices in a phantom in the presence of electron and photon beams. Most published research has used commercial devices and apparatus, some of them prototypes. Table 1 shows a sample[a] of the available literature on the use of MOSFETs in photon-based EBRT. As can be seen from the table, there is very little published research discussing the use of these dosimeters in vivo.

Commercial vendors of MOSFET dosimeters include Best Medical Canada, Ltd. (Ottawa, Ontario, Canada), Sicel Technologies, Inc. (Morrisville, North Carolina, U.S.), and REM Oxford, Ltd. (Eynsham, Oxford, U.K.). Best Medical produces MOSFETs and supporting apparatus formerly marketed by Thomson-Nielsen (Ottawa, Canada). The Best dosimeters are primarily intended for entrance and exit dosimetry, whereas Sicel Technologies produces MOSFET for entrance dosimetry (OneDose[TM]) and for implantable dosimetry [Dose Verification System (DVS[®]) dosimeters that are wireless and can be implanted directly into the tumor volume, then read telemetrically]. Details of the operation and clinical application of the DVS implantable dosimeter will be presented later in this chapter.

---

[a]We only present relatively new papers on the use of MOSFET dosimeters in high-energy external photon beams. Older papers are not discussed because their results, although interesting with respect to the evolution of MOSFET dosimeter technology, may not be clinically applicable.

Table 1 A Sample of the Current MOSFET Dosimeter Literature

Reference	Company	Model	Phantom	In vivo	Source/Energy
Beddar et al. (32)	Sicel	DVS	Yes	No	^{60}Co
Bharanidharan et al. (33)	Best	TN502RD	Yes	No	^{60}Co, 6 MV, 15 MV
Black et al. (34)	Sicel	DVS	Yes	Yes	6 MV, 18 MV, electrons
Briere et al. (35)	Sicel	DVS	Yes	No	^{60}Co
Butson et al. (36)	REM	TOT500	Yes	No	6 MV, 18 MV
Cheung et al. (37)	REM	TOT500	Yes	No	6 MV
Chuang et al. (38)	Best	TN502RD	Yes	No	6 MV
Halvorsen (39)	Sicel	OneDose	Yes	No	6 MV
Jornet et al. (40)	Best	TN502RD	Yes	No	18 MV
Marcie et al. (41)	Best	TN502RD	Yes	Yes	6 MV
Ramani et al. (20)	Best	TN502RD	Yes	No	^{60}Co, 6, 18, 25 MV, electrons
Ramaseshan et al. (42)	Best	TN RDM 502	Yes	No	^{60}Co, 4, 6, 10, 18 MV, electron
Rowbottom (43)	Best	TN RDM 502	Yes	No	6 MV
Scalchi 1998 (44)	Best	TN502RD	Yes	No	6 MV
Scalchi et al. (45)	Best	TN502RD	Yes	No	6 MV
Scarantino et al. (46)	Sicel	DVS	Yes	Yes[a]	6 MV, 18 MV
Scarantino et al. (47)	Sicel	DVS	No	Yes	6 MV, 18 MV
Soubra et al. (31)	Best	TN502RD[a]	Yes	No	^{60}Co, electrons

[a]In vivo measurements were done in canines.
Abbreviations: MOSFET, metal oxide semiconductor field effect transistor; DVS, Dose Verification System.

In Vivo Usage

The following discussion is limited to the use of MOSFET dosimeters in high-energy, photon-based radiation treatments. MOSFET dosimeters have been used to monitor kilovoltage (48–50), electron (51–53), and brachytherapy (24,54–58) treatments. The use of MOSFET dosimeters in the context of brachytherapy will be discussed later in this chapter.

In vivo dosimetry can be divided into several subareas: surface, transit, intraluminal, and implanted. The term in situ has been used for intraluminal and implanted dosimetry. Surface dosimetry involves the use of dosimeters on the patient surface at well-specified entrance and exit points along the path of a beam. Transit dosimetry requires the use of an external measurement device, like an EPID, not in contact with the patient surface. Intraluminal dosimetry involves placing the dosimeter inside a lumen, that is, in proximity to the area to be treated; in the case of prostate irradiation, measurements have been done with dosimeters placed in the urethra (58,59) and rectum (6). Implanted dosimetry involves the placement of the dosimeter directly into the tissue at a point of interest in either target or organ at risk. Implanted dosimeters can be either permanent (46,47) or temporary (24,25). MOSFET dosimeters can be used for all types of in vivo dosimetry, except transit dosimetry.

In both surface and transit dosimetry, an external dose measurement is used to infer correctness of treatment dose in the patient. If the dose measurements at the patient surface or at a detector panel agree with predicted values

from a treatment planning system (TPS), then the dose delivered to target or normal tissues is potentially correct. If predicted and measured values do not agree, dose to target or normal tissues is probably incorrect. With intraluminal dosimetry used in prostate treatments, the dosimeter is placed in tissues that are of interest (i.e., rectum, urethra) and dosimetry to the prostate is inferred. The dosimeter may be volumetrically imaged during CT simulation, and dose to the dosimeter can be calculated by the TPS. If the dose measured by the dosimeter during treatment agrees with predicted dose, then the delivered dose is potentially, but not guaranteed to be, correct. The only direct means of measuring dose at an arbitrary point in target or normal tissue is through dosimeter implantation.

Because of their small size and the fact that they do not need an immediate external connection to a power supply or reader, MOSFETs are extremely versatile and ideal for implantation. They can also be used for almost any type of measurement in which TLDs and diodes have been used, including very low energy radiation treatments where photoelectric interactions predominate. Because of their high atomic number silicon-based composition, diodes and MOSFETs exhibit overresponse to very low energy photons. It has been shown for some MOSFET detectors that the maximum overresponse is on the order of about fourfold for energies of 33 keV. No energy dependencies are seen for energies greater than 120 keV for some MOSFET dosimeters (60), yet others have shown an overresponse by a factor of two to three at 120 keV. Possibly because of these photoelectric effects, lower energy applications may require calibration more often than those employing higher energy (61).

Dosimeter Placement

For surface dosimeters, placement on the central axis of a beam or along a weight point ray is the norm. Typically, doses measured at the surface of the patient are used to estimate dose at the depth of maximum dose by multiplying raw dosimeter readings by calibration factors, field size correction factors, dose rate factors, and so forth (TG62) (62).

Intraluminal or implanted dosimeter placement must be more thoughtfully considered. There are issues of patient comfort and safety, dosimeter location stability, as well as dosimetric considerations. One source of guidance for dosimeter placement in target tissues is the International Commission on Radiation Units and Measurements (ICRU) "reference point" recommendations (62,63). The ICRU recommends point placement in tissue that is clinically relevant and representative of the dose distribution throughout the planning target volume (PTV), easy to define in a clear and unambiguous way, and in a location where the dose can be accurately determined. Additionally, the point should be in a region where there are no large dose gradients. A point located at the center (or central part) of the PTV generally fulfills these requirements and is recommended as the ICRU reference point. Dosimeter placement in normal tissue may be challenging, as the clinician is often most interested in dose to normal tissues near the edge of the PTV, where dose gradients are likely to be significant.

Characterization and Dependencies

What follows is an overview of important MOSFET dosimeter characteristics and dependencies. In general, all commercial devices have properties that make them a good choice for high-energy photon dosimetry applications that have previously employed TLDs and diodes. Before using MOSFET dosimeters in the clinic, the medical physicist should validate them under the conditions in which they will be used.

Accuracy

MOSFET dosimeters have shown an achievable accuracy of 3% to 5% with respect to phantom measurements (34–36,38,39,41,42,47). Practical accuracy during patient treatments (the difference from TPS estimation) may

be affected by cumulative errors from patient setup, patient motion, and dose calculation (34,41,47). With implantable dosimeters, migration after implantation has been reported (46,47), which may be an additional source of error.[b] Signal drift, known as fade, is present in all MOSFET dosimeters and must be taken into account by reading dosimeters in the time frame recommended by the manufacturer.

Temperature Independence

Some MOSFET dosimeters have been shown to be practically free of temperature dependency over a wide range of temperatures (e.g., 20–40°C) (31,44). Other dosimeters show modest dependencies that can be controlled by taking preirradiation and postirradiation readings at the same temperature (37). This can be accomplished by placing the dosimeter on the patient and allowing its temperature to equilibrate to that of the patient over a period of about two minutes. This is probably good clinical practice, in general, for dosimeters.

Angular Variation

Angular variation in dosimeter readings is due to interactions between beam orientation and asymmetries in dosimeter design or construction. The clearest example of a design asymmetry is with regard to surface dosimeters that have a bulb side for build up and a flat side meant to be in contact with the patient's skin. In practice, it is difficult to make a dosimeter that is totally symmetric from both a design and construction standpoint, and angular variation has been seen from 2% to over 27%, depending on dosimeter model (33,38,42–45). Most dosimeters have angular dependencies in the 2% to 8% range. Angular variation effects may be difficult to avoid both in surface applications, where an unavoidable sloping patient surface may exist, and in implanted applications, where multiple beam angles make it impossible to eliminate angular variations between device orientation and beam incidence. Implantable dosimeters may exhibit reduced angular dependency due to full buildup provided by surrounding tissue.

Dose and Energy Effects

A critical aspect of a good dosimeter is that it exhibits a predictable response to a specific quantity of dose, its response is independent of dose rate, and it is relatively independent of energy spectrum changes within the energy range of clinical interest. The response of modern

---

[b]Dosimeter migration with respect to the DVS dosimeter can be eliminated if the dosimeter is used according to updated manufacturer's guidelines.

MOSFET dosimeters has been shown to be linear with dose (31,33,38–40,42) and independent of dose rate (33,39,42). Chuang et al. (38) found no systematic deviation from depth doses measured with an ion chamber for a 6 MV beam indicating that there may be no significant energy spectrum effects for the type of dosimeter that was tested. There are two methods for achieving linear response: use of the dual bias MOSFET circuit (e.g., Thomson-Nielsen/Best Medical) or use of a nonlinear calibration curve to effectively linearize the dosimeter response (e.g., Sicel Technologies).

Calibration Factors

A calibration factor is a proportionality constant with units of Gy/mV required to convert raw voltage readings in millivolts to dose. Some dosimeters may come precalibrated from the manufacturer (e.g., Sicel Technologies), while others are calibrated by the physicist (e.g., Best Medical). The dose response of some MOSFET dosimeters is affected by field size and energy spectrum and may need to be individually calibrated for specific applications (33,44). For others MOSFET dosimeters, a single calibration factor may suffice with a maximum of 5% error over a broad range of field sizes, energies, orientation, and depths (42). MOSFETs have a limited lifetime because of the increase of trapped charge in the oxide layer. Saturation occurs after a specific amount of dose. For example, DVS implantable dosimeters can be used up to a cumulative dose of approximately 80 Gy.

THE USE OF MOSFET DOSIMETRY IN IMAGE-GUIDED RADIATION THERAPY

The use of implantable MOSFET dosimeters with image-guided radiation therapy (IGRT) systems can serve two purposes. The first purpose is to investigate the precision, accuracy, and possible performance issues of IGRT systems. The second purpose is to use the MOSFET dosimeter as a fiducial marker. For example, the DVS is known as a Smartmarker™ because of its ability to be used both as a dosimeter and a marker for certain IGRT treatments. The IGRT technique introduces an X-ray imaging system integrated to medical linear accelerators, allowing patient imaging at the time of treatment. IGRT imaging systems that are in use today may include: (*i*) megavolt EPID, (*ii*) Megavolt computed tomography (MVCT), (*iii*) accelerator-mounted kilovolt (kV) imagers, (*iv*) kilovolt cone-beam computed tomography (CBCT), (*v*) ultrasound imaging systems, and (*vi*) imageless localization via "beacons" (53).

In IGRT, the errors due to movement between imaging and dose delivery are minimized because of the imaging system being available just before irradiation. This new technique requires new quality assurance (QA) procedures to examine the precision and overall targeting accuracy of the integrated system, which is related to uncertainties in leaf placement and linear accelerator, isocenter stability with gantry, and coach rotation (43,64). An ideal detector for IGRT should be visible under radiological examinations and should have a very small active volume in order not to perturb the dose distribution. It should be possible to easily compare the measured dose with point-dose calculations in TPSs. Moreover, immediate readout and reuse of the detector should allow for repeated measurements without disturbing the experimental setup (43,64).

The imaging capabilities, overall precision, and accuracy of an IGRT system must be known before safe clinical implementation can take place. The investigation of IGRT system accuracy and precision requires the use of a dosimeter, which can be seen in images produced by the system. Such dosimeters must be very small, exhibit minimal angular sensitivity, and be capable of detecting small doses of radiation (~1 cGy). They must also have measurement precision higher than that of the imaging and the delivery system (43).

It has been reported that MOSFETs are clearly visible on CBCT image (43,65). Other IGRT systems, which are capable of visualizing MOSFETs, are MVCT, megavolt EPID, kilovolt EPID, and ultrasound (34). Currently, in the prostate, placement of MOSFET dosimeters is most commonly performed with aid of ultrasound imaging.

Rowbottom et al. used MOSFET dosimeters in a phantom to study the precision and accuracy of CBCT (64). Their study focused on the capability of the CBCT system to determine the effects of parameters such as gantry rotation accuracy and multileaf collimator (MLC) position accuracy. These parameters, in turn, can affect the size of the smallest margin required for treatment delivery. The stationary unambiguous phantom that was used means that patient positioning and movement were not taken into consideration. The authors concluded that with the aid of image guidance, imaging and delivery can be achieved with submillimeter accuracy in the anterior-posterior (AP) and lateral directions and to within a millimeter in the superior-inferior direction. The uncertainty in the delivery of dose was approximately 0.2 mm in the axial plane and 1.0 mm for the superior-inferior plane. These additional margins may be added to PTV margins to account for systematic uncertainty.

In addition to being able to be used for dose verification, MOSFET dosimeters have great potential of being employed as a fiducial marker. If so used, they may eliminate the need for conventional fiducial markers, such as gold seeds, for target localization. The challenge of using a MOSFET dosimeter as a fiducial maker lies in its relatively small size. For example, typical dimensions of the

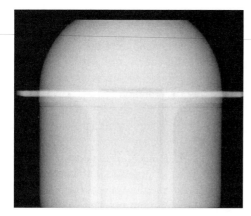

Figure 3 Megavolt EPID image of a phantom containing 2-MOSFET dosimeters. With EPID imager used in "clinical" mode exposed to 2 monitor units (MU), it was not possible to visualize any of the dosimeter. *Abbreviations*: EPID, electronic portal imaging device; MOSFET, metal oxide semiconductor field effect transistor.

DVS dosimeter, including structural material (the capsule), are 20- to 30-mm long and 1 to 3 mm in diameter; however, the metal oxide or the active area is less than 1 mm^2 (34) and may not be in the region that is best imaged (e.g., the coil). The use of MOSFETs as fiducial markers is relatively recent, and there is very little published research on the subject. Because literature on using MOSFET as fiducial marker is so scarce, the following experiment was designed to investigate the possibility of visualizing MOSFETs using different IGRT imaging systems (Figs. 3–5). Two DVS MOSFET dosimeters were placed in a phantom. The phantom is a polystyrene cylinder measuring 20 cm in diameter and 20-cm long. With EPID imager used in "clinical" mode with 2 monitor unit (MU), it was not possible to visualize any of the dosimeter as shown in Figure 3. However, using the imager in "service" mode with high quality image option being selected, the dosimeters were poorly visible. Figure 4 shows a kilovolt on-board imager (OBI) image of the same phantom. Both

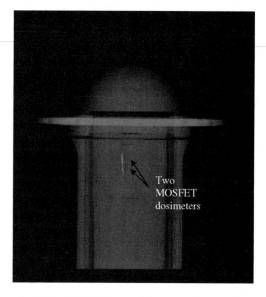

Figure 4 Kilovolt OBI image of the same phantom in Figure 3 containing 2-MOSFET dosimeters. Both dosimeters are visible in the image. *Abbreviations*: OBI, on-board imager; MOSFET, metal oxide semiconductor field effect transistor.

dosimeters are visible in the image. Figure 5 is CBCT image of the phantom. The dosimeters are clearly visible in all three views: axial, sagittal, and coronal. Suffice it to say that in both the kilovolt EPID image and the kV CBCT image the whole MOSFET dosimeters were visible rather than the active volume only.

QA USING MOSFET DOSIMETERS

MOSFET dosimeters can be used as a QA tool in radiation therapy. Their use may include both patient-specific QA and equipment QA. Patient QA refers to practice of comparing measurements of predicted TPS dose to patient dose measurements. These measurements may either occur on a daily basis or one to several times during treatment.

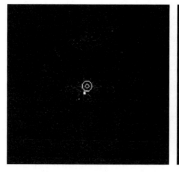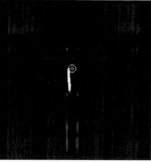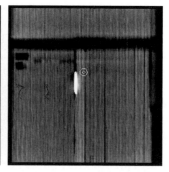

Figure 5 Kilovolt CBCT image of the same phantom in Figures 3 and 4, containing 2-MOSFET dosimeters. The dosimeters are clearly visible in all three views: axial, sagittal, and coronal. *Abbreviations*: CBCT, cone-beam computed tomography; MOSFET, metal oxide semiconductor field effect transistor.

There are several factors that make MOSFET dosimeters an attractive choice for intensity-modulated radiation therapy (IMRT) QA. These factors are: fast and simple dose reading procedures, the small size of the detector especially when used in small homogenous dose regions, and dose linearity. The disadvantage of using MOSFET for IMRT QA lies in the fact that many dosimeters would be necessary to obtain a complete isodose distribution. Chuang et al. used MOSFET dosimeters for clinical IMRT dose verification concurrently with ion chambers (38). It was reported that the difference between calculated dose and measured dose is 5% when using MOSFET dosimeters, while the difference is 3% using ion chamber measurements.

The microMOSFET (TN-502RDM) has been characterized for its application to integral system tests for IGRT (43,64). The position of peak response to a 0.08-mm slit of radiation was determined, and the dosimeter was found clearly visible on the CBCT images with no added artifacts (43). The ability to locate the MOSFET active volume to within 0.2 mm by CBCT allows their use in an integral system test in a phantom containing an array of micro-MOSFETs, to investigate the precision of the IGRT system components in absence of patient-related errors (64). The practically isotropic angular response of microMOSFETs allows their application for noncoplanar beams (42). High-sensitivity TN microMOSFETs (TN-1002RDM) were used to measure dose on patients undergoing CBCT using the X-ray volume imaging (XVI®) system integrated with a medical accelerator (Synergy, ELEKTA). The average agreement between measured and estimated skin doses of five patients were found to be within ±5% (66). Micro-MOSFETs with radiopaque markers have been introduced in tomotherapy patient QA (67) to verify the skin doses and to check the skin sparing approach achieved by a new treatment planning technique.

MOSFET dosimeters can also be used to perform QA measurements for linear accelerator output. The versatility and accuracy of these dosimeters facilitate a quick check of the output of the accelerator, which might be important if machine output is reported to be out of specification during daily QA. Normally, absolute output measurements require elaborate and time-consuming equipment setup (ionization chambers) and measurements using the TG-51 calibration protocol (63). With MOSFET dosimeters, a rapid QA check of output measurements might be performed much more easily.

A typical measurement setup would be a 10×10 cm^2 beam, 100-cm source-to-surface distance, water or solid phantom as medium, and 200-cGy dose. Dosimeters would be placed at depth of maximum dose, which is the typical calibration point for linear accelerators. Briere et al. reported the use of MOSFET dosimeters for performing accelerator output QA (35). The measurements were performed for both 6 and 18 MV. Halvorsen also used MOSFET dosimeter to measure "absolute" outputs for both 6 and 18 MV beams. They observed an average difference of less than 2% compared to manufacturer's calibration when measured at the depth of maximum dose (39). In summary, IGRT systems alone cannot detect misadministrations that might occur, such as improper dose calibration, incomplete IMRT QA, or MLC leaf sequence errors. However, when IGRT systems are used in combination with an implantable dosimeter, such as MOSFET, this may help to facilitate more accurate dose delivery.

DESIGN AND OPERATION OF AN IN SITU DOSIMETER SYSTEM

Until recently, it has been impractical to measure actual delivered dose for each treatment session at a tumor site below the skin surface. Now, however, the first wireless, permanently implantable dosimeter has been developed to measure external beam radiation dose received at the target tissue. This dosimeter has been clinically implemented for prostate and breast cancer treatments, with other target sites likely to follow. The implantable dosimeter, DVS, uses a p-channel MOSFET as the radiation-sensing element. MOSFET's require minimal power to operate making it possible to provide enough power by inductive coupling from an outside coil directly to an antenna contained within the dosimeter. The DVS implantable dosimeter can be used as an adjunct to treatment planning and radiation delivery techniques to verify that the actual dose received at the tumor volume on a daily basis is within the acceptable dose range prescribed.

Dosimeter Design

The DVS dosimeter is encapsulated in a hermetic, biocompatible glass capsule (Fig. 6). The implantable dosimeter consists of an antenna and a microelectronic hybrid

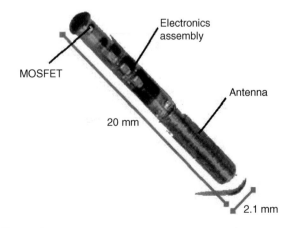

Figure 6 Implantable dosimeter DVS and internal components.

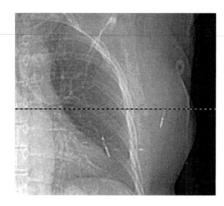

Figure 7 Radiographic image showing two DVS dosimeters. *Source*: From Ref. 68.

assembly that contains the MOSFET radiation sensors, customized circuitry, and several passive components (Fig. 6). After the antenna is connected to the hybrid, the antenna/hybrid assembly is inserted into an epoxy-filled capsule prior to laser sealing. To prevent moisture ingress into the capsule, the open end of the capsule is laser-sealed and the hermetic seal is tested using a helium leak detection process.

The dosimeter is commercially available in a capsule dimension of 2.1 mm in diameter and 20 mm in length. Clinical trials on patients were performed with a larger dosimeter design (3.25 mm × 25 mm). The dosimeter and components are visible on kV images, CT, and ultrasound (Fig. 7). The detailed structure of the MOSFET as well as the technical aspects of the dosimeter system has previously been described (34,46,47).

The DVS system consists of an implantable, telemetric radiation dosimeter and an external reader system to communicate with the dosimeter (Fig. 8). Dose is communicated to the external reader using a reader wand (reader antenna) by radio frequency identification (RFID) technology. A customized application-specific integrated circuit (ASIC) was developed to digitize the MOSFET voltage readings and transmit the data to a reader system.

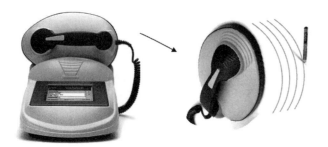

Figure 8 DVS reader system and reader wand. *Abbreviation*: DVS, dose verification system.

The dosimeter RFID system transmits radiation dose data that is utilized by the reader to convert the voltage shift into absorbed dose-to-tissue at the MOSFET location using dosimeter specific calibration values.

Telemetric Data Acquisition System

Although the DVS dosimeter requires power to operate, it is often referred to as a passive device since it contains no battery. As with many RFID products, dosimeter power is derived from the low frequency magnetic field generated by the DVS reader antenna. The magnetic field is coupled to the ferrite core antenna inside the dosimeter capsule, which generates a voltage proportional to the magnetic field intensity. To maximize the antenna voltage and improve reading range, the antenna is tuned to the frequency generated by the reader.

In addition to providing dosimeter power, the magnetic field generated by the reader provides the bidirectional communications interface between the reader and dosimeter. To facilitate communication with multiple dosimeters, the reader uniquely addresses each dosimeter via a 32-bit identification (ID) number. Once the DVS reader broadcasts the ID to all dosimeters in the magnetic field, only the dosimeter with a matching ID number responds with sensor data. The reader can also request data from multiple radiation sensors and an onboard temperature sensor. The reader transmits packets to the implantable dosimeter by amplitude modulation of the magnetic field. The amplitude modulation is decoded by the dosimeter ASIC receiver circuitry. After each valid bit is received, the ASIC receiver determines if the dosimeter is being addressed. Once a dosimeter is addressed, the ASIC state machine begins the data acquisition and packet transmission process. The ASIC contains a 14-bit sigma delta analog-to-digital converter (ADC) to digitize the MOSFET radiation sensor threshold voltage. Once the analog-to-digital conversion process is complete, the ASIC state machine creates a transmit packet consisting of the 32-bit ID, 14-bit sensor data, and a 16-bit CRC (cyclic redundancy check sum) value to ensure packet transmission integrity (68).

The dosimeter data packet is transmitted to the reader using a method commonly referred to as backscatter modulation. Unlike a traditional radio transmitter that produces a modulated radio frequency signal to transmit information, backscatter modulation utilizes the magnetic field generated by the reader to transmit data. The link between the reader antenna and the dosimeter antenna can be modeled as a loosely coupled transformer with the reader antenna forming the primary winding and the dosimeter antenna forming the secondary winding. The dosimeter transmits data by loading and unloading the antenna circuit. The load variations are reflected to the transformer primary (reader antenna) where sensitive receiver circuitry located in the reader can detect and demodulate the data transmitted by the dosimeter. The dosimeter-induced voltage perturbation on the reader receive antenna is usually in the range of 10 to 100 mV depending on transmit power and the distance between the dosimeter and the reader antenna. The reader antenna voltage that produces the magnetic field is greater than 600 V, which mandates the use of a sensitive receiver to detect the 10 to 100 mV data modulation signal superimposed in the 600 V drive voltage. The reader receive circuitry contains filters to mitigate the effect of external noise sources from electronic equipment.

Dosimeter Calibration

Since calibration of the implanted dosimeter cannot be accomplished once it is inside a patient, precise methods for precalibrating these devices have been developed and tested. The DVS dosimeter is currently calibrated for use with typical EBRT doses and irradiation protocols: doses of 150 to 250 cGy once per day. The calibration protocol takes into account the variables that can affect this type of dose delivery to increase the performance and accuracy of the dosimeter response in a patient. New calibration protocols are being developed for use of the dosimeter with hypofractionated doses and other radiation sources (Ir-192).

Since the amount of trapped charge is proportional to the ionizing radiation dose, the MOSFET threshold voltage shift may be used to measure dose. A MOSFET's radiation sensitivity is the term used to describe the change in threshold voltage caused by a given amount of radiation. More precisely, the radiation sensitivity of a MOSFET is defined as the change in threshold voltage per unit of dose applied, expressed typically in mV/cGy.

Ionizing radiation affects a MOSFET by changing the threshold voltage required to enable current flow from the source to the drain of the MOSFET (Fig. 1). To determine the radiation sensitivity (Rad_{sens}) of the MOSFET, the threshold voltage is measured before and after dose is applied (Eq. 1):

$$Rad_{sens} = \frac{(V_{post} - V_{pre})}{D},$$ (1)

where V_{post} is the threshold voltage after the dose is applied (mV), V_{pre} is the threshold voltage before the dose is applied (mV), and D is the dose applied (cGy).

As radiation exposure increases, more charge is trapped in the gate oxide. The positive space charge resulting from the trapped charge repels holes and thus decreases the chance of the positively charged holes being trapped near the Si/SiO_2 interface. The net effect is a reduction in voltage radiation sensitivity (V_{TH}/D) for increasing

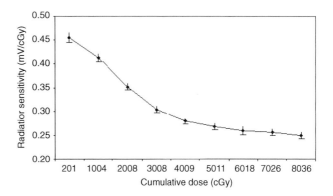

Figure 9 Relationship between radiation sensitivity and cumulative dose. *Source*: From Ref. 68.

cumulative dose. This change in threshold voltage of the MOSFET is cumulative as a function of dose. As a result, the radiation sensitivity is not constant for the life of the MOSFET and becomes a nonlinear function of the threshold voltage (Fig. 9). The DVS dosimeter "saturates" at around 80 Gy.

A ^{60}Co source is used for calibration because of its consistent dose. As part of the manufacturing process, the nominal radiation sensitivity of each DVS dosimeter is measured using ^{60}Co. These values are used to correct the voltage response of each individual dosimeter. This process allows each dosimeter to be "fine-tuned" to improve its accuracy. The calibration of the DVS also requires knowledge of the dose response curve up to 80 Gy to determine the relationship between the radiation dose applied and the change in threshold voltage. This response curve is determined for each dosimeter lot production, since small changes in production can affect the dosimeter response. Sample dosimeters from each lot are tested over the full-dose range to develop this dose response curve. An independent radiation calibration laboratory verifies the resulting calibration for each lot. Once verified, the calibration coefficients are applied to each dosimeter within a lot. Each dosimeter has a calibration certificate detailing the specific accuracy as a function of cumulative dose based on its lot production. The dosimeter performance has been validated by in vitro studies (32,35,68).

The factory calibration protocol determines the calibration curve for each dosimeter used in a typical external beam radiation treatment regime. In addition, the curve characterizes the response of the MOSFET, including fade effects, for daily radiation delivery. Fade is the term used to describe the decrease in the trapped charge in a MOSFET as a function of time after radiation exposure. Test measurements on the MOSFET yield less than 2% fade over 20 minutes. The dosimeters are read within two to three minutes after exposure during calibration. Since the MOSFET response can be affected by temperature, the dosimeters are calibrated for use at 37°C (human body temperature). Each DVS dosimeter also contains a thermal sensor. This sensor is calibrated during the manufacturing process and can be used to monitor the temperature during the calibration process.

To measure absorbed dose by the dosimeter, a predose and postdose reading is acquired. The predose reading is acquired prior to radiation delivery using the hand-held reader wand, which contains the antenna (Fig. 8). Similarly, the postdose reading is acquired after radiation delivery. To minimize fade effects, the postdose readings need to be acquired within 10 minutes after irradiation. These readings are then used to calculate the daily dose fraction that is reported for each treatment session by relating the voltage shift in the calibration curve. The daily fractional dose values are stored in a database and are summed to calculate a cumulative dose.

Radiation Characteristics

The dosimeter's radiation characteristics have been set forth in several published studies. A summary of the basic response of the dosimeter as a function of angular incidence, temperature, attenuation, and energy is provided in this section. Additional details on the relevant methodology and test data can be found in each of the references provided below.

The dosimeter angular dependency has been found to be very small (<1.5%) for radiation incident perpendicular (radial) to the dosimeter long axis. The maximum angular dependence of approximately 6% is obtained for radiation that is incident parallel to the dosimeter axis traveling through the coil and electronics (Fig. 10). This larger deviation is expected since the coil and electronics are in the direct path between the radiation beam and the MOSFETs and can be eliminated for traditional clinical radiation treatments by implanting the dosimeter in close parallel alignment with the body axis (<30° off axis, as has been done in the pilot studies and clinical trial patients) (46,47,68).

Previous in vitro studies for the implantable dosimeter have shown a large sensitivity to temperature variations during irradiations (32). This relationship did not pose a problem during temperature controlled in vitro testing or in vivo applications since the body regulates temperature to a constant 37°C. The previous DVS dosimeter used a MOSFET with a large threshold voltage temperature coefficient, resulting in approximately an 8 to 20 cGy variation for each 1°C difference in predose and postdose reading temperature during a 200-cGy irradiation (46). The new commercially available DVS utilizes a MOSFET with a low threshold voltage temperature coefficient,

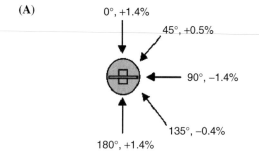

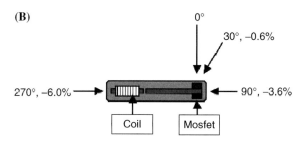

Figure 10 DVS radiation (**A**) radial and (**B**) longitudinal angular dependency. *Source*: From Ref. 68.

resulting in approximately 1.0 to 3.3 cGy variation for each 1°C difference during a 200-cGy irradiation.

Due to the lower temperature variation dependency of the current dosimeter, it is possible to perform measurements in a well-insulated phantom at room temperature. Testing has shown that the DVS dosimeter is approximately 3.32% more sensitive (higher dose reading for same applied dose) when irradiated at 37°C versus 23°C (68). The testing methodology used to develop this correction factor was validated up to 8 to 10 sessions of radiation dose (16–20 Gy). Additional studies would have to be performed to validate the room temperature correction and simulate a complete course of radiation therapy (20–50 sessions) at room temperature. Nevertheless, this correction factor provides a useful mechanism to perform testing in a simple water equivalent phantom at room temperature.

The components of the DVS dosimeter (ferrite, copper coil, analog circuit board) could cause some attenuation of radiation dose on the side of the dosimeter opposite the radiation field (68). It has been found that the attenuation is similar to surgical suture or gold seed markers. Testing showed that the maximum dose reduction for 6 MV radiation occurs right next to the dosimeter, as with any other metallic surgical marker or implant. At 2 mm below the dosimeter, a maximum dose reduction of 3.7% is encountered directly under the antenna. The dose recovers to less than 1% reduction at 7.5 mm below the dosimeter. At the depth of 9.4 mm, no dose perturbation was measured. This data was the result from only one beam of radiation. In clinical practice, radiation is directed to the body from different angles, further reducing the overall effect of dose attenuation around the dosimeter.

The dosimeter has shown small energy dependency within the clinical MV energy range if implanted at depths beyond d_{max}. The ratio of sensitivities between ^{60}Co and 6 MV has also shown a small energy dependency (~0.5%). The DVS has decreased sensitivity (~1%) when irradiating with 18 MV as compared with 6 MV. Because of this small energy dependence, the calibration of the dosimeter is set such that the 6-MV dose response is biased to read 0.5% higher while the 18-MV dose response is biased 0.5% lower. Phantom testing has been performed to confirm the performance of a calibrated dosimeter for different energy ranges (68,69).

Studies have shown that MOSFETs have a stronger energy dependency below 130 kV, increasing three to four times as the energy decreases below the 100 kV range (70). A recent report demonstrated that the DVS MOSFET dosimeter can overrespond by a factor of 2 to 3 in the kV energy range due to the predominance of the photoelectric effect (71).

It has been documented that pelvic kV CBCT images can deliver additional dose to patients in the range of 3 to 6 cGy (72). This dose can be detected and measured by the DVS dosimeter, resulting in additional dose reading in the range of 12 to 16 cGy to the center of a 30 cm square shaped phantom (68). Additional data has showed that standard two-dimensional kV portal images deliver negligible or nonmeasurable dose to the DVS. Therefore, if CBCT is used on a frequent basis for patient treatment, this dose can be considered for the final dose calculation or can be eliminated by taking the predose reading after the CBCT imaging is performed. For MV CBCT or MV planar images, the dosimeter could easily track the additional dose delivered to a patient due to its linear response in this energy range.

ANIMAL STUDIES OF IN SITU DOSIMETRY

Relatively little in situ dosimetry has been performed in animal models. Gladstone et al. (25) tested a miniature implantable MOSFET dosimeter in mice during RIT trials. More recently, Scarantino et al. (46) have tested an implantable telemetric MOSFET dosimeter in vitro and in 10 dogs. Each canine subject presented with a spontaneous, malignant tumor to be treated in 16 fractions with EBRT. One telemetric sensor was implanted in each tumor. In three dogs a second sensor was implanted in nearby normal tissue. The experiments were designed to observe (*i*) stability/mobility of the implanted devices in vivo, (*ii*) successful readout, and (*iii*) biocompatibility with a tissue environment. During the experiments, two of the sensors in two different subjects were observed to

migrate by 3.5 and 7 cm, respectively. This underscores the importance of anchoring the devices securely. Dosimetric measurements showed instances of daily variation in excess of 10%, which the authors attributed to inaccuracies in the calibration procedure used for the tests. In one of the three canine subjects with two redundant dosimeters, an instance of daily fractional underdosage on the order of 20% to 30% was indicated by both dosimeters. The authors suggested that the coincident measurement of underdose in both sensors was indicative of a true dose delivery error, but in the absence of corroborating entrance/exit dose measurements, this would not have been provable.

HUMAN STUDIES OF IN SITU DOSIMETRY

Although the ability to measure radiation doses in vivo has been in existence for many years, it has only recently become possible to measure actual doses at the tumor/target site. Thus, for the purposes of this discussion, it may be helpful to distinguish in vivo dosimetry from in situ dosimetry. Historically, in the former case, dose measurements are determined with detectors, which are placed on the skin to measure entrance and/or exit dose of a beam, and the dose to the target within this beam is calculated using dose reconstruction algorithms (73–76). The reports claim an accuracy of less than or equal to 5%, but utilizing the method of entrance and exit can be time consuming and may not be able to identify the effect of specific uncertainties such as organ movement or deformation and treatment or patient setup errors. More recently, EPIDs were developed for verification and correction of daily radiotherapy treatment alignment (77–80). The portal images can be used to verify two-dimensional dose distributions (77,78), since the pixel signals are related to the amount of radiation transmitted through the patient. The available in vivo methods described do not provide an actual measured dose, but rather an extrapolation of dose.

In situ intracavitary dosimetry, involving the placement of probes into the bladder and/or rectum prior to treatment, has recently been described (6,81,82). The probes may contain diodes, which can transmit normal tissue dose data electronically (6,81), or they may contain ionization chambers (82). Accurate repositioning of the probe prior to each treatment fraction is critical and requires onboard imaging capabilities for maximum accuracy (82). These approaches may be useful for normal tissue dose measurements immediately adjacent to the prostate, but do not provide information on dose to the malignant target volume. They typically have been utilized during only a few fractions per patient, rather than throughout an entire course of treatment.

Weber et al. (81) assessed the dose delivered to the anal canal using thermoluminescent dosimetry (TLD) during the initial dose of external beam irradiation in 31 patients. TLD values differed by a mean of 5.8%; however, differences of at least 10% were noted in eight (26%) patients and 15% in three patients. Hayne et al. (6) measured the in situ dose using a rectal probe placed in the anorectum in nine patients (during the first five fractions in five patients and two fractions in four patients) with cancers of the prostate, bladder, cervix, or uterus. The probe contained five n-type photon-detecting diodes placed at 2-cm intervals from the anal verge. The average measured doses in the target volume (center) were all within 7% of predicted doses, whereas the dose at the edge of the target volume varied significantly (–68% to +68%). Outside the target volume, doses up to 0.3 Gy were measured, which were not predicted by their planning system. One of the difficulties encountered with these methods was to insure consistency in the daily placement of the dosimeters. More recently, Wertz et al. (82) addressed this problem by using CBCT and anatomical landmarks to insure consistent placement of ionization chambers in the rectum. They measured the in situ dose in seven patients (21 dose measurements) undergoing IMRT for prostate cancer. They found that there was good agreement (1.4 ± 4.9%) between measured doses and predicted doses when the dose was compared with a point relative to the isocenter. However, the mean dose deviation at corresponding anatomic positions was 6.5 ± 21.6%. The daily use of probes described above can be problematic, since it is possible, due to rectal irritation developing as treatment progresses, that probe insertion may become too uncomfortable for some patients. Therefore, a more convenient method, as described below, would appear more suited to daily use, especially considering the influences of long treatment times with IMRT and the potential for intrafractional variation in delivered dose.

In recent years, high dose per fraction EBRT has experienced resurgence, and several early trials have been published using this approach in the treatment of prostate cancer. High-dose single-fraction EBRT has not been reported, to our knowledge, as a treatment for prostate cancer. It has been used in the intraoperative setting for the treatment of several different malignancies. Ciocca et al. (83) reported on the use of in situ dosimetry using radiochromic film placed in the operative bed in a series of 54 patients with early stage breast cancer, who received 21 Gy in a single fraction to the surgical bed following quadrantectomy. In general, they found good agreement between measured and expected dose (mean deviation = 1.8 ± 4.7%), with deviations larger than 7% in 23% of cases. They used dosimetry information to define an action plan if errors of greater than or equal to 7% were detected in two consecutive patients, or greater than or equal to 10% in one patient. Comparable results were recently reported using a MOSFET system (51). These

authors reported the results of in situ dosimetry in a group of 12 patients treated with single fraction intraoperative electron beam radiotherapy for breast cancer. Measured values were within 5% of calculated doses in all but one case, and the one discrepancy was felt to be due to improper positioning of the dosimeter.

The characteristics of dual MOSFETs such as small size, full buildup isotropy, instant readout, waterproof design, and temperature independent response make these detectors suitable for measurements in high-dose gradient fields present in both low dose rate (LDR) and HDR brachytherapy treatments. The high sensitivity microMOSFET dosimeter (TN-1002RDM) with the high sensitivity bias supply was used for in vivo dosimetry during LDR prostate brachytherapy (58). The MOSFET has been inserted inside a urinary catheter placed in urethra. The dosimeter sensitivity was found to be about 31 to 33 mV/cGy for a low-energy ^{125}I source. Patient data demonstrated that the maximum initial dose rate at the urethra varied between 10 and 16 cGy/hr, corresponding to a total absorbed dose of 205 to 328 Gy. The intraurethra initial dose rate measurements with MOSFETs provided evaluation of the overall quality of the implant, by analyzing the maximum dose received by the urethra, the prostate base and apex coverage, and the length of the prostatic urethra being irradiated.

The standard sensitivity 5-MOSFET linear array (TN-252LA5) was also used for patient urethral dose verification in prostate HDR brachytherapy for single and multiple fractions (600 cGy per fraction) (84). An excellent correlation of 2.8% was found between the MOSFET readings and the treatment planning dose calculations. In vivo dosimetry with MOSFETs in brachytherapy has been proven effective to indicate possible treatment complications due to excessive dose to the urethra.

Scarantino et al. (46) reported the first permanently implantable in situ dosimeter. This device uses a MOSFET dosimeter and is read telemetrically each day after treatment as described in the section "Design and Operation of an in situ Dosimeter System". The design and operation of the device are reviewed above. Its use in patients was first reported by Scarantino et al. (47) in 2005 and was updated by Black et al. (34) that same year. Initial FDA-approved pilot studies contained a total of 18 patients who underwent implantation of one or two dosimeters into the gross tumor volume and/or surrounding normal tissues. Sites implanted were lung ($n = 3$), rectum (pelvis) ($n = 4$), prostate ($n = 4$), breast ($n = 6$), and thigh ($n = 1$). A total of 31 sensors were implanted. Treatment planning CTs were obtained after implantation, and the dosimeters were included as anatomic structures in the treatment plans for the purpose of calculating the expected dose. The accuracy of the system was confirmed via in vitro phantom experiments, and it was determined that under idealized conditions, an uncertainty level of ±5%, consistent with machine commissioning, is achievable. Considerable variability, however, between observed versus expected dose was observed in the patients. In two-thirds of the patients, dose deviations of more than 5% were recorded for at least 40% of treatments. Since significant movement of the dosimeter was noted in only one patient in whom the device was implanted in necrotic tissue, this was not felt to be the cause of the dose deviations. Patients were not treated using image-guided techniques, but rather were aligned using skin tattoos and bony landmarks. The near-Gaussian distribution of dose readings suggested random rather than systematic error as the cause.

On the basis of the results of the pilot studies, a pivotal study was instituted (85). The objectives as well as study parameters were similar to the pilot study except that the study was limited to prostate and breast cancer patients. A total of 59 patients were entered and 119 dosimeters implanted. The protocol recommended that each patient receive two dosimeters, one associated with the tumor (prostate capsule) and one in normal tissue (1–2 cm from capsule in prostate). A transperineal approach, employing a specially designed canula and trochar, was used when inserting the DVS into the prostate.

A total of 1749 daily readings were obtained from prostate cancer patients; 1308 during treatment of the primary field and 441 during reduced field. A variability of greater than 7% between observed and expected daily readings was noted in 23% of patients during large field irradiation and in 35% during treatment of the boost field. IMRT was utilized during the boost field. More importantly, a difference of greater than or equal to 7% variability in the cumulative dose occurred in 27% (8 of 29) of the patients during large field and in 38% (7 of 18) during boost-field irradiation. Finally, a total of 18 out of 29 patients were treated with IGRT techniques; two with transabdominal ultrasound (BAT, B-mode acquisition and targeting), three with CBCT, and 13 with implanted gold fiducials and MV imaging. The use of IGRT techniques did not result in any appreciable difference in the degree of variability between measured and expected dose (86). Further, in most patients the pattern of dose measurements was consistent (either overdose or underdose), which was consistent from day to day and observed throughout the treatment, especially during irradiation of the boost field. The pattern in the first three to five fractions was indicative of the treatment course. The high variability in dose observed during irradiation of the boost field is probably related to both the tight fields and organ movement and could be compounded if patient is not properly positioned for treatment.

Errors in treatment delivery can occur for several reasons including organ movement and deformity, which are difficult to control, and patient positioning and treatment planning errors, which are more controllable. Regardless of the cause, unless there is documentation of the dose measurement, the physician will not be aware of the variability and its possible impact on patient treatment.

PRACTICAL GUIDELINES FOR IMPLEMENTATION OF IN SITU DOSIMETRY IN THE CLINIC

The DVS is intended for use in radiation therapy to verify treatment planning and radiation dose to target tissues and organs in or near the irradiated areas of a patient. The accuracy of the DVS is less than or equal to 5.5% (±2%) up to 20 Gy and less than or equal to 6.5% (±2%) up to 74 Gy. The accuracy decreases slightly for doses beyond 74 Gy. The lot-specific accuracy is detailed in the calibration certificate included with each dosimeter. Readings deviating from the prescribed dose by more than the specified accuracy could indicate a trend that should be noted. The physician should decide the maximum acceptable percent discrepancy between the prescribed and measured dose.

On the basis of the inherent accuracy of the device, guidelines have been developed to provide the physician a frame of reference checklist to help with the clinical implementation and data analysis. The guidelines for clinical implementation detailed below should act as a reference point only since each clinical site should review and implement their own guidelines for DVS clinical data analysis.

Guidelines for clinical implementation:

I. Dose measurements should be made after every dose of radiation within 10 minutes of dose delivery (optimally 2–3 minutes after dose delivery).

   a. Daily dose measurements help identify a pattern for the patient's radiation treatment.

II. The recorded dose measurements should be reviewed by the physician at least once every week.

   a. The medical physicist should also include a review of the DVS data as part of their weekly chart checks.

   b. It is recommended to carefully review the data obtained during the first three to five fractions of a new patient treatment.

III. Systematic dose deviations of greater than or equal to 7% over a number of fractions should result in a reevaluation of the treatment plan, patient setup, and equipment function to determine the reason for the variation. Replanning and/or resimulation of the patient should be considered after careful evaluation of the above-mentioned parameters. The following steps can be referenced if a systematic errant daily dose reading pattern is obtained:

a. Treatment plan:

1. Verify that the MOSFET area of the DVS is properly identified on the treatment plan. Use diagnostic film, kV CT scout images to verify exact position of the DVS.
2. Verify that the appropriate predicted dose value has been entered into the DVS system.
3. Verify that the prescription isodose line has been incorporated in the predicted dose value.
4. Include and/or review effects of heterogeneity corrections.
5. Evaluate dose gradient around the DVS (~3 mm).
6. Verify plan transfer to record and verify (R&V) system.
7. Review IMRT QA results, if applicable.

b. Patient setup:

1. Verify that the patient setup position corresponds to patient simulation position.
2. Evaluate patient source-skin distance (SSD) parameters, AP separation, patient weight changes.
3. Verify digitally reconstructed radiographs (DRRs) and port films.
4. Verify appropriate blocks or MLC shape are being used, wedges, etc.
5. Evaluate patient treatment preparation (bladder/bowel filling if applicable).
6. Evaluate treatment margins and replan, if needed.
7. If using IGRT:
   i. Verify that shift or patient adjustment did not exceed department limits.
   ii. Compare distance of adjustment with distance to agreement on treatment plan.
   iii. Identify if there is a correlation between adjustment of patient and significant variance.

c. Equipment function:

1. Verify any previous machine repairs performed.
2. Review linear accelerator daily output and beam performance records.
3. Verify that the treatment and verification system are working properly.
4. Verify IGRT equipment QA and functionality.

d. If necessary, repeat CT simulation:

1. Verify DVS position is within same isodose region as planned (include heterogeneity factors, if appropriate).
2. Compare current DVS position with original pretreatment position.

IV. Random variations of greater than or equal to 7% observed over a number of fractions should result in an evaluation of positioning consistency, patient movement and/or organ movement during treatment. Replanning and/or resimulation of the patient should be considered after careful evaluation of the above-mentioned parameters. The following steps can be referenced if a random errant daily dose reading pattern is obtained:

a. Evaluate patient positioning consistency.

1. Verify that treatment position corresponds to patient position during simulation.
2. Verify day-to-day patient skin SSD parameters and anatomic changes because of weight.
3. Verify DRRs and port films. It is recommended to repeat port films as an initial troubleshooting maneuver.
4. Evaluate patient daily treatment preparation (bladder/bowel filling, if applicable).
5. For IGRT:
   i. Verify shift or patient adjustment daily for consistency and operator accuracy.
   ii. Verify that patient adjustment did not exceed clinic limits.

b. Evaluate patient movement during treatment.

1. Evaluate immobilization devices used.
2. Evaluate: deep breathing or coughing during treatment, irritable patient.
3. Evaluate treatment margins.

c. Organ movement during treatment.

1. Reevaluate treatment margins.
2. Review treatment plan.
3. Re-CT, if necessary.

V. A single error reading of greater than or equal to 10% should be immediately reported to the radiation oncologist, and it is recommended that an evaluation of the patient setup, treatment plan, setup images, and equipment should be undertaken prior to the next patient treatment.

a. Notify the physician in case error readings exceed a certain threshold (10% recommended).

VI. During highly conformal radiation therapy, significant variation in measured dose may be observed with dosimeters placed outside the prescription dose area due to possible high dose gradients around the dosimeter.

a. If the dosimeter is within or very close (<3 mm) to the field edge or in normal tissue outside the field, the DVS readings could vary due to the field dose gradient.
b. Dosimeters placed in dose gradient regions should be evaluated with a similar process as that used for

IMRT QA evaluation, that is, taking into account that very small positioning errors (<3 mm) could lead to high dose reading variations (gamma analysis function: local dose difference, and the distance to agreement).

FUTURE DEVELOPMENTS

Internal in situ dosimetry presents two new opportunities: (*i*) the direct verification of dose delivery for those patients amenable to the procedure, and (*ii*) more accurate validation of conventional entrance/exit dosimetry techniques. Once there is sufficient confidence in the accuracy of implanted telemetric sensors, they can be used as a "ground truth" to evaluate external dosimetry. This would extend some of the benefits of internal dosimetry to those patients who are not suited to the invasive procedure.

Recently, a novel concept of MOSFET-based four-dimensional in vivo dosimetry in radiotherapy has been conceived (87). A prototype of a new system capable of simultaneous measurement of dose and spatial position is being developed. The device, controlled by a computer, consists of a probe combining two technologies: a MOSFET radiation detector coupled with a magnetic positioning device. Special software that provides sampling position and dose in user-defined time intervals has been developed. Tests conducted in a 6 MV beam indicate that there is no interference from the linear accelerator electromagnetic field on the performance of this new four-dimensional dosimetry system. The new system can be used in IGRT to complement the information not only about the dosimeter position during entire treatment time, but also about the dose accumulation as a function of irradiation time.

SUMMARY OF PERTINENT CONCLUSIONS

- In situ dosimetry should become an important and integral part of the QA programs of institutions adopting the sophisticated treatment planning approaches required for IMRT and/or IGRT.
- These devices may provide important patient treatment data complementary to image-guided localization (34), if used regularly in these patients, since the device is imagable using kilovoltage and megavoltage EPIDs, CBCT, and ultrasound.
- The daily dose measurements also allow for the development and implementation of QA procedures, should deviations be detected on a regular basis, which exceed a predetermined comfort level.

- Target dose measurements can provide the final confirmation of the dose received in the target by measuring the net effect of all the variables that can affect accurate dose delivery, such as organ motion and patient movement during treatment. This information can assist the radiation oncologist in optimizing the radiation treatment for each patient.
- Daily in vivo dose measurements may be especially valuable as radiation oncologists develop plans with tighter margins, higher total doses, or hypofractionation, requiring increasingly complex delivery methods, for which localization devices such as ultrasound or CBCT may not provide optimal pretreatment visualization.
- Future versions of these devices will likely combine simultaneous measurement of dose with spatial position transmission, which should be available in real time.

REFERENCES

1. Emami B, Lyman J, Brown A, et al. Tolerance of normal tissue to therapeutic irradiation. Int J Radiat Oncol Biol Phys 1991; 21:109–122.
2. Pollack A, Zagars GK, Starkschall G, et al. Prostate cancer radiation dose response: results of the M. D. Anderson phase III randomized trial. Int J Radiat Oncol Biol Phys 2002; 53:1097–1105.
3. Zelefsky MJ, Fuks Z, Happersett L, et al. Clinical experience with intensity modulated radiation therapy (IMRT) in prostate cancer. Radiother Oncol 2000; 55:241–249.
4. Dawson LA, Mah K, Franssen E, et al. Target position variability throughout prostate radiotherapy. Int J Radiat Oncol Biol Phys 1998; 42:1155–1161.
5. Zelefsky MJ, Crean D, Mageras GS, et al. Quantification and predictors of prostate position variability in 50 patients evaluated with multiple CT scans during conformal radiotherapy. Radiother Oncol 1999; 50:225–234.
6. Hayne D, Johnson U, D'Souza D, et al. Anorectal irradiation in pelvic radiotherapy: an assessment using in-vivo dosimetry. Clin Oncol (R Coll Radiol) 2001; 13:126–129.
7. Christie A. Roentgen diagnosis and therapy. Philadelphia: Lippincott, 1924.
8. Knox R. Radiography and radio-therapeutics. New York: McMillan, 1918.
9. Hassan M, Pearce G. A radiotelemetry pill for the measurement of ionizing radiation using a mercuric iodide detector. Phys Med Biol 1978; 23:302–308.
10. Heukelom S, Lanson JH, Mijnheer BJ. In vivo dosimetry during pelvic treatment. Radiother Oncol 1992; 25:111–120.
11. Loncol T, Greffe JL, Vynckier S, et al. Entrance and exit dose measurements with semiconductors and thermoluminescent dosemeters: a comparison of methods and in vivo results. Radiother Oncol 1996; 41:179–187.
12. Alecu R, Alecu M, Ochran TG. A method to improve the effectiveness of diode in vivo dosimetry. Med Phys 1998; 25:746–749.

13. Meiler RJ, Podgorsak MB. Characterization of the response of commercial diode detectors used for in vivo dosimetry. Med Dosim 1997; 22:31–37.

14. Van Dam J, Vaerman C, Blanckaert N, et al. Are port films reliable for in vivo exit dose measurements? Radiother Oncol 1992; 25:67–72.

15. Boellaard R, Essers M, van Herk M, et al. New method to obtain the midplane dose using portal in vivo dosimetry. Int J Radiat Oncol Biol Phys 1998; 41:465–474.

16. Huyskens D, Van Dam J, Dutreix A. Midplane dose determination using in vivo dose measurements in combination with portal imaging. Phys Med Biol 1994; 39:1089–1101.

17. Lilienfeld J. U.S. Patent 1 877 140. U.S. Patent Office, 1933.

18. Holmes-Siedle A. A space charge dosimeter. Nucl Instrum Methods 1974; 121:169–179.

19. Thomson I, Thomson R, Berndt L. Radiation dosimetry with MOS sensors. Radiat Prot Dosimetry 1984; 6:121–124.

20. Ramani R, Russell S, O'Brien P. Clinical dosimetry using MOSFETs. Int J Radiat Oncol Biol Phys 1997; 37:959–964.

21. Webb S. The physics of three-dimensional radiation therapy. Bristol: Institute of Physics Publishing, 1993.

22. United States Nuclear Regulatory Commission. Report NUREG/CR-5223: Scintillating Fiber Detector For In Vivo Endoscopic Internal Dosimetry, 1988.

23. Pai S, Reinstein LE, Gluckman G, et al. The use of improved radiochromic film for in vivo quality assurance of high dose rate brachytherapy. Med Phys 1998; 25:1217–1221.

24. Gladstone DJ, Lu XQ, Humm JL, et al. A miniature MOSFET radiation dosimeter probe. Med Phys 1994; 21:1721–1728.

25. Gladstone DJ, Chin LM. Real-time, in vivo measurement of radiation dose during radioimmunotherapy in mice using a miniature MOSFET dosimeter probe. Radiat Res 1995; 141:330–335.

26. Yorke ED, Williams LE, Demidecki AJ, et al. Multicellular dosimetry for beta-emitting radionuclides: autoradiography, thermoluminescent dosimetry and three-dimensional dose calculations. Med Phys 1993; 20:543–550.

27. Demidecki AJ, Williams LE, Wong JY, et al. Considerations on the calibration of small thermoluminescent dosimeters used for measurement of beta particle absorbed doses in liquid environments. Med Phys 1993; 20:1079–1087.

28. Paans A, Schippers J. Proton therapy in combination with PET as monitor: a feasibility study. IEEE Nuclear Science Symposium and Medical Imaging Conference. Vol 2; 1992,:957–959.

29. Ishikawa A, Takeda N, Ahn S, et al. Radiation dosimetry system. In: Office USP, ed. U.S. patent 6398710, 2002.

30. Hughes R. Charge-carrier transport phenomena in amorphous SiO2. Phys Rev Lett 1973; 30:1333.

31. Soubra M, Cygler J, Mackay G. Evaluation of a dual bias dual metal oxide-silicon semiconductor field effect transistor detector as radiation dosimeter. Med Phys 1994; 21:567–572.

32. Beddar AS, Salehpour M, Briere TM, et al. Preliminary evaluation of implantable MOSFET radiation dosimeters. Phys Med Biol 2005; 50:141–149.

33. Bharanidharan G, Manigandan D, Devan K, et al. Characterization of responses and comparison of calibration factor for commercial MOSFET detectors. Med Dosim 2005; 30:213–218.

34. Black RD, Scarantino CW, Mann GG, et al. An analysis of an implantable dosimeter system for external beam therapy. Int J Radiat Oncol Biol Phys 2005; 63:290–300.

35. Briere TM, Beddar AS, Gillin MT. Evaluation of precalibrated implantable MOSFET radiation dosimeters for megavoltage photon beams. Med Phys 2005; 32:3346–3349.

36. Butson MJ, Cheung T, Yu PK. Peripheral dose measurement with a MOSFET detector. Appl Radiat Isot 2005; 62:631–634.

37. Cheung T, Butson MJ, Yu PK. Effects of temperature variation on MOSFET dosimetry. Phys Med Biol 2004; 49:N191–N196.

38. Chuang CF, Verhey LJ, Xia P. Investigation of the use of MOSFET for clinical IMRT dosimetric verification. Med Phys 2002; 29:1109–1115.

39. Halvorsen PH. Dosimetric evaluation of a new design MOSFET in vivo dosimeter. Med Phys 2005; 32:110–117.

40. Jornet N, Carrasco P, Jurado D, et al. Comparison study of MOSFET detectors and diodes for entrance in vivo dosimetry in 18 MV x-ray beams. Med Phys 2004; 31:2534–2542.

41. Marcie S, Charpiot E, Bensadoun RJ, et al. In vivo measurements with MOSFET detectors in oropharynx and nasopharynx intensity-modulated radiation therapy. Int J Radiat Oncol Biol Phys 2005; 61:1603–1606.

42. Ramaseshan R, Kohli KS, Zhang TJ, et al. Performance characteristics of a microMOSFET as an in vivo dosimeter in radiation therapy. Phys Med Biol 2004; 49:4031–4048.

43. Rowbottom CG, Jaffray DA. Characteristics and performance of a micro-MOSFET: an "imageable" dosimeter for image-guided radiotherapy. Med Phys 2004; 31:609–615.

44. Scalchi P, Francescon P. Calibration of a mosfet detection system for 6-MV in vivo dosimetry. Int J Radiat Oncol Biol Phys 1998; 40:987–993.

45. Scalchi P, Francescon P, Rajaguru P. Characterization of a new MOSFET detector configuration for in vivo skin dosimetry. Med Phys 2005; 32:1571–1578.

46. Scarantino CW, Ruslander DM, Rini CJ, et al. An implantable radiation dosimeter for use in external beam radiation therapy. Med Phys 2004; 31:2658–2671.

47. Scarantino CW, Rini CJ, Aquino M, et al. Initial clinical results of an in vivo dosimeter during external beam radiation therapy. Int J Radiat Oncol Biol Phys 2005; 62:606–613.

48. Peet DJ, Pryor MD. Evaluation of a MOSFET radiation sensor for the measurement of entrance surface dose in diagnostic radiology. Br J Radiol 1999; 72:562–568.

49. Kaplan GI, Rosenfeld AB, Allen BJ, et al. Improved spatial resolution by MOSFET dosimetry of an x-ray microbeam. Med Phys 2000; 27:239–244.

50. Ehringfeld C, Schmid S, Poljanc K, et al. Application of commercial MOSFET detectors for in vivo dosimetry in

the therapeutic x-ray range from 80 kV to 250 kV. Phys Med Biol 2005; 50:289–303.

51. Consorti R, Petrucci A, Fortunato F, et al. In vivo dosimetry with MOSFETs: dosimetric characterization and first clinical results in intraoperative radiotherapy. Int J Radiat Oncol Biol Phys 2005; 63:952–960.

52. Ciocca M, Piazzi V, Lazzari R, et al. Real-time in vivo dosimetry using micro-MOSFET detectors during intraoperative electron beam radiation therapy in early-stage breast cancer. Radiother Oncol 2006; 78:213–216.

53. Bloemen-van Gurp EJ, Minken AW, Mijnheer BJ, et al. Clinical implementation of MOSFET detectors for dosimetry in electron beams. Radiother Oncol 2006; 80:288–295.

54. Zilio VO, Joneja OP, Popowski Y, et al. Absolute depth-dose-rate measurements for an 192Ir HDR brachytherapy source in water using MOSFET detectors. Med Phys 2006; 33:1532–1539.

55. Kinhikar RA, Sharma PK, Tambe CM, et al. Dosimetric evaluation of a new OneDose MOSFET for Ir-192 energy. Phys Med Biol 2006; 51:1261–1268.

56. Kinhikar RA, Sharma PK, Tambe CM, et al. Clinical application of a OneDose MOSFET for skin dose measurements during internal mammary chain irradiation with high dose rate brachytherapy in carcinoma of the breast. Phys Med Biol 2006; 51:N263–N268.

57. Gladstone DJ, Chin LM. Automated data collection and analysis system for MOSFET radiation detectors. Med Phys 1991; 18:542–548.

58. Cygler JE, Saoudi A, Perry G, et al. Feasibility study of using MOSFET detectors for in vivo dosimetry during permanent low-dose-rate prostate implants. Radiother Oncol 2006; 80:296–301.

59. Brezovich IA, Duan J, Pareek PN, et al. In vivo urethral dose measurements: a method to verify high dose rate prostate treatments. Med Phys 2000; 27:2297–2301.

60. Edwards CR, Green S, Palethorpe JE, et al. The response of a MOSFET, p-type semiconductor and LiF TLD to quasi-monoenergetic x-rays. Phys Med Biol 1997; 42:2383–2391.

61. Lavallee MC, Gingras L, Beaulieu L. Energy and integrated dose dependence of MOSFET dosimeter sensitivity for irradiation energies between 30 kV and 60Co. Med Phys 2006; 33:3683–3689.

62. Task Group 62 AAPM Radiation Therapy Committee. AAPM Reprot No. 87: Diode in vivo dosimetry for patients receiving external beam radiation therapy. Report of Task Group 62 of the Radiation Therapy Committee. Madison: American Association of Physicists in Medicine, 2005:1–84.

63. Almond PR, Biggs PJ, Coursey BM, et al. AAPM's TG-51 protocol for clinical reference dosimetry of high-energy photon and electron beams. Med Phys 1999; 26:1847–1870.

64. Rowbottom C, Jaffray D. Development of an integral system test for image-guided radiotherapy. Med Phys 2004; 31:3500–3505.

65. Siewerdsen JH, Jaffray DA. Cone-beam computed tomography with a flat-panel imager: effects of image lag. Med Phys 1999; 26:2635–2647.

66. Islam MK, Purdie TG, Norrlinger BD, et al. Patient dose from kilovoltage cone beam computed tomography imaging in radiation therapy. Med Phys 2006; 33:1573–1582.

67. Cherpak A, Studinski R, Cygler J. MOSFET detectors in quality assurance of tomotherapy treatments. Radiother Oncol 2008; 86:242–250.

68. Beyer G, Mann G, Pursley J, et al. An implantable dosimeter for the measurement of radiation dose in tissue during cancer therapy. IEEE Sens J 2007 (Special issue on in vivo sensors for medicine).

69. Briere T, Gillin M, Beddar A. Characterization of the dose response of a new implantable MOSFET detector. 49th Annual Meeting of the American Association of Physicists in Medicine, 2007.

70. Wang B, Xu XG, Kim CH. Monte Carlo study of MOSFET dosemeter characteristics: dose dependence on photon energy, direction and dosemeter composition. Radiat Prot Dosimetry 2005; 113:40–46.

71. Fagerstrom J, Micka M, DeWerd L. DVS MOSFET dosimeter response to kilovoltage radiation. 49th Annual Meeting of the American Association of physicists in medicine, 2007.

72. Wen N, Guan H, Hammond R, et al. Skin and body dose measurements for Varian cone-beam CT (CBCT) during IMRT for prostate cancer. Med Phys 2006; 33:2280.

73. Adeyemi A, Lord J. An audit of radiotherapy patient doses measured with in vivo semiconductor detectors. Br J Radiol 1997; 70:399–408.

74. Fiorino C, Corletto D, Mangili P, et al. Quality assurance by systematic in vivo dosimetry: results on a large cohort of patients. Radiother Oncol 2000; 56:85–95.

75. Shakeshaft JT, Morgan HM, Simpson PD. In vivo dosimetry using diodes as a quality control tool–experience of 2 years and 2000 patients. Br J Radiol 1999; 72:891–895.

76. Meijer GJ, Minken AW, van Ingen KM, et al. Accurate in vivo dosimetry of a randomized trial of prostate cancer irradiation. Int J Radiat Oncol Biol Phys 2001; 49:1409–1418.

77. Boellaard R, van Herk M, Uiterwaal H, et al. First clinical tests using a liquid-filled electronic portal imaging device and a convolution model for the verification of the midplane dose. Radiother Oncol 1998; 47:303–312.

78. Kroonwijk M, Pasma KL, Quint S, et al. In vivo dosimetry for prostate cancer patients using an electronic portal imaging device (EPID); demonstration of internal organ motion. Radiother Oncol 1998; 49:125–132.

79. Louwe RJ, Tielenburg R, van Ingen KM, et al. The stability of liquid-filled matrix ionization chamber electronic portal imaging devices for dosimetry purposes. Med Phys 2004; 31:819–827.

80. Piermattei A, Fidanzio A, Stimato G, et al. In vivo dosimetry by an aSi-based EPID. Med Phys 2006; 33:4414–4422.

81. Weber DC, Nouet P, Kurtz JM, et al. Assessment of target dose delivery in anal cancer using in vivo thermoluminescent dosimetry. Radiother Oncol 2001; 59:39–43.

82. Wertz H, Boda-Heggemann J, Walter C, et al. Image-guided in vivo dosimetry for quality assurance of IMRT treatment for prostate cancer. Int J Radiat Oncol Biol Phys 2007; 67:288–295.

83. Ciocca M, Orecchia R, Garibaldi C, et al. In vivo dosimetry using radiochromic films during intraoperative electron beam radiation therapy in early-stage breast cancer. Radiother Oncol 2003; 69:285–289.

84. Sadeghi A, Prestidge B, Lee J, et al. Clinical use of linear array MOSFET for urethral dose verification in prostate high dose rate brachytherapy. Med Phys 2006; 33:2146.

85. Scarantino C, Prestidge B, Anscher M, et al. The observed variance between predicted and measured radiation dose in breast and prostate patients utilizing an in-vivo dosimeter. 2008 (Submitted for publication).

86. Beyer G, Scarantino C, Prestidge B. Technical evaluation of radiation dose delivered in prostate patients as measured by an implantable MOSFET dosimeter. Int J Radiat Oncol Biol Phys 2007; 69(3):925–935.

87. Cygler J, Saoudi A, Cherpak A, et al. 4-D in vivo dosimetry in radiotherapy. Med Phys 2008 (in press).

21

Future Developments II: Dose Painting with Functional Imaging, Online Dose Tracking and Adaptation, IMRT with Robotic Brachytherapy, and Other Nonradiation Modalities

YING XIAO, TARUN PODDER, ADAM P. DICKER, AND YAN YU

Department of Radiation Oncology, Kimmel Cancer Center, Thomas Jefferson University, Philadelphia, Pennsylvania, U.S.A.

DOSE PAINTING WITH INTENSITY-MODULATED RADIATION THERAPY: THE RADIOBIOLOGICAL TARGET

The latest available technology in radiation therapy, intensity-modulated radiation therapy (IMRT), offers more precise radiation delivery with high dose to target volume while sparing nearby critical structures. IMRT is defined as the radiation delivery technique that uses radiation fields of various sizes whose intensity could be varied to control the dose distributions that could be tailored to fit complex geometric arrangement of targets and for avoidance of critical structures. By allowing the intensity within the target to vary opened the door to the possibility of protecting critical structures that were positioned near the target and fell within one or more of the different treatment fields, as well as "paint" or "sculpt" high-/low-dose regions within the target.

IMRT delivery technology has advanced rapidly over the recent years. Figure 1 depicts various multileaf collimator (MLC)-based IMRT delivery technologies (1).

Other IMRT delivery techniques include physical attenuators and robotic delivery with collimators. With the ability of IMRT to deliver, by design, nonuniform dose across the target, the question arises as to how to optimize the radiation delivery, taking into account all the information available to us regarding the tumor location, tumor extent, and the response of tumor to radiation dose to achieve maximum kill of tumor cells and maximum protection of normal structures. The advent of imaging capabilities in the area of nuclear magnetic resonance imaging (MRI) and spectroscopy, positron emission tomography (PET), and molecular imaging promises to provide physiology and functional information, as well as tumor biology at the genotype and phenotype levels.

The significance of MRI in cancer detection and staging lies in its soft tissue contrast because of the differences in the T1 and T2 relaxation parameters of normal and abnormal states. Developments of contrast-enhancement techniques can yield physiological and microenvironmental information such as blood flow, water molecule mobility, oxygen concentration, etc. Nuclear magnetic resonance (NMR) can provide ample biological information in the level of biomolecules. Proton (^{1}H) spectroscopy is one of the NMR spectroscopy techniques that offers sensitivity, spatial resolution, sufficient signal-to-noise ratio, and reasonable image acquisition time. MR spectroscopy (MRS) is able to detect signals from low molecular weight

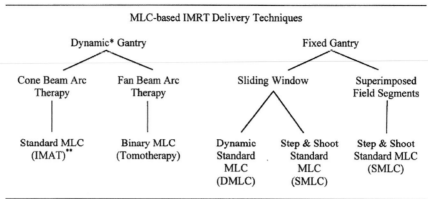

Figure 1 MLC-based IMRT delivery techniques. *Abbreviations*: MLC, multileaf collimator; IMRT, intensity-modulated radiation therapy; DMLC, dynamic multileaf collimation; SMLC, segmental multileaf collimation; IMAT, intensity-modulated arc therapy. *Source*: From Ref. 1.

metabolites such as choline and creatine that are present at concentrations of a few millimeters in tissue. The contrast achieved with MRS provides a promising alternative for identifying tumor extent and regions of high metabolic activity. Spectra may be acquired from single voxels or from a two-dimensional or three-dimensional array of voxels using spectroscopic imaging. The current state of the art achieves a spatial resolution of 6 to 10 mm in a scan time of about 10 to 15 minutes. Coregistered MR images can be acquired in the same examination. MR spectroscopic imaging (MRSI) provides a noninvasive method of evaluating metabolic markers of prostate cancer or healthy prostatic tissue. Multiple studies have showed the incremental role of MRSI combined with the anatomical information provided by MRI for assessment of cancer location and extent within the prostate, staging, and cancer aggressiveness. Further developments—including new 3T technology—will likely provide improved spectral resolution for better prostate cancer detection and characterization. It is anticipated that MRS will become an essential tool for treatment planning where other modalities lack the necessary contrast (2–4).

T2-weighted MRI for imaging prostate has much superior contrast to CT, transrectal ultrasound, and digital rectal examinations. However, the sensitivity and specificity are still 83% and 50%, respectively by MRI alone (5). The use of ^{1}H MRSI in the prostate is needed to aid target definition. The main spectral peaks observed in normal prostate are those of the choline-containing compounds, creatine and phosphocreatine, and a large peak from citrate. Choline compounds are associated primarily with membrane synthesis, while creatine is involved in energy metabolism. Citrate is a product of normal epithelial

cell metabolism in the prostate, where high levels of zinc inhibit the enzyme aconitase and hence prevent the oxidation of citrate in the Krebs cycle that occurs in other cells. In prostate cancer, choline is elevated and the normal production of citrate is reduced. Benign prostatic hyperplasia, on the other hand, is characterized by high levels of citrate. Hence, the choline/citrate ratio is a fairly reliable measure of the presence of cancer. A strong correlation has been found between negative MRSI and negative biopsy findings and between positive MRSI and positive biopsy findings (6). However, there is only a weak correlation between the concentration of prostate-specific antigen (PSA, the current "gold standard") and either biopsy or MRSI findings (6). Step-section pathological examination of radical prostatectomy specimens demonstrated that MRI combined with MRSI yielded a significant improvement in cancer localization to a prostate sextant (left or right; base, mid-gland, or apex) compared with MRI alone (7). There is strong evidence that MRS has a valuable role to play in radiotherapy treatment planning. MRSI has been used in combination with MRI to define regions for dose escalation within the prostate (8–11), permitting a dose of greater than 90 Gy to the high-risk region while treating the remainder of the prostate to about 70 Gy.

^{1}H MRSI data may be acquired from the prostate using an external phased-array coil. However, the best signal-to-noise ratio is achieved using an endorectal coil. The main disadvantage of the endorectal approach is slight deformation of the prostate, which needs to be allowed for in using the images for radiotherapy treatment planning. Deformation will be discussed in the following section. Another concern with MRS is that voxel sizes of typically 8 to 10 mm are required to achieve an adequate signal-to-noise ratio, with a large part of this volume needing to be occupied by abnormal tissue for a change in signal to be detected. Thus, small infiltrating lesions are unlikely to be detectable. While some improvement in sensitivity and spectral specificity is expected with higher field scanners and improved sensitivity coils, this is likely to yield only a small improvement in spatial resolution. However, while in principle both MRI and CT have much better spatial resolution, MRS has the potential to improve identification of the gross tumor volume and hence improve treatment using radiotherapy.

Fluorodeoxyglucose (FDG) is shown not to be a suitable PET tracer for diagnosing prostate cancer. Unlike other tumor types, prostate cancer often does not display increased glucose metabolism (12). Studies showed little difference between FDG uptake in prostate cancer and benign prostatic hyperplasia (13,14), and that there is limited additional information from FDG-PET in diagnosis and staging of prostate cancer (15–18). However, due to the fact that tissue uptake of radiolabeled choline corresponds to an increase in membrane lipid synthesis, [C-11]-choline-PET have comparable or even better sensitivities than with MRI and MRS for primary lesions (19). Initial preclinical and clinical studies showed that [F-18]-fluorocholine is a promising tracer for the evaluation of primary and metastatic prostate cancer (20–22). The coregistered functional and anatomical information of PET/CT appears to be particularly helpful in the evaluation of PET tracers in the abdomen and pelvis. [C-11]-choline-PET/CT revealed a sensitivity of 83% for localization of nodules greater than 5 mm, which was comparable to transrectal ultrasound-guided biopsy (23). Because of the limited resolution of PET imaging, information regarding the detection of extraprostatic tumor extension could not be found. The same group performed a direct comparison of [C-11]-choline-PET/CT with sextant results of step-section histopathology and found a sensitivity, specificity, and accuracy of 66%, 81%, and 71%, respectively (24). Choline PET and acetate PET are promising tracers in the diagnosis of prostate cancer, but their validity in local tumor demarcation, lymph node diagnosis, and detection of recurrence has to be defined in future clinical trials (25).

Combined radiotherapy and gene therapy is a novel therapeutic approach for prostate cancer (26–28). There are various potential benefits in combining ionizing radiation with gene therapy to achieve enhanced antitumor effects: (*i*) ionizing radiation improves transfection/transduction efficiency, transgene integration, and possibly, the "bystander effect" of gene therapy; (*ii*) gene therapy, on the other hand, may interfere with repair of radiation-induced DNA damage and increase DNA susceptibility to radiation damage in cancer cells; and (*iii*) radiotherapy and gene therapy target at different parts of the cell cycle. Preclinical data have demonstrated the enhanced antitumor

effects of this combined approach in local tumor control, prolongation of survival, as well as systemic control. The goal of this combined approach is to enhance cancer cure without an increase in treatment-related toxicity. This approach also offers a new paradigm in spatial cooperation, whereby two local therapies are combined to elicit both local and systemic effects. Early clinical results showed the safety of this approach.

ONLINE DOSE TRACKING AND ADAPTATION

Deformable Target and Structures

Image-guided radiation therapy (IGRT) for the treatment of cancer has become a reality with the availability of imaging capabilities in the radiation treatment room with the patient in the actual treatment position, where volume images can be acquired on a daily basis. Commercially available in-room image devices now include CT/volumetric CT. It is reasonable to expect even more sophisticated functional imaging modalities, e.g., PET, available for the patient in treatment position, in the future. These images can potentially guide radiation therapy in the following two aspects. First, the direct reference of the images obtained with the patient in the treatment position to the treatment machine coordinates can substantially reduce the geometric uncertainty of internal structures. With the additional real-time tracking and adjustment capabilities, more precise radiation will then be delivered with high dose to target volume while sparing nearby critical structures, taking advantage of the latest available technology in radiation therapy, i.e., IMRT. Second, with the images available on a more frequent basis, analysis will yield tumor response during radiation treatments in the early stages that will allow adjustment of treatment techniques (fraction size, radiation modality, radiation treatment plan modification, etc.).

IGRT has limited implementation, mostly for localization for the time being, especially for the radiotherapy of the cancer of the prostate. However, mainly developments are made in research of strategies and tools for image analysis and/or for adjusting treatments when image/dose analysis indicates the need for change. Fully integrated package that includes image/dose analysis methods and radiation treatment adjustment tools are being developed to make these new imaging capabilities truly helpful.

Among the developments for efficient image analysis, initially for target localization with the potential for target delineation and critical structure definition for the images, some of the tools acquired images online with patient in the treatment position daily (e.g., daily cone-beam CT) and adopted rigid body gray-scale registration (29–31) and deformable image–registration approach (32,33). These tools and approaches are reported to improve upon the efficiency and to reduce the variation among observers, which is an issue in prostate radiotherapy (34).

Among the most widely implemented deformable registration algorithms is Thirion's "demons" algorithm (35). In its implementation, each image is viewed as a set of isointensity contours. The main idea is that a regular grid of forces deforms an image by pushing the contours in the normal direction. The orientation and magnitude of the displacement is derived from the instantaneous optical flow equation that contains the information from the fixed image and the moving image to be registered and the displacement or optical flow between the images. For registration, the projection of the vector on the direction of the intensity gradient becomes unstable for small values of the image gradient, resulting in large displacement values. To overcome this problem, Thirion renormalized the equation. Reconstruction of the deformation field is an ill-posed problem where matching the fixed and moving images has many solutions. For example, since each image pixel is free to move independently, it is possible that all pixels of one particular value in the moving image could map to a single image pixel in the fixed image of the same value. The resulting deformation field may be unrealistic for real-world applications. An option to solve for the field uniquely is to enforce an elastic-like behavior, smoothing the deformation field with a Gaussian filter between iterations.

In Vivo Dose Verification and Reconstruction

Electronic Portal Imaging Device Dose Verification and Reconstruction

Electronic portal imaging device (EPID) have been widely used for verification of patient positioning in place of film because of its efficiency in obtaining instantaneous digital images of the patient anatomy, and the treatment field can be compared with digital reconstructed radiographs (DRRs) from the planning system. Besides utility in positioning verification, studies have been ongoing to obtain dosimetric information from the EPID for treatment delivery verification without (pretreatment) or with (in vivo) patient (36–44). In vivo EPID dosimetry has the following advantages: the hardware is already fixed to the linear accelerator, providing instantaneous high-resolution digital images. EPID image acquisition can be part of the actual patient treatment procedure, which does not require additional time and dose to the patient. If one is able to obtain three-dimensional reconstructed delivered dose information, adaptive plans can be generated on the basis of the delivered dose to the patient.

EPID images were acquired either with camera, ion chamber matrix, or with solid-state (e.g., a-Si) flat panel imager. They generally have large enough detection area

that can contain most radiation treatment field sizes with submillimeter resolutions.

Verification of the delivered dose with EPID falls into two categories. One compared the dose at the EPID plane (40,45) and the other made comparisons between the reconstructed dose to the voxels delivered inside the patient and the dose predicted by the treatment planning system (38,46). With the second approach, however, it is potentially feasible to adjust dose based not just on the anatomy variation but also delivered dose variation during the treatment, especially with the three-dimensional reconstructed dose information (47–49).

There are a number of methods applied to derive two-dimensional planar dose for a certain plane in the patient intersecting the beam (46,50). The two-dimensional planar back-projected dose reconstruction method starts from conversion of segment images to an absolute two-dimensional dose distribution in the plane of the patient, defined as the plane perpendicular to the beam axis intersecting the isocenter. Pixel values of the transit dose image are processed using scatter kernels (for scatter within the EPID and scatter from the patient to the EPID), the scatter-to-primary ratio (for scattered radiation within the patient), the inverse square law, and the measured transmission to obtain the absolute dose distribution in the isocentric plane of the patient. The measured transmission of the beam through the patient is determined from images acquired for each field (or segment), both with and without the patient. The location of the reconstruction plane is arbitrary, so a correction is required to account for attenuation of the beam from the isocentric plane to the exit surface. The external contour of the patient CT scan is used to obtain the ratio of geometrical path lengths, which is used to calculate the attenuation per pixel. The density of the transmission medium is assumed to be homogeneous; therefore, the dose may be incorrect for areas on the plane where the beam passed through media of non-tissue equivalent density. Reconstructed two-dimensional dose distributions for each field are then the sum of the reconstructed dose distributions of all segments belonging to that field. The second two-dimensional planar dose derivation method first calculates the two-dimensional contribution of the primary and scattered dose component at the exit side of the patient or phantom from the measured transmission dose. Then, a correction is applied for the difference in contribution for both dose components between exit side and midplane, yielding the midplane dose.

These two-dimensional methods have been adopted for clinical in vivo dosimetric verifications, especially when IMRT is involved. In one example of using this back-projection algorithm (46), two-dimensional dose distributions inside a phantom or patient are reconstructed from portal images. The method requires the primary dose component at the position of the EPID. A parameterized description of the lateral scatter within the imager was obtained from measurements with an ionization chamber in a mini phantom. In addition to point dose measurements on the central axis of square fields of different size, dose profiles of those fields are used as reference input data. This method yielded a better description of the lateral scatter within the EPID, which resulted in a higher accuracy in the back-projected, two-dimensional dose distributions. The accuracy was tested for pretreatment verification of IMRT plans for the treatment of prostate cancer. All segments are evaluated by comparing the back-projected, two-dimensional EPID dose distribution with a film measurement inside a homogeneous slab phantom. The γ-evaluation method was used with a dose-difference criterion of 2% of dose maximum and a distance-to-agreement criterion of 2 mm. Excellent agreement was found between EPID and film measurements for each field, both in the central part of the beam and in the penumbra and low-dose regions.

Simple two-dimensional dose reconstruction has been extended to three dimensions in the vicinity of the isocenter plane with reasonable accuracy (47). However, with the availability of online CT data from cone-beam and other techniques, more sophisticated and potentially more accurate three-dimensional reconstruction methods can be applied. In one concept originally presented by McNutt et al. (49), an iterative superposition/convolution method was used to obtain the primary energy fluence. The three-dimensional patient dose was then calculated applying predefined scatter kernels. Another effort by Patridge et al. (48) also used iterative method for primary energy fluence prediction. Instead of a direct dose calculation using predefined scatter kernels, they proposed Monte Carlo method or the calculation engine from a treatment planning system. Three-dimensional dose reconstruction is an area that deserves a great deal of research efforts. An accurate three-dimensional in vivo dose construction for radiotherapy delivery is essential for any successful dose-adaptive treatment protocol.

In order for the dose information to be derived from EPID signals, properties of the EPID response behavior need to be well understood. Studies have identified characteristics of EPID that need to be considered and correction factors applied to obtain dose accuracy from EPID measurements to be within 1% (51). The over-response of the EPID signal can be significant over the patient-detector distance. Addition of a certain thickness of material could reduce this over response. The response of EPID varies over dose per pulse, pulse repetition frequency, and number of monitor units. Ghosting effects, in which under-response is found for shorter beam times, also contribute to the variation of EPID response. The long-term stability of some of the EPID panels are studied and found to be suitable for dosimetry acquisition after applying a dynamic correction (52).

Three-Dimensional In Vivo Dosimetry with PET-CT

With the increasingly wider implementation of heavy particle therapy, along with high energy photon radiotherapy, it is possible to take advantage of the photonuclear and direct nuclear interactions in tissue for in-vivo dosimetric imaging with PET-CT. Ion beams produce PET emitters through nuclear interactions. Radioactive beams could also consist of intrinsic PET emitters. These would allow direct imaging of Bragg peak distribution which is related to the absorbed dose. The high energy photons, on the other hand, produce positron emitters with energies above 20 MeV. The intensities are proportional to the photon fluence which is intimately related to absorbed dose. With the prior delivered dose information, it is then possible to adapt the future treatment plan basing upon not only the target and structural variation, but also the exact dose still needed for target, adding more to or subtracting from the delivered dose. With the help from multiple image modalities, future re-planning process would include information from numerous aspects: radiation responsiveness (resistance) considering hypoxia, possible planning and delivery errors, general deformation of patient anatomy throughout the treatment course (53).

RADIOTHERAPY TREATMENT PLANNING WITH TARGET MOTION

Online Imaging, Dose Tracking, Real-Time Planning, Parallel Optimization

With online target definition and prior in vivo dose derived, it is conceivable for real-time planning to be used as an adjustment strategy. Accuracy and precision are the qualities of the treatment plans that have improved immensely in the past 20 years, especially since the advent of IMRT. Yet, new developments in imaging technologies provide us with a possibility to augment, quantitatively and qualitatively, the treatment planning process in a way that was not previously clinically viable. However, concomitant to that is also the growth of complexities of reported solutions and their implementations.

Treatment planning computation (TPC) is a mathematical inverse problem predicated on the prescription expressed either as physical and/or biological stipulations. In principle, the latter are more relevant but they are not mature enough to replace the former constraints. However, the biological goals' preponderance makes it imperative for a modern TPC to accommodate a relevant component, at least in terms of the research capabilities or the extensibility of the system. Another tacit facet of the TPC is the technological constraints that impinge indirectly on the domain of realizable treatments. These constraints may address issues that are transparent for therapeutic goals, for instance, the modeling of the resultant intensity map that could be computationally amenable to the given leaf sequencing algorithm or in general to this phase of plan preparation (54). TPC employs some optimization schemes or related methods.

The computation of beam weights includes dose-based voxel dependent and dose-volume constraints [dose-volume histogram (DVH) equivalent] as articulated by prescriptions. Another concept used in modeling is the equivalent uniform dose (EUD) (55). Its most popular version $EUD = (1/N \sum_i^N D_i^a)^{1/a}$ (56) can be viewed as a handy modeling construct because of the mathematical characteristics of the function. However, there is still a nexus with the biological underlining [e.g., tumor control probability (TCP) and normal tissue complication probability (NTCP)] via the power law behavior of the effective dose used for the reduction of the DVH (57–61); a is a structure-dependent parameter, negative for targets and positive for organs at risk (OARs). The EUD addresses the inhomogeneity of the dose distribution in structures. It is important to model the computation with criteria that are also used for the plan evaluation.

Another aspect that we want to control is the complexity of the intensity patterns. This can be addressed by either the exogenous way of adding a smoothing constraint (62) to the optimization or endogenously using smoothing component (63) within the optimization. These solutions allow us to keep the therapeutic aspect of the sought dose distribution in sync with the technological limitations of the dose delivery.

With the online acquired image data available and the dose reconstructed via one method or another, ideally one would be able to optimize the radiotherapy treatment plan on a day-to-day basis. This planning problem poses a rather stringent request on the speed of the computation.

The algorithms that could accommodate the above modeling and computational characteristics and could be implemented with parallelization to take advantage of the ever-increasing computing power are investigated. Among those are the subgradient projection method and the component averaging projection technique (64–74). The usefulness of these algorithms is outlined in computational context (70–74). They are fast and inherently parallel, which allows us to use modern multiprocessor computers. They can provide solutions within one to two minutes. The findings also indicate that they inherently strive to produce relatively smooth patterns (71), yet the explicit constraint of this type can be applied as well. The dose-based and dose volume-based constraints (70,71) were prototyped. The EUD α-sublevel set (75)-based constraints

can be defined as convex for OARs and targets. The proposed iterative algorithms must use convex functions as constraints. The accommodation of the EUD for target and critical structures will be realized with the EUD supra- and sublevel sets (75) that comply with the convexity requirement. The other methods are the (quasi) Newton method and conjugate gradient methods (76,77) that are often reported in the IMRT optimization (78–81). They are fast and amenable to accommodate constraints. They might be combined with the feasibility search methods for hybrid optimization approach.

Robust Optimization

Another treatment planning optimization approach that addresses the target motion is incorporating motion information into the initial formation of the optimization problem. The recent development of planning optimization involves the idea of a "motion pdf" (82–86), which uses a probability density function (pdf) to define what proportion of time the tumor spends in each breathing phase (in reality, discretization leads to a probability mass function or pmf). Similar pmf models exist for interfraction motion (87). This pmf approach requires that the motion is reproducible and stable during the treatment delivery (82). Using a pmf to account for tumor motion produces acceptable dose distributions, provided the motion does not deviate significantly from what is expected. The uncertainty associated with pmf however can also be modeled and formulated with mathematical approaches (88). These solutions are found to deliver fewer doses to nearby critical structures than the conventional margin solutions, which typically overcompensate for the target motion (89,90). It is also possible to vary the level of concern for various structures and for individual patient cases.

IMAGE- AND DOSE-GUIDED ROBOTIC DELIVERY

The word "robot" was introduced in English language in 1921 by the play writer Karl Cape. Now we use it very commonly in our daily life. But what is really meant by a robot? The most complete definition is "A robot is a reprogrammable multifunctional manipulator designed to move materials, parts, tools, or specialized devices through variable programmed motions for performance of a variety of tasks" (91). Of the four branches of robotics, namely, medical robotics, land-based or industrial robotics, space robotics, and underwater robotics, the medical robotics is the latest one and now gaining significant momentum. Presently, there are various applications of robots in the medical field. The application of robotic technology has undergone rapid growth in the field of endoscopic surgery in the past several years, particularly in robotic-assisted radical prostatectomy. Increasingly, robotic devices are coming into the radiotherapy clinic as potential solutions to online adaptive treatment delivery. When coupled with close-loop control strategies, image and physiological sensor guidance, predictive and feedforward tracking algorithms, and real-time dose-guided IMRT, robotic assistance promises to catalyze the next paradigm change in high-precision radiation delivery.

In prostate brachytherapy, accuracy of radioactive seed placement is important for optimal dose delivery to the target tissue while sparing the critical organs and structures. But accurate placement of needles in soft tissue is challenging because of tissue heterogeneity and elastic stiffness, tissue deformation and movement, unfavorable anatomic structures, needle bending, inadequate sensing, and poor maneuverability. In contemporary prostate brachytherapy procedures, the needles are inserted manually using ultrasound guidance through fixed holes of a physical template. Therefore, flexibility and maneuverability of needle insertion is severely limited. Sometimes it is difficult to avoid pubic arch (especially for patients with larger prostates) because the needles can only be inserted straight through the template's holes. The consistency and efficiency of the treatment procedure are highly dependent on the skills of the clinicians. A robotic system can potentially improve the accuracy and consistency of operation by assisting the clinicians.

In the past several years, researchers have been developing ultrasound-guided robotic systems for prostate brachytherapy (92–99). Fichtinger *et al.* (92) and Stoianovici *et al.* (93) have developed a needle placement robotic system that is comprised of a 3 degree-of-freedom (DOF) Cartesian bridge over the patient, a 2DOF remote center of motion (RCM), and a 1DOF needle insertion with friction transmission. They have employed a 7DOF passive arm between the Cartesian stage and the remaining two modules, namely RCM and needle inserter, to position and orient the needle in imaging instruments such as CT imager. In this system, the brachytherapy seeds can be deposited manually. Using a 5DOF industrial robot, Wei *et al.* (94,95) were successful in positioning and orienting a single hole template for prostate brachytherapy. Through this accurately positioned template a needle can be inserted manually. A motorized needle rotation module was integrated with the robot and ultrasound probe rotation was motorized for 3D image reconstruction. Kronreif *et al.* (96,97) developed a 4DOF needle placement robotic system which consisted of two offset x-y stages allowing positioning and orienting the needle over the perineum. In this system the needles can be manually inserted through a needle guiding attachment. Needle insertion depth is monitored in ultrasound images. Meltsner et al. (98) developed a custom-built 6 DOF robotic system for

prostate brachytherapy and reported about 2.1 mm (about 7 mm without rotation) accuracy in seed delivery into gel phantom at 10-cm depth. Kennedy et al. (99) designed a 4 DOF prototype, which was intended to replace the conventional fixed template. The commercially available robotic system for prostate seed delivery is the Nucletron's FIRST system (100). This system has two motorized motions: one for rotating the transrectal ultrasound (TRUS) probe and the other for pushing the seeds and spacer from the cartridges. All other motions including needle placement using conventional template are manual.

Recently, Yu et al. (101) have developed a fully automated robotic system for prostate seed implant (Figs. 2 and 3). Numerous techniques such as needle rotation and angulation during insertion, force-torque detection, which were perfected by a variety of proof-of-principle experiments, have been implemented in the system design. Experimental results revealed that velocity modulation, especially rotation [partial rotation (102) or continuous (103,104)], significantly improves needle insertion and targeting accuracy. Reduction in force also minimizes tissue/organ deformation and target deflection (Figs. 4 and 5) and thus is expected to improve seed implantation accuracy. During automated robotic mode of operation, in the absence of human tactile sensing, the needle insertion force must be monitored for safety. To measure and monitor force profiles during the operational procedures, two single-axis force sensors (model M13, Honeywell Sensotech, Columbus, Ohio, U.S.) were

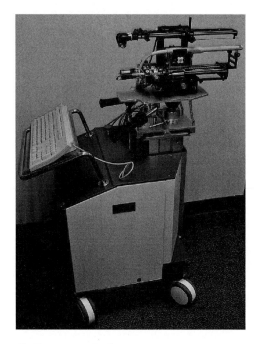

Figure 2 Prototype robotic system.

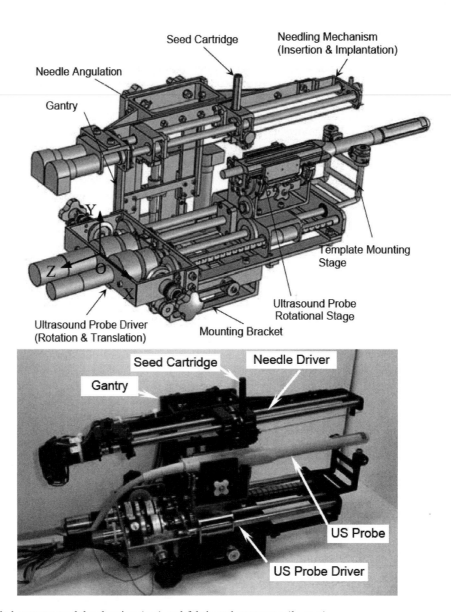

Figure 3   Assembled surgery module: drawing (*top*) and fabricated prototype (*bottom*).

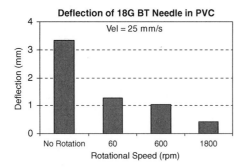

Figure 4   Reduction of needle deflection (bevel-tip brachytherapy needle in PVC phantom). *Abbreviation*: PVC, polyvinyl chloride.

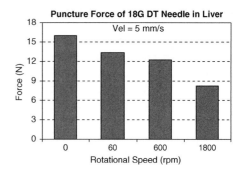

Figure 5   Reduction in insertion force on needle (diamond-tip brachytherapy needle in bovine liver phantom).

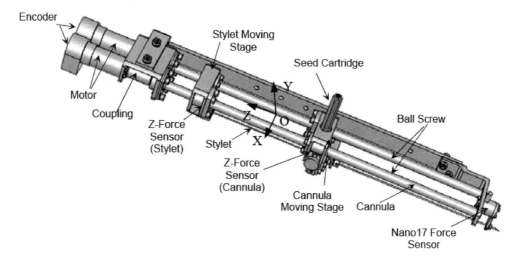

Figure 6 Needle driver.

installed each at the proximal ends of the stylet and cannula, and one six-axis force-torque sensor (model Nano17, ATI Industrial Automation, Apex, North Carolina, U.S.) was installed at the distal end of the cannula (Fig. 6). Monitoring of these forces is useful in detecting pubic arch interference (PAI) and will help in assessing needle bending due to transverse forces. Preliminary seed implant experiments using tissue equivalent soft material phantom prepared from polyvinyl chloride exhibited (Fig. 7) seed placement error (root mean square) of about 0.5 mm, which is quite encouraging.

Robot-assisted therapeutic delivery system is attractive for several reasons. The main advantages are increased accuracy, reduced human variability, and possible reduction of operation time and clinician's fatigue. There can be two methods of robotic needle insertion and seed deposition: (*i*) singe-channel technique and (*ii*) multi-channel technique. In single-channel mode, one needle

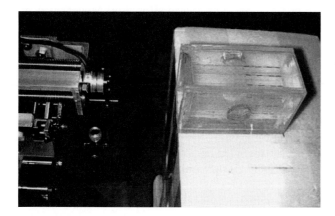

Figure 7 Seed delivery in soft material (PVC) phantom. *Abbreviation*: PVC, polyvinyl chloride.

can be inserted at a time and typically, two to five seeds along a needle track are deposited in the prostate according to the dosimetric plan. Drawbacks of this modality are (*i*) it is a slow process because one needle is used at a time (typically, 15–25 needles are required); (*ii*) every time the needle is inserted, the prostate and other organs are deformed and displaced, thereby incurring seed placement inaccuracy; (*iii*) there is a chance of a needle colliding with already deposited seeds and displacing the seed; and (*iv*) needle deflection and its relative position in the prostate cannot be predicted in advance for interactive (or dynamic) dosimetric planning. In contrast, the multi-channel system is capable of placing several needles or even all needles at a time, and thereby, it will be faster to deliver the seeds required for the treatment. A multichannel delivery system can effectively avoid the problem of gradual prostate swelling (i.e., edema) and deformation, which occurs while depositing the seeds by a single needle. Since the prostate is not rigidly mounted, it can move and rotate as well as deform quite unpredictably each time a needle is inserted. However, when several needles are inserted concurrently, the prostate will be uniformly pushed back symmetrically to a more stable position and the deformation can better be estimated for precise delivery of seeds. Thus, the multichannel system can overcome the drawbacks that may be encountered by the single-channel systems.

Currently, Podder et al. (105) are developing a multichannel robotic system that will be, unlike a single-channel robotic system or conventional manual technique, capable of inserting a large number of needles concurrently (Figs. 8 and 9). This system possesses several potential added advantages such as reduced target displacement, reduced edema, and less operating time as compared with single-needle insertion technique. This multichannel system has been designed to insert multiple

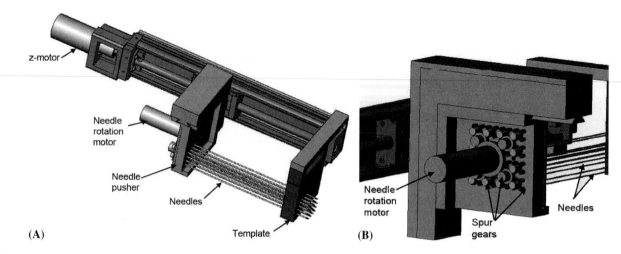

Figure 8 Needle insertion module of the multichannel robotic system—simultaneous rotation and insertion of multiple needles. (**A**) Front-end and side view. (**B**) Back-end and side view.

needles simultaneously into the prostate. As shown in Figure 8, all 16 needles can be inserted simultaneously while all the needles can be rotated by using a single motor (Fig. 8B). This provision of needle rotation will reduce the insertion force as well as organ (or target) deflection and deformation. After inserting the needles at the desired positions and depths, they will be fixed into position using a locking mechanism in the template. Then,

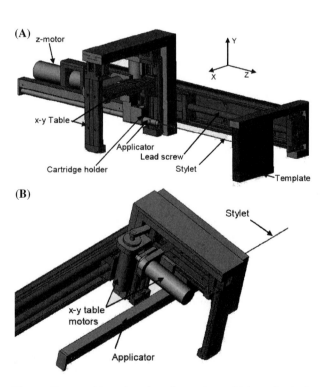

Figure 9 x-y table and seed applicator for multichannel robotic system. (**A**) Front-end and side view. (**B**) Back-end and side view.

the insertion module will be replaced by the x-y table module (Fig. 9) using the dove-tail joint, while the applicator is used to deliver the radioactive seeds needle-by-needle at the desired coordinates based on the dosimetric plan. The x-y table moves in the transverse plane to position the seed applicator at the desired location while the main translational actuator activates the stylet to push the seed into the prostate. The entire procedure will be performed under ultrasound image guidance.

It is known that among the available imaging modalities, MRI is the best modality for differentiating the soft tissue boundaries between the prostate and its surrounding anatomy. Therefore, by utilizing MRI in prostate brachytherapy, the ability of delivering a precisely shaped treatment may be improved, and it may be possible to achieve more targeted therapy while sparing normal tissues and critical structures. Robot-assisted brachytherapy system can enhance needle placement accuracy and consistency of treatment. Thus, a robotic system guided by MRI has the potential to further improve the delivery of radiation treatment for prostate cancer. Recently, Muntener et al. (106) and Patriciu et al. (107) reported an MR compatible robotic system for prostate seed implant. This system was able to deliver seeds in tissue-mimicking phantom under 0.5T to 3T MR environment with an accuracy of 0.72 ± 0.36 mm. As high-dose-rate (HDR) brachytherapy is attracting increased attention in clinical circles, an MR-guided HDR robotic system aided by powerful optimization engine like the genetic algorithm (GA) would be the next state-of-the-art technology in this frontier field. Further improvement may be possible if adaptive dosimetric planning is integrated with patient-specific predictive models (108) of tissue deformation and displacement aided by artificial neural networks. However, in the near future, ultrasound may remain as

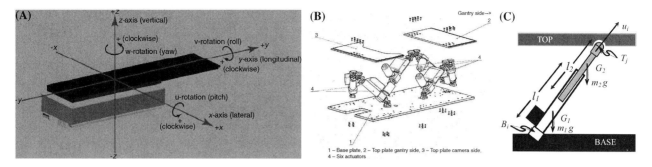

Figure 10 HexaPOD robotic couch. (**A**) External isometric view. (**B**) Internal isometric view. (**C**) Schematic of the leg.

the common modality for imaging because of its cost and convenience.

Various internal organs including prostate move because of respiratory and cardiac motions. Among different available techniques, the MLC gating is commonly used to compensate the undesired motion of the target. However, MLC-gating technique has several disadvantages. For example, use of internal fiducials for motion monitoring requires kilovoltage X-ray, which delivers unwanted radiation dose to the patient. Gating suffers from severely low duty cycle (only 30–50%) and IMRT efficiency (only 20–50%). All these lead to a 4- to 15-fold increase in delivery time over conventional treatment (109).

Presently available commercial robotic systems for external beam radiation therapy include the CyberKnife Radiosurgery System (Accuray, Sunnyvale, California, U.S.), and 6 DOF HexaPOD patient positioning system (Elekta AB, Stockholm, Sweden). These systems have the potential to enable position and motion compensation with promising speed and accuracy. Coordinated control between high-speed MLCs and robotic couch offers another intriguing opportunity. Recently, a group of researchers have investigated the feasibility of using the treatment couch (HexaPOD and Dynatrac) for intrafraction motion tracking (110). Their study concluded that the achievable speed was much less than that required for compensating respiration-induced tumor motion in the realm of clinically relevant motion amplitudes. Such a robotic system, which is subjected to a large load and operating at moderate frequency and amplitude, requires not only robust electromechanical design but also stable closed-loop dynamic control that can produce a high degree of repeatability and accuracy with varying external perturbations.

The movement of target-volume (internal organ/tumor) can be measured either using a combination of various sensory systems such as (*i*) surrogate breathing motion signals from external markers, (*ii*) implanted electromagnetic transponders, and (*iii*) four-dimensional CT (and/or X-ray) images of implanted fiducial markers. In the former

case, a robust three-dimensional model correlating the tumor motion and the external markers signal can be developed. In the later cases, the coordinates of the tumor volume can be periodically extracted from the direct measurement of the transponder's position. A closed-loop dynamic control of the 6 DOF robotic couch can be employed to continuously reposition the patient reciprocatively to the tumor motion so that the treatment beam always finds the target-volume stationary.

Recently, Podder et al. (111) reported a decentralized closed-loop dynamic controller for adjusting the MLC-bank and robotic couch on the basis of their dynamic response bandwidth, so that the target-volume appears to be stationary to the radiation beam and that the beam can be delivered close to 100% duty cycle. To track the tumor for optimal dose delivery to the clinical target volume (CTV) with minimal planning target volume (PTV), it was proposed to control both the MLC-bank and the HexaPOD (which is a special type of Stewart platform, i.e., a parallel robotic manipulator, Fig. 10) simultaneously (112,113). These two subsystems (MLC-bank and HexaPOD couch) have vastly different dynamic responses, i.e., natural frequency bandwidths. The trajectory of the tumor movement due to respiratory and cardiac motions is decomposed into two segments (high- and low-frequency segments) using the wavelet technique. The high-frequency component is assigned to the lighter subsystem, i.e., the MLC or MLC-bank, and the low-frequency component with larger amplitude is allocated to the heavier subsystem, i.e., the couch (Fig. 11). Simulated tumor motion was decomposed using wavelet technique into two segments, where the low-frequency component was allocated to the HexaPOD couch and the high-frequency component was allocated to MLC-bank, as shown in Figure 12. Significant improvement in the tracking of tumor was observed when the decomposed trajectories were allocated to both the MLC-bank and the HexaPOD couch (Fig. 13, blue line), whereas when only the HexaPOD couch was used, large residual fluctuating error in tumor tracking was found (Fig. 13, green line).

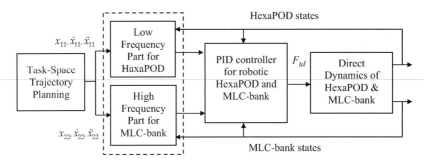

Figure 11 Block diagram of the decentralized coordinated dynamics-based closed-loop controller for HexaPOD robotic couch and linear accelerator's MLC-bank. *Abbreviation*: MLC, multileaf collimator.

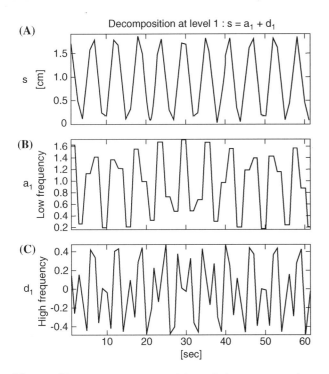

Figure 12 Wavelet decomposition of the tumor motion. (**A**) Resultant motion. (**B**) Low-frequency component. (**C**) High-frequency component.

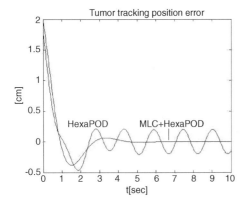

Figure 13 Tumor tracking errors—using MLC-bank and HexaPOD (*blue line*) and using HexaPOD only (*wavy green line*). *Abbreviation*: MLC, multileaf collimator.

Thus, it appears in numerical simulation that decentralized dynamics-based controller can track the tumor motion more accurately.

Implementation of the proposed technique can potentially improve real-time tracking of the tumor-volume to deliver precise radiation dose at almost 100% duty cycle while minimizing irradiation to surrounding normal tissues and sparing critical organs. This, in turn, will potentially improve the quality of patient treatment by lowering the toxicity level and increasing survival. In this study, a relatively simple but elegant closed-loop proportional integral derivative (PID) control algorithm has been deployed, and the results are quite promising. However, more sophisticated control strategies such as adaptive learning control aided by artificial neural network may yield the next higher level solution that can potentially accommodate the dynamics of surgical and therapeutic environment. One of the main challenges and research opportunities is to synchronize the respiratory motion with the robotic couch and/or IMRT delivery considering system latency, patient's physiodynamics, and target-volume deformation in addition to target movement.

SUMMARY OF PERTINENT CONCLUSIONS

- Physiological and functional information in addition to tumor biology at the genotype and phenotype level may enable "dose painting," taking advantage of the latest planning and delivery technologies.
- Efficient and accurate target definition tools and strategies, for example, deformable registration, can greatly facilitate the IGRT process.
- Three-dimensional in vivo dosimetry is an essential component of successful image- and dose-guided radiation treatment process.
- Real-time online treatment will be possible once treatment planning can be achieved within minutes with online target defined and prior dosimetric information.
- Robot-assisted brachytherapy can increase accuracy, reduce human variability, and potentially reduce operation time and clinician's fatigue.

- Multichannel robotic brachytherapy system may be able to reduce edema and symmetric deformation or displacement of the prostate and can eventually enhance seed delivery accuracy.
- MR-guided HDR/low-dose rate (LDR) robotic system aided by powerful optimization engine like the genetic algorithm can be the next state-of-the-art technology for more targeted therapy.
- Further improvement may be possible if the adaptive dosimetric planning is integrated with the patient-specific predictive model of tissue deformation and displacement aided by artificial neural network.
- Dynamics-based coordinated control strategy using MLC and robotic couch has the potential to deliver radiation therapy to any moving organ with near 100% duty cycle.

REFERENCES

1. Galvin JM, Ezzell G, Eisbrauch A, et al. Implementing IMRT in clinical practice: a joint document of the American Society for Therapeutic Radiology and Oncology and the American Association of Physicists in Medicine. Int J Radiat Oncol Biol Phys 2004; 58:1616–1634.
2. Payne GS, Leach MO. Applications of magnetic resonance spectroscopy in radiotherapy treatment planning. Br J Radiol 2006; 79:S16–S26.
3. Taouli B. MR spectroscopic imaging for evaluation of prostate cancer. J Radiol 2006; 87:222–227.
4. Hricak H. MR imaging and MR spectroscopic imaging in the pre-treatment evaluation of prostate cancer. Br J Radiol 2005; 78:S103–S111.
5. Beyersdorff D, Taupitz M, Winkelmann B, et al. Patients with a history of elevated prostate-specific antigen levels and negative transrectal US-guided quadrant or sextant biopsy results: value of MR imaging. Radiology 2002; 224:701–706.
6. Pickett B, Kurhanewicz J, Coakley F, et al. Use of MRI and spectroscopy in evaluation of external beam radiotherapy for prostate cancer. Int J Radiat Oncol Biol Phys 2004; 60:1047–1055.
7. Scheidler J, Hricak H, Vigneron DB, et al. Prostate cancer: localization with three-dimensional proton MR spectroscopic imaging—clinicopathologic study. Radiology 1999; 213:473–480.
8. Xia P, Pickett B, Vigneault E, et al. Forward or inversely planned segmental multileaf collimator IMRT and sequential tomotherapy to treat multiple dominant intraprostatic lesions of prostate cancer to 90 Gy. Int J Radiat Oncol Biol Phys 2001; 51:244–254.
9. Pouliot J, Kim Y, Lessard E, et al. Inverse planning for HDR prostate brachytherapy used to boost dominant intraprostatic lesions defined by magnetic resonance spectroscopy imaging. Int J Radiat Oncol Biol Phys 2004; 59:1196–1207.
10. Pickett B, Kurhanewicz J, Pouliot J, et al. Three-dimensional conformal external beam radiotherapy compared with permanent prostate implantation in low-risk prostate cancer based on endorectal magnetic resonance spectroscopy imaging and prostate-specific antigen level. Int J Radiat Oncol Biol Phys 2006; 65:65–72.
11. Pickett B, Vigneault E, Kurhanewicz J, et al. Static field intensity modulation to treat a dominant intra-prostatic lesion to 90 gy compared to seven field 3-dimensional radiotherapy. Int J Radiat Oncol Biol Phys 1999; 44:921–929.
12. Powles T, Murray I, Brock C, et al. Molecular positron emission tomography and PET/CT imaging in urological malignancies. Eur Urol 2007; 51:1511–1521.
13. Effert PJ, Bares R, Handt S, et al. Metabolic imaging of untreated prostate cancer by positron emission tomography with sup 18 fluorine-labeled deoxyglucose. J Urol 1996; 155:994–998.
14. Hofer C, Laubenbacher C, Block T, et al. Fluorine-18-fluorodeoxyglucose positron emission tomography is useless for the detection of local recurrence after radical prostatectomy. Eur Urol 1999; 36:31–35.
15. Haseman MK, Reed NL, Rosenthal SA. Monoclonal antibody imaging of occult prostate cancer in patients with elevated prostate-specific antigen. Positron emission tomography and biopsy correlation. Clin Nucl Med 1996; 21:704–713.
16. Shreve PD, Grossman HB, Gross MD, et al. Metastatic prostate cancer: initial findings of PET with 2-deoxy-2-[F-18]fluoro-D-glucose. Radiology 1996; 199:751–756.
17. Yeh SDJ, Imbriaco M, Larson SM, et al. Detection of bony metastases of androgen-independent prostate cancer by PET-FDG. Nucl Med Biol 1996; 23:693–697.
18. Schoöder H, Herrmann K, Goönen M, et al. 2-[18F]fluoro-2-deoxyglucose positron emission tomography for the detection of disease in patients with prostate-specific antigen relapse after radical prostatectomy. Clin Cancer Res 2005; 11:4761–4769.
19. Yamaguchi T, Lee J, Uemura H, et al. Prostate cancer: a comparative study of 11C-choline PET and MR imaging combined with proton MR spectroscopy. Eur J Nucl Med Mol Imaging 2005; 32:742–748.
20. DeGrado TR, Baldwin SW, Wang S, et al. Synthesis and evaluation of 18F-labeled choline analogs as oncologic PET tracers. J Nucl Med 2001; 42:1805–1814.
21. Coleman RE, DeGrado TR, Wang S, et al. Preliminary evaluation of F-18 fluorocholine (FCH) as a PET tumor imaging agent. Clin Positron Imaging (Netherlands). 2000; 3:147.
22. Price DT, Coleman RE, Liao RP, et al. Comparison of [18F]fluorocholine and [18F]fluorodeoxyglucose for positron emission tomography of androgen dependent and androgen independent prostate cancer. J Urol 2002; 168:273–280.
23. Martorana G, Schiavina R, Corti B, et al. 11C-choline positron emission Tomography/Computerized tomography for tumor localization of primary prostate cancer in comparison with 12-core biopsy. J Urol 2006; 176:954–960.
24. Farsad M, Schiavina R, Castellucci P, et al. Detection and localization of prostate cancer: correlation of 11C-choline

PET/CT with histopathologic step-section analysis. J Nucl Med 2005; 46:1642–1649.

25. Grosu AL, Piert M, Weber WA, et al. Positron emission tomography for radiation treatment planning. Strahlenther Onkol 2005; 181:483–499.

26. Teh BS, Aguilar-Cordova E, Vlachaki MT, et al. Combining radiotherapy with gene therapy (from the bench to the bedside): a novel treatment strategy for prostate cancer. Oncologist 2002; 7:458–466.

27. Parry R, Schneider D, Hudson D, et al. Identification of a novel prostate tumor target, Mindin/RG-1, for antibody-based radiotherapy of prostate cancer. Cancer Res 2005; 65: 8397–8405.

28. Dilley J, Reddy S, Ko D, et al. Oncolytic adenovirus CG7870 in combination with radiation demonstrates synergistic enhancements of antitumor efficacy without loss of specificity. Cancer Gene Ther 2005; 12:715–722.

29. Court LE, Dong L. Automatic registration of the prostate for computed-tomography-guided radiotherapy. Med Phys 2003; 30:2750–2757.

30. Smitsmans MH, de Bois J, Sonke JJ, et al. Automatic prostate localization on cone-beam CT scans for high precision image-guided radiotherapy. Int J Radiat Oncol Biol Phys 2005; 63:975–984.

31. Smitsmans MHP, Wolthaus JWH, Artignan X, et al. Automatic localization of the prostate for on-line or off-line image-guided radiotherapy. Int J Radiat. Oncol. Biol Phys 2004; 60:623–635.

32. Wang H, Dong L, Lii MF, et al. Implementation and validation of a three-dimensional deformable registration algorithm for targeted prostate cancer radiotherapy. Int J Radiat Oncol Biol Phys 2005; 61:725–735.

33. Chao KSC, Bhide S, Chen H, et al. Reduce in variation and improve efficiency of target volume delineation by a computer-assisted system using a deformable image registration approach. Int J Radiat Oncol Biol Phys 2007; 68: 1512–1521.

34. Fiorino C, Reni M, Bolognesi A, et al. Intra- and inter-observer variability in contouring prostate and seminal vesicles: implications for conformal treatment planning. Radiother Oncol 1998; 47:285–292.

35. Thirion J. Image matching as a diffusion process: an analogy with maxwell's demons. Med Image Anal 1998; 2: 243–260.

36. Engstrom PE, Haraldsson P, Landberg T, et al. In vivo dose verification of IMRT treated head and neck cancer patients. Acta Oncol 2005; 44:572–578.

37. Kroonwijk M, Pasma KL, Quint S, et al. In vivo dosimetry for prostate cancer patients using an electronic portal imaging device (EPID); demonstration of internal organ motion. Radiother Oncol 1998; 49:125–132.

38. McDermott LN, Wendling M, Sonke JJ, et al. Replacing pretreatment verification with in vivo EPID dosimetry for prostate IMRT. Int J Radiat Oncol Biol Phys 2007; 67: 1568–1577.

39. McDermott LN, Wendling M, van Asselen B, et al. Clinical experience with EPID dosimetry for prostate IMRT pretreatment dose verification. Med Phys 2006; 33:3921–3930.

40. Nijsten SM, Mijnheer BJ, Dekker AL, et al. Routine individualised patient dosimetry using electronic portal imaging devices. Radiother Oncol 2007; 83:65–75.

41. Pasma KL, Kroonwijk M, Quint S, et al. Transit dosimetry with an electronic portal imaging device (EPID) for 115 prostate cancer patients. Int J Radiat Oncol Biol Phys 1999; 45:1297–1303.

42. Piermattei A, Fidanzio A, Stimato G, et al. In vivo dosimetry by an aSi-based EPID. Med Phys 2006; 33:4414–4422.

43. Talamonti C, Casati M, Bucciolini M. Pretreatment verification of IMRT absolute dose distributions using a commercial a-si EPID. Med Phys 2006; 33:4367–4378.

44. Van Esch A, Vanstraelen B, Verstraete J, et al. Pre-treatment dosimetric verification by means of a liquid-filled electronic portal imaging device during dynamic delivery of intensity modulated treatment fields. Radiother Oncol 2001; 60: 181–190.

45. Dahlgren CV, Eilertsen K, Jørgensen TD, et al. Portal dose image verification: the collapsed cone superposition method applied with different electronic portal imaging devices. Phys Med Biol 2006; 51:335–349.

46. Wendling M, Louwe RJ, McDermott LN, et al. Accurate two-dimensional IMRT verification using a back-projection EPID dosimetry method. Med Phys 2006; 33:259–273.

47. Louwe RJ, Damen EM, van Herk M, et al. Three-dimensional dose reconstruction of breast cancer treatment using portal imaging. Med Phys 2003; 30:2376–2389.

48. Partridge M, Ebert M, Hesse BM. IMRT verification by three-dimensional dose reconstruction from portal beam measurements. Med Phys 2002; 29:1847–1858.

49. McNutt TR, Mackie TR, Reckwerdt P, et al. Modeling dose distributions from portal dose images using the convolution/superposition method. Med Phys 1996; 23: 1381–1392.

50. Boellaard R, Essers M, van Herk M, et al. New method to obtain the midplane dose using portal in vivo dosimetry. Int J Radiat Oncol Biol Phys 1998; 41:465–474.

51. McDermott LN, Louwe RJW, Sonke JJ, et al. Dose-response and ghosting effects of an amorphous silicon electronic portal imaging device. Med Phys 2004; 31:285–295.

52. Louwe RJ, McDermott LN, Sonke JJ, et al. The long-term stability of amorphous silicon flat panel imaging devices for dosimetry purposes. Med Phys 2004; 31: 2989–2995.

53. Brahme A. Biologically optimized 3-dimensional in vivo predictive assay-based radiation therapy using positron emission tomography-computerized tomography imaging. Acta Oncol 2003; 42:123–136.

54. Spirou SV, Fournier-Bidoz N, Yang J, et al. Smoothing intensity-modulated beam profiles to improve the efficiency of delivery. Med Phys 2001; 28 (10):2015–2112.

55. Andrzej N. Reporting, and analyzing dose distributions: a concept of equivalent uniform dose. 1997; 24:103–110.

56. Niemierko A. A generalized concept of equivalent uniform dose (EUD). Med Phys 1999; 26:1100.

57. Webb S. The physics of three-dimensional radiation therapy: conformal radiotherapy, radiosurgery, and treatment planning. Philadelphia: Institute of Physics Publishing, 1993.

58. Webb S. The physics of conformal radiotherapy: advances in technology. Philadelphia: Institute of Physics Publishing, 1997:382.

59. Webb S. Intensity-modulated radiation therapy. Bristol and Philadelphia: Institute of Physics Publishing, 2001.

60. Palta JR, Mackie TR, eds. Intensity-modulated radiation therapy: the state of art. Madison WI: Medical Physics Pub Corp, 2003.

61. Center MotMS-C. A practical guide to intensity-modulated radiation therapy. Medical Physics Pub Corp, 2003.

62. Cho PS, Marks RJ II. Hardware-sensitive optimization for intensity modulated radiotherapy. Phys Med Biol 2000; 45:429–440.

63. Webb S, Convey DJ, Evans PM. Inverse planning with constraints to generate smoothed intensity-modulated beams. Phys Med Biol 1998; 43:2785–2794.

64. Censor Y, Altschuler MD, Powlis WD. A computational solution of the inverse problem in radiation therapy treatment planning. Appl Math Comput 1988; 25:57–87.

65. Censor Y, Gordon D, Gordon R. Component averaging: an efficient iterative parallel algorithms for large and sparse unstructured problems. Parallel Computing 2001; 27:777–808.

66. Hoffner JH, Decker P, Schmidt EL, et al. Development of a fast optimization preview in radiation treatment planning. Strahlenther Onkol 1996; 172:384–394.

67. Iusem AN, Moledo L. A finitely convergent method of simultaneously subgradient projections for the convex feasibility problem. Mat Appl Comput 1986; 5:169–184.

68. Lee S, Cho PS, Marks RJ II, et al. Conformal radiotherapy computation by the method of alternating projections onto convex sets. Phys Med Biol 1997; 42:1065–1086.

69. Stark H, Yang Y. Vector space projections: a numerical approach to signal and image processing, neural nets, and optics. New York: John Wiley, 1998.

70. Michalski D, Xiao Y, Censor Y, et al. The dose-volume constraint satisfaction problem with simultaneous subgradient projection method for inverse treatment planning with field segments. Phys Med Biol 2004; 49:601–616.

71. Xiao Y, Michalski D, Censor Y, et al. Inherent smoothness of intensity patterns for intensity modulated radiation therapy generated by simultaneous projection algorithms. Phys Med Biol 2004; 49:3227–3245.

72. Xiao Y, Censor Y, Michalski D, et al. The least-intensity feasible solution for aperture-based inverse planning in radiation therapy. Annals of Operations Research 2003; 119:183–203.

73. Xiao Y, Galvin J, Hossain M, et al. An optimized forward-planning technique for intensity modulated radiation therapy. Med Phys 2000; 9:2093–2099.

74. Xiao Y, Werner-Wasik M, Michalski D, et al. Comparison of three IMRT inverse planning techniques that allow for partial esophagus sparing in patients receiving thoracic radiation therapy for lung cancer. Med Dosim 2004; 29: 210–216.

75. Boyd S, Vandenberghe L. Convex optimization. Cambridge: Cambridge University Press, 2004:730.

76. Bazaraa MS, Sherali HD, Shetty CM. Nonlinear Programming: Theory and Algorithms. New York: Wiley, 1993.

77. Jorge N, Stephen JW. Numerical Optimization. Berlin, Germany: Springer; 1999.

78. Wu Q, Mohan R. Multiple local minima in IMRT optimization based on dose-volume criteria. Med Phys 2002; 29(7): 1514–1527.

79. Wu Q, Mohan R. Algorithm and functionality of an intensity modulated radiotherapy. Med Phys 2000; 27(4): 701–711.

80. Wu Q, Mohan R, Niemierko A, et al. Optimization of intensity-modulated radiotherapy plans based on the equivalent uniform dose. Int J Radiat Oncol Biol Phys 2002; 52(1):224–235.

81. Zhang X, Liu H, Wang X, et al. Speed and convergence properties of gradient algorithms for optimization of IMRT. Med Phys 2004; 31(5):1141–1152.

82. Trofimov A, Rietzel E, Lu HM, et al. Temporo-spatial IMRT optimization: concepts, implementation and initial results. Phys Med Biol 2005; 50:2779–2798.

83. Bortfeld T, Jokivarsi K, Goitein M, et al. Effects of intra-fraction motion on IMRT dose delivery: statistical analysis and simulation. Phys Med Biol 2002; 47: 2203–2220.

84. Zhang T, Jeraj R, Keller H, et al. Treatment plan optimization incorporating respiratory motion. Med Phys 2004; 31: 1576–1586.

85. Li JG, Xing L. Inverse planning incorporating organ motion. Med Phys 2000; 27:1573–1578.

86. Engelsman M, Sharp GC, Bortfeld T, et al. How much margin reduction is possible through gating or breath hold? Phys Med Biol 2005; 50:477–490.

87. Unkelbach J, Oelfke U. Inclusion of organ movements in IMRT treatment planning via inverse planning based on probability distributions. Phys Med Biol 2004; 49: 4005–4029.

88. Chan TC, Bortfeld T, Tsitsiklis JN. A robust approach to IMRT optimization. Phys Med Biol 2006; 51:2567–2583.

89. Baum C, Alber M, Birkner M, et al. Robust treatment planning for intensity modulated radiotherapy of prostate cancer based on coverage probabilities. Radiother Oncol 2006; 78:27–35.

90. Unkelbach J, Oelfke U. Incorporating organ movements in IMRT treatment planning for prostate cancer: minimizing uncertainties in the inverse planning process. Med Phys 2005; 32:2471–2483.

91. Fu KS, Gonzalez RC, Lee CSG. Robotics: control, sensing, vision, and intelligence. New York: McGraw Hill International, 1988.

92. Fichtinger G, DeWeese TL, Patriciu A, et al. System for robotically assisted prostate biopsy and therapy with intraoperative CT guidance. Acad Radiol 2002; 9:60–74.

93. Stoianovici D, Cleary K, Patriciu A, et al. AcuBot: a robot for radiological interventions. In: IEEE Transactions on Robotics and Automation 2003; 19(5):927–930.

94. Wei Z, Wan G, Gardi L, et al. Robot-assisted 3D-TRUS guided prostate brachytherapy: system integration and validation. Med Phys 2004; 31(3):539–548.

95. Wei Z, Wan Z, Gardi L, et al. Robotic aided 3D TRUS guided intraoperative prostate brachytherapy. SPIE 2004; 5367:361–370.

96. Kettenbach J, Kronreif G, Figl M, et al. Robot-assisted biopsy using computed tomography-guidance: initial results from in vitro tests. Invest Radiol 2005; 40:219–228.

97. Kettenbach J, Kronreif G, Figl M, et al. Robot-assisted biopsy using ultrasound guidance: initial results from in vitro tests. Eur Radiol 2005; 15:765–771.

98. Meltsner M, Ferrier N, Thomadsen B. Performance evaluation of a novel brachytherapy robot. Florida, AAPM, 2006:2264.

99. Kennedy C, Iordachita I, Burdette C, et al. Robotically assisted needle placement for prostate brachytherapy. Med Phys 2006; 33:2264.

100. Nucletron's FIRST system. Available at: http://www.nucletron.com/. Accessed October 18, 2007.

101. Yu Y, Podder TK, Zhang Y, et al. Robot-assisted prostate brachytherapy. In: Proceedings of International Conference on Medical Image Computing and Computer Assisted Intervention (MICCAI), Copenhagen, Denmark, 2006:41–49.

102. Wan G, Wei Z, Gardi L, et al. Brachytherapy needle deflection evaluation and correction. Mcd Phys 2005; 32(4): 902–909.

103. Podder TK, Liao L, Sherman J, et al. Assessment of prostate brachytherapy and breast biopsy needle insertions and methods to improve targeting accuracy. In: Proceedings of IFMBE International Conference on Biomedical Engineering (ICBME), Singapore, 2005.

104. Yan K, Ng WS, Yu Y, et al. Needle steering modeling and analysis using unconstrained modal analysis. In: Proceedings of the IEEE International Conference on Biomedical Robotics and Biomechatronics, Pisa, Italy, 2006:65–70.

105. Podder TK, Ng WS, Yu Y. Multi-channel robotic system for prostate brachytherapy. Proceedings, IEEE Engineering in Medicine and Biology Society (EMBS/EMBC), Lyon, France, 2007:1233–1236.

106. Muntener M, Patriciu A, Petrisor D, et al. Magnetic resonance imaging compatible robotic system for gully automated brachytherapy seed placement. Urology 2006; 68(6):1313–1317.

107. Patriciu A, Petrisor D, Muntener M, et al. Automated brachytherapy seed placement under MRI guidance. IEEE Trans Biomed Eng 2007; 54(8):1499–1506.

108. Podder TK, Sherman J, Fuller D, et al. Needle insertion force estimation model using procedure-specific and patient-specific criteria. Proceedings, IEEE Engineering in Medicine and Biology Society (EMBS/EMBC), New York, NY, 2006:555–558.

109. Keall PJ, Mageras GS, Balter JM, et al. The management of respiratory motion in radiation oncology report of AAPM Task Group 76. Med Phys 2006; 33(10):3874–3900.

110. D'Souza W, Naqvi SA, Yu CX. Real-time intra-fraction-motion tracking using the treatment couch: a feasibility study. Phys Med Biol 2005; 50:4021–4033.

111. Podder TK, Buzurovic I, Yu Y. Coordinated dynamics-based control of robotic couch and MLC-bank for feedforward radiation therapy. CARS 2007; 2:S49–S52.

112. Podder TK, Sarkar N. Dynamic trajectory planning for autonomous underwater vehicle-manipulator systems. In: Proceedings of the IEEE International Conference on Robotics and Automation (ICRA), San Francisco, CA, 2000:3461–3466.

113. Podder TK, Sarkar N. A unified dynamics-based motion planning algorithm for autonomous underwater vehicle-manipulator systems. Robotica 2004; 2(1):117–128.

Index